VOLUME NINETY FIVE

VITAMINS AND HORMONES

The Pancreatic Beta Cell

VOLUME NINETY FIVE

VITAMINS AND HORMONES

The Pancreatic Beta Cell

Series Editor

GERALD LITWACK, PhD

Toluca Lake, North Hollywood, California

ELSEVIER

AMSTERDAM • BOSTON • HEIDELBERG • LONDON
NEW YORK • OXFORD • PARIS • SAN DIEGO
SAN FRANCISCO • SINGAPORE • SYDNEY • TOKYO
Academic Press is an imprint of Elsevier

AP

Cover photo credit:
Squires, P. E., Jones, P. M., Younis, M. Y. G., and Hills, C. E.
The Calcium-Sensing Receptor and β-Cell Function
Vitamins and Hormones (2014) 95, pp. 249–268

Academic Press is an imprint of Elsevier
32 Jamestown Road, London, NW1 7BY, UK
The Boulevard, Langford Lane, Kidlington, Oxford, OX5 1GB, UK
Linacre House, Jordan Hill, Oxford OX2 8DP, UK
225 Wyman Street, Waltham, MA 02451, USA
525 B Street, Suite 1800, San Diego, CA 92101-4495, USA

First edition 2014

ISBN: 978-0-12-800174-5
ISSN: 0083-6729

Printed and bound by CPI Group (UK) Ltd, Croydon, CR0 4YY

CONTENTS

CONTRIBUTORS

Muhammad Rizwan Alam
Institute of Molecular Biology and Biochemistry, Center of Molecular Medicine, Medical University of Graz, Graz, Austria

Peter Arvan
Division of Metabolism, Endocrinology & Diabetes, The University of Michigan Medical School, Ann Arbor, Michigan, USA

Yael Bar
Department of Human Molecular Genetics and Biochemistry, Sackler School of Medicine, Tel Aviv University, Tel Aviv, Israel

Andreas Barthel
Department of Medicine III, University Hospital Carl Gustav Carus, Dresden, and Endokrinologikum Ruhr, Bochum, Germany

Alberto Bartolome
Departamento de Bioquímica y Biología Molecular II, Facultad de Farmacia, Universidad Complutense; Centro de Investigación Biomédica en Red de Diabetes y Enfermedades Metabólicas Asociadas (CIBERDEM), Barcelona, and Instituto de Investigación Sanitaria del Hospital Clínico San Carlos de Madrid (IdISSC), Madrid, Spain

Norman L. Block
Department of Pathology, University of Miami Miller School of Medicine; Department of Medicine, Division of Hematology-Oncology, University of Miami Miller School of Medicine, and Veterans Administration Medical Center, Miami, Florida, USA

Stefan R. Bornstein
Department of Medicine III, University Hospital Carl Gustav Carus; The Paul Langerhans Institute, and Center for Regenerative Therapies Dresden, Dresden University of Technology, Dresden, Germany

Bipasha Bose
Nanyang Technological University, School of Biological Sciences, NTU Lab Location @ Level 2 Singapore Institute for Clinical Sciences, Brenner Centre for Molecular Medicine, Singapore, Singapore

Matthias Braun
Alberta Diabetes Institute, Department of Pharmacology, Faculty of Medicine and Dentistry, University of Alberta, Edmonton, Alberta, Canada

Katarzyna A. Broniowska
Department of Biochemistry, Medical College of Wisconsin, Milwaukee, Wisconsin, USA

John A. Corbett
Department of Biochemistry, Medical College of Wisconsin, Milwaukee, Wisconsin, USA

Nadine L. Dudek
Department of Biochemistry and Molecular Biology, Monash University, Clayton, Victoria, Australia

Carlos Manlio Diaz-Garcia
Department of Neural Development and Physiology, Neuroscience Division, Instituto de Fisiología Celular, Universidad Nacional Autónoma de México, Mexico, Mexico

Shimon Efrat
Department of Human Molecular Genetics and Biochemistry, Sackler School of Medicine, Tel Aviv University, Tel Aviv, Israel

Wolfgang F. Graier
Institute of Molecular Biology and Biochemistry, Center of Molecular Medicine, Medical University of Graz, Graz, Austria

Lukas N. Groschner
Institute of Molecular Biology and Biochemistry, Center of Molecular Medicine, Medical University of Graz, Graz, Austria

Carlos Guillén
Departamento de Bioquímica y Biología Molecular II, Facultad de Farmacia, Universidad Complutense; Centro de Investigación Biomédica en Red de Diabetes y Enfermedades Metabólicas Asociadas (CIBERDEM), Barcelona, and Instituto de Investigación Sanitaria del Hospital Clínico San Carlos de Madrid (IdISSC), Madrid, Spain

Huan Guo
Division of Metabolism, Endocrinology & Diabetes, The University of Michigan Medical School, Ann Arbor, Michigan, USA

Claire E. Hills
School of Life Sciences, University of Warwick, Coventry, United Kingdom

Marcia Hiriart
Department of Neural Development and Physiology, Neuroscience Division, Instituto de Fisiología Celular, Universidad Nacional Autónoma de México, Mexico, Mexico

Liping Huang
United States Department of Agriculture/Agricultural Research Service/Western Human Nutrition Research Center, Obesity and Metabolism Research Unit, and Department of Nutrition, University of California Davis, Davis, California, USA

Christopher J. Jackson
Sutton Arthritis Research Laboratories, Kolling Institute of Medical Research, The University of Sydney at Royal North Shore Hospital, St Leonards, New South Wales, Australia

Peter M. Jones
Diabetes & Nutritional Sciences Division, School of Medicine, King's College London, London, United Kingdom

Kishore Reddy Katikireddy
Schepens Eye Research Institute, Harvard Medical School, Boston, Massachusetts, USA

Kevin Keane
School of Biomedical Sciences, CHIRI Biosciences Research Precinct, Faculty of Health Sciences, Curtin University, GPO Box U1987, Perth, Western Australia, Australia

Carlos Larqué
Department of Neural Development and Physiology, Neuroscience Division, Instituto de Fisiología Celular, Universidad Nacional Autónoma de México, Mexico, Mexico

Ming Liu
Division of Metabolism, Endocrinology & Diabetes, The University of Michigan Medical School, Ann Arbor, Michigan, USA, and Department of Metabolism, Tianjin Medical University General Hospital, Tianjin, PR China

Barbara Ludwig
Department of Medicine III, University Hospital Carl Gustav Carus; The Paul Langerhans Institute, and Center for Regenerative Therapies Dresden, Dresden University of Technology, Dresden, Germany

Stefan Ludwig
Department of Visceral, Thorax and Vascular Surgery, University Hospital Carl Gustav Carus, Dresden, Germany

Tania Maffucci
Queen Mary University of London, Barts and The London School of Medicine and Dentistry, Blizard Institute, Centre for Diabetes, Inositide Signalling Group, London, United Kingdom

Simona Mazza
Queen Mary University of London, Barts and The London School of Medicine and Dentistry, Blizard Institute, Centre for Diabetes, Inositide Signalling Group, London, United Kingdom

Philip Newsholme
School of Biomedical Sciences, CHIRI Biosciences Research Precinct, Faculty of Health Sciences, Curtin University, GPO Box U1987, Perth, Western Australia, Australia

Bryndon J. Oleson
Department of Biochemistry, Medical College of Wisconsin, Milwaukee, Wisconsin, USA

Anthony W. Purcell
Department of Biochemistry and Molecular Biology, Monash University, Clayton, Victoria, Australia

Yanfei Qi
Signal Transduction Program, Centenary Institute, Sydney, Australia

Andreas Reichel
Department of Medicine III, University Hospital Carl Gustav Carus, Dresden, Germany

Andrew V. Schally
Department of Pathology, University of Miami Miller School of Medicine; Department of Medicine, Division of Endocrinology, University of Miami Miller School of Medicine; Department of Medicine, Division of Hematology-Oncology, University of

Miami MillerSchool of Medicine, and Veterans Administration Medical Center, Miami, Florida, USA

Paul E. Squires
School of Life Sciences, University of Warwick, Coventry, United Kingdom

Sudheer Shenoy P
Nanyang Technological University, School of Biological Sciences, NTU Lab Location @ Level 2 Singapore Institute for Clinical Sciences, Brenner Centre for Molecular Medicine, Singapore, Singapore

Myrian Velasco
Department of Neural Development and Physiology, Neuroscience Division, Instituto de Fisiología Celular, Universidad Nacional Autónoma de México, Mexico, Mexico

Jordan Wright
Division of Metabolism, Endocrinology & Diabetes, The University of Michigan Medical School, Ann Arbor, Michigan, USA

Pu Xia
Signal Transduction Program, Centenary Institute, Sydney, Australia, and Department of Endocrinology and Metabolism, Zhongshan Hospital, Fudan University, Shanghai, PR China

Yi Xiong
Division of Metabolism, Endocrinology & Diabetes, The University of Michigan Medical School, Ann Arbor, Michigan, USA

Meilang Xue
Sutton Arthritis Research Laboratories, Kolling Institute of Medical Research, The University of Sydney at Royal North Shore Hospital, St Leonards, New South Wales, Australia

Kazuya Yamagata
Department of Medical Biochemistry, Faculty of Life Sciences, Kumamoto University, Kumamoto, Japan

Mustafa Y.G. Younis
School of Life Sciences, University of Warwick, Coventry, United Kingdom

PREFACE

The pancreatic beta cell is the only source of insulin in the human body, and its destruction by a variety of causations, including autoimmunity, infection, and/or genetic mutations, leads to type 1 diabetes in the very young and to type 2 diabetes, especially in adults but, increasingly, in earlier age groups because of poor diet, obesity, and lack of exercise. The incidence of type 2 diabetes is reaching epidemic proportions in the West, and its severe impact stresses the health care system and the economy. It is vital to understand the basic science of the functioning of the beta cell and the gene products that regulate the functionality of the beta cell and the synthesis of insulin, not to mention the critical need for therapies of type 2 diabetes. This volume, in up-to-date knowledge, reviews all of these considerations from basic science to present and future treatment of this disease.

Chapter 1 of these contributions is entitled "Metabolic regulation of insulin secretion" by K. Keane and P. Newsholme. This is followed by "Proinsulin entry and transit through the endoplasmic reticulum in pancreatic beta cells" by M. Liu, J. Wright, H. Guo, Y. Xiong, and P. Arvan. "Metabolism–secretion coupling and mitochondrial calcium activities in clonal pancreatic β-cells" is the product of L.N. Groschner, M.R. Alam, and W.F. Graier. M. Hiriart, M. Velasco, C. Larqué, and C.M. Diaz-Garcia offer "Metabolic syndrome and ionic channels in pancreatic beta cells." Considering the autoimmune causation of disease, N.L. Dudek and A.W. Purcell contribute "The beta-cell immunopeptidome." S. Mazza and T. Maffucci report on "Autophagy and pancreatic β-cells." M. Braun reviews "The somatostatin receptor in human pancreatic β-cells." We have learned of the death of Dr. Matthias Braun before the issue of galley proofs for his correction. The Series Editor takes responsibility for answering the Publisher's queries concerning the manuscript. Dr. Braun was the author of Chapter 7 titled "The Somatostatin Receptor in Human Pancreatic β-Cells".

Two papers consider treatments for diabetes. The first is by B. Ludwig, A. Barthel, A. Reichel, N.L. Block, S. Ludwig, A.V. Schally, and S.R. Bornstein: "Modulation of the pancreatic islet-stress axis as a novel potential therapeutic target in diabetes mellitus." The second offering is by B. Bose, K.R. Katikireddy, and S. Shenoy entitled "Regenerative medicine for diabetes: differentiation of human pluripotent stem cells into functional β-cells *in vitro* and their proposed journey to clinical translation."

In the vein of specific factors in the functioning of the beta cell, a number of contributions follow. "The calcium-sensing receptor and β-cell function" is the topic of P.E. Squires, P.M. Jones, M.Y.G. Younis, and C.E. Hills. P. Xia and Y. Qi cover "Cellular inhibitor of apoptosis protein-1 and survival of beta cells undergoing endoplasmic reticulum stress." "β-Cell responses to nitric oxide" is the subject of K.A. Broniowska, B.J. Oleson, and J.A. Corbett. M. Xue and C.J. Jackson review "Activated protein C and its potential applications in prevention of islet β-cell damage and diabetes." "Zinc and its transporters, pancreatic β-cells, and insulin metabolism" is discussed by L. Huang. Y. Bar and S. Efrat consider "The NOTCH pathway in β-cell growth and differentiation." "Roles of HNF1α and HNF4α in pancreatic β-cells: lessons from a monogenic form of diabetes (MODY)" is the topic of K. Yamagata. The final contribution by A. Bartolome and C. Guillén is "Role of the mammalian target of rapamycin (mTOR) complexes in pancreatic β-cell mass regulation."

I am indebted to Helene Kabes for her diligent monitoring of this collection to the point of publication.

The cover illustration is reproduced from Figure 10.1 of Chapter 10 by P.E. Squires, P.M. Jones, M.Y.G. Younis, and C.E. Hills entitled: "The Calcium-Sensing Receptor and β-Cell Function".

Gerald Litwack
Toluca Lake, North Hollywood, California
September 20, 2013

CHAPTER ONE

Metabolic Regulation of Insulin Secretion

Kevin Keane, Philip Newsholme[1]
School of Biomedical Sciences, CHIRI Biosciences Research Precinct, Faculty of Health Sciences, Curtin University, GPO Box U1987, Perth, Western Australia, Australia
[1]Corresponding author: e-mail address: philip.newsholme@curtin.edu.au

Contents

Abstract

Regulation of metabolic fuel homeostasis is a critical function of β-cells, which are located in the islets of Langerhans of the animal pancreas. Impairment of this β-cell function is a hallmark of pancreatic β-cell failure and may lead to development of type 2 diabetes mellitus. β-Cells are essentially "fuel sensors" that monitor and react to elevated nutrient load by releasing insulin. This response involves metabolic activation and generation of metabolic coupling factors (MCFs) that relay the nutrient signal throughout the cell and induce insulin biosynthesis and secretion. Glucose is the most important insulin secretagogue as it is the primary fuel source in food. Glucose metabolism is central to generation of MCFs that lead to insulin release, most notably ATP. In addition, other classes of nutrients are able to augment insulin secretion and these include members of the lipid and amino acid family of nutrients. Therefore, it is important to investigate the interplay between glucose, lipid, and amino acid metabolism, as it is this mixed nutrient sensing that generate the MCFs required for insulin exocytosis. The mechanisms by which these nutrients are metabolized to generate MCFs, and how they impact on β-cell insulin release and function, are discussed in detail in this article.

Vitamins and Hormones, Volume 95
ISSN 0083-6729
http://dx.doi.org/10.1016/B978-0-12-800174-5.00001-6

1. INTRODUCTION

Secretion of the metabolic hormone insulin is central to the regulation of fuel homeostasis in animals. Insulin is released into the vasculature by specialized cells, known as β-cells, which are located in the islets of Langerhans of the animal pancreas. These "fuel-sensing" β-cells are stimulated to circulate insulin in response to elevated blood glucose levels, which generally occurs following ingestion of a carbohydrate containing meal. The primary role of insulin is to interact with and activate key membrane-bound receptors in cells that store surplus carbohydrate in the form of glycogen (liver and muscle) or as fatty acids (adipose tissue). On the other hand, the pancreas is also partly responsible for enhancing the blood glucose concentration in nutrient-deprived states (i.e., starvation), by secreting the hormone glucagon. The main function of this protein is to promote conversion of stored glycogen to free glucose by the process of glycogenolysis. Blood glucose concentrations are significantly affected by changes in nutrient intake and/or expenditure (e.g., exercise) and consequently are sustained within a tight range by rotating the release of insulin and glucagon from the pancreas.

The pancreatic islets of Langerhans are exquisitely designed to respond to physiological changes in plasma glucose. There are approximately 1 million individual islets in the human pancreas and collectively they receive about 10% of the body's blood supply (Hellman, 1959; Rorsman & Braun, 2013). Furthermore, with the aid of capillary fenestrations, islets receive 10 × more blood than the surrounding exocrine cells and are allowed unobstructed contact with the vasculature enabling rapid nutrient-sensing and direct secretion of glucagon/insulin into the bloodstream (Fu, Gilbert, & Liu, 2013). Each islet is composed of a selection of specialized cells that are responsible for glycaemic homeostasis. The glucagon-producing α-cells comprise about 35–40% of the islet cell population, while insulin-producing β-cells account for approximately 50% (Cabrera et al., 2006; Rorsman & Braun, 2013). The remainder of cells in pancreatic islets are somatostatin-releasing δ-cells and pancreatic peptide (PP)-secreting PP-cells (10–15%) (Rorsman & Braun, 2013). Somatostatin plays a regulatory function in islets and can inhibit both insulin and glucagon secretion, while the role of PP remains unclear (Newsholme et al., 2011). β-Cells are the most extensively studied of this cell type collection due to their commitment to insulin biosynthesis, insulin release and the consequential implications for diabetes mellitus (DM). It is well established that the impairment of glucose homeostasis control and subsequent β-cell failure correlates with DM development, particularly in type 2 manifestations of the disease (T2DM) (Jensen et al., 2008; Newsholme & Krause, 2012). Therefore, current research is attempting to clarify the elements (dietary, molecular, and pharmacological) that affect the process of insulin biosynthesis and exocytosis, as a means to develop novel treatments for patients with these disorders.

β-Cell insulin secretion is a highly controlled process and is subject to a variety of regulatory mechanisms. There are many insulin secretagogues that induce insulin release. Some of these include glucose, fatty acids, amino acids, incretins, hormones, nucleotides, calcium/potassium electrochemical gradient, metabolic coupling factors (MCFs), and the cellular level of reactive oxygen/nitrogen species (ROS/RNS). However, glucose is the principle insulin stimulant as it is the primary source of fuel in food (Fu et al., 2013). Metabolism of glucose by β-cells leads directly to the generation of ATP via glycolysis and to reducing equivalents such as NADH and $FADH_2$ via the tricarboxylic acid (TCA) cycle. NADH and $FADH_2$ contribute to the total level of ATP when they are oxidized by the electron transport chain (ETC) in the mitochondria. The net result of this high-energy environment is an enhanced ATP/ADP ratio in the β-cell, which promotes plasma membrane depolarization by inhibition of K^+_{ATP}-sensitive channels (Jensen et al., 2008; Newsholme & Krause, 2012). This depolarization leads to simultaneous opening of voltage-gated Ca^{2+} channels, promoting an intracellular flux of calcium ions that ultimately induces insulin granule exocytosis (Fig. 1.1) (Newsholme et al., 2010; Newsholme & Krause, 2012). Glucose-stimulated insulin secretion (GSIS) is fundamental to normoglycaemic control and dysregulation of this process results in metabolic disorders such as DM (Newsholme & Krause, 2012).

Pancreatic β-cell failure is a major contributing factor to onset and progression of both T1 and T2DM, even though the etiology of each may superficially appear different (Cnop et al., 2005). β-Cell failure or loss of function refers to a reduction in insulin secretion and/or a failure of cells to respond to plasma glucose (i.e., insulin resistance), eventually leading to reduced β-cell mass by initiation of apoptotic cell death (Cnop et al., 2005). In T1DM, an autoimmunological attack of β-cells is the primary cause of reduced insulin secretion and decreased β-cell mass (Cnop et al., 2005). In contrast, the development of T2DM is more complex, with the process of initiating and propagating dysfunction and destruction of β-cells occurring over a greater period of time and dependent on several key stages of progression (Cnop et al., 2005). Weir and Bonner-Weir proposed five

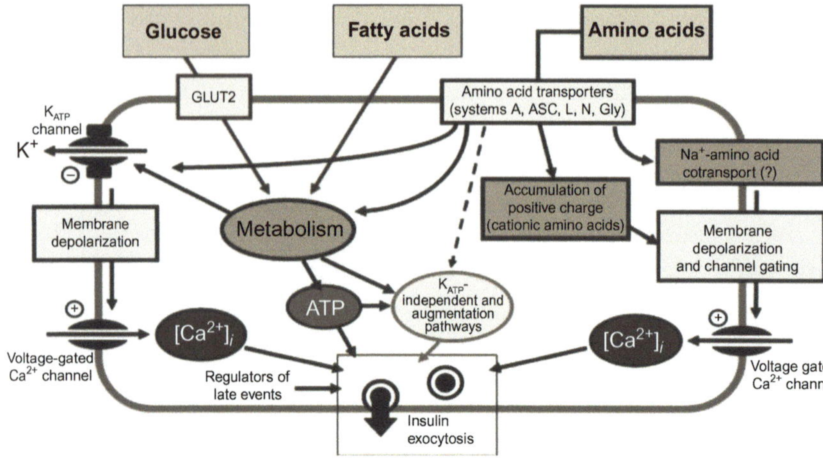

Figure 1.1 Mechanisms of nutrient-stimulated insulin secretion. Glucose metabolism is essential for stimulation of insulin secretion (impacting on K^+_{ATP} channel closure prompting membrane depolarization). Amino acid metabolism enhances insulin secretion via (a) direct depolarization of the plasma membrane (e.g., cationic amino acid, L-arginine); (b) metabolism (e.g., alanine, glutamine, leucine); and (c) cotransport with Na^+ and cell membrane depolarization (e.g., alanine). Fatty acid metabolism enhances basal insulin secretion in glucose absence through generation of ATP. *Taken from Newsholme, Gaudel, and McClenaghan (2010).* (See the color plate.)

distinct stages of development in T2DM and these were based on changes in β-cell mass, phenotype and function (Weir & Bonner-Weir, 2004). Briefly, the first stage, Compensation, involves a compensatory response to increased metabolic load, where insulin release is elevated to maintain normoglycaemia and may stem from increased β-cell mass or increased β-cell hypertrophy (Lee & Pervaiz, 2007; Weir & Bonner-Weir, 2004). Stage 2, Stable Adaption, here there is a loss of acute GSIS and the fasting glucose range increases (5–7.3 mM). The previous compensatory mechanism has failed to maintain normoglycaemic concentrations in this phase (Weir & Bonner-Weir, 2004). Stage 3 refers to Unstable Early Decompensation that comprises elevation of fasting plasma glucose above 7.3 mM. This phase follows initiation of β-cell death and reduced β-cell mass due to glucotoxicity and lipotoxicity. Progression to stage 4, Stable Decompensation, depends on sustained glucolipotoxicity and a further reduction in β-cell mass, typically ~50% in T2DM patients (Weir & Bonner-Weir, 2004). This period is considered stable and patients can remain here without developing ketosis, although islet β-cells become severely dedifferentiated. The final phase, stage 5 Severe Decompensation, is characterized by a complete loss of β-cell mass and consequently function, with plasma glucose concentrations exceeding 22 mM (Weir & Bonner-Weir, 2004). Patients can fluctuate between stages 1 and 4 depending on diet, exercise, and drugs, but those at stage 5 are dependent on exogenous insulin and are in danger of developing ketosis (Weir & Bonner-Weir, 2004). These periods of disease progression mainly relate to T2DM, but there are commonalities that can be imparted upon the evolution of T1DM. However, the key exception is that the upward shift between specific phases can occur at rapid rates in T1DM patients, given the swift autoimmune destruction of β-cells (Weir & Bonner-Weir, 2004).

Although T2DM is generally related to dysfunctional metabolism, immune cell infiltration, and inflammation are becoming important features in T2DM islets (Donath et al., 2008; Ehses et al., 2007). Likewise, elements of metabolic dysfunction are becoming increasingly evident in T1DM due to impaired insulin release. Hyperglycaemia and dyslipidaemia from lack of insulin secretion appear to exacerbate the disease, and some T1DM patients can often present with characteristics that are commonly observed in T2DM (Odegaard & Chawla, 2012). Furthermore, high-glucose load has been linked to engagement of the immune system as shown by secretion of IL-1β from *in vitro* culture of nondiabetic islets in elevated glucose (Donath et al., 2008). *In vivo*, this could lead to NFκB activation, Fas upregulation, reduced insulin secretion, and β-cell DNA fragmentation, along with promoting immune cell infiltration (Donath et al., 2008; Wang, Guan, & Yang, 2010). Consequently, understanding the molecular regulation of glucose and fatty acid metabolism, and their impact on insulin secretion under physiological conditions, is critical to dissecting factors that contribute to hyperglycaemia and dyslipidaemia in both T1 and T2DM patients. In addition, it is also prudent to consider the metabolic effects of another large group of macronutrients that are available from the diet, amino acids, in order to fully delineate the limits and benefits of nutrients on metabolic regulation of insulin secretion. Therefore, the precise way in which glucose, fatty and amino acid metabolism affects β-cell insulin secretion, proliferation, and survival will be discussed in the following sections.

2. GLUCOSE METABOLISM AND INSULIN SECRETION

2.1. Glycolysis

Glucose is the main insulin secretagogue and induces β-cell insulin exocytosis via its chemical degradation (glycolysis), but also by mitochondrial metabolism of glycolytic products (i.e., pyruvate) (Newsholme & Krause, 2012). Glucose is transported into the β-cells via specialized, insulin-independent membrane transporter proteins called GLUT's. There are several isoforms of these proteins, with GLUT1 and GLUT3 the main transporters in human β-cells, while GLUT2 is the principal transporter in rodent β-cells (De Vos et al., 1995; McCulloch et al., 2011; Rorsman & Braun, 2013). The K_m values of GLUT1 and GLUT2 for glucose are 6 and 11 mM, respectively, while the K_m of GLUT3 is 1 mM. The relatively high values for GLUT1 and 2 proposes that these transporters are activated only when significantly high levels of glucose are detected in the blood stream, for example following ingestion of food. However, the high affinity of GLUT3 for glucose would suggest that it plays a role in β-cell metabolic fuel homeostasis during periods of glucose deprivation. Interestingly, the difference in affinity between GLUT1 and 2 appears to correlate with the difference in basal plasma glucose concentrations in healthy humans (around 5 mM) and mice (7–10 mM) (Li et al., 2009; Remedi, Agapova, Vyas, Hruz, & Nichols, 2011; Rorsman & Braun, 2013). These insulin-independent control mechanisms allow β-cell sensing of nutrients, and also intracellular transport of free glucose molecules when levels are elevated enough to justify insulin release.

Upon internalization of glucose, glycolysis is quickly initiated and glucose is phosphorylated in a series of steps to create the nucleotide ATP, an important insulin releasing factor as outlined above. The first reaction is rapid and is catalyzed by the enzyme glucokinase (GCK). This yields glucose-6-phosphate and the speed of conversion prevents undesirable shuttling of free glucose out of the cell by GLUT transporters. GCK is an intricately designed hexokinase that has low affinity (high K_m) for glucose of approximately 6 mM (Fu et al., 2013; Newsholme & Krause, 2012). Similar to the GLUT proteins mentioned previously, GCK will only operate when a sufficient amount of glucose has entered the β-cell. Therefore, this glycolytic enzyme is rate-limiting and is not inhibited by its product which is normally a common metabolic regulatory mechanism (Fu et al., 2013). The combination of these two features indicates that GCK can maintain glycolytic flux in the face of high-glucose load (Fu et al., 2013). Interestingly, it has been suggested that changes in GCK function resulted in decreased GSIS that could possibly lead to DM, thus highlighting the importance of this metabolic step (Gloyn et al., 2005; Rorsman & Braun, 2013). In addition, another glycolytic enzyme, phosphofructokinase (PFK), is also an important regulatory site in glycolysis and is allosterically controlled by ATP levels

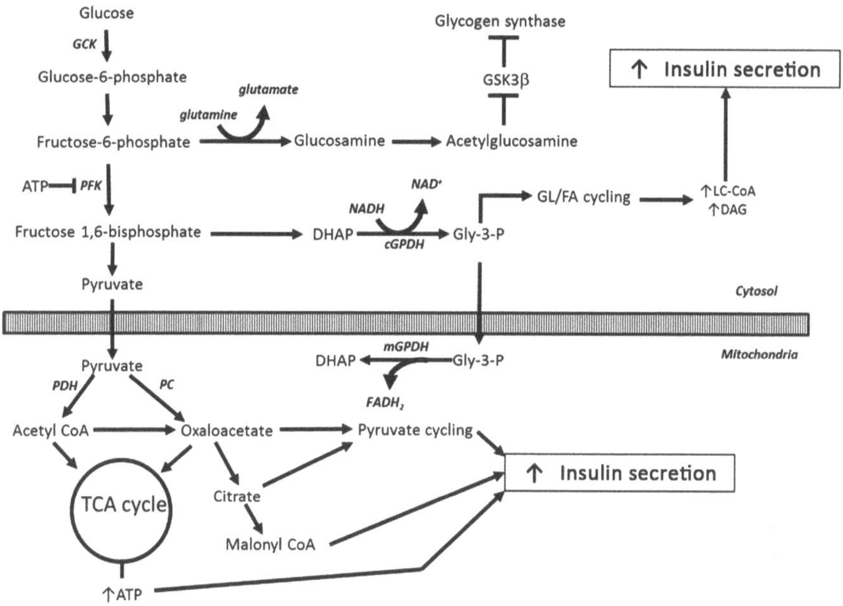

Figure 1.2 Overview of the interplay between glycolytic, TCA, and insulin secretion pathways in pancreatic β-cells. Glycolytic intermediates may be diverted away from glycolysis leading to glycogen synthesis. TCA metabolism results in elevated ATP production and insulin secretion. GL/FA cycling leads to enhanced insulin secretion via formation of signaling lipids. GCK, glucokinase; PFK, phosphofructokinase; PC, pyruvate carboxylase; PDH, pyruvate dehydrogenase; DHAP, dihydroxyacetone phosphate; Gly-3-P, glycerol-3-phosphate; GPDH, glycerol-3-phosphate dehydrogenase; GL/FA, glycerolipid/fatty acid; DAG, diacylglycerol; LC-CoA, long-chain CoA.

(Fig. 1.2). Alterations in PFK activity can also lead to fluctuations in glycolytic flux toward pyruvate (Nielsen, Sorensen, Hynne, & Busse, 1998; Westermark & Lansner, 2003).

However, there are glycolytic intermediates that may be deviated away from the process of glycolysis. For example, reaction of fructose-6-phosphate with glutamine via the hexosamine biochemical pathway (HBP), may lead to increased glycogen synthesis, but may also lead to increased endoplasmic reticulum (ER) stress (Fig. 1.2). This pathway has been associated with development of insulin resistance (Srinivasan, Tatu, Mohan, & Balasubramanyam, 2009). In addition, formation of dihydoxyacetone phosphate (DHAP) and glycerol-3-phosphate (Gly-3-P) from fructose 1, 6-bisphosphate, influences glycerolipid (GL)/free fatty acid (FFA) cycling and metabolism (Fig. 1.2) (Nolan & Prentki, 2008). In this shuttle, two enzymes isoforms (cytosolic and mitochondrial Gly-3-P dehydrogenase, GPDH) act sequentially in order to derive $FADH_2$ from conversion of Gly-3-P back to DHAP in the mitochondria (Jitrapakdee, Wutthisathapornchai, Wallace, & MacDonald, 2010). Production of $FADH_2$ subsequently leads to ATP synthesis and insulin release (Fig. 1.2).

2.2. Downstream of glycolysis

If glucose carbons avoid Gly-3-P shuttling and the HBP pathway, the glycolytic end product, pyruvate, generates additional MCF's via the TCA cycle that enhance the ATP/ADP ratio and insulin release. Pyruvate is converted to either acetyl-CoA or oxaloacetate by pyruvate dehydrogenase (PDH; glucose oxidation pathway) and pyruvate carboxylase (PC; anaplerosis/cataplerosis pathway), respectively, and these intermediates enter the TCA cycle leading to increased $FADH_2$ and NADPH formation, and consequently ATP production via oxidative phosphorylation in the mitochondria (Fig. 1.2). Previously, it has been shown that PC and PDH are both highly expressed in β-cells (Jitrapakdee et al., 2010). However, PC is also highly expressed in tissues that participate in gluconeogenesis (e.g., liver), but β-cells do not possess the necessary enzyme compliment to perform gluconeogenesis (i.e., phosphoenolpyruvate carboxykinase), and therefore it must play an anaplerotic function in islets (MacDonald, 1995a, 1995b). Interestingly, studies in murine models have indicated that siRNA knock-down of PC reduces β-cell proliferation and GSIS in insulinoma cells and rat islets (Hasan et al., 2008; Xu, Han, Long, Epstein, & Liu, 2008), while upregulation of PC enhanced these characteristics (Xu et al., 2008). In contrast, recent reports have suggested that there was a marked difference in PC activity between rodent and human islets. MacDonald et al. has demonstrated that PC expression was significantly lower (80–90%) in human islets, compared to both mouse and rat islets (MacDonald et al., 2011). These researchers also found that human islets expressed significantly higher levels of succinyl-CoA:3-ketoacid-CoA transferase (SCOT) and acetoacetyl-CoA synthase, which may operate in tandem to create cytosolic acyl-CoAs from acetoacetate (MacDonald et al., 2011). Therefore, human β-cells may employ this alternative enzymatic mechanism more regularly than utilizing PC and citrate to generate acyl-CoA (MacDonald et al., 2011). However, further studies are required to verify this hypothesis.

Similarly, the complete function of PDH has not been fully clarified, but it is understood to assist PC action by generating acetyl-CoA (Jitrapakdee et al., 2010). It is known that PDH activity is rigorously controlled by various inhibitory end products such as acetyl-CoA, NADH, and ATP, and by several PDH kinase enzymes (Sugden & Holness, 2011). The rationale behind such stringent regulation is that the action of PDH irreversibly commits glucose-derived carbon to oxidation (Sugden & Holness, 2011). Moreover, the role played by PDH in regulating GSIS is also not fully elucidated. Current reports have suggested that inhibition of PDH by overexpression of PDH kinase 4 in INS-1 cells, did not negatively impact on insulin secretion (Xu et al., 2008). However, these data do not entirely reject an important regulatory function of PDH, given its characterized action of generating acetyl-CoA (Jitrapakdee et al., 2010). Therefore, the position of PDH in β-cell metabolism and insulin secretion is still to be determined.

2.3. β-Cell shuttles

Pancreatic β-cells express very low levels of lactate dehydrogenase (LDH), and mainly regenerate NAD^+ for glycolysis through high expression of mitochondrial NADH/NADPH (redox) shuttles such as pyruvate/malate, pyruvate/citrate, malate/aspartate, and Gly-3-P (Maassen et al., 2006). Production of oxaloacetate from PC is a key modulator of both pyruvate/malate and pyruvate/citrate shuttles. PC-derived oxaloacetate is converted to malate and traverses the mitochondrial membrane to the cytosol via the malate carrier, where malic enzyme1 (ME1) reconverts it to pyruvate, simultaneously creating NADPH. Pyruvate can then reenter the mitochondria repeating the process with more NADPH produced (Fig. 1.3) (Jitrapakdee et al., 2010). Alternatively, PC-derived oxaloacetate can condense with acetyl-CoA (possibly provided by PDH) in mitochondria to produce citrate (Fig. 1.3). This intermediate can enter the cytosol and ATP-citrate lyase (ACL) may regenerate oxaloacetate and acetyl-CoA from citrate (Jitrapakdee et al., 2010). Cytosolic malate dehydrogenase then creates malate from oxaloacetate, and NADPH can be produced from the ME1 reaction as detailed above (Fig. 1.3). Simultaneously, acetyl-CoA regenerated from citrate can be carboxylated to malonyl-CoA by acetyl-CoA carboxylase (ACC), and this has important implications in fatty acid metabolism and amplification of GSIS (Fig. 1.3) (Jitrapakdee et al., 2010).

The malate/aspartate shuttle also has a significant impact on generation of reducing equivalents and consequently ATP production/insulin secretion in β-cells. This shuttle is the primary shuttle that transfers glycolytic reducing equivalents from the cytoplasm to the mitochondria in the β-cell, and eloquently links glycolysis to mitochondrial and amino acid metabolism

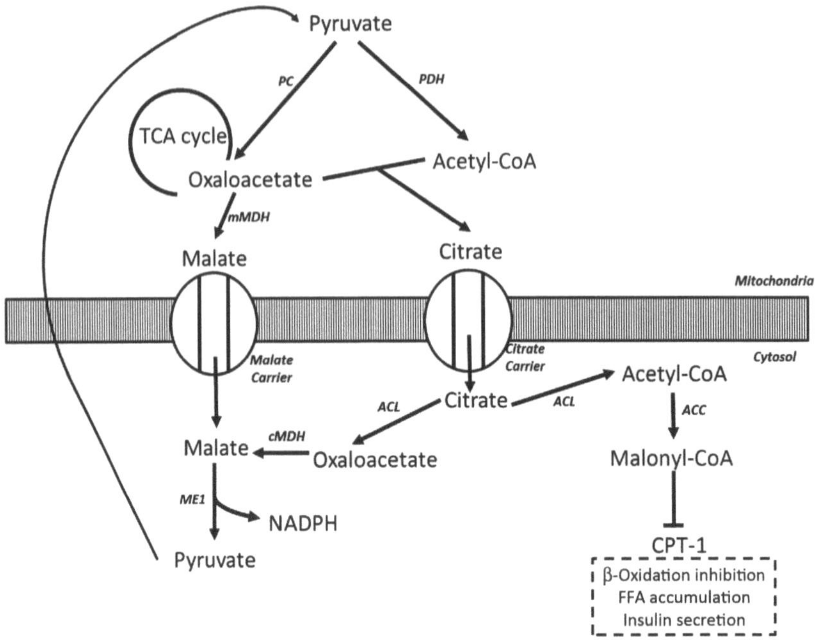

Figure 1.3 The pyruvate/malate and pyruvate/citrate shuttles are important mechanisms for producing NADPH in β-cells. Pyruvate-derived oxaloacetate is converted to malate by mitochondrial malate dehydrogenase (mMDH) and passes into the cytosol. Malate is converted back to pyruvate by maleic enzyme-1 (ME1) producing NADPH, while pyruvate is cycled back across the mitochondrial membrane. Pyruvate-derived oxaloacetate can condense with acetyl-CoA to generate citrate that is transferred to the cytosol and separated into oxaloacetate and acetyl-CoA. Oxaloacetate is then converted to malate by cytosolic malate dehydrogenase (cMDH) and forms NADPH by ME1. Acetyl-CoA is converted to malonyl-CoA and inhibits FFA oxidation. PC, pyruvate carboxylase; PDH, pyruvate dehydrogenase; ACL, ATP-citrate lyase; ACC, acetyl-CoA carboxylase.

(Newsholme, Bender, Kiely, & Brennan, 2007). In this process, cytosolic malate dehydrogenase (cMDH) reduces oxaloacetate to malate and NAD^+, so that it can cross the mitochondrial membrane (Fig. 1.4). The reaction is then reversed by mitochondrial MDH (mMDH), along with the generation of NADH. Mitochondrial oxaloacetate is moved back to the cytosol by transamination to aspartate in the presence of glutamate (Fig. 1.4). This movement allows rotation of the shuttle, while the generated NADH produces ATP via the ETC (Newsholme, Bender, et al., 2007). Furthermore, Aralar1, a mitochondrial aspartate–glutamate carrier that participates in malate–aspartate cycling, has been shown to play a significant function in GSIS. Deletion of Aralar1 in INS-1 cells results in a complete loss of

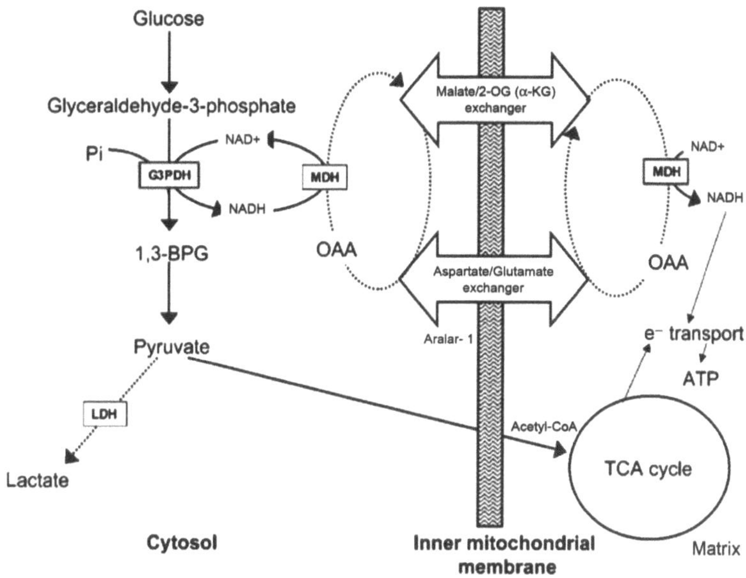

Figure 1.4 The malate–aspartate shuttle is central to the movement of reducing equivalents in the form of NADH, from the cytoplasm to the mitochondrion in β-cells. Cytoplasmic malate dehydrogenase reduces (MDH) oxaloacetate (OAA) to malate, while generating NAD^+ from NADH. Malate enters the mitochondrion and is converted back to OAA producing NADH via mitochondrial MDH. Transamination of OAA to 2-oxoglutarate via the aspartate/glutamate exchanger subsequently transports OAA back to the cytosol and maintains this cycle event. *Taken from Newsholme, Bender, et al. (2007).*

malate–aspartate shuttle activity, and a subsequent 25% reduction in insulin secretion (Marmol et al., 2009). Conversely, upregulation of Aralar1 improves GSIS and amino acid-stimulated insulin secretion in BRIN-BD11 cells (Bender, Maechler, McClenaghan, Flatt, & Newsholme, 2009).

The generation of reducing equivalents and/or ATP by the described mechanisms, are central to glucose metabolism, and as outlined previously, it is this ATP signal that is primarily responsible for insulin granule exocytosis in β-cells. There are several important and remarkable adaptions of β-cells that ensure continued oxidative and anaplerotic metabolism of glucose and pyruvate, that maximize ATP output against the backdrop of limited lactate resources (Bender et al., 2009; Jensen et al., 2008; McClenaghan et al., 2009; Newsholme, Bender, et al., 2007; Newsholme, Keane, Welters, & Morgan, 2007; Newsholme & Krause, 2012). These adaptions include the ability to "sense" glucose in a physiologically relevant range of 2–20 mmol/L, low expression of LDH with a corresponding high-expression redox shuttles, along with increased PDH and PC activity (Newsholme & Krause, 2012). However, given the biphasic insulin response in animals, where there is an immediately releasable pool of insulin following exposure to increased blood glucose (over 8 min), and a subsequent slow, gradual release over 36 min (Jitrapakdee et al., 2010; Straub & Sharp, 2002), there remains the possibility that other processes are involved and these may be K^{+}_{ATP} channel independent. Studies have demonstrated that K^{+}_{ATP}-independent GSIS was evident in mice with disrupted or deleted K^{+}_{ATP} channels (Miki et al., 1998; Remedi et al., 2011) and in animals treated with diazoxide (Gembal, Gilon, & Henquin, 1992). Although the K^{+}_{ATP}-independent method of insulin secretion has not been fully clarified, it is reasonable to assume that a plethora of factors, which may include fatty and amino acids, regulate the interplay between mixed nutrient-sensing and insulin exocytosis. This is particularly evident if one considers the physical and mechanical mechanisms that govern insulin granule release, which are subject to vesicle manufacture, recruitment, and plasma membrane docking. Therefore, in the following sections, we will discuss the impact of both fatty and amino acids metabolism on insulin secretion.

3. FATTY ACID METABOLISM AND INSULIN SECRETION

In addition to carbohydrates, FFAs are also critical metabolic constituents for normal β-cell function and insulin release, but they have also been implicated in β-cell failure and insulin resistance (Nolan, Madiraju, Delghingaro-Augusto, Peyot, & Prentki, 2006). Access of FFA to the cytosol is not strictly regulated by specific membrane transporters, such as the GLUT proteins for glucose. Instead, FFAs gain entry to the β-cell by freely diffusing through the plasma membrane, due to their lipophilic profile (Hamilton & Kamp, 1999). Consequently, admission to the cytosol is primarily subject to the local availability of FFAs (Newsholme, Keane, et al., 2007). Under energy-reduced conditions, internalized FFAs are metabolized to long-chain acyl-CoA (LC-CoA) by acyl-CoA synthase (ACS) in the cytosol and then transported to the interior of the mitochondria by Carnitine Palmitoyl Transferase-1 (CPT-1) (Berne, 1975; Newsholme & Krause, 2012). Here, LC-CoA is oxidized by a process known as β-oxidation, as a means to replenish ATP in the energy-reduced state of the cell. This method of ATP generation sustains a basal release of insulin, in a K^{+}_{ATP}-dependent manner (Newsholme et al., 2010). However, following ingestion of a carbohydrate containing meal, citrate, produced by glycolytic metabolism and generation of TCA intermediates, is converted to malonyl-CoA by acetyl-CoA carboxylase (ACC), and this allosterically inhibits the action of CPT-1, thus preventing further FFA transport into the mitochondria (Fig. 1.5) (Carpentier, Mittelman, Bergman, Giacca, & Lewis, 2000; Nolan, Madiraju, et al., 2006). The net effect is suppression of β-oxidation and enhancement of lipid signaling by accrual of cytosolic FFA. This FFA partitioning significantly amplifies insulin granule exocytosis by altering the acylation state of regulatory ion channel proteins, increasing Ca^{2+} influx, generation of insulinotropic lipids (LC-CoA; diacylglycerol [DAG]) and enhancing insulin vesicle docking with the plasma membrane (Fig. 1.5) (Deeney et al., 2000; Haber et al., 2006; Newsholme et al., 2010; Newsholme & Krause, 2012). Therefore, FFAs do not stimulate insulin secretion directly, but rather potentiate GSIS in β-cells (Fig. 1.5) (Keane & Newsholme, 2008; Nolan & Prentki, 2008).

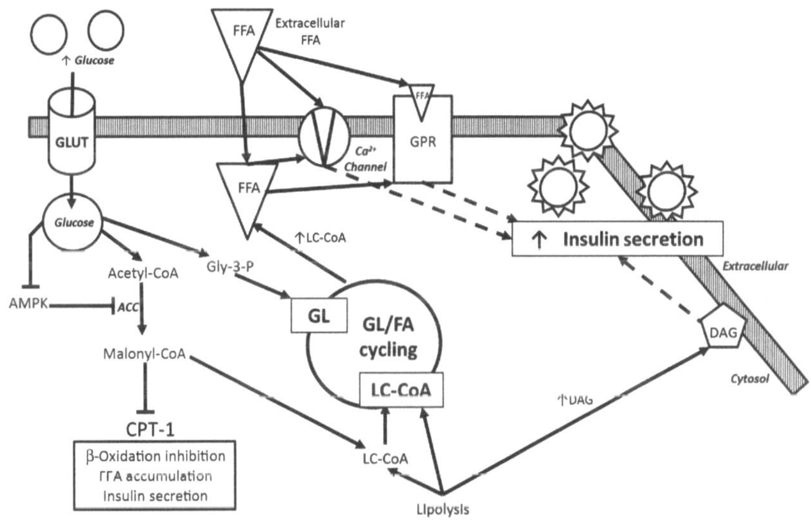

Figure 1.5 Overview of the interplay between glucose and free fatty acid (FFA) metabolism, glycerolipid/fatty acid (GL/FA) cycling, lipolysis, and insulin secretion. Increased glucose can induce FFA accumulation in the cytosol via malonyl-CoA inhibition of β-oxidation, initiation of GL/FA cycling through generation of glycerol-3-P (Gly-3-P) and glycerol and lipolysis. Increased FFA partitioning to the cytosol amplifies insulin granule exocytosis by altering the acylation state of regulatory ion channel proteins, increasing Ca^{2+} influx, generation of insulinotropic lipids (long-chain, CoA; diacylglycerol, DAG), and enhancing insulin vesicle docking with the plasma membrane. Dashed lines indicate routes to insulin secretion. ACC, acetyl-CoA carboxylase; GPR, G-protein-couple receptor.

The activity of malonyl-CoA is mainly regulated by AMP-activated kinase (AMPK), which has the ability to inhibit ACC by phosphorylation, leading to reduced conversion of citrate to malonyl-CoA (Newsholme & Krause, 2012). In addition, AMPK can enhance the catalytic ability of malonyl-CoA decarboxylase (MCD), also by phosphorylation, and this results in increased decarboxylation and inactivation of malonyl-CoA (Nolan, Madiraju, et al., 2006). Both processes reduce the expression of active malonyl-CoA, thus they facilitate reduced FFA esterification, increased FFA entry to the mitochondria and consequently enhanced β-oxidation (Fig. 1.5) (Nolan, Madiraju, et al., 2006; Ruderman & Prentki, 2004). Interestingly, it has been demonstrated that the combination of malonyl-CoA and FFA, are key factors for regulating GSIS. Using MCD overexpression, it was found that reduced malonyl-CoA had no significant effect on GSIS. However, in the presence of FFA, MCD overexpression and consequently malonyl-CoA suppression, significantly reduced GSIS in INS832/13 β-cells and islets (Mulder et al., 2001; Nolan, Madiraju, et al., 2006; Roduit et al., 2004). As such, AMPK, who regulates malonyl-CoA, is sensitive to the energy status of the cell and is stimulated by a high-AMP/ATP ratio in nutrient-deprived conditions (Nolan, Madiraju, et al., 2006). Interestingly, AMPK can also augment the expression status of important transcription factors, like sterol-regulatory-element-binding protein-1c (SREBP-1c) and hepatocyte nuclear factor-4α (HNF-4α), that are associated with regulation of additional lipogenic and glycolytic proteins (Newsholme & Krause, 2012).

Another glucose-responsive element of FFA signaling and metabolism is the cycling of glycerolipids/fatty acids (GL/FA) in β-cells. Central to this pathway is the formation of Gly-3-P from a side reaction of glycolysis (from inbound glucose) and generation of glycerol and FFAs from triglycerides by lipolysis. Although it may seem contradictory, it has been shown that both FA esterification and lipolysis can be stimulated in β-cells by glucose challenge in the presence of FFA, while β-oxidation is inhibited (Nolan, Madiraju, et al., 2006). The purpose of this cycle may be to provide insulinotropic lipid signaling molecules, by lipolysis (e.g., LC-CoA, DAG) that aid insulin vesicle manufacture and exocytosis, while simultaneously restocking the fatty acid stores. Production of DAG activates protein kinase C (PKC) and also Munc-13, which is a synaptic vesicle priming protein involved in granule exocytosis (Newsholme et al., 2010; Newsholme, Keane, et al., 2007; Nolan, Madiraju, et al., 2006; Nolan & Prentki, 2008). Additionally, LC-CoA can acylate other docking proteins, such as synaptosomal-associated protein-25 (SNAP25) and synaptogamin, and this enhances their ability to interact with the plasma membrane, thus facilitating increased exocytosis (Nolan, Madiraju, et al., 2006; Rorsman & Braun, 2013). GL/FA cycling may offer several advantages to β-cells over typical glycolytic flux. A significant share of inbound glucose (25%) is converted to Gly-3-P and this could potentially facilitate production of NAD^+ that is required for swift glycolysis of the remaining glucose (Nolan & Prentki, 2008). Furthermore, this route deviates some of the glucose carbon away from mitochondrial metabolism and therefore may offer an alternative mechanism to generate MCF's that is independent of the TCA cycle and oxidative phosphorylation (Nolan & Prentki, 2008). In addition, this process may also protect the β-cell by reducing mitochondrial dysfunction, protein glycation, and ER stress resulting from oxidative metabolism (Nolan & Prentki, 2008).

Another suggested mechanism by which lipids augment insulin secretion is via interaction with G-protein coupled receptors (GPR) (Shapiro, Shachar, Sekler, Hershfinkel, & Walker, 2005). This is the third segment of the "trident model" hypothesis proposed by Nolan, Madiraju, et al. (2006) for FFA-mediated amplification of GSIS, and follows the TCA/malonyl-CoA signaling and GL/FA cycling pathways (Fig. 1.5) (Nolan, Madiraju, et al., 2006). Recent reports have shown that GPR's are abundantly expressed in β-cells and were associated with insulinogenic index (Newsholme & Krause, 2012; Tomita et al., 2006). Several GPR isoforms, including GPR40, GPR41, GPR119, and GPR120 are important in β-cell physiology (Newsholme & Krause, 2012). For instance, downregulation of GPR40 (or free fatty acid receptor-1, FFAR-1) in rat β-cells and islets, reduced FFA-amplification of GSIS (Itoh et al., 2003), while studies in GPR40-deficient mice showed a decrease in GSIS by about 50% (Latour et al., 2007). This latter finding suggested that FFA can potentiate GSIS by an alternative mechanism, such as malonyl-CoA signaling or GL/FA cycling (Nolan & Prentki, 2008). It is thought that GPR's transduce the FFA interaction to GSIS-amplification by enhancing Ca^{2+} efflux from the ER (Nolan & Prentki, 2008). However, this appears to be dependent on glucose-mediated activation of L-type calcium channels, which further explains the enhancement role of FFA's, rather than direct stimulation of insulin release (Nolan & Prentki, 2008). GPRs can be activated by a range of FFA molecules varying in chain length, although the exact mechanisms of GSIS-amplification are still not entirely understood (Newsholme & Krause, 2012; Ulven, 2012). Nonetheless, current evidence has pointed to the use of GPR receptor agonists as potential therapeutic agents to control hyperglycaemia in T2DM patients (Burant et al., 2012). An example of which is TAK-875, that reduced glycated hemoglobin and hypoglycaemic effects in DM patients, in comparison with glimepiride and placebo (Burant et al., 2012). Other research has demonstrated that omega-3 fatty acids can promote insulin-sensitization and antiinflammatory effects in obese mice models, and this appeared to be mediated through the GPR120 receptor (Oh et al., 2010).

The effects of FFAs on insulin exocytosis are also dependent on several other aspects including, the type of lipid, the level of hydrogen saturation, the length of the carbon chain, and whether exposure is under acute or chronic settings (Newsholme & Krause, 2012). For example, saturated fatty acids such as palmitic and stearic acid acutely enhance GSIS, but chronically decrease GSIS *in vitro* (Hosokawa, Corkey, & Leahy, 1997; Keane et al., 2011). In contrast, monounsaturated oleic acid and polyunsaturated arachidonic acid can elevate insulin secretion in β-cell lines following chronic exposure (Keane et al., 2011; Vassiliou et al., 2009). However, chronic exposure of β-cells to high-circulatory lipid levels, such as occurs in T2DM, can also impair glucose oxidation and consequently result in a decreased ATP/AMP ratio, with a subsequent activation of AMPK (Newsholme & Krause, 2012). This will inhibit fatty acid synthesis, while driving fatty acid oxidation. Thus, further inhibition of GSIS can occur via metabolic inactivation of TCA enzymes like PDH and activation of inhibitory PDH kinases (Newsholme & Krause, 2012). In addition, the level of insulinotropic lipid signaling molecules such as DAG may decrease, leading to reduced insulin exocytosis (Haber et al., 2006). The detrimental outputs of FFA metabolism in terms of promoting cell death will be described later in reference to increased lipotoxicity from fuel surfeit. However, we will now discuss the impact of amino acids on β-cell metabolism, and how amino acids are intrinsically connected to glucose and fatty acid metabolism.

4. AMINO ACID METABOLISM AND INSULIN SECRETION

Amino acids are the third major class of nutrients that are required for cell survival, along with carbohydrates and lipids. Amino acid metabolism is essential for protein and nucleotide synthesis, as well as participating in nutrient- and glucose-stimulated insulin secretion. Several amino acids are known to elicit positive and/or negative effects on β-cell insulin release *in vitro* and *in vivo*. Similar to FFA, these effects are dependent on whether exposure is acute or chronic, and also dependent on cytosolic/mitochondrial metabolism and stimulation/suppression of gene expression (Newsholme & Krause, 2012). However, individual amino acids alone at physiological concentrations do not enhance GSIS, but rather amino acids at elevated concentrations, or in specific combinations at physiological levels can enhance GSIS (Newsholme & Krause, 2012). They impact on both the triggering and amplification cascades of insulin secretion, and do so through three distinct mechanisms (Nolan & Prentki, 2008). These include, (a) ATP generation via TCA metabolism and/or shuttle exchanges, (b) direct depolarization of plasma membrane by interaction with amino acid transporters and (c) membrane depolarization via cotransport of Na^+ ions along with the amino acid (Newsholme et al., 2010). The insulinotropic and noninsulinotropic characteristics of selected amino acids in β-cells will now be discussed.

The most abundant amino acids in plasma and extracellular fluid are L-alanine and L-glutamine (Newsholme et al., 2010; Nolan & Prentki, 2008). Therefore, it is reasonable to assume that they may influence insulin exocytosis. Numerous studies have demonstrated the positive effects of alanine on insulin secretion and in a variety of β-cell models. The authors have shown that alanine was consumed at rapid rates and increased insulin release in BRIN-BD11 cell lines and rat islets (Dixon, Nolan, McClenaghan, Flatt, & Newsholme, 2003; Newsholme et al., 2010; Newsholme & Krause, 2012). Others have shown that alanine has insulinotropic properties in rat RINm5f cells (Dunne, Yule, Gallacher, & Petersen, 1990), and in the newly deposited 1.1B4 human insulin secreting cell line (McCluskey et al., 2011). More recently, the authors have constructed an integrated mathematical modeling system that allowed determination of alanine metabolism and Ca^{2+}-handling in β-cells, with monitoring of subsequent effects on GSIS and amino acid-stimulated insulin secretion (Salvucci, Neufeld, & Newsholme, 2013). From these studies, we have discovered that elevated intracellular ATP and Ca^{2+} levels were required for complete insulin secretory responses in BRIN-BD11 cells, and this was confirmed *in vitro* using the BRIN-BD11 cell line (Salvucci et al., 2013). In addition, other analyses revealed that alanine-mediated Na^+ cotransport acted synergistically with membrane depolarization leading to K^+_{ATP}-independent Ca^{2+} influx and insulin secretion (McClenaghan, Barnett, & Flatt, 1998; Newsholme & Krause, 2012; Salvucci et al., 2013). Other insulinotropic mechanisms of alanine metabolism include, conversion to pyruvate (Salvucci et al., 2013), glutamate, aspartate, and lactate (Newsholme et al., 2010). These metabolic transformations may generate further MCFs that enhance ATP and consequently K^+_{ATP}-dependent insulin secretion, and may occur via pyruvate cycling, increasing TCA activity or by enhancing metabolic shuttling (Fig. 1.6) (Newsholme et al., 2006). However, some reports have suggested that β-cells can become desensitized to the insulinotropic effects of alanine, but simultaneously reported that it could protect β-cells from cytokine-induced apoptosis (Cunningham, McClenaghan, Flatt, & Newsholme, 2005). This is obviously an advantageous characteristic in the T1DM setting, but may be equally applicable in T2DM.

Similarly, glutamine is consumed by β-cells at rapid rates (Dixon et al., 2003) and is believed to be essential for maintaining β-cell metabolism and function. However, glutamine does not induce insulin exocytosis when administered individually (Dixon et al., 2003; Newsholme et al., 2010; Newsholme & Krause, 2012). The high utilization of glutamine suggests that it participates in other β-cells functions, such as a raw material for protein, purine, and pyrimidine manufacture (Newsholme & Krause, 2012). However, inhibition of glutamine synthesis using chemical inhibitors was demonstrated to abrogate GSIS, and suggested a significant role in GSIS potentiation (Li et al., 2004; Newsholme et al., 2010). Interestingly, coadministration of glutamine with leucine significantly enhanced insulin release (Henquin, 2000; Newsholme, Bender, et al., 2007), and was

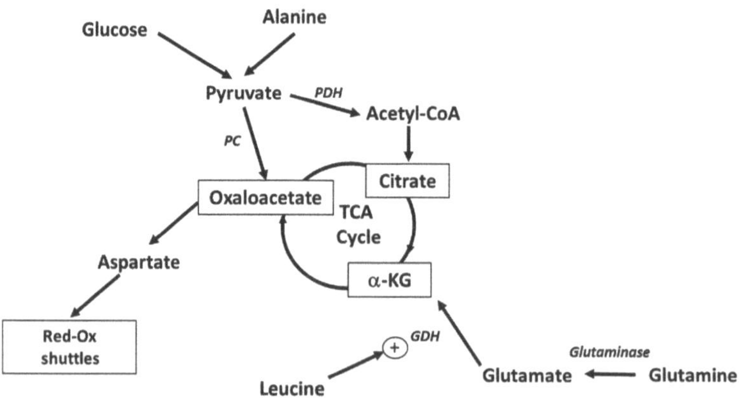

Figure 1.6 Schematic diagram following the metabolism of selected amino acids and the subsequent interplay with components of the TCA cycle. Glutamine carbons enter the TCA cycle via glutaminase and GDH, while alanine enters via pyruvate metabolism. The regulation of GDH activity by leucine is also shown. α-KG, α-ketoglutarate; PC, pyruvate carboxylase; GDH, glutamate dehydrogenase; PDH, pyruvate dehydrogenase. *Adapted from Newsholme, Brennan, and Bender (2006).*

understood to involve activation of glutamate dehydrogenase (GDH), which allowed entry of glutamine into the TCA cycle (Fig. 1.6) (Nolan & Prentki, 2008; Sener & Malaisse, 1980). The reason as to why glutamine does not induce insulin secretion alone is not clear but it is thought to arise from its metabolism. Utilizing carbon tracer technology and NMR analysis, glutamine was shown to increase aspartate and glutamate production (Fig. 1.6) (Brennan et al., 2003). Therefore, glutamine metabolism may feed into MCF-generating pathways like the aspartate/malate shuttle and the TCA cycle via α-ketoglutarate formation (Fig. 1.6) (Brennan et al., 2003; Newsholme & Krause, 2012; Nolan & Prentki, 2008). In addition, glutamine may contribute to β-cell antioxidant defense by glutamate conversion, with subsequent entry to γ-glutamyl cycle (Brennan et al., 2003; Newsholme & Krause, 2012). This may result in increased glutathione synthesis and elevated antioxidant levels may stabilize ROS formation during enhanced β-cell oxidative phosphorylation in response to glucose load. Indeed, glutamate production from glutamine also plays a role in activation of the aspartate/glutamate carrier (Aralar1) and converts mitochondrial oxaloacetate to aspartate allowing transfer back to the cytosol (Fig. 1.4). This allows continuation of the aspartate/malate exchanger and consequently NADH production (Newsholme, Bender, et al., 2007). Although glutamine does not individually impact on insulin release, its metabolism appears to be coupled to several mechanisms that can augment insulin secretion.

Interestingly, intracellular glutamate concentration appears to be intimately correlated with insulin exocytosis. However, the connection between glutamate and insulin secretion is still not entirely clear. Some researchers have demonstrated that total intracellular glutamate levels were increased in response to glucose in islets and β-cell lines (Brennan et al., 2002; Broca, Brennan, Petit, Newsholme, & Maechler, 2003), while others showed no significant change (Danielsson, Hellman, & Idahl, 1970; MacDonald & Fahien, 2000). Other studies have demonstrated that glutamate accumulated in insulin vesicles and could be potentially transported into the surrounding matrix during insulin release (Hoy et al., 2002; Newsholme & Krause, 2012). Recent evidence indicated that glutamate could promote Ca^{2+}-dependent insulin secretion following transportation into these insulin-containing vesicles (Gammelsaeter et al., 2011). Furthermore, externalized glutamate may impact on β-cell glutamate receptor activation and could possibly induce receptor desensitization in an autocrine fashion, if the release is over extended periods of time (Corless, Kiely, McClenaghan, Flatt, & Newsholme, 2006). Similarly, glutamate release may reduce glucagon secretion from neighboring glutamate-sensitive pancreatic α-cells, and indicate a new paracrine regulatory mechanism for controlling blood carbohydrate levels (Corless et al., 2006).

Other amino acids, such as arginine, have been suggested to promote insulin release. Arginine is a positively charged amino acid and gains entry to the β-cell via the electrogenic transporter mCAT2A (Newsholme & Krause, 2012). This causes changes in plasma membrane potential that results in opening of Ca^{2+} ion channels, with a subsequent Ca^{2+} influx and insulin exocytosis (McClenaghan et al., 1998; Newsholme & Krause, 2012; Sener et al., 2000). It has been shown that arginine enhanced β-cell function when β-cell lines and rat islets were subjected to cytokine insult (Krause et al., 2011). Exogenously added amino acid protected cells from cytokine-induced apoptosis, while it partially boosted insulin secretion (Krause et al., 2011). Furthermore, arginine increased the levels of antioxidants and glutamate in these cells, which suggested that it may protect β-cells from oxidative stress in addition to inducing insulin secretion (Krause et al., 2011). In contrast, negative effects of arginine have also been observed from its reaction with inducible nitric oxide synthase (iNOS) (Newsholme & Krause, 2012). This reaction can potentially produce nitric oxide (NO), which at elevated levels, may be harmful to the antioxidant compromised β-cell (Newsholme & Krause, 2012).

Interestingly, homocysteine metabolism to asymmetric dimethylarginine (ADMA) can inhibit neuronal NOS and to a lesser extent iNOS. However, this effect is detrimental to the β-cell as NO is important in cell signaling and is required for glucose uptake at low basal levels (Higaki, Hirshman, Fujii, & Goodyear, 2001; Krause et al., 2012). Therefore, homocysteine may reduce the level of NO production and impact on β-cell function (Baylis, 2008; Newsholme & Krause, 2012). Indeed, it has been reported that homocysteine levels are elevated in obese hyperinsulinaemic T2DM patients, while they are also increased in T1DM patients, but only after disease-related complications, such as diabetic nephropathy (Newsholme, Bender, et al., 2007; Sanchez-Margalet et al., 2002). Homocysteine is a sulfur-containing amino acid and has been reported to reduce GSIS and amino acid-stimulated insulin secretion in rat pancreatic β-cells (Patterson, Flatt, & McClenaghan, 2006). The exact mechanism by which homocysteine exerts this negative effect is still not fully elucidated, but it is believed that it alters enzyme/protein activity, or induces oxidative stress (Medina, Urdiales, & Amores-Sanchez, 2001; Patterson, Flatt, & McClenaghan, 2007).

Conversely, cysteine at low concentrations has been reported to potentiate GSIS (Ammon, Hehl, Enz, Setiadi-Ranti, & Verspohl, 1986). Cysteine is one of three amino acids (along with glycine and glutamate) that make up glutathione, and is consequently an important raw material for antioxidant synthesis (Rasilainen, Nieminen, Levonen, Otonkoski, & Lapatto, 2002). Added cysteine was shown to protect β-cells from hydrogen peroxide (H_2O_2) insult (Rasilainen et al., 2002) and also protected mouse β-cells from glucotoxicity (Kaneko et al., 2009). However, in mouse islets and MIN65 β-cells, cysteine was converted to hydrogen sulfide (H_2S) and it appeared to reduce GSIS (Kaneko, Kimura, Kimura, & Niki, 2006). Therefore, depending on the context, cysteine may have beneficial or detrimental effects on β-cell function.

On the other hand, branched-chain amino acids (BCAA), consisting of leucine, isoleucine and valine, have been reported to play a beneficial role in insulin exocytosis but elevated plasma levels are correlated with increased insulin resistance (Lu, Xie, Jia, & Jia, 2013; Newsholme & Krause, 2012). Dairy product consumption has been linked to improvements in obesity and T2DM management, and milk-derived products, such as whey protein, are an excellent source of BCAA (Jakubowicz & Froy, 2013; Tremblay & Gilbert, 2009). Whey protein and whey protein hydrolysates have been suggested to improve glycaemic control and insulin release in *in vitro* and *in vivo* animal models (Gaudel et al., 2013), as well decreasing fasting insulin levels and hyperglycaemia in obese and T2DM human subjects (Jakubowicz & Froy, 2013). The mechanism of action of BCAA is not quite clear, but they are proposed to increase protein synthesis and thermogenesis via activation of mTOR signaling (Jakubowicz & Froy, 2013). In addition, these amino acids may also participate in TCA cycling by providing α-ketoglutarate substrates, and enhancing ATP turnover (Jakubowicz & Froy, 2013). Interestingly, leucine is a major component of whey protein and whey has 50–70% more leucine in comparison with other dietary protein sources (Jakubowicz & Froy, 2013). Leucine may have several mechanisms that mediate its insulinotropic effects. These include production of α-ketoglutarate and increased allosteric activation of GDH leading to increased TCA activity (Fig. 1.6) (Newsholme et al., 2010), enhanced ATP synthase and GCK expression (Yang et al., 2006), inhibition of K^+_{ATP} ion channels by α-keto acids including α-ketoglutarate (Newsholme et al., 2010) and by decreasing the activity of AMPK resulting in cytosolic FFA accumulation (Jakubowicz & Froy, 2013). In fact, recent research evidence has revealed that the positive effects of leucine on GDH activity, stems from an increase in substrate affinity, that leads to enhanced TCA cycling and is linked to a component of FFA metabolism, short-chain

L-3-hydroxyacyl-CoA dehydrogenase (SCHAD) (Heslegrave & Hussain, 2013). SCHAD catalyses one of the final reactions of β-oxidation, and is thought to regulate the activity of GDH by reducing its substrate affinity (Heslegrave & Hussain, 2013). Leucine tolerance tests were performed in patients with mutations in gene coding for SCHAD, and severe hyper-insulinaemia hypoglycaemia was observed. This work highlights a novel regulatory pathway that connects FFA to amino acid metabolism (Heslegrave & Hussain, 2013).

Taken together, there is a large body of evidence to suggest that amino acids potentiate GSIS in a variety of β-cell models. Furthermore, these findings also indicate that amino acids mediate these effects via several metabolic processes. However, even though some specific amino acids exert detrimental effects on β-cell function, the majority of these molecules positively influence insulin release, and may potentially be harnessed as treatments to aid DM management or to combat DM progression.

5. ASSOCIATION OF NUTRIENT METABOLISM WITH PANCREATIC β-CELL DYSFUNCTION

Incessant fuel surfeit is known to have detrimental effects on β-cell insulin release and is correlated with onset of insulin resistance (Newsholme et al., 2010). Elevated plasma glucose promotes insulin secretion from healthy islets, but in the diabetic state, hyperglycaemia can reduce insulin biosynthesis and secretion if glucose load is prolonged and exceeds the compensatory response. This phenomenon is known as glucotoxicity and is a significant contributor to DM progression and resultant β-cell apoptosis. Some of the reported mechanisms by which glucotoxicity may lead to β-cell dysfunction include, generation of excessive reactive oxygen/nitrogen species (ROS/PNS) due to increased oxidative phosphorylation, reduced expression of insulin-related genes, elevated intracellular Ca^{2+} and initiation of ER stress (Chang-Chen, Mullur, & Bernal-Mizrachi, 2008). It is understood that increased glycolytic flux in response to increased glucose levels will enhance ETC activity and ATP production, but may also lead to increased superoxide ($O_2^{\cdot-}$) anion leakage (Schoonbroodt & Piette, 2000). Superoxide is an important ROS, as it can potentially generate other forms of ROS/RNS including, the less reactive H_2O_2 via superoxide dismutase (SOD), or the highly reactive hydroxyl anion by the iron-catalyzed Fenton reaction (Gehrmann, Elsner, & Lenzen, 2010; Newsholme et al., 2012; Schoonbroodt & Piette, 2000). Additionally, $O_2^{\cdot-}$ can produce

RNS via interaction with NO, which subsequently forms the nitrogen free radical, peroxynitrite ($ONOO^-$) (Newsholme et al., 2012). It has been suggested that $ONOO^-$ is more cytotoxic than NO or O_2^- individually, and is extremely harmful to rat and human islet cells *in vitro* (Crow & Beckman, 1995; Delaney et al., 1996). Furthermore, this RNS has been detected in pancreatic islets in NOD mice and suggested it may play a role in the pathogenesis of T1DM (Rabinovitch & Suarez-Pinzon, 2003). These highly reactive molecules exert their negative effects by causing oxidative damage to β-cell DNA, lipids and proteins, and consequently may promote mitochondrial-mediated apoptosis (Newsholme et al., 2012). In addition, they may activate stress-induced signaling pathways such as, NFκB (nuclear factor kappa B) or JNK (c-Jun-N-terminal kinase), leading to proinflammatory cytokine release and/or cell death (Chang-Chen et al., 2008). β-Cells are built to sense nutrients in the physiological range, but have a limited antioxidant arsenal and are considered vulnerable to oxidative stress (Chang-Chen et al., 2008; Newsholme et al., 2012; Rahier, Guiot, Goebbels, Sempoux, & Henquin, 2008). Therefore, it is not surprising that markers of oxidative stress have been detected in the islets of hyperglycaemic T2DM patients (Chang-Chen et al., 2008; Tanaka, Tran, Harmon, & Robertson, 2002).

Interestingly, high glucose can also impact upon the expression of glycolytic and insulin-related genes. *In vivo* and *in vitro* β-cell models have demonstrated that excessive glucose negatively regulates expression of GLUT2, GCK, Ca^{2+} channels, and the insulin gene via decreased binding of transcription factors, pancreatic and duodenal homeobox 1 (Pdx1), neurogenic differentiation 1 (NeuroD1), and V-maf musculoaponeurotic fibrosarcoma oncogene homolog A (MafA) to the insulin promoter (Cnop et al., 2005; Newsholme et al., 2010). Downregulated transcription of these genes resulted in an ineffective response to extracellular glucose, reduced glycolysis and ATP production, diminished exocytotic signaling, and reduced insulin content and secretion. Conversely, elevated glucose may also upregulate genes that deviate carbon from the traditional β-cell glycolytic and TCA pathways, such as LDH, glucose-6-phosphatase, and hexokinase 1 (Cnop et al., 2005). Taken together, these changes in gene transcription may perturb the level of ATP production that is required for efficient insulin exocytosis and may decrease the sensitivity of β-cells to glucose and consequently reduce GSIS.

A persistent increase in intracellular Ca^{2+} in response to hyperglycaemia may also impact on insulin secretion. Intracellular β-cell Ca^{2+} is mainly derived from two sources, extracellular influx (from cell membrane depolarization) and efflux from organelles like the ER. Enhanced mitochondrial $O_2^{\cdot -}$ generation, and NO production from the β-cell, can lead to activation of Ca^{2+}-release channels in the ER, causing Ca^{2+} depletion which may promote ER-mediated apoptosis (Back, Kang, Han, & Chung, 2012; Chang-Chen et al., 2008; Mekahli, Bultynck, Parys, De Smedt, & Missiaen, 2011), along with the unfolded protein response (UPR) (refer to review, Chakrabarti, Chen, & Varner, 2011). There is a substantial demand for protein/insulin production in pancreatic β-cells. Therefore, they have a very active and well developed ER. However, this may suggest that β-cells are more susceptible to ER stress during the extended periods of protein synthesis (Cnop et al., 2005; Cunha et al., 2008). Previously, inhibition of proinsulin processing and transport has been implicated in DM (Guest, Bailyes, & Hutton, 1997; Mekahli et al., 2011), and accumulation of native or unfolded proteins in the ER activates caspase enzymes, such as caspase-12 (Kaufman, 1999; Szegezdi, Logue, Gorman, & Samali, 2006). Consequently, major changes in ER function, arising from glucose-induced ROS/RNS and intracellular Ca^{2+}, may lead to impaired insulin release, β-cell dysfunction, and ultimately β-cell apoptosis.

Lipid accumulation (lipotoxicity) in the β-cell is also a possible player in mediating ER stress. Obesity is associated with increased plasma glucose and lipid levels due to high-carbohydrate- and fat-based intake and is a primary risk factor in relation to T2DM (Cunha et al., 2008). Therefore, the detrimental effects of excess FFA are often discussed against the backdrop of hyperglycaemia, given that these negative effects occur predominantly in the presence of elevated glucose (Chang-Chen et al., 2008). The term for this concept is glucolipotoxicity, and the mechanisms by which FFAs amplify this process is not entirely known (Back et al., 2012). However, studies have demonstrated that palmitic acid elicited a deleterious effect on β-cell ER morphology and depleted ER Ca^{2+} levels, leading to induction of ER stress (Cnop, 2008; Cunha et al., 2008). In addition, fatty acid esterification in the ER may also cause increased competition for the ER machinery with newly synthesized or unfolded proteins, thus impeding the processing and transport of vital proteins from the ER (Cunha et al., 2008).

Another important mechanism of lipid-induced toxicity arises from the impairment of FFA oxidation, with subsequent lipid partitioning to the cytosol and ceramide formation. We have previously described the inhibitory effect of glucose-derived malonyl-CoA on β-oxidation that results in FFA accumulation in the cytosol. Therefore, hyperglycaemic conditions may prevent the detoxification of lipids in the β-cell and this lipotoxicity may manifest as increased ceramide production and contribute to insulin resistance (Lang, Ullrich, & Gulbins, 2011). It has been shown that ceramide formation, induced by FFA's, is certainly toxic to human islets (Lang et al., 2011; Lupi et al., 2002). Palmitic acid, a saturated FFA, is synthesized *de novo* in the liver and is the most common FFA found in the human diet (Keane et al., 2011). Furthermore, this molecule can be converted to palmitoyl CoA, which is a substrate for ceramide generation, along with the amino acid serine (Lang et al., 2011). The mechanisms by which ceramide induces β-cell dysfunction and apoptosis are not clear. However, it is understood that ceramide acts as a second messenger and participates in multiple signaling pathways by accumulating in the plasma membrane and in organelles, particularly the mitochondria (Lang et al., 2011). These ceramide microdomains become large enough to interact with key signaling receptors and may prevent the association of said receptors with their corresponding regulatory molecules (Lang et al., 2011). Examples include inhibition of PI3K/Akt (phosphatidyl inositol-3 kinase/protein kinase B) signaling, activation of cytokine release and induction of proapoptotic molecules such as PKC, caspases, and cathepsin D (Cowart, 2009; Hannun & Obeid, 2008; Ruvolo, 2003). Consequently, ceramide lipid rafts may activate or inhibit a wide variety of signaling pathways that could reduce insulin secretion, induce β-cell dysfunction and possibly β-cell death.

AMPK is also a principal signaling hub in metabolic regulation, and is sensitive to the energy status of the β-cell. The role of AMPK in mediating FFA and insulin secretion is not fully elucidated. In the energy-reduced state, active AMPK enhances β-oxidation and detoxifies lipids, mirroring the effect of increased physical activity (Towler & Hardie, 2007). Interestingly, chronic exposure to high-circulatory glucose and lipids, as occurs in T2DM also induces AMPK activation, but this may result in decreased insulin release via reduced expression of insulinotropic lipid signaling molecules, like DAG and acyl CoA (Haber et al., 2006; Newsholme & Krause, 2012). However, pharmacological activators of AMPK (e.g., metformin), have been reported to improve glucose and lipid profiles in insulin-resistant rodent models (Viollet et al., 2010). Consequently, hyperinsulinaemia may be reduced in these models and this may improve insulin sensitivity, β-cell function and possibly protect β-cell mass (Viollet et al., 2010).

Taken together, it is apparent that oxidative and ER stresses are critical mechanisms that facilitate the gluco-, lipo- or glucolipotoxicity features that are observed in the metabolic syndrome, and may possibly contribute to β-cell failure and death (Cunha et al., 2008). However, it should be emphasized that metabolism of glucose, FFA, and amino acids are intricately linked. We have clearly described the current understanding of how amino acid metabolism impacts upon glucose and FFA metabolism, which is principally through alterations in glycolytic and TCA pathways. Therefore, further investigation into these processes may aid development of novel nutrient-based therapies for the metabolic syndrome.

6. CONCLUSIONS

Carbohydrate, lipid, and amino acid metabolism plays a significant role in regulation of insulin secretion and GSIS. Pancreatic β-cells are specifically designed to respond to metabolic fuel input, and adapt to nutrient surfeit in order to maintain glucose homeostasis in the body. Glucose is the most important insulin secretagogue and its metabolism is central to regulation of insulin secretion. In addition, both fatty and amino acids participate intimately in the control of insulin release. However, β-cells forfeit protection from excess nutrient, for nutrient-sensing capabilities, and are consequently in danger from constant nutrient overload. In the westernized world, diminished physical activity and excess consumption of high-fat and high-carbohydrate containing foods, has led to an astonishing rise in T2DM (Odegaard & Chawla, 2012). Overconsumption manifests as the metabolic syndrome, characterized by impaired glucose tolerance (IGT), hyperglycaemia, hyperinsulinaemia, and ultimately T2DM. However, even though diet and exercise remains the most effective (and cheapest) therapy, novel treatment strategies may be required in the future. Therefore, a better insight into the complexities of β-cell function, demise, and destruction are required. In this chapter, we have presented work that highlights the recent advances in understanding the detrimental and beneficial effects of nutrient classes on insulin release and β-cell function. It is clear that nutrient-derived generation of ROS/RNS and ER stress are significant players leading to inhibited β-cell function. However, several amino acids appear to have advantageous attributes and these alone, or in specific combinations, may be harnessed in the development of novel antidiabetic modalities.

REFERENCES

Ammon, H. P., Hehl, K. H., Enz, G., Setiadi-Ranti, A., & Verspohl, E. J. (1986). Cysteine analogues potentiate glucose-induced insulin release in vitro. *Diabetes*, *35*(12), 1390–1396.

Back, S. H., Kang, S.-W., Han, J., & Chung, H.-T. (2012). Endoplasmic reticulum stress in the β-cell pathogenesis of type 2 diabetes. *Experimental Diabetes Research*, *2012*(21915177), 618396–618407.

Baylis, C. (2008). Nitric oxide deficiency in chronic kidney disease. *American Journal of Physiology. Renal Physiology*, *294*(1), F1–F9.

Bender, K., Maechler, P., McClenaghan, N. H., Flatt, P. R., & Newsholme, P. (2009). Overexpression of the malate-aspartate NADH shuttle member Aralar1 in the clonal beta-cell line BRIN-BD11 enhances amino-acid-stimulated insulin secretion and cell metabolism. *Clinical Science (London, England)*, *117*(9), 321–330.

Berne, C. (1975). The metabolism of lipids in mouse pancreatic islets. The biosynthesis of triacylglycerols and phospholipids. *The Biochemical Journal*, *152*(3), 667–673.

Brennan, L., Corless, M., Hewage, C., Malthouse, J. P., McClenaghan, N. H., Flatt, P. R., et al. (2003). 13C NMR analysis reveals a link between L-glutamine metabolism, D-glucose metabolism and gamma-glutamyl cycle activity in a clonal pancreatic beta-cell line. *Diabetologia*, *46*(11), 1512–1521.

Brennan, L., Shine, A., Hewage, C., Malthouse, J. P., Brindle, K. M., McClenaghan, N., et al. (2002). A nuclear magnetic resonance-based demonstration of substantial oxidative L-alanine metabolism and L-alanine-enhanced glucose metabolism in a clonal pancreatic beta-cell line: Metabolism of L-alanine is important to the regulation of insulin secretion. *Diabetes*, *51*(6), 1714–1721.

Broca, C., Brennan, L., Petit, P., Newsholme, P., & Maechler, P. (2003). Mitochondria-derived glutamate at the interplay between branched-chain amino acid and glucose-induced insulin secretion. *FEBS Letters*, *545*(2–3), 167–172.

Burant, C. F., Viswanathan, P., Marcinak, J., Cao, C., Vakilynejad, M., Xie, B., et al. (2012). TAK-875 versus placebo or glimepiride in type 2 diabetes mellitus: A phase 2, randomised, double-blind, placebo-controlled trial. *Lancet*, *379*(9824), 1403–1411.

Cabrera, O., Berman, D. M., Kenyon, N. S., Ricordi, C., Berggren, P. O., & Caicedo, A. (2006). The unique cytoarchitecture of human pancreatic islets has implications for islet cell function. *Proceedings of the National Academy of Sciences of the United States of America*, *103*(7), 2334–2339.

Carpentier, A., Mittelman, S. D., Bergman, R. N., Giacca, A., & Lewis, G. F. (2000). Prolonged elevation of plasma free fatty acids impairs pancreatic beta-cell function in obese nondiabetic humans but not in individuals with type 2 diabetes. *Diabetes*, *49*(3), 399–408.

Chakrabarti, A., Chen, A. W., & Varner, J. D. (2011). A review of the mammalian unfolded protein response. *Biotechnology and Bioengineering*, *108*(12), 2777–2793.

Chang-Chen, K. J., Mullur, R., & Bernal-Mizrachi, E. (2008). Beta-cell failure as a complication of diabetes. *Reviews in Endocrine & Metabolic Disorders*, *9*(4), 329–343.

Cnop, M. (2008). Fatty acids and glucolipotoxicity in the pathogenesis of Type 2 diabetes. *Biochemical Society Transactions*, *36*(Pt 3), 348–352.

Cnop, M., Welsh, N., Jonas, J.-C., Jorns, A., Lenzen, S., & Eizirik, D. L. (2005). Mechanisms of pancreatic beta-cell death in type 1 and type 2 diabetes: Many differences, few similarities. *Diabetes*, *54*(Suppl. 2), 97–9107.

Corless, M., Kiely, A., McClenaghan, N. H., Flatt, P. R., & Newsholme, P. (2006). Glutamine regulates expression of key transcription factor, signal transduction, metabolic gene, and protein expression in a clonal pancreatic beta-cell line. *The Journal of Endocrinology*, *190*(3), 719–727.

Cowart, L. A. (2009). Sphingolipids: Players in the pathology of metabolic disease. *Trends in Endocrinology and Metabolism: TEM, 20*(1), 34–42.
Crow, J. P., & Beckman, J. S. (1995). The role of peroxynitrite in nitric oxide-mediated toxicity. *Current Topics in Microbiology and Immunology, 196*, 57–73.
Cunha, D. A., Hekerman, P., Ladriere, L., Bazarra-Castro, A., Ortis, F., Wakeham, M. C., et al. (2008). Initiation and execution of lipotoxic ER stress in pancreatic beta-cells. *Journal of Cell Science, 121*(Pt 14), 2308–2318.
Cunningham, G. A., McClenaghan, N. H., Flatt, P. R., & Newsholme, P. (2005). L-Alanine induces changes in metabolic and signal transduction gene expression in a clonal rat pancreatic beta-cell line and protects from pro-inflammatory cytokine-induced apoptosis. *Clinical Science (London, England), 109*(5), 447–455.
Danielsson, A., Hellman, B., & Idahl, L. A. (1970). Levels of -ketoglutarate and glutamate in stimulated pancreatic -cells. *Hormone and Metabolic Research = Hormon- und Stoffwechselforschung = Hormones et metabolisme, 2*(1), 28–31.
Deeney, J. T., Gromada, J., Hoy, M., Olsen, H. L., Rhodes, C. J., Prentki, M., et al. (2000). Acute stimulation with long chain acyl-CoA enhances exocytosis in insulin-secreting cells (HIT T-15 and NMRI beta-cells). *The Journal of Biological Chemistry, 275*(13), 9363–9368.
Delaney, C. A., Tyrberg, B., Bouwens, L., Vaghef, H., Hellman, B., & Eizirik, D. L. (1996). Sensitivity of human pancreatic islets to peroxynitrite-induced cell dysfunction and death. *FEBS Letters, 394*(8830662), 300–306.
De Vos, A., Heimberg, H., Quartier, E., Huypens, P., Bouwens, L., Pipeleers, D., et al. (1995). Human and rat beta cells differ in glucose transporter but not in glucokinase gene expression. *The Journal of Clinical Investigation, 96*(5), 2489–2495.
Dixon, G., Nolan, J., McClenaghan, N., Flatt, P. R., & Newsholme, P. (2003). A comparative study of amino acid consumption by rat islet cells and the clonal beta-cell line BRIN-BD11—The functional significance of L-alanine. *The Journal of Endocrinology, 179*(3), 447–454.
Donath, M. Y., Schumann, D. M., Faulenbach, M., Ellingsgaard, H., Perren, A., & Ehses, J. A. (2008). Islet inflammation in type 2 diabetes: From metabolic stress to therapy. *Diabetes Care, 31*(Suppl. 2), 161–164.
Dunne, M. J., Yule, D. I., Gallacher, D. V., & Petersen, O. H. (1990). Effects of alanine on insulin-secreting cells: Patch-clamp and single cell intracellular Ca2+ measurements. *Biochimica et Biophysica Acta, 1055*(2), 157–164.
Ehses, J. A., Perren, A., Eppler, E., Ribaux, P., Pospisilik, J. A., Maor-Cahn, R., et al. (2007). Increased number of islet-associated macrophages in type 2 diabetes. *Diabetes, 56*(9), 2356–2370.
Fu, Z., Gilbert, E. R., & Liu, D. (2013). Regulation of insulin synthesis and secretion and pancreatic Beta-cell dysfunction in diabetes. *Current Diabetes Reviews, 9*(1), 25–53.
Gammelsaeter, R., Coppola, T., Marcaggi, P., Storm-Mathisen, J., Chaudhry, F. A., Attwell, D., et al. (2011). A role for glutamate transporters in the regulation of insulin secretion. *PloS One, 6*(8), e22960.
Gaudel, C., Nongonierma, A. B., Maher, S., Flynn, S., Krause, M., Murray, B. A., et al. (2013). A whey protein hydrolysate promotes insulinotropic activity in a clonal pancreatic beta-cell line and enhances glycemic function in ob/ob mice. *The Journal of Nutrition, 143*(7), 1109–1114.
Gehrmann, W., Elsner, M., & Lenzen, S. (2010). Role of metabolically generated reactive oxygen species for lipotoxicity in pancreatic β-cells. *Diabetes, Obesity & Metabolism, 12*(Suppl. 2), 149–158.
Gembal, M., Gilon, P., & Henquin, J. C. (1992). Evidence that glucose can control insulin release independently from its action on ATP-sensitive K+channels in mouse B cells. *The Journal of Clinical Investigation, 89*(4), 1288–1295.

Gloyn, A. L., Odili, S., Zelent, D., Buettger, C., Castleden, H. A., Steele, A. M., et al. (2005). Insights into the structure and regulation of glucokinase from a novel mutation (V62M), which causes maturity-onset diabetes of the young. *The Journal of Biological Chemistry*, *280*(14), 14105–14113.

Guest, P. C., Bailyes, E. M., & Hutton, J. C. (1997). Endoplasmic reticulum Ca2+ is important for the proteolytic processing and intracellular transport of proinsulin in the pancreatic beta-cell. *The Biochemical Journal*, *323*(Pt 2), 445–450.

Haber, E. P., Procopio, J., Carvalho, C. R., Carpinelli, A. R., Newsholme, P., & Curi, R. (2006). New insights into fatty acid modulation of pancreatic beta-cell function. *International Review of Cytology*, *248*, 1–41.

Hamilton, J. A., & Kamp, F. (1999). How are free fatty acids transported in membranes? Is it by proteins or by free diffusion through the lipids? *Diabetes*, *48*(12), 2255–2269.

Hannun, Y. A., & Obeid, L. M. (2008). Principles of bioactive lipid signalling: Lessons from sphingolipids. *Nature Reviews. Molecular Cell Biology*, *9*(2), 139–150.

Hasan, N. M., Longacre, M. J., Stoker, S. W., Boonsaen, T., Jitrapakdee, S., Kendrick, M. A., et al. (2008). Impaired anaplerosis and insulin secretion in insulinoma cells caused by small interfering RNA-mediated suppression of pyruvate carboxylase. *The Journal of Biological Chemistry*, *283*(42), 28048–28059.

Hellman, B. (1959). The frequency distribution of the number and volume of the islets Langerhans in man. I. Studies on non-diabetic adults. *Acta Societatis Medicorum Upsaliensis*, *64*, 432–460.

Henquin, J. C. (2000). Triggering and amplifying pathways of regulation of insulin secretion by glucose. *Diabetes*, *49*(11), 1751–1760.

Heslegrave, A. J., & Hussain, K. (2013). Novel insights into fatty acid oxidation, amino acid metabolism, and insulin secretion from studying patients with loss of function mutations in 3-hydroxyacyl-CoA dehydrogenase. *The Journal of Clinical Endocrinology and Metabolism*, *98*(2), 496–501.

Higaki, Y., Hirshman, M. F., Fujii, N., & Goodyear, L. J. (2001). Nitric oxide increases glucose uptake through a mechanism that is distinct from the insulin and contraction pathways in rat skeletal muscle. *Diabetes*, *50*(2), 241–247.

Hosokawa, H., Corkey, B. E., & Leahy, J. L. (1997). Beta-cell hypersensitivity to glucose following 24-h exposure of rat islets to fatty acids. *Diabetologia*, *40*(4), 392–397.

Hoy, M., Maechler, P., Efanov, A. M., Wollheim, C. B., Berggren, P. O., & Gromada, J. (2002). Increase in cellular glutamate levels stimulates exocytosis in pancreatic beta-cells. *FEBS Letters*, *531*(2), 199–203.

Itoh, Y., Kawamata, Y., Harada, M., Kobayashi, M., Fujii, R., Fukusumi, S., et al. (2003). Free fatty acids regulate insulin secretion from pancreatic beta cells through GPR40. *Nature*, *422*(6928), 173–176.

Jakubowicz, D., & Froy, O. (2013). Biochemical and metabolic mechanisms by which dietary whey protein may combat obesity and Type 2 diabetes. *The Journal of Nutritional Biochemistry*, *24*(1), 1–5.

Jensen, M. V., Joseph, J. W., Ronnebaum, S. M., Burgess, S. C., Sherry, A. D., & Newgard, C. B. (2008). Metabolic cycling in control of glucose-stimulated insulin secretion. *American Journal of Physiology, Endocrinology and Metabolism*, *295*(6), E1287–E1297.

Jitrapakdee, S., Wutthisathapornchai, A., Wallace, J. C., & MacDonald, M. J. (2010). Regulation of insulin secretion: Role of mitochondrial signalling. *Diabetologia*, *53*(20225132), 1019–1032.

Kaneko, Y., Kimura, Y., Kimura, H., & Niki, I. (2006). L-cysteine inhibits insulin release from the pancreatic beta-cell: Possible involvement of metabolic production of hydrogen sulfide, a novel gasotransmitter. *Diabetes*, *55*(5), 1391–1397.

Kaneko, Y., Kimura, T., Taniguchi, S., Souma, M., Kojima, Y., Kimura, Y., et al. (2009). Glucose-induced production of hydrogen sulfide may protect the pancreatic beta-cells from apoptotic cell death by high glucose. *FEBS Letters*, *583*(2), 377–382.

Kaufman, R. J. (1999). Stress signaling from the lumen of the endoplasmic reticulum: Coordination of gene transcriptional and translational controls. *Genes & Development*, *13*(10), 1211–1233.

Keane, D., & Newsholme, P. (2008). Saturated and unsaturated (including arachidonic acid) non-esterified fatty acid modulation of insulin secretion from pancreatic beta-cells. *Biochemical Society Transactions*, *36*(Pt 5), 955–958.

Keane, D. C., Takahashi, H. K., Dhayal, S., Morgan, N. G., Curi, R., & Newsholme, P. (2011). Arachidonic acid actions on functional integrity and attenuation of the negative effects of palmitic acid in a clonal pancreatic β-cell line. *Clinical Science (London, England)*, *120*(5), 195–206.

Krause, M. S., McClenaghan, N. H., Flatt, P. R., de Bittencourt, P. I. H., Murphy, C., & Newsholme, P. (2011). L-arginine is essential for pancreatic β-cell functional integrity, metabolism and defense from inflammatory challenge. *The Journal of Endocrinology*, *211*(1), 87–97.

Krause, M., Rodrigues-Krause, J., O'Hagan, C., De Vito, G., Boreham, C., Susta, D., et al. (2012). Differential nitric oxide levels in the blood and skeletal muscle of type 2 diabetic subjects may be consequence of adiposity: A preliminary study. *Metabolism, Clinical and Experimental*, *61*(11), 1528–1537.

Lang, F., Ullrich, S., & Gulbins, E. (2011). Ceramide formation as a target in beta-cell survival and function. *Expert Opinion on Therapeutic Targets*, *15*(9), 1061–1071.

Latour, M. G., Alquier, T., Oseid, E., Tremblay, C., Jetton, T. L., Luo, J., et al. (2007). GPR40 is necessary but not sufficient for fatty acid stimulation of insulin secretion in vivo. *Diabetes*, *56*(4), 1087–1094.

Lee, S. C., & Pervaiz, S. (2007). Apoptosis in the pathophysiology of diabetes mellitus. *The International Journal of Biochemistry & Cell Biology*, *39*(3), 497–504.

Li, C., Buettger, C., Kwagh, J., Matter, A., Daikhin, Y., Nissim, I. B., et al. (2004). A signaling role of glutamine in insulin secretion. *The Journal of Biological Chemistry*, *279*(14), 13393–13401.

Li, D. Q., Jing, X., Salehi, A., Collins, S. C., Hoppa, M. B., Rosengren, A. H., et al. (2009). Suppression of sulfonylurea- and glucose-induced insulin secretion in vitro and in vivo in mice lacking the chloride transport protein ClC-3. *Cell Metabolism*, *10*(4), 309–315.

Lu, J., Xie, G., Jia, W., & Jia, W. (2013). Insulin resistance and the metabolism of branched-chain amino acids. *Frontiers of Medicine*, 7(1), 53–59.

Lupi, R., Dotta, F., Marselli, L., Del Guerra, S., Masini, M., Santangelo, C., et al. (2002). Prolonged exposure to free fatty acids has cytostatic and pro-apoptotic effects on human pancreatic islets: Evidence that beta-cell death is caspase mediated, partially dependent on ceramide pathway, and Bcl-2 regulated. *Diabetes*, *51*(5), 1437–1442.

Maassen, J. A., t Hart, L. M., Janssen, G. M. C., Reiling, E., Romijn, J. A., & Lemkes, H. H. (2006). Mitochondrial diabetes and its lessons for common Type 2 diabetes. *Biochemical Society Transactions*, *34*(Pt 5), 819–823.

MacDonald, M. J. (1995a). Influence of glucose on pyruvate carboxylase expression in pancreatic islets. *Archives of Biochemistry and Biophysics*, *319*(1), 128–132.

MacDonald, M. J. (1995b). Feasibility of a mitochondrial pyruvate malate shuttle in pancreatic islets. Further implication of cytosolic NADPH in insulin secretion. *The Journal of Biological Chemistry*, *270*(34), 20051–20058.

MacDonald, M. J., & Fahien, L. A. (2000). Glutamate is not a messenger in insulin secretion. *The Journal of Biological Chemistry*, *275*(44), 34025–34027.

MacDonald, M. J., Longacre, M. J., Stoker, S. W., Kendrick, M., Thonpho, A., Brown, L. J., et al. (2011). Differences between human and rodent pancreatic islets: Low pyruvate carboxylase, atp citrate lyase, and pyruvate carboxylation and high glucose-stimulated acetoacetate in human pancreatic islets. *The Journal of Biological Chemistry, 286*(21), 18383–18396.

Marmol, P., Pardo, B., Wiederkehr, A., del Arco, A., Wollheim, C. B., & Satrustegui, J. (2009). Requirement for aralar and its Ca2+-binding sites in Ca2+ signal transduction in mitochondria from INS-1 clonal beta-cells. *The Journal of Biological Chemistry, 284*(1), 515–524.

McClenaghan, N. H., Barnett, C. R., & Flatt, P. R. (1998). Na+cotransport by metabolizable and nonmetabolizable amino acids stimulates a glucose-regulated insulin-secretory response. *Biochemical and Biophysical Research Communications, 249*(2), 299–303.

McClenaghan, N. H., Scullion, S. M., Mion, B., Hewage, C., Malthouse, J. P. G., Flatt, P. R., et al. (2009). Prolonged L-alanine exposure induces changes in metabolism, Ca(2+) handling and desensitization of insulin secretion in clonal pancreatic beta-cells. *Clinical Science (London, England), 116*(4), 341–351.

McCluskey, J. T., Hamid, M., Guo-Parke, H., McClenaghan, N. H., Gomis, R., & Flatt, P. R. (2011). Development and functional characterization of insulin-releasing human pancreatic beta cell lines produced by electrofusion. *The Journal of Biological Chemistry, 286*(25), 21982–21992.

McCulloch, L. J., van de Bunt, M., Braun, M., Frayn, K. N., Clark, A., & Gloyn, A. L. (2011). GLUT2 (SLC2A2) is not the principal glucose transporter in human pancreatic beta cells: Implications for understanding genetic association signals at this locus. *Molecular Genetics and Metabolism, 104*(4), 648–653.

Medina, M., Urdiales, J. L., & Amores-Sanchez, M. I. (2001). Roles of homocysteine in cell metabolism: Old and new functions. *European Journal of Biochemistry/FEBS, 268*(14), 3871–3882.

Mekahli, D., Bultynck, G., Parys, J. B., De Smedt, H., & Missiaen, L. (2011). Endoplasmic-reticulum calcium depletion and disease. *Cold Spring Harbor Perspectives in Biology, 3*(6), a004317.

Miki, T., Nagashima, K., Tashiro, F., Kotake, K., Yoshitomi, H., Tamamoto, A., et al. (1998). Defective insulin secretion and enhanced insulin action in KATP channel-deficient mice. *Proceedings of the National Academy of Sciences, 95*(18), 10402–10406.

Mulder, H., Lu, D., Finley, J. T., An, J., Cohen, J., Antinozzi, P. A., et al. (2001). Overexpression of a modified human malonyl-CoA decarboxylase blocks the glucose-induced increase in malonyl-CoA level but has no impact on insulin secretion in INS-1-derived (832/13) beta-cells. *The Journal of Biological Chemistry, 276*(9), 6479–6484.

Newsholme, P., Abdulkader, F., Rebelato, E., Romanatto, T., Pinheiro, C. H. J., Vitzel, K. F., et al. (2011). Amino acids and diabetes: Implications for endocrine, metabolic and immune function. *Frontiers in Bioscience, 16*, 315–339.

Newsholme, P., Bender, K., Kiely, A., & Brennan, L. (2007). Amino acid metabolism, insulin secretion and diabetes. *Biochemical Society Transactions, 35*(Pt 5), 1180–1186.

Newsholme, P., Brennan, L., & Bender, K. (2006). Amino acid metabolism, β-cell function, and diabetes. *Diabetes, 55*(Suppl. 2), S39–S47.

Newsholme, P., Gaudel, C., & McClenaghan, N. H. (2010). Nutrient regulation of insulin secretion and beta-cell functional integrity. *Advances in Experimental Medicine and Biology, 654*, 91–114.

Newsholme, P., Keane, D., Welters, H. J., & Morgan, N. G. (2007). Life and death decisions of the pancreatic beta-cell: The role of fatty acids. *Clinical Science (London, England), 112*(1), 27–42.

Newsholme, P., & Krause, M. (2012). Nutritional regulation of insulin secretion: Implications for diabetes. *The Clinical Biochemist. Reviews/Australian Association of Clinical Biochemists, 33*(2), 35–47.

Newsholme, P., Rebelato, E., Abdulkader, F., Krause, M., Carpinelli, A., & Curi, R. (2012). Reactive oxygen and nitrogen species generation, antioxidant defenses, and β-cell function: A critical role for amino acids. *The Journal of Endocrinology*, *214*(1), 11–20.

Nielsen, K., Sorensen, P. G., Hynne, F., & Busse, H. G. (1998). Sustained oscillations in glycolysis: An experimental and theoretical study of chaotic and complex periodic behavior and of quenching of simple oscillations. *Biophysical Chemistry*, *72*(1–2), 49–62.

Nolan, C. J., Madiraju, M. S., Delghingaro-Augusto, V., Peyot, M. L., & Prentki, M. (2006). Fatty acid signaling in the beta-cell and insulin secretion. *Diabetes*, *55*(Suppl. 2), S16–S23.

Nolan, C. J., & Prentki, M. (2008). The islet beta-cell: Fuel responsive and vulnerable. *Trends in Endocrinology and Metabolism: TEM*, *19*(8), 285–291.

Odegaard, J. I., & Chawla, A. (2012). Connecting type 1 and type 2 diabetes through innate immunity. *Cold Spring Harbor Perspectives in Medicine*, *2*(3), a007724.

Oh, D. Y., Talukdar, S., Bae, E. J., Imamura, T., Morinaga, H., Fan, W., et al. (2010). GPR120 is an omega-3 fatty acid receptor mediating potent anti-inflammatory and insulin-sensitizing effects. *Cell*, *142*(5), 687–698.

Patterson, S., Flatt, P. R., & McClenaghan, N. H. (2006). Homocysteine and other structurally-diverse amino thiols can alter pancreatic beta cell function without evoking cellular damage. *Biochimica et Biophysica Acta*, *1760*(7), 1109–1114.

Patterson, S., Flatt, P. R., & McClenaghan, N. H. (2007). Homocysteine-induced impairment of insulin secretion from clonal pancreatic BRIN-BD11 beta-cells is not prevented by catalase. *Pancreas*, *34*(1), 144–151.

Rabinovitch, A., & Suarez-Pinzon, W. L. (2003). Role of cytokines in the pathogenesis of autoimmune diabetes mellitus. *Reviews in Endocrine & Metabolic Disorders*, *4*(3), 291–299.

Rahier, J., Guiot, Y., Goebbels, R. M., Sempoux, C., & Henquin, J. C. (2008). Pancreatic beta-cell mass in European subjects with type 2 diabetes. *Diabetes, Obesity & Metabolism*, *10*(Suppl. 4), 32–42.

Rasilainen, S., Nieminen, J. M., Levonen, A.-L., Otonkoski, T., & Lapatto, R. (2002). Dose-dependent cysteine-mediated protection of insulin-producing cells from damage by hydrogen peroxide. *Biochemical Pharmacology*, *63*(7), 1297–1304.

Remedi, M. S., Agapova, S. E., Vyas, A. K., Hruz, P. W., & Nichols, C. G. (2011). Acute sulfonylurea therapy at disease onset can cause permanent remission of KATP-induced diabetes. *Diabetes*, *60*(10), 2515–2522.

Roduit, R., Nolan, C., Alarcon, C., Moore, P., Barbeau, A., Delghingaro-Augusto, V., et al. (2004). A role for the malonyl-CoA/long-chain acyl-CoA pathway of lipid signaling in the regulation of insulin secretion in response to both fuel and nonfuel stimuli. *Diabetes*, *53*(4), 1007–1019.

Rorsman, P., & Braun, M. (2013). Regulation of insulin secretion in human pancreatic islets. *Annual Review of Physiology*, *75*, 155–179.

Ruderman, N., & Prentki, M. (2004). AMP kinase and malonyl-CoA: Targets for therapy of the metabolic syndrome. *Nature Reviews. Drug Discovery*, *3*(4), 340–351.

Ruvolo, P. P. (2003). Intracellular signal transduction pathways activated by ceramide and its metabolites. *Pharmacological Research: The Official Journal of the Italian Pharmacological Society*, *47*(5), 383–392.

Salvucci, M., Neufeld, Z., & Newsholme, P. (2013). Mathematical model of metabolism and electrophysiology of amino acid and glucose stimulated insulin secretion: In vitro validation using a beta-cell line. *PloS One*, *8*(3), e52611.

Sanchez-Margalet, V., Valle, M., Ruz, F. J., Gascon, F., Mateo, J., & Goberna, R. (2002). Elevated plasma total homocysteine levels in hyperinsulinemic obese subjects. *The Journal of Nutritional Biochemistry*, *13*(2), 75–79.

Schoonbroodt, S., & Piette, J. (2000). Oxidative stress interference with the nuclear factor-kappa B activation pathways. *Biochemical Pharmacology*, *60*(8), 1075–1083.

Sener, A., Best, L. C., Yates, A. P., Kadiata, M. M., Olivares, E., Louchami, K., et al. (2000). Stimulus-secretion coupling of arginine-induced insulin release: Comparison between the cationic amino acid and its methyl ester. *Endocrine*, *13*(3), 329–340.

Sener, A., & Malaisse, W. J. (1980). L-leucine and a nonmetabolized analogue activate pancreatic islet glutamate dehydrogenase. *Nature*, *288*(5787), 187–189.

Shapiro, H., Shachar, S., Sekler, I., Hershfinkel, M., & Walker, M. D. (2005). Role of GPR40 in fatty acid action on the beta cell line INS-1E. *Biochemical and Biophysical Research Communications*, *335*(1), 97–9104.

Srinivasan, V., Tatu, U., Mohan, V., & Balasubramanyam, M. (2009). Molecular convergence of hexosamine biosynthetic pathway and ER stress leading to insulin resistance in L6 skeletal muscle cells. *Molecular and Cellular Biochemistry*, *328*(1–2), 217–224.

Straub, S. G., & Sharp, G. W. (2002). Glucose-stimulated signaling pathways in biphasic insulin secretion. *Diabetes/Metabolism Research and Reviews*, *18*(6), 451–463.

Sugden, M. C., & Holness, M. J. (2011). The pyruvate carboxylase-pyruvate dehydrogenase axis in islet pyruvate metabolism: Going round in circles? *Islets*, *3*(6), 302–319.

Szegezdi, E., Logue, S. E., Gorman, A. M., & Samali, A. (2006). Mediators of endoplasmic reticulum stress-induced apoptosis. *EMBO Reports*, *7*(9), 880–885.

Tanaka, Y., Tran, P. O. T., Harmon, J., & Robertson, R. P. (2002). A role for glutathione peroxidase in protecting pancreatic β cells against oxidative stress in a model of glucose toxicity. *Proceedings of the National Academy of Sciences*, *99*(19), 12363–12368.

Tomita, T., Masuzaki, H., Iwakura, H., Fujikura, J., Noguchi, M., Tanaka, T., et al. (2006). Expression of the gene for a membrane-bound fatty acid receptor in the pancreas and islet cell tumours in humans: Evidence for GPR40 expression in pancreatic beta cells and implications for insulin secretion. *Diabetologia*, *49*(5), 962–968.

Towler, M. C., & Hardie, D. G. (2007). AMP-activated protein kinase in metabolic control and insulin signaling. *Circulation Research*, *100*(3), 328–341.

Tremblay, A., & Gilbert, J. A. (2009). Milk products, insulin resistance syndrome and type 2 diabetes. *Journal of the American College of Nutrition*, *28*(Suppl. 1), 91S–102S.

Ulven, T. (2012). Short-chain free fatty acid receptors FFA2/GPR43 and FFA3/GPR41 as new potential therapeutic targets. *Frontiers in Endocrinology*, *3*, 111.

Vassiliou, E., Gonzalez, A., Garcia, C., Tadros, J., Chakraborty, G., & Toney, J. (2009). Oleic acid and peanut oil high in oleic acid reverse the inhibitory effect of insulin production of the inflammatory cytokine TNF-alpha both in vitro and in vivo systems. *Lipids in Health and Disease*, *8*(1), 25.

Viollet, B., Horman, S., Leclerc, J., Lantier, L., Foretz, M., Billaud, M., et al. (2010). AMPK inhibition in health and disease. *Critical Reviews in Biochemistry and Molecular Biology*, *45*(4), 276–295.

Wang, C., Guan, Y., & Yang, J. (2010). Cytokines in the progression of pancreatic β-cell dysfunction. *International Journal of Endocrinology*, *2010*.

Weir, G. C., & Bonner-Weir, S. (2004). Five stages of evolving beta-cell dysfunction during progression to diabetes. *Diabetes*, *53*(Suppl. 3), S16 S21.

Westermark, P. O., & Lansner, A. (2003). A model of phosphofructokinase and glycolytic oscillations in the pancreatic beta-cell. *Biophysical Journal*, *85*(1), 126–139.

Xu, J., Han, J., Long, Y. S., Epstein, P. N., & Liu, Y. Q. (2008). The role of pyruvate carboxylase in insulin secretion and proliferation in rat pancreatic beta cells. *Diabetologia*, *51*(11), 2022–2030.

Yang, J., Wong, R. K., Park, M., Wu, J., Cook, J. R., York, D. A., et al. (2006). Leucine regulation of glucokinase and ATP synthase sensitizes glucose-induced insulin secretion in pancreatic beta-cells. *Diabetes*, *55*(1), 193–201.

CHAPTER TWO

Proinsulin Entry and Transit Through the Endoplasmic Reticulum in Pancreatic Beta Cells

Ming Liu*,†,1, Jordan Wright*, Huan Guo*, Yi Xiong*, Peter Arvan*,1

*Division of Metabolism, Endocrinology & Diabetes, The University of Michigan Medical School, Ann Arbor, Michigan, USA

†Department of Metabolism, Tianjin Medical University General Hospital, Tianjin, PR China

[1]Corresponding authors: e-mail address: mingli@umich.edu; parvan@umich.edu

Contents

Abstract

Insulin is an essential hormone for maintaining metabolic homeostasis in the body. To make fully bioactive insulin, pancreatic beta cells initiate synthesis of the insulin precursor, preproinsulin, at the cytosolic side of the endoplasmic reticulum (ER), whereupon it undergoes co- and post-translational translocation across the ER membrane. Preproinsulin is cleaved by signal peptidase to form proinsulin that folds on the luminal side of the ER, forming three evolutionarily conserved disulfide bonds. Properly folded proinsulin forms dimers and exits from the ER, trafficking through Golgi complex into immature secretory granules wherein C-peptide is endoproteolytically excised, allowing fully bioactive two-chain insulin to ultimately be stored in mature granules for insulin secretion. Although insulin biosynthesis has been intensely studied in recent decades,

Vitamins and Hormones, Volume 95
ISSN 0083-6729
http://dx.doi.org/10.1016/B978-0-12-800174-5.00002-8

the earliest events, including proinsulin entry and exit from the ER, have been relatively understudied. However, over the past 5 years, more than 20 new insulin gene mutations have been reported to cause a new syndrome termed ***M**utant *INS*-gene-induced **D**iabetes of Youth (MIDY). Although these mutants have not been completely characterized, most of them affect proinsulin entry and exit from the ER. Here, we summarize our current knowledge about the early events of insulin biosynthesis and review recent advances in understanding how defects in these events may lead to pancreatic beta cell failure.

1. OVERVIEW OF INSULIN BIOSYNTHESIS IN PANCREATIC BETA CELLS

In pancreatic beta cells, insulin biosynthesis is initiated in the cytosol as the insulin mRNA begins to be translated into the precursor, preproinsulin (Liu et al., 2012; Patzelt et al., 1978). Preproinsulin is a single-chain molecule comprising the signal peptide, insulin B-chain, C-peptide, and insulin A-chain (Fig. 2.1). The N-terminal signal peptide drives newly synthesized preproinsulin to and across the ER membrane, where the signal peptide is removed by signal peptidase, forming proinsulin. In the oxidizing environment of the endoplasmic reticulum (ER) lumen, proinsulin rapidly folds, forming three evolutionarily conserved disulfide bonds, including two interchain disulfide bonds B7–A7 and B19–A20, and one intrachain disulfide bond A6–A11 (Huang & Arvan, 1995; Liu, Li, Cavener, & Arvan, 2005; Liu, Ramos-Castañeda, & Arvan, 2003; Zhang, Ming, & Arvan, 2003). Properly folded proinsulin dimerizes and exits the ER for delivery to the Golgi apparatus. As Zn^{2+} concentration begins to rise in the trans-Golgi network (TGN; Dunn, 2005), proinsulin is thought to form hexamers around central coordinating Zn^{2+} ions.

After translation, complete conversion of preproinsulin to mature insulin (Fig. 2.1) takes between 30 and 150 min. Among the early events of insulin biosynthesis, it has long been believed that proinsulin folding leading to ER exit is rate-limiting for proinsulin delivery to secretory granules (Aridor, Guzik, Bielli, & Fish, 2004; Lodish, 1988). However, using specific antibodies against proinsulin, recent evidence suggests that in resting beta cells, proinsulin molecules primarily accumulate in the Golgi apparatus rather than the ER (Haataja et al., 2012). Indeed, such Golgi accumulation is also visible in live beta cells expressing a GFP-fused proinsulin, even though the GFP moiety adds incremental folding time for proinsulin in the ER. Modification of N-linked glycans on glycoproteins is generally

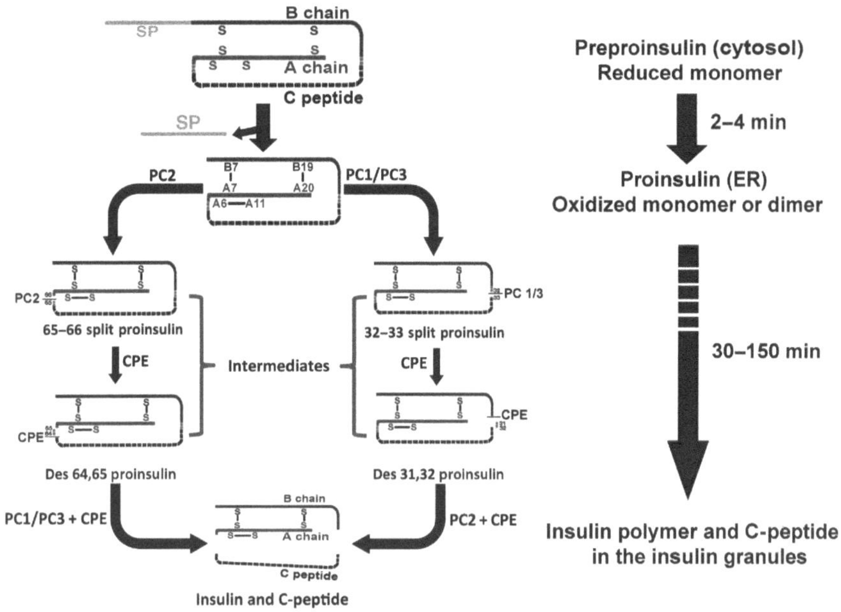

Figure 2.1 Insulin biosynthesis in pancreatic beta cells. Insulin biosynthesis begins as a precursor, preproinsulin, within the cytosol. Preproinsulin is comprised of sequentially as signal peptide (magenta), insulin B-chain (blue), C-peptide (black), and insulin A-chain (red). Newly synthesized preproinsulin undergoes co- and posttranslational translocation into the endoplasmic reticulum (ER), where it is cleaved by signal peptidase, forming proinsulin. The proinsulin folds in the ER, forming three evolutionarily conserved disulfide bonds, including two interchain disulfide bonds B7–A7 and B19–A20 and one intrachain disulfide bond A6–A11. Properly folded proinsulin forms dimers and exits from the ER, trafficking through Golgi complex into secretory granules where prohormone convertases (PC1/3 and PC2) in concert with carboxypeptidase E (CPE) to process proinsulin to C-peptide and two-chain mature insulin stored in the insulin granules. *Liu et al.* (See the color plate.)

thought of as a major contribution of the Golgi apparatus to secretory protein processing and trafficking—however, proinsulin (which is not a glycoprotein) in the Golgi is thought to undergo only zinc-dependent hexamerization (Dodson & Steiner, 1998; Huang & Arvan, 1995; Orci et al., 1986). Curiously, the Golgi pool of proinsulin appears to increase further in the pancreatic islets of mice lacking the ZnT8 zinc transporter (Haataja et al., 2012), suggesting that the time needed for hexamerization may delay proinsulin intracellular transport in the Golgi apparatus.

Proinsulin endoproteolytic processing can begin as early as in the TGN (Jamieson & Palade, 1967), but most proinsulin processing occurs in immature secretory granules (Kemmler, Steiner, & Borg, 1973; Kuliawat & Arvan, 1992; Orci et al., 1985) where the prohormone convertases (PC1/3 and PC2) in concert with carboxypeptidase E (CPE) process proinsulin to insulin and C-peptide (Davidson, 2004; Dodson & Steiner, 1998; Fricker, Evans, Esch, & Herbert, 1986; Steiner, 1998), as shall now be described.

Of the steps in processing proinsulin to insulin (Fig. 2.1), endoproteolytic cleavage tends to occur first at the B–C junction by PC1/3, producing 32–33 split proinsulin, exposing dibasic residues Arg31/32 that are removed by CPE to form the processing intermediate called des-31,32 proinsulin. PC2 can cleave intact proinsulin, but des-31,32 proinsulin is a preferred PC2 substrate (Furuta et al., 1998; Rhodes, Lincoln, & Shoelson, 1992; Zhu et al., 2002) such that PC2-based endoproteolysis tends to follow that of PC1/3. Sequential actions of PC1/3 and PC2 may also be favored by the relative rates of maturation/activation of these enzymes and the optimal ionic conditions for their activity (Davidson, 2004). For example, PC1/3 becomes functional in the TGN or early secretory granules when the pH is around 6.0 and the calcium concentration exceeds 0.2–0.5 mM (Bailyes et al., 1992; Demaurex, Furuya, D'Souza, Bonifacino, & Grinstein, 1998), whereas PC2 is thought to be nonfunctional at the time of its initial arrival in the TGN or newly formed granules (Bailyes et al., 1995; Lamango, Apletalina, Liu, & Lindberg, 1999).

Following cleavages by both PC1/3 and PC2, proinsulin intermediates undergo exopeptidase cleavage by CPE to remove their C-terminal dibasic (Arg-Arg or Lys-Arg) residues to complete the formation of mature insulin and C-peptide. CPE has no enzymatic activity on intact proinsulin, but it can convert the two split proinsulin intermediates, 32–33 split proinsulin or 64–65 split proinsulin, into their appropriate des-31,32 or des-63,64 proinsulin products, respectively—and convert diarginyl insulin to mature insulin (Davidson & Hutton, 1987). Direct *in vivo* proof of the role of CPE in proinsulin processing came from the discovery of the $CPE^{fat/fat}$ mouse with a homozygous point mutation in CPE. The mouse develops mild diabetes with severe obesity along with elevated circulating proinsulin intermediates and accumulated C-terminally extended diarginyl insulin in islets (Naggert et al., 1995; Varlamov et al., 1997). Subsequently, it has been shown that C-terminal processing of bioactive peptides is inhibited by only 80% in $CPE^{fat/fat}$ mice (Fricker, Berman, Leiter, & Devi, 1996), suggesting that other enzymes including carboxypeptidase D may partially compensate for CPE deficiency (Dong, Fricker, & Day, 1999).

CPE is expressed widely in neuroendocrine tissues (e.g., pancreatic islets, pituitary, adrenal, brain) where it is involved in the biosynthesis of many neuropeptides and peptide hormones (Fricker, 1988; Fricker et al., 1986). As a glycoprotein that exists in both membrane-associated and soluble forms, CPE is delivered to secretory granules along with its peptide substrates. In addition to its catalytic activity, although it remains to be further resolved, membrane-associated CPE has been proposed to function as a sorting receptor to capture secretory proteins into the regulated secretory pathway—and thus might be important for proinsulin delivery into insulin secretory granules (Cawley et al., 2012; Cool & Loh, 1998; Cool et al., 1997).

Fully processed insulin is stored along with C-peptide in insulin granules. It has been estimated that there are about 5000–6000 insulin granules per beta cell (Fava et al., 2012) with each granule containing up to 250,000 insulin molecules (Uchizono, Alarcón, Wicksteed, Marsh, & Rhodes, 2007). Upon short glucose stimulation, relatively few insulin granules need to undergo exocytosis so that a large majority remains in beta cells. However, upon more prolonged stimulation, significant depletion of insulin secretory granules is detected, especially from beta cells near the central region of islets (at least in rodents). Accompanying this granule depletion is an expansion of the early secretory pathway including the ER and Golgi apparatus (Stefan, Meda, Neufeld, & Orci, 1987). Even under unstimulated conditions, insulin granules are constantly turning over with a half-life of about 3–5 days (Halban, 1991; Halban & Wollheim, 1980; Rhodes & Halban, 1987). Granules that do not undergo exocytosis are eventually retired by crinophagy/autophagy (Halban, 1991). For detailed reviews about the regulation of insulin secretion, see the review articles (Rorsman & Braun, 2013; Rorsman & Renstrom, 2003).

2. PROINSULIN ENTRY INTO THE ER

2.1. Secretory protein translocation into the ER

For secretory proteins including preproinsulin, it is the signal peptide that drives the targeting of nascent polypeptides from the cytosol to the ER, the entry point into the secretory pathway (Blobel & Dobberstein, 1975; Rapoport, 2007). Signal peptides are typically located at the N-terminus of secretory proteins and are on average 20–30 residues in length. Signal peptides generally comprise three regions: an n-region with hydrophilic and positive charge residues; a central core h-region with 5–15 hydrophobic residues; and a more polar c-region containing a signal peptidase cleavage site (von Heijne, 1998; Zheng & Gierasch, 1996). Early studies showed that, except for the h-region, signal sequences were simple, interchangeable, tolerant of a wide range of mutations, and even able to direct the ER targeting of proteins expressed in evolutionarily distant organisms (Gierasch, 1989; Talmadge, Stahl, & Gilbert, 1980). These early studies implied that, besides directing the nascent polypeptide to the secretory pathway, signal sequences might not play an important role in regulating protein biosynthesis. However, more recent evidence indicates that variation of signal sequences can indeed affect protein targeting and translocation, signal peptide cleavage, as well as postcleavage events (Hegde & Bernstein, 2006; Rane, Chakrabarti, Feigenbaum, & Hegde, 2010; Swanton & High, 2006; Zhang, Rashid, Wang, & Shan, 2010). Indeed, variation of signal sequences may underlie a more complex role in regulating protein synthesis and targeting under certain pathophysiological conditions, for example, ER stress (Hegde & Bernstein, 2006; Swanton & High, 2006).

Protein translocation into the ER can occur either cotranslationally, during which translocation is concomitant with protein synthesis, or posttranslationally, in which translocation occurs after a polypeptide has been fully translated in the cytosol (Mitra, Frank, & Driessen, 2006). In mammalian cells, it appears that the efficiency of translocation of preproteins less than 100 amino acids in length relies strongly on Sec62-dependent posttranslational translocation mechanisms. Conversely, preproteins larger than 160 residues undergo exclusively signal recognition particle (SRP)-dependent cotranslational translocation, whereas preproteins of intermediate (120–160 residues) length can use both the SRP pathway and Sec62 (Lakkaraju et al., 2012). At least three steps are involved in protein translocation from the cytosol to the ER: (1) recognition and targeting of nascent polypeptides to the ER membrane; (2) translocation of proteins across the ER membrane; and (3) signal peptide cleavage, protein folding, and maturation in the ER. Here, rather than more extensive reviews of protein targeting and translocation across the ER membrane (Cross, Sinning, Luirink, & High, 2009; Driessen & Nouwen, 2008; Rapoport, 2007), we focus on key events likely to be important for preproinsulin, highlighting recent advances in understanding how defects in these events may cause pancreatic beta cell failure and diabetes.

2.2. Preproinsulin recognition and targeting to the ER

Early studies indicated that the ER targeting of preproinsulin occurs before completion of its synthesis and that the SRP was absolutely required, suggesting that the translocation of preproinsulin is mainly through SRP-dependent cotranslational translocation (Eskridge & Shields, 1983; Okun & Shields, 1992; Wolin & Walter, 1993). For this, the signal peptide of newly synthesized preproinsulin is first recognized and bound by SRP as it emerges from the ribosome. This binding results in a slowing down or pause of preproinsulin translation known as "elongation arrest," a conserved function of SRP that facilitates the coupling of protein translation and translocation processes (Walter & Blobel, 1983). SRP then targets the entire ribosome–preproinsulin complex to the Sec61 translocon by docking to the SRP receptor (SR) on the ER membrane (Fig. 2.2).

In mammalian cells, SRP is a ribonucleoprotein complex, comprising six proteins and a 7S SRP RNA. It has two functionally and structurally dissectible domains: the Alu domain and the S-domain. The Alu domain confers peptide elongation arrest activity, while the S-domain mediates both

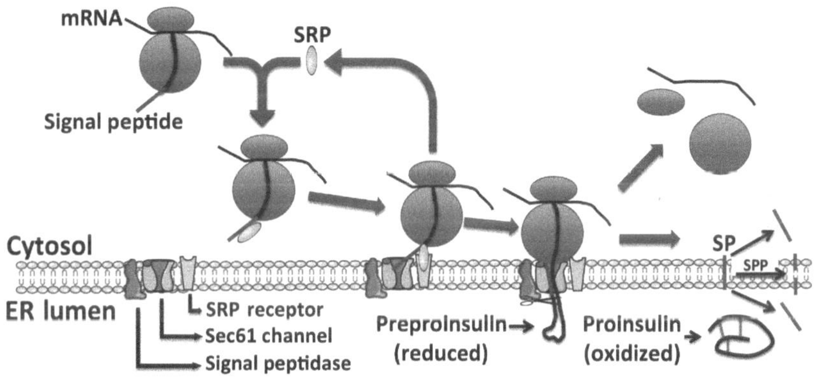

Figure 2.2 The earliest events of insulin biosynthesis: cotranslational translocation of newly synthesized preproinsulin from the cytosol to the ER. The signal peptide (SP) of newly synthesized preproinsulin is first recognized and bound by signal recognition particle (SRP) as it emerges from the ribosome. This binding results in a slowing down or pause of preproinsulin translation known as "elongation arrest." SRP then targets the entire ribosome–preproinsulin complex to the Sec61 translocon by docking to SRP receptor (SR) on the ER membrane. SP interacts with Sec61 channel, SRP is released, preproinsulin translation resumes and its proinsulin domain begins to be translocated into the ER, where SP is cleaved by signal peptidase at the ER luminal side, forming proinsulin, which rapidly folds in the ER. *Figures were produced using Servier Medical Art www.servier.com; Liu et al.* (See the color plate.)

signal sequence binding and SR docking to the ER membrane (Halic & Beckmann, 2005). The most conserved subunit, SRP54, locates in the S-domain. It contains a methionine-rich M-domain that binds the signal sequences and an NG-domain that interacts with SR at the ER membrane (Cross et al., 2009; Focia, Shepotinovskaya, Seidler, & Freymann, 2004; Saraogi & Shan, 2011). SR is a heterodimeric complex of SRα and SRβ subunits. SRβ is an ER transmembrane protein binding to the soluble SRα at the cytosolic side of the ER membrane. During recognition, the M-domain of SRP54 binds to the preproinsulin signal sequence emerging from the ribosome and slows down protein synthesis, which can prevent the premature initiation of preproinsulin folding prior to nascent chain targeting to the ER membrane. At least 60 amino acids of preproinsulin need to be synthesized for efficient SRP binding and targeting (Eskridge & Shields, 1983). Upon arriving at the ER membrane, SRP interacts with SR and docks to the α subunit of SR. At that point, SRP is released and translation of preproinsulin resumes. The docking and release of SRP from SR at the ER membrane requires GTP and is tightly controlled by conformational changes of GTPases on both subunits.

Recently, several studies revealed that posttranslational translocation exists not only in yeast but also in mammalian cells, especially for small secretory proteins (Bionda et al., 2010; Johnson et al., 2012; Shao & Hegde, 2011). Indeed, for preproinsulin, at 110 amino acids in length, cotranslational translocation is expected to be inefficient due to a short time window for signal sequence recognition by SRP. Therefore, posttranslational translocation may provide a backup mechanism to facilitate translocation of preproinsulin. In fact, a recent study shows that about 5–10% of newly synthesized preproinsulin is fully reduced, indicative of molecules that have not yet been exposed to the oxidizing environment of the ER lumen (Liu et al., 2012). The data support that translation of at least a subset of preproinsulin molecules may be completed before exposure to the ER lumen; thus, these fully translated preproinsulin molecules may follow a Sec62-dependent posttranslational translocation across the ER membrane (Lakkaraju et al., 2012).

2.3. Preproinsulin translocation across the ER membrane

Once the ribosome–nascent chain complexes are targeted to the ER membrane by SRP, the ribosome attaches to the Sec61 translocon. The h-region of the signal peptide is then transferred to Sec61 translocon complexes and translation resumes. In mammalian cells, Sec61 complexes are composed of three subunits, Sec61α, Sec61β, and Sec61γ (Johnson & van Waes, 1999; Zimmermann, Eyrisch, Ahmad, & Helms, 2011). The core of the translocon channel appears to be mainly formed by α- and γ-subunits (Osborne, Rapoport, & van den Berg, 2005). Cross-linking experiments have established that signal sequences of secretory proteins (and signal anchors of membrane proteins) are in contact with Sec61α during translocation (Pilon, Romisch, Quach, & Schekman, 1998; Plath, Mothes, Wilkinson, Stirling, & Rapoport, 1998). This contact determines the orientation of signal sequence in the ER membrane. At least three factors play roles in determining the orientation of the signal sequence within the Sec61 channel: the length of the h-region; the charge gradient of the translocon channel spanning the ER membrane; and the charge gradient of signal sequence flanking the h-region (Goder, Junne, & Spiess, 2004; Hartmann, Rapoport, & Lodish, 1989; Parks & Lamb, 1991; von Heijne, 1986; Wahlberg & Spiess, 1997). A study of yeast Sec61P (mammalian homolog of Sec61α) showed that conserved positively charged residues are located mostly on the side of the bilayer nearest to the ER lumen, while negatively charged residues tend to reside in loops on the cytosolic side.

The signal sequence of preproinsulin has a positively charged arginine six residue from the initiator methionine. During translocation, this R6 charged residue interacts with the Sec61 channel to position the N-terminus of the signal peptide toward the cytosol. Interestingly, two mutations affecting this positively charged R6 residue of preproinsulin, which may affect the orientation of their signal sequences in the Sec61 translocon during the translocation (detailed below), have been recently reported to cause late-onset diabetes in humans (Boesgaard et al., 2010; Edghill et al., 2008; Meur et al., 2010).

2.4. Coordination between preproinsulin signal peptide cleavage and downstream proinsulin folding

When the nascent polypeptide chain enters the Sec61 translocon at the ER, preproteins largely remain unfolded (although short α-helices may form). The unfolded conformation of preproteins allows signal peptidase to efficiently recognize the cleavage site of preproteins as they emerge into the ER lumen (Fewell & Brodsky, 2000; Hebert & Molinari, 2007). Cleavage by signal peptidase generally requires that 60–80 amino acids of the nascent polypeptide are translated (Okun & Shields, 1992; Okun, Eskridge, &

Shields, 1990; Wolin & Walter, 1993). Among those translated residues, ~40 amino acids may reside within the ~100-Å-long tunnel of the ribosome (Ban, Nissen, Hansen, Moore, & Steitz, 2000; Matlack & Walter, 1995) and ~30 amino acids are threaded through Sec61 translocon (Fewell & Brodsky, 2000; Haigh & Johnson, 2002; Liao, Lin, Do, & Johnson, 1997). Preproinsulin is a small protein comprising 110 amino acids. Therefore, although two-thirds of the preproinsulin peptide chain may already be translated as it emerges into the ER, most of those translated residues are still in the ribosome and Sec61 channel rather than being exposed within the ER lumen. Without question, cleavage of the signal peptide can affect normal downstream folding proinsulin—exposure of proinsulin domains to the ER lumen with folding initiated prematurely (prior to signal peptide cleavage) is very detrimental to the subsequent conformational maturation of proinsulin to the native state (Liu et al., 2012).

The ER lumen possesses a unique environment (e.g., one that is more oxidizing than the cytosol)—designed co- and posttranslational modifications of proteins—favoring disulfide bond formation (Hwang, Sinskey, & Lodish, 1992; Sevier et al., 2007) and N-linked glycosylation (Spiro, 2002). As noted earlier, proinsulin is not glycosylated, so its most important folding process in the ER involves disulfide maturation (Huang & Arvan, 1995; Liu et al., 2005). During translocation across the ER membrane, as proinsulin begins to emerge into the ER lumen, the first cysteine residue exposed is the seventh residue of the insulin B-chain known as C(B7), which needs to pair with the subsequent C(A7) to make a bond that will ultimately serve as an interchain disulfide bond within mature insulin. However, during the process of translocation, the next cysteinyl residue to emerge within the ER lumen after C(B7) is C(B19), with a time delay estimated at approximately 3 s (assuming translation/translocation at five amino acids per second; Braakman, Hoover-Litty, Wagner, & Helenius, 1991). Conceivably, cleavage of the signal peptide of preproinsulin might allow B7 to "move away" from incoming B19 before this second cysteine residue becomes available in the ER lumen.

It is still quite unclear whether, which, and how ER chaperones and oxidoreductases may participate in the resolution of mispaired preproinsulin disulfide bonds and the formation of proper disulfide pairs within the ER. So far, all that is known is that protein disulfide isomerase (PDI) does not facilitate the process of proinsulin disulfide maturation (Rajpal, Schuiki, Liu, Volchuk, & Arvan, 2012). However, an efficient and faithful signal peptide cleavage that tightly coordinates preproinsulin translocation with proinsulin folding is certainly one crucial step for proper disulfide pairing of proinsulin (Liu et al., 2012).

2.5. Pancreatic beta cell failure and diabetes caused by defects in some of the earliest events of insulin biosynthesis

In pancreatic beta cells, the half-life of preproinsulin is only about 1–2 min (Patzelt et al., 1978). This short half-life has been a technical challenge to investigate the biological behavior of preproinsulin in living cells. Therefore, most early studies focused on preproinsulin were carried out using *in vitro* translation systems (Eskridge & Shields, 1983; Okun et al., 1990; Okun & Shields, 1992; Wolin & Walter, 1993). Since the studies of Steiner and colleagues who first reported the time-dependent disappearance of preproinsulin (Patzelt et al., 1978), the sequential events allowing nascent preproinsulin to be converted to folded proinsulin in the ER of β-cells have been largely unexplored. Yet the question of how preproinsulin translocation, signal peptide cleavage, oxidative proinsulin folding, and proinsulin dimerization are coordinated has never had more pathophysiological significance than at present. Over the past 5 years, five new preproinsulin signal peptide mutations have been reported to cause diabetes in humans (Bonfanti et al., 2009; Edghill et al., 2008; Garin et al., 2010; Meur et al., 2010; Stoy et al., 2007), indicating serious adverse consequences when these early processes are not properly executed. Interestingly, although all these mutations are located in the preproinsulin signal peptide, the clinical diabetes phenotypes vary widely. In particular, A24D causes severe autosomal-dominant neonatal-onset diabetes, whereas R6C and R6H cause mild late-onset autosomal-dominant diabetes, and M1I causes autosomal-recessive diabetes (Fig. 2.3). These observations suggest that different molecular mechanisms may underlie the insulin deficiency in each case. Here, we review available data about the cellular defects caused by these mutants and discuss how these defects may lead to beta cell failure and insulin-deficient diabetes.

Preproinsulin-A24D is one of the most common insulin gene mutations causing Mutant *INS*-gene-induced Diabetes of Youth (MIDY) and is the most studied of all the preproinsulin signal peptide mutations. Although all patients are heterozygous, most reported patients carrying this mutation develop severe insulin-deficient diabetes in the first 6 months of life (Edghill et al., 2008; Stoy et al., 2007). This fact alone suggests that the mutant preproinsulin severely damages beta cell insulin production or survival. Preproinsulin-A24D causes loss of the highly conserved signal peptide cleavage site (residue "−1" relative to the first residue of the insulin B-chain) and

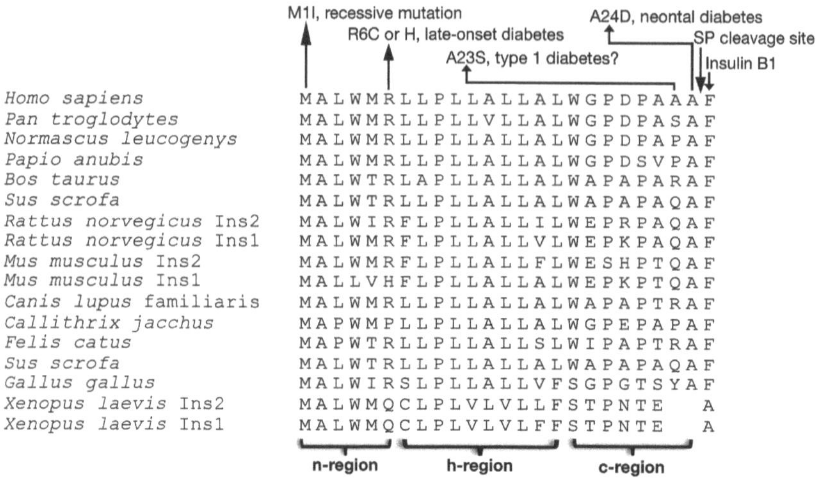

Figure 2.3 The homology of preproinsulin signal sequences and the mutations associated with diabetes in humans. As with other secretory preproteins, preproinsulin signal peptides have three characteristic regions: an n-region with hydrophilic and positively charged residues; a central core h-region with 9–10 hydrophobic residues; and a more polar c-region containing a signal peptidase cleavage site. M1I is a recessive mutation, which affects the first methionine residue and abolishes the native translation initiation site for the preproinsulin. R6C or H is associated with late-onset diabetes. The mutation is located at a well-conserved positively charged residue in the n-region of the signal peptide. It results in a loss of the N-terminal positive charge, which may affect normal targeting and translocation of mutant preproinsulin. A23S is located at −2 position relative to the first residue of the insulin B-chain. This position exhibits significant evolutionary variation. Available evidence suggests that A23 is likely a polymorphic variant rather a pathogenic mutation (see text). The A24D mutant is at the highly conserved signal peptidase cleavage site. It disrupts normal signal peptide cleavage, causing downstream proinsulin misfolding, leading to neonatal diabetes. *Liu et al.*

affects the cleavage of preproinsulin. Thus, preproinsulin-A24D largely presents as an uncleaved form (Sohma et al., 2010) that is retained in the ER and induces ER stress (Liu et al., 2012; Park, Ye, Steiner, & Bell, 2010). Interestingly, about 5–10% of human preproinsulin-A24D does get cleaved. However, the proinsulin derived from the A24D mutant is unable to be exported from the ER, suggesting that it is misfolded. Misfolding of the resultant proinsulin is caused both by a delay of signal peptide cleavage in the ER and by a cleavage that ultimately occurs at the wrong site, thereby altering the N-terminus of proinsulin which normally plays a key role in the proinsulin folding process (Liu, Hua, et al., 2010; Sohma et al., 2010).

In addition to inducing ER stress, preproinsulin-A24D can interact with coexpressed wild-type proinsulin in the ER, blocking its intracellular transport and decreasing wild-type insulin production. This initial mechanism has been suggested to account for the onset of insulin deficiency leading to diabetes in heterozygous patients carrying the A24D mutation. Importantly, upregulating ER oxidoreducin-1 (ERO1, see Section 3.1, below) partially rescues wild-type proinsulin from the blockade caused by coexpressed preproinsulin-A24D, thereby increasing insulin production (Liu et al., 2012). These findings may open the door to new treatments to prevent or limit diabetes in these patients and other patients with proinsulin misfolding. Specifically, instead of trying to "fix" misfolded preproinsulin or proinsulin, it may be feasible to "rescue" the remaining wild-type proinsulin from blockade, that is, allowing wild-type proinsulin to exit from the ER and produce bioactive insulin. It is important to note that a single expressed allele of wild-type insulin is sufficient to maintain normoglycemia, both in humans and animal models (Duvillie et al., 1997; Garin et al., 2010; Leroux et al., 2001). Thus, rescuing only a portion of proinsulin may be sufficient able to produce enough insulin to prevent/delay the development of insulin-deficient diabetes.

Preproinsulin-A23S was originally found in a patient who was diagnosed with type 1 diabetes, and had been proposed to trigger to the MIDY syndrome (Bonfanti et al., 2009). However, based on genetic and biological data, it seems unlikely that preproinsulin-A23S is an authentically diabetogenic mutation. This 23rd residue of preproinsulin (residue "−2" relative to the first residue of the insulin B-chain) is near the signal peptide cleavage site. However, unlike the conserved feature of small uncharged amino acids at positions −1 and −3, the −2 position exhibits significant evolutionary variation (Fikes, Barkocy-Gallagher, Klapper, & Bassford, 1990; Palzkill, Le, Wong, & Botstein, 1994). In fact, as shown in Fig. 2.3, serine is the native residue at the −2 position of chimpanzee preproinsulin. There is polymorphic variation at this position even in the human genome (Naohisa et al., 2001). Moreover, biochemical studies have been unable to demonstrate that preproinsulin-A23S exhibits any defect in signal peptide cleavage, downstream proinsulin folding, or insulin production (Liu et al., 2012). Thus, A23S is most likely a polymorphic variant rather a pathogenic mutation—although it remains possible that preproinsulin-A23S might cause diabetes through an as yet unknown mechanism.

The expression of preproinsulin-R6C or -R6H is associated with milder diabetes. The age of onset of diabetes in these patients has ranged from 15 to 65 years of age, and most patients have been treated with diet and oral hypoglycemic agents (Boesgaard et al., 2010; Edghill et al., 2008; Meur et al.,

2010). Available clinical data from two patients expressing preproinsulin-R6H show a ~30% reduction in beta cell function (Boesgaard et al., 2010). The R6C or R6H mutation is located within the n-region of the preproinsulin signal sequence. This residue is well conserved across mammalian species and chickens but is not conserved in Xenopus (Fig. 2.3). Loss of the R6 positive charge at the N-terminus of the preproinsulin signal peptide can impact on the ability of the signal peptide N-terminus to guide and position the signal sequence upon contact with the Sec61 translocon. Since the more positively charged residues of the Sec61 channel reside close to the luminal side of the ER membrane, signal sequences with N-terminal positive charge tend to make a "loop" during preprotein translocation (i.e., with N-terminus of the signal sequence positioned toward the cytosolic side and the C-terminus oriented toward the ER lumen). Loss of N-terminal positive charge of preproinsulin-R6C or -R6H may result in a disorientation of the signal sequence during preproinsulin translocation. However, a recent study using GFP-tagged preproinsulin reported that the R6C or R6H mutations have no significant defect in proinsulin targeting in the secretory pathway based on the finding of green fluorescent puncta representing insulin granules. Moreover, this study suggested that preproinsulin-R6C or -R6H does not cause ER stress yet promote significant induction of CHOP expression, which is a generally recognized cell stress marker (Meur et al., 2010). These interesting findings suggest that the preproinsulin mutation of R6 may possibly utilize a distinct mechanism to bring about diabetes—for which further investigation is clearly warranted.

Preproinsulin-M1I is considered a recessive mutation linked to neonatal diabetes (Garin et al., 2010). The mutation affects the first methionyl residue and abolishes the native translational initiation site for the preproinsulin. Interestingly, there is an ATG encoding another methionine that normally resides at the fifth residue of preproinsulin (Fig. 2.3), and this might be postulated to function as an alternative start codon. However, the nucleotide sequence surrounding this ATG does not favor translational initiation because nucleotide position −3 relative to this ATG is a pyrimidine rather than a purine (adenine or guanine)—failing to conform to the Kozak consensus for translational initiation (Kozak, 1989). Data from *in vitro* experiments indicate that the preproinsulin-M1I substitution results in ~80% reduction in proinsulin production compared to that derived from wild-type preproinsulin (Garin et al., 2010). The decreased proinsulin content is not caused by affecting the transcription of mutant insulin gene nor by decreasing stability of mutant mRNA, suggesting that the translation of preproinsulin-M1I mRNA is likely to be defective due to a failure to be initiated at the site of the native start codon.

3. PROINSULIN TRANSIT THROUGH THE ER

3.1. Proinsulin oxidative folding in the ER

As with many secretory proteins, disulfide bonds help to stabilize proinsulin (and insulin) molecules before and after secretion. Disulfide bond formation in many secretory proteins is catalyzed by members of the PDI protein family, of which there are approximately 20 members. As illustrated in Fig. 2.4, a disulfide bond within PDI is shuttled to the substrate protein, resulting in reduction of the PDI active site. PDI is then reoxidized by ERO1, which forms disulfide bonds *de novo* using molecular oxygen as a terminal electron receptor.

ERO1 has two mammalian homologs, ERO1α, which is expressed ubiquitously, and ERO1β, the expression of which is limited largely to pancreatic β cells (Zito, Chin, Blais, Harding, & Ron, 2010). Though the ERO1 pathway is of great significance in mammalian cells, recent evidence suggests that several ERO1-independent pathways may also contribute to disulfide bond formation in secretory protein substrates. These include peroxiredoxin 4, glutathione peroxidase 7 and 8 (GPX7 and GPX8), quiescin sulfhydryl oxidase, and vitamin K epoxide reductase. For a more detailed

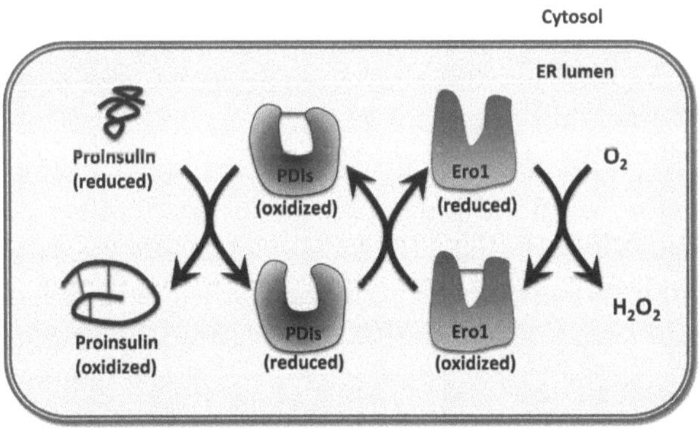

Figure 2.4 Proinsulin disulfide bond formation. Within the ER, proinsulin must form three intramolecular disulfide bonds. Members of the PDI protein family (green) transfer disulfide bonds (orange line) to the proinsulin molecule, and then must be reoxidized by Ero1 (purple). Ero1 in turn forms *de novo* disulfide bonds by reducing molecular oxygen. This cycle must repeat three times to form the required proinsulin disulfide bonds. *Liu et al.* (See the color plate.)

description of these gene products and their catalytic activities, please see Bulleid and Ellgaard (2011).

PDI family proteins are defined by the presence of an NH2-terminal ER signal peptide and at least one thioredoxin-like domain (Appenzeller-Herzog & Ellgaard, 2008). The first-identified member of the family, PDI, is known to catalyze formation (oxidation), breakage (reduction), and reshuffling (isomerization) of disulfide bonds, as well as nonredox-dependent chaperone activity to assist in protein folding. Though the name of the group suggests that all members act as isomerases, the actual functions of these proteins vary widely, with some lacking an active site (i.e., including the necessary CXXC motif; Galligan & Petersen, 2012) and thus these cannot catalyze disulfide bond formation. For detailed reviews of this protein family, please see Appenzeller-Herzog and Ellgaard (2008), Ellgaard and Ruddock (2005), and Galligan and Petersen (2012).

The specific pathway(s) responsible for proinsulin oxidation in pancreatic beta cells remains an active area of investigation. Proinsulin is expressed almost exclusively in beta cells (although proinsulin expression in the thymus is needed to avoid beta cell autoimmune disease; Eisenbarth, 2003) wherein Ero1β has been proposed to be a major source of oxidizing equivalents in the ER. Indeed, knockdown of Ero1β in beta cell lines decreases insulin content and secretion (Khoo et al., 2011). Furthermore, mice with reduced Ero1β expression have delayed proinsulin oxidation and impaired insulin synthesis (Zito et al., 2010). Interestingly, double mutant mice with reduced Ero1α and Ero1β are still able to oxidize proinsulin (although at a reduced rate), suggesting that at least one Ero1-independent oxidation pathway (Sevier, 2010) must also be able to contribute to proinsulin disulfide bond formation, for which further studies are still needed.

Until recently, PDI was thought to be the enzyme that directly catalyzes disulfide bond formation in proinsulin. *In vitro* studies have demonstrated that PDI catalyzes refolding and disulfide bond formation of reduced denatured proinsulin (Winter, Klappa, Freedman, Lilie, & Rudolph, 2002) and insulin (Tang & Tsou, 1990; Tang, Wang, & Tsou, 1988). Recent studies, however, suggest that PDI does not catalyze proinsulin disulfide bond formation and, if anything, acts more as an "unfoldase" or isomerase that delays proinsulin maturation. A few of the other PDI family members have been studied with respect to insulin (summarized below), but much work remains to determine if another member of the PDI family may be the principle enzyme responsible for proinsulin oxidation. Two proteins, TMX4 (Sugiura et al., 2010) and Erp57 (Bourdi et al., 1995), have the ability to reduce insulin *in vitro*, but as these proteins interact more readily with glycoprotein substrates (Oliver, van der Wal, Bulleid, & High, 1997), their role in proinsulin oxidation remains questionable. An important consideration is that proinsulin is so abundantly expressed that unless a putative proinsulin oxidase were superactive, the oxidase would itself need to be sufficiently highly expressed to handle the load of proinsulin disulfide bonds in the beta cell ER that has been estimated as high as 3 million per minute (Scheuner & Kaufman, 2008). One PDI family member, Erp46, is highly expressed in beta cells, and siRNA knockdown has been found to cause a decrease in insulin content and secretion (Alberti et al., 2009). Clearly, more work is needed to understand pathways of proinsulin oxidation within the ER.

3.2. Quality control and ER exit

Before exiting the ER, proteins must pass ER quality control (QC), which helps prevent potentially toxic misfolded proteins from reaching other compartments of the cell or being secreted (Ellgaard & Helenius, 2003; Ellgaard, Molinari, & Helenius, 1999). The primary mechanism of QC is based on ER chaperone binding to unfolded or misfolded proteins. These chaperones, which include members of the Hsp70 family (mainly BiP), Hsp40s (ERdj1–5), Hsp90s (GRP94), lectin chaperones (calnexin and calreticulin), and the PDI family members, recognize, bind, and retain unfolded proteins in the ER. One consequence of this binding is to limit inappropriate (often hydrophobic) interactions between unfolded species, and thereby to assist cargo proteins in reaching their native state. The mechanism by which different ER chaperones recognize their unfolded protein substrates may vary. For example, BiP binds aliphatic peptides (Flynn, Pohl, Flocco, & Rothman, 1991) that are normally buried internally within well-folded globular proteins; lectin chaperones bind to specific forms of N-linked oligosaccharides (Molinari & Helenius, 1999); and PDI family members form mixed disulfide bonds with substrate proteins bearing exposed, unpaired cysteinyl residues. Additionally, the PDI family members may have classical chaperone activity that is independent of disulfide bond formation (Puig & Gilbert, 1994). For many oligomeric proteins, proper subunit assembly is also a prerequisite for ER exit (Hurtley & Helenius, 1989) as the subunits help to conceal hydrophobic patches and thiols that otherwise would have attracted chaperone and oxidoreductase binding.

In pancreatic islets and in cell culture models, BiP interacts strongly with proinsulin, especially with misfolded forms (Liu, Haataja, et al., 2010; Liu et al., 2005; Scheuner et al., 2005; Schmitz, Maintz, Kehle, & Herzog, 1995). Thus, BiP likely plays a major role in proinsulin ER QC. Likewise, PDI and other PDI family members have been shown to directly interact with proinsulin, and overexpression of PDI delays ER exit of proinsulin, suggesting that PDI may also play a role in proinsulin QC rather than in disulfide bond formation. As proinsulin is not glycosylated, calreticulin and calnexin are not expected to affect proinsulin QC, but other chaperones such as GRP94 and ERdj1–5 remain to be investigated.

In the ER, proinsulin is thought to form noncovalent homodimers (Haataja et al., 2012) that proceed to the distal secretory pathway to form homohexamers for processing to mature insulin. The proinsulin monomer has two extensive nonpolar surfaces, one of which is buried upon dimerization. Although dimerization may not be absolutely required for proinsulin exit from the ER and transport to the Golgi (Quinn, Orci, Ravazzola, & Moore, 1991), dimerization may play a significant role in proinsulin QC and trafficking.

3.3. Proinsulin misfolding and degradation

Protein folding is an imperfect process, and even under normal conditions, a significant fraction of wild-type proteins may not reach the native state (Schubert et al., 2000). If misfolded proteins accumulate to a high enough degree in the ER, they may form toxic aggregates (Stefani & Dobson, 2003). To prevent aggregation, the cell can either attempt to refold the protein or degrade it. As discussed earlier, ER chaperones bind to misfolded proteins, isolating them from interaction with other molecules. PDI family members break aberrant disulfide bonds and facilitate disulfide (re)formation, providing an opportunity for substrate proteins to progress toward a native configuration. If refolding fails, degradation of the aberrant molecule proceeds via a process termed ER-associated degradation (ERAD). In ERAD, the misfolded protein is first recognized by binding to ER chaperones. The misfolded protein is then retrotranslocated from the ER to the cytosol (Fig. 2.5; Pilon, Schekman, & Romisch, 1997; Plemper, Bohmler, Bordallo, Sommer, & Wolf, 1997; Scott & Schekman, 2008). If disulfide bonds have been formed, it is believed that they must be broken before retrotranslocation, a process that is likely to involve the reductase function of some of the PDI family members (Grubb, Guo, Fisher, & Brodsky, 2012; Moore, Bernardi, & Tsai, 2010; Walczak, Bernardi, & Tsai, 2012). Ubiquitination of ERAD substrate proteins during retrotranslocation,

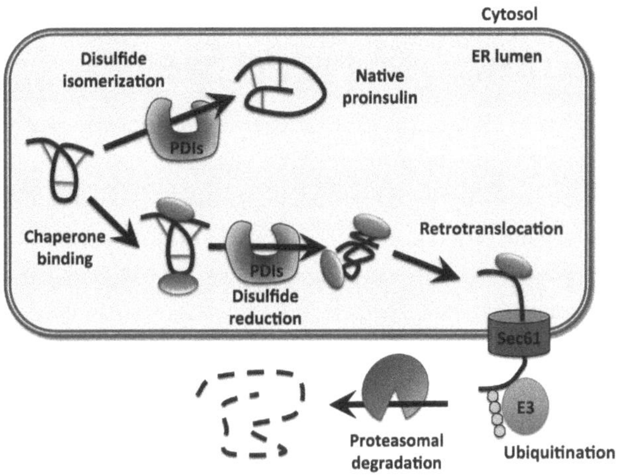

Figure 2.5 Disposal of misfolded proinsulin: isomerization and ERAD. When proinsulin misfolds and forms nonnative disulfide bonds, PDI family proteins act as isomerases to shuffle the disulfide bonds and allow the molecule to potentially reach its native conformation. When molecules remain misfolded, they are targeted for ERAD. Chaperones such as BiP (red) recognize the misfolded protein, and PDI family proteins (green) reduce the disulfide bonds prior to proinsulin retrotranslocation through the Sec61 translocon. During retrotranslocation, E3 ligases (orange) ubiquitinate the reduced proinsulin, targeting it for proteasomal degradation in the cytosol. *Liu et al.* (See the color plate.)

through the concerted action of Hrd1, gp78, RMA1, TEB4, and CHIP (Guerriero & Brodsky, 2012), targets the misfolded substrate to the cytosolic 26s proteasome for degradation (Finley, 2009). For a detailed review of ERAD, please see Guerriero and Brodsky (2012).

Proinsulin is surprisingly prone to misfolding (Wang et al., 2011; Wang & Osei, 2011), which has been hypothesized to contribute to the pathogenesis of type 2 diabetes. As described earlier, in MIDY, mutant proinsulins misfold and accumulate in the ER, preventing efficient secretion of wild-type proinsulin, and eventually leading to ER stress-mediated beta cell death (Liu, Haataja, et al., 2010; Liu, Hodish, et al., 2010; Liu, Hodish, Rhodes, & Arvan, 2007; Liu et al., 2005; Park et al., 2010; Rajan et al., 2010). Both wild-type and mutant proinsulin molecules have been found to be ERAD substrates (Allen et al., 2004; Hartley et al., 2010). Given that ERAD may be important for mitigating the effects of misfolded proinsulin, ERAD may also be a potential therapeutic target, both for MIDY and for more common forms of type 2 diabetes in which proinsulin misfolded has been postulated.

4. CONCLUSION AND PERSPECTIVE

The discovery of insulin gene mutations associated with diabetes in humans had drawn increasing attention to the earliest events in insulin biosynthesis. Although some progress has been made in better understanding proinsulin folding and misfolding in the ER, and how misfolded proinsulin leads to pancreatic beta failure and diabetes, many questions regarding preproinsulin entry and exit from the ER remain unanswered. Specifically, is ER entry of proinsulin regulated, and if so, how? How is misfolded proinsulin recognized and degraded? How can we prevent pancreatic beta cell failure and diabetes caused by misfolded proinsulin? Are mutant proinsulins associated with diabetes "rescuable" or "fixable"? How can we prevent misfolded mutant proinsulin from negatively interacting with coexisting wild-type proinsulin? Although insulin gene mutations only account for rare cases of diabetes, they provide excellent models to study the pathogenesis of diabetes caused by defects in ER entry and exit of proinsulin. Addressing these questions will help not only to develop novel strategies to enhance proinsulin folding and ER exit but also to gain new insights in thinking about pancreatic beta cell secretory function, beta cell survival, and new treatments for the most common forms of diabetes.

ACKNOWLEDGMENTS

This work was supported primarily by NIH RO1-DK088856 (to M. L.) and NIH RO1-DK-48280 (to P. A.), and also by a research grant from The National Natural Science Foundation of China 81070629 (to M. L.) and a research grant from March Dimes foundation 6-FY11-357 (to M. L.)

REFERENCES

Alberti, A., Karamessinis, P., Peroulis, M., Kypreou, K., Kavvadas, P., Pagakis, S., et al. (2009). ERp46 is reduced by high glucose and regulates insulin content in pancreatic beta-cells. *American Journal of Physiology Endocrinology and Metabolism*, *297*(3), E812–E821.

Allen, J. R., Nguyen, L. X., Sargent, K. E., Lipson, K. L., Hackett, A., & Urano, F. (2004). High ER stress in beta-cells stimulates intracellular degradation of misfolded insulin. *Biochemical and Biophysical Research Communications*, *324*(1), 166–170.

Appenzeller-Herzog, C., & Ellgaard, L. (2008). The human PDI family: Versatility packed into a single fold. *Biochimica et Biophysica Acta*, *1783*(4), 535–548.

Aridor, M., Guzik, A. K., Bielli, A., & Fish, K. N. (2004). Endoplasmic reticulum export site formation and function in dendrites. *The Journal of Neuroscience*, *24*(15), 3770–3776.

Bailyes, E. M., Shennan, K. I., Seal, A. J., Smeekens, S. P., Steiner, D. F., Hutton, J. C., et al. (1992). A member of the eukaryotic subtilisin family (PC3) has the enzymic properties of the type 1 proinsulin-converting endopeptidase. *The Biochemical Journal, 285*(2), 391–394.

Bailyes, E. M., Shennan, K. I., Usac, E. F., Arden, S. D., Guest, P. C., Docherty, K., et al. (1995). Differences between the catalytic properties of recombinant human PC2 and endogenous rat PC2. *The Biochemical Journal, 309*(2), 587–594.

Ban, N., Nissen, P., Hansen, J., Moore, P. B., & Steitz, T. A. (2000). The complete atomic structure of the large ribosomal subunit at 2.4Å resolution. *Science, 289*(5481), 905–920.

Bionda, T., Tillmann, B., Simm, S., Beilstein, K., Ruprecht, M., & Schleiff, E. (2010). Chloroplast import signals: The length requirement for translocation in vitro and in vivo. *Journal of Molecular Biology, 402*(3), 510–523.

Blobel, G., & Dobberstein, B. (1975). Transfer of proteins across membranes. I. Presence of proteolytically processed and unprocessed nascent immunoglobulin light chains on membrane-bound ribosomes of murine myeloma. *The Journal of Cell Biology, 67*(3), 835–851.

Boesgaard, T., Pruhova, S., Andersson, E., Cinek, O., Obermannova, B., Lauenborg, J., et al. (2010). Further evidence that mutations in INS can be a rare cause of maturity-onset diabetes of the young (MODY). *BMC Medical Genetics, 11*(1), 42.

Bonfanti, R., Colombo, C., Nocerino, V., Massa, O., Lampasona, V., Iafusco, D., et al. (2009). Insulin gene mutations as cause of diabetes in children negative for five type 1 diabetes autoantibodies. *Diabetes Care, 32*(1), 123–125.

Bourdi, M., Demady, D., Martin, J. L., Jabbour, S. K., Martin, B. M., George, J. W., et al. (1995). cDNA cloning and baculovirus expression of the human liver endoplasmic reticulum P58: Characterization as a protein disulfide isomerase isoform, but not as a protease or a carnitine acyltransferase. *Archives of Biochemistry and Biophysics, 323*(2), 397–403.

Braakman, I., Hoover-Litty, H., Wagner, K. R., & Helenius, A. (1991). Folding of influenza hemagglutinin in the endoplasmic reticulum. *The Journal of Cell Biology, 114*(3), 401–411.

Bulleid, N. J., & Ellgaard, L. (2011). Multiple ways to make disulfides. *Trends in Biochemical Sciences, 36*(9), 485–492.

Cawley, N. X., Wetsel, W. C., Murthy, S. R. K., Park, J. J., Pacak, K., & Loh, Y. P. (2012). New roles of carboxypeptidase E in endocrine and neural function and cancer. *Endocrine Reviews, 33*(2), 216–253.

Cool, D. R., & Loh, Y. P. (1998). Carboxypeptidase E is a sorting receptor for prohormones: Binding and kinetic studies. *Molecular and Cellular Endocrinology, 139*(1–2), 7–13.

Cool, D. R., Normant, E., Shen, F.-S., Chen, H.-C., Pannell, L., Zhang, Y., et al. (1997). Carboxypeptidase E is a regulated secretory pathway sorting receptor: Genetic obliteration leads to endocrine disorders in Cpefat mice. *Cell, 88*(1), 73–83.

Cross, B. C. S., Sinning, I., Luirink, J., & High, S. (2009). Delivering proteins for export from the cytosol. *Nature Reviews. Molecular Cell Biology, 10*(4), 255–264. http://dx.doi.org/10.1038/nrm2657.

Davidson, H. (2004). (Pro)Insulin processing. *Cell Biochemistry and Biophysics, 40*(3), 143–157.

Davidson, H. W., & Hutton, J. C. (1987). The insulin-secretory-granule carboxypeptidase H. Purification and demonstration of involvement in proinsulin processing. *The Biochemical Journal, 245*(2), 575–582.

Demaurex, N., Furuya, W., D'Souza, S., Bonifacino, J. S., & Grinstein, S. (1998). Mechanism of acidification of the trans-Golgi network (TGN). *Journal of Biological Chemistry, 273*(4), 2044–2051.

Dodson, G., & Steiner, D. (1998). The role of assembly in insulin's biosynthesis. *Current Opinion in Structural Biology, 8*(2), 189–194.

Dong, W., Fricker, L. D., & Day, R. (1999). Carboxypeptidase D is a potential candidate to carry out redundant processing functions of carboxypeptidase E based on comparative distribution studies in the rat central nervous system. *Neuroscience, 89*(4), 1301–1317.

Driessen, A. J. M., & Nouwen, N. (2008). Protein translocation across the bacterial cytoplasmic membrane. *Annual Review of Biochemistry*, 77(1), 643–667.
Dunn, M. (2005). Zinc, ligand interactions modulate assembly and stability of the insulin hexamer. *Biometals*, *18*(4), 295–303.
Duvillie, B., Cordonnier, N., Deltour, L., Dandoy-Dron, F., Itier, J.-M., Monthioux, E., et al. (1997). Phenotypic alterations in insulin-deficient mutant mice. *Proceedings of the National Academy of Sciences of the United States of America*, *94*(10), 5137–5140.
Edghill, E. L., Flanagan, S. E., Patch, A.-M., Boustred, C., Parrish, A., Shields, B., et al. (2008). Insulin mutation screening in 1,044 patients with diabetes. *Diabetes*, *57*(4), 1034–1042.
Eisenbarth, G. S. (2003). Insulin autoimmunity. *Annals of the New York Academy of Sciences*, *1005*(1), 109–118.
Ellgaard, L., & Helenius, A. (2003). Quality control in the endoplasmic reticulum. *Nature Reviews. Molecular Cell Biology*, *4*(3), 181–191. http://dx.doi.org/10.1038/nrm1052.
Ellgaard, L., Molinari, M., & Helenius, A. (1999). Setting the standards: Quality control in the secretory pathway. *Science*, *286*(5446), 1882–1888.
Ellgaard, L., & Ruddock, L. W. (2005). The human protein disulphide isomerase family: Substrate interactions and functional properties. *EMBO Reports*, *6*(1), 28–32.
Eskridge, E., & Shields, D. (1983). Cell-free processing and segregation of insulin precursors. *The Journal of Biological Chemistry*, *258*(19), 11487–11491.
Fava, E., Dehghany, J., Ouwendijk, J., Muller, A., Niederlein, A., Verkade, P., et al. (2012). Novel standards in the measurement of rat insulin granules combining electron microscopy, high-content image analysis and in silico modelling. *Diabetologia*, *55*(4), 1013–1023.
Fewell, S., & Brodsky, J. (2000). *Entry into the Endoplasmic Reticulum: Protein Translocation, Folding and Quality Control. Madame Curie Bioscience Database [Internet]*. Austin, TX: Landes Bioscience.
Fikes, J. D., Barkocy-Gallagher, G. A., Klapper, D. G., & Bassford, P. J. (1990). Maturation of Escherichia coli maltose-binding protein by signal peptidase I in vivo. Sequence requirements for efficient processing and demonstration of an alternate cleavage site. *Journal of Biological Chemistry*, *265*(6), 3417–3423.
Finley, D. (2009). Recognition and processing of ubiquitin-protein conjugates by the proteasome. *Annual Review of Biochemistry*, *78*, 477–513.
Flynn, G. C., Pohl, J., Flocco, M. T., & Rothman, J. E. (1991). Peptide-binding specificity of the molecular chaperone BiP. *Nature*, *353*(6346), 726–730. http://dx.doi.org/10.1038/353726a0.
Focia, P. J., Shepotinovskaya, I. V., Seidler, J. A., & Freymann, D. M. (2004). Heterodimeric GTPase core of the SRP targeting complex. *Science*, *303*(5656), 373–377.
Fricker, L. D. (1988). Carboxypeptidase E. *Annual Review of Physiology*, *50*(1), 309–321.
Fricker, L. D., Berman, Y. L., Leiter, E. H., & Devi, L. A. (1996). Carboxypeptidase E activity is deficient in mice with the fat mutation: Effect on peptide processing. *Journal of Biological Chemistry*, *271*(48), 30619–30624.
Fricker, L. D., Evans, C. J., Esch, F. S., & Herbert, E. (1986). Cloning and sequence analysis of cDNA for bovine carboxypeptidase E. *Nature*, *323*(6087), 461–464.
Furuta, M., Carroll, R., Martin, S., Swift, H. H., Ravazzola, M., Orci, L., et al. (1998). Incomplete processing of proinsulin to insulin accompanied by elevation of Des-31,32 proinsulin intermediates in islets of mice lacking active PC2. *Journal of Biological Chemistry*, *273*(6), 3431–3437.
Galligan, J. J., & Petersen, D. R. (2012). The human protein disulfide isomerase gene family. *Human Genomics*, *6*, 6.
Garin, I., Edghill, E. L., Akerman, I., Rubio-Cabezas, O., Rica, I., Locke, J. M., et al. (2010). Recessive mutations in the INS gene result in neonatal diabetes through reduced insulin

biosynthesis. *Proceedings of the National Academy of Sciences of the United States of America, 107*(7), 3105–3110.

Gierasch, L. M. (1989). Signal sequences. *Biochemistry, 28*(3), 923–930.

Goder, V., Junne, T., & Spiess, M. (2004). Sec61p contributes to signal sequence orientation according to the positive-inside rule. *Molecular Biology of the Cell, 15*(3), 1470–1478.

Grubb, S., Guo, L., Fisher, E. A., & Brodsky, J. L. (2012). Protein disulfide isomerases contribute differentially to the endoplasmic reticulum-associated degradation of apolipoprotein B and other substrates. *Molecular Biology of the Cell, 23*(4), 520–532.

Guerriero, C. J., & Brodsky, J. L. (2012). The delicate balance between secreted protein folding and endoplasmic reticulum-associated degradation in human physiology. *Physiological Reviews, 92*(2), 537–576.

Haataja, L., Snapp, E., Wright, J., Liu, M., Hardy, A. B., Wheeler, M. B., et al. (2013). Proinsulin intermolecular interactions during secretory trafficking in pancreatic beta cells. *Journal of Biological Chemistry, 288*, 1896–1906.

Haigh, N. G., & Johnson, A. E. (2002). A new role for BiP: Closing the aqueous translocon pore during protein integration into the ER membrane. *The Journal of Cell Biology, 156*(2), 261–270.

Halban, P. A. (1991). Structural domains and molecular lifestyles of insulin and its precursors in the pancreatic beta cell. *Diabetologia, 34*(11), 767–778.

Halban, P. A., & Wollheim, C. B. (1980). Intracellular degradation of insulin stores by rat pancreatic islets in vitro. An alternative pathway for homeostasis of pancreatic insulin content. *Journal of Biological Chemistry, 255*(13), 6003–6006.

Halic, M., & Beckmann, R. (2005). The signal recognition particle and its interactions during protein targeting. *Current Opinion in Structural Biology, 15*(1), 116–125.

Hartley, T., Siva, M., Lai, E., Teodoro, T., Zhang, L., & Volchuk, A. (2010). Endoplasmic reticulum stress response in an INS-1 pancreatic beta-cell line with inducible expression of a folding-deficient proinsulin. *BMC Cell Biology, 11*(1), 59.

Hartmann, E., Rapoport, T. A., & Lodish, H. F. (1989). Predicting the orientation of eukaryotic membrane-spanning proteins. *Proceedings of the National Academy of Sciences of the United States of America, 86*(15), 5786–5790.

Hebert, D. N., & Molinari, M. (2007). In and out of the ER. Protein folding, quality control, degradation, and related human diseases. *Physiological Reviews, 87*(4), 1377–1408. http://dx.doi.org/10.1152/physrev.00050.2006.

Hegde, R. S., & Bernstein, H. D. (2006). The surprising complexity of signal sequences. *Trends in Biochemical Sciences, 31*(10), 563–571.

Huang, X. F., & Arvan, P. (1995). Intracellular transport of proinsulin in pancreatic beta-cells. Structural maturation probed by disulfide accessibility. *The Journal of Biological Chemistry, 270*(35), 20417–20423.

Hurtley, S. M., & Helenius, A. (1989). Protein oligomerization in the endoplasmic reticulum. *Annual Review of Cell Biology, 5*, 277–307.

Hwang, C., Sinskey, A., & Lodish, H. (1992). Oxidized redox state of glutathione in the endoplasmic reticulum. *Science, 257*(5076), 1496–1502.

Jamieson, J. D., & Palade, G. E. (1967). Intracellular transport of secretory proteins in the pancreatic exocrine cell: I. Role of the peripheral elements of the Golgi complex. *The Journal of Cell Biology, 34*(2), 577–596.

Johnson, A. E., & van Waes, M. A. (1999). The translocon: A dynamic gateway at the er membrane. *Annual Review of Cell and Developmental Biology, 15*(1), 799–842.

Johnson, N., Vilardi, F., Lang, S., Leznicki, P., Zimmermann, R., & High, S. (2012). TRC40 can deliver short secretory proteins to the Sec61 translocon. *Journal of Cell Science, 125*(15), 3612–3620.

Kemmler, W., Steiner, D. F., & Borg, J. (1973). Studies on the conversion of proinsulin to insulin: III. Studies in vitro with a crude secretion granule fraction isolated from rat Islets of Langerhans. *Journal of Biological Chemistry*, *248*(13), 4544–4551.

Khoo, C., Yang, J., Rajpal, G., Wang, Y., Liu, J., Arvan, P., et al. (2011). Endoplasmic reticulum oxidoreductin-1-like beta (ero1l{beta}) regulates susceptibility to endoplasmic reticulum stress and is induced by insulin flux in {beta}-cells. *Endocrinology*, *152*(7), 2599–2608.

Kozak, M. (1989). Circumstances and mechanisms of inhibition of translation by secondary structure in eucaryotic mRNAs. *Molecular and Cellular Biology*, *9*(11), 5134–5142.

Kuliawat, R., & Arvan, P. (1992). Protein targeting via the "constitutive-like" secretory pathway in isolated pancreatic islets: Passive sorting in the immature granule compartment. *The Journal of Cell Biology*, *118*(3), 521–529.

Lakkaraju, A. K. K., Thankappan, R., Mary, C., Garrison, J. L., Taunton, J., & Strub, K. (2012). Efficient secretion of small proteins in mammalian cells relies on Sec62-dependent posttranslational translocation. *Molecular Biology of the Cell*, *23*(14), 2712–2722.

Lamango, N. S., Apletalina, E., Liu, J., & Lindberg, I. (1999). The proteolytic maturation of prohormone convertase 2 (PC2) is a pH-driven process. *Archives of Biochemistry and Biophysics*, *362*(2), 275–282.

Leroux, L., Desbois, P., Lamotte, L., Duvillié, B., Cordonnier, N., Jackerott, M., et al. (2001). Compensatory responses in mice carrying a null mutation for Ins1 or Ins2. *Diabetes*, *50*(90001), S150–S153.

Liao, S., Lin, J., Do, H., & Johnson, A. E. (1997). Both lumenal and cytosolic gating of the aqueous er translocon pore are regulated from inside the ribosome during membrane protein integration. *Cell*, *90*(1), 31–41.

Liu, M., Haataja, L., Wright, J., Wickramasinghe, N. P., Hua, Q. X., Phillips, N. F., et al. (2010). Mutant INS-gene induced diabetes of youth: Proinsulin cysteine residues impose dominant-negative inhibition on wild-type proinsulin transport. *PLoS One*, *5*(10), e13333.

Liu, M., Hodish, I., Haataja, L., Lara-Lemus, R., Rajpal, G., Wright, J., et al. (2010). Proinsulin misfolding and diabetes: Mutant INS gene-induced diabetes of youth. *Trends in Endocrinology and Metabolism*, *21*(11), 652–659.

Liu, M., Hodish, I., Rhodes, C. J., & Arvan, P. (2007). Proinsulin maturation, misfolding, and proteotoxicity. *Proceedings of the National Academy of Sciences of the United States of America*, *104*(40), 15841–15846.

Liu, M., Hua, Q.-X., Hu, S.-Q., Jia, W., Yang, Y., Saith, S. E., et al. (2010). Deciphering the hidden informational content of protein sequences. *Journal of Biological Chemistry*, *285*(40), 30989–31001.

Liu, M., Lara-Lemus, R., Shan, S.-O., Wright, J., Haataja, L., Barbetti, F., et al. (2012). Impaired cleavage of preproinsulin signal peptide linked to autosomal-dominant diabetes. *Diabetes*, *61*, 828–837.

Liu, M., Li, Y., Cavener, D., & Arvan, P. (2005). Proinsulin disulfide maturation and misfolding in the endoplasmic reticulum. *Journal of Biological Chemistry*, *280*(14), 13209–13212.

Liu, M., Ramos-Castaneda, J., & Arvan, P. (2003). Role of the connecting peptide in insulin biosynthesis. *The Journal of Biological Chemistry*, *278*(17), 14798–14805.

Lodish, H. F. (1988). Transport of secretory and membrane glycoproteins from the rough endoplasmic reticulum to the Golgi. A rate-limiting step in protein maturation and secretion. *Journal of Biological Chemistry*, *263*(5), 2107–2110.

Matlack, K. E. S., & Walter, P. (1995). The 70 carboxyl-terminal amino acids of nascent secretory proteins are protected from proteolysis by the ribosome and the protein

translocation apparatus of the endoplasmic reticulum membrane. *Journal of Biological Chemistry, 270*(11), 6170–6180.
Meur, G., Simon, A., Harun, N., Virally, M., Dechaume, A., Bonnefond, A., et al. (2010). Insulin gene mutations resulting in early-onset diabetes: Marked differences in clinical presentation, metabolic status, and pathogenic effect through endoplasmic reticulum retention. *Diabetes, 59*(3), 653–661.
Mitra, K., Frank, J., & Driessen, A. (2006). Co- and post-translational translocation through the protein-conducting channel: Analogous mechanisms at work? *Nature Structural & Molecular Biology, 13*(11), 957–964. http://dx.doi.org/10.1038/nsmb1166.
Molinari, M., & Helenius, A. (1999). Glycoproteins form mixed disulphides with oxidoreductases during folding in living cells. *Nature, 402*(6757), 90–93.
Moore, P., Bernardi, K. M., & Tsai, B. (2010). The Ero1alpha-PDI redox cycle regulates retro-translocation of cholera toxin. *Molecular Biology of the Cell, 21*(7), 1305–1313.
Naggert, J. K., Fricker, L. D., Varlamov, O., Nishina, P. M., Rouille, Y., Steiner, D. F., et al. (1995). Hyperproinsulinaemia in obese fat/fat mice associated with a carboxypeptidase E mutation which reduces enzyme activity. *Nature Genetics, 10*(2), 135–142.
Naohisa, O., Akira, N., Kentaro, F., Shigeo, I., Takashi, F., Manami, H., et al. (2001). Polymorphisms of the insulin gene among Japanese subjects. *Metabolism, Clinical and Experimental, 50*(6), 631–634.
Okun, M. M., Eskridge, E. M., & Shields, D. (1990). Truncations of a secretory protein define minimum lengths required for binding to signal recognition particle and translocation across the endoplasmic reticulum membrane. *Journal of Biological Chemistry, 265*(13), 7478–7484.
Okun, M., & Shields, D. (1992). Translocation of preproinsulin across the endoplasmic reticulum membrane. The relationship between nascent polypeptide size and extent of signal recognition particle-mediated inhibition of protein synthesis. *The Journal of Biological Chemistry, 267*(16), 11476–11482.
Oliver, J. D., van der Wal, F. J., Bulleid, N. J., & High, S. (1997). Interaction of the thiol-dependent reductase ERp57 with nascent glycoproteins. *Science, 275*(5296), 86–88.
Orci, L., Ravazzola, M., Amherdt, M., Madsen, O., Perrelet, A., Vassalli, J. D., et al. (1986). Conversion of proinsulin to insulin occurs coordinately with acidification of maturing secretory vesicles. *The Journal of Cell Biology, 103*(6), 2273–2281.
Orci, L., Ravazzola, M., Amherdt, M. N., Madsen, O., Vassalli, J.-D., & Perrelet, A. (1985). Direct identification of prohormone conversion site in insulin-secreting cells. *Cell, 42*(2), 671–681.
Osborne, A. R., Rapoport, T. A., & van den Berg, B. (2005). Protein translocation by the sec61/secy channel. *Annual Review of Cell and Developmental Biology, 21*(1), 529–550.
Palzkill, T., Le, Q. Q., Wong, A., & Botstein, D. (1994). Selection of functional signal peptide cleavage sites from a library of random sequences. *Journal of Bacteriology, 176*(3), 563–568.
Park, S.-Y., Ye, H., Steiner, D. F., & Bell, G. I. (2010). Mutant proinsulin proteins associated with neonatal diabetes are retained in the endoplasmic reticulum and not efficiently secreted. *Biochemical and Biophysical Research Communications, 391*(3), 1449–1454.
Parks, G. D., & Lamb, R. A. (1991). Topology of eukaryotic type II membrane proteins: Importance of N-terminal positively charged residues flanking the hydrophobic domain. *Cell, 64*(4), 777–787.
Patzelt, C., Labrecque, A. D., Duguid, J. R., Carroll, R. J., Keim, P. S., Heinrikson, R. L., et al. (1978). Detection and kinetic behavior of preproinsulin in pancreatic islets. *Proceedings of the National Academy of Sciences of the United States of America, 75*(3), 1260–1264.
Pilon, M., Romisch, K., Quach, D., & Schekman, R. (1998). Sec61p serves multiple roles in secretory precursor binding and translocation into the endoplasmic reticulum membrane. *Molecular Biology of the Cell, 9*(12), 3455–3473.

Pilon, M., Schekman, R., & Romisch, K. (1997). Sec61p mediates export of a misfolded secretory protein from the endoplasmic reticulum to the cytosol for degradation. *The EMBO Journal, 16*(15), 4540–4548.

Plath, K., Mothes, W., Wilkinson, B. M., Stirling, C. J., & Rapoport, T. A. (1998). Signal sequence recognition in posttranslational protein transport across the yeast ER membrane. *Cell, 94*(6), 795–807.

Plemper, R. K., Bohmler, S., Bordallo, J., Sommer, T., & Wolf, D. H. (1997). Mutant analysis links the translocon and BiP to retrograde protein transport for ER degradation. *Nature, 388*(6645), 891–895.

Puig, A., & Gilbert, H. F. (1994). Protein disulfide isomerase exhibits chaperone and anti-chaperone activity in the oxidative refolding of lysozyme. *Journal of Biological Chemistry, 269*(10), 7764–7771.

Quinn, D., Orci, L., Ravazzola, M., & Moore, H. (1991). Intracellular transport and sorting of mutant human proinsulins that fail to form hexamers. *The Journal of Cell Biology, 113*(5), 987–996.

Rajan, S., Eames, S. C., Park, S. Y., Labno, C., Bell, G. I., Prince, V. E., et al. (2010). In vitro processing and secretion of mutant insulin proteins that cause permanent neonatal diabetes. *American Journal of Physiology Endocrinology and Metabolism, 298*(3), E403–E410.

Rajpal, G., Schuiki, I., Liu, M., Volchuk, A., & Arvan, P. (2012). Action of protein disulfide isomerase on proinsulin exit from endoplasmic reticulum of pancreatic β-cells. *Journal of Biological Chemistry, 287*(1), 43–47.

Rane, N. S., Chakrabarti, O., Feigenbaum, L., & Hegde, R. S. (2010). Signal sequence insufficiency contributes to neurodegeneration caused by transmembrane prion protein. *The Journal of Cell Biology, 188*(4), 515–526.

Rapoport, T. A. (2007). Protein translocation across the eukaryotic endoplasmic reticulum and bacterial plasma membranes. *Nature, 450*(7170), 663–669.

Rhodes, C. J., & Halban, P. A. (1987). Newly synthesized proinsulin/insulin and stored insulin are released from pancreatic B cells predominantly via a regulated, rather than a constitutive, pathway. *The Journal of Cell Biology, 105*(1), 145–153.

Rhodes, C. J., Lincoln, B., & Shoelson, S. E. (1992). Preferential cleavage of des-31,32-proinsulin over intact proinsulin by the insulin secretory granule type II endopeptidase. Implication of a favored route for prohormone processing. *Journal of Biological Chemistry, 267*(32), 22719–22727.

Rorsman, P., & Braun, M. (2013). Regulation of insulin secretion in human pancreatic islets. *Annual Review of Physiology, 75*(1), 155–179.

Rorsman, P., & Renstrom, E. (2003). Insulin granule dynamics in pancreatic beta cells. *Diabetologia, 46*(8), 1029–1045.

Saraogi, I., & Shan, S.-O. (2011). Molecular mechanism of co-translational protein targeting by the signal recognition particle. *Traffic, 12*(5), 535–542.

Scheuner, D., & Kaufman, R. J. (2008). The unfolded protein response: A pathway that links insulin demand with {beta}-cell failure and diabetes. *Endocrine Reviews, 29*(3), 317–333.

Scheuner, D., Vander Mierde, D., Song, B., Flamez, D., Creemers, J. W., Tsukamoto, K., et al. (2005). Control of mRNA translation preserves endoplasmic reticulum function in beta cells and maintains glucose homeostasis. *Nature Medicine, 11*(7), 757–764.

Schmitz, A., Maintz, M., Kehle, T., & Herzog, V. (1995). In vivo iodination of a misfolded proinsulin reveals co-localized signals for Bip binding and for degradation in the ER. *The EMBO Journal, 14*(6), 1091–1098.

Schubert, U., Antón, L. C., Gibbs, J., Norbury, C. C., Yewdell, J. W., & Bennink, J. R. (2000). Rapid degradation of a large fraction of newly synthesized proteins by proteasomes. *Nature, 404*(6779), 770–774.

Scott, D. C., & Schekman, R. (2008). Role of Sec61p in the ER-associated degradation of short-lived transmembrane proteins. *The Journal of Cell Biology, 181*(7), 1095–1105.

Sevier, C. S. (2010). New insights into oxidative folding. *The Journal of Cell Biology, 188*(6), 757–758.
Sevier, C. S., Qu, H., Heldman, N., Gross, E., Fass, D., & Kaiser, C. A. (2007). Modulation of cellular disulfide-bond formation and the Er redox environment by feedback regulation of Ero1. *Cell, 129*(2), 333–344.
Shao, S., & Hegde, R. S. (2011). A calmodulin-dependent translocation pathway for small secretory proteins. *Cell, 147*(7), 1576–1588.
Sohma, Y., Hua, Q. X., Liu, M., Phillips, N. B., Hu, S. Q., Whittaker, J., et al. (2010). Contribution of residue B5 to the folding and function of insulin and IGF-I: Constraints and fine-tuning in the evolution of a protein family. *The Journal of Biological Chemistry, 285*(7), 5040–5055.
Spiro, R. G. (2002). Protein glycosylation: Nature, distribution, enzymatic formation, and disease implications of glycopeptide bonds. *Glycobiology, 12*(4), 43R–56R.
Stefan, Y., Meda, P., Neufeld, M., & Orci, L. (1987). Stimulation of insulin secretion reveals heterogeneity of pancreatic B cells in vivo. *The Journal of Clinical Investigation, 80*(1), 175–183.
Stefani, M., & Dobson, C. M. (2003). Protein aggregation and aggregate toxicity: New insights into protein folding, misfolding diseases and biological evolution. *Journal of Molecular Medicine (Berlin), 81*(11), 678–699.
Steiner, D. F. (1998). The proprotein convertases. *Current Opinion in Chemical Biology, 2*(1), 31–39.
Stoy, J., Edghill, E. L., Flanagan, S. E., Ye, H., Paz, V. P., Pluzhnikov, A., et al. (2007). Insulin gene mutations as a cause of permanent neonatal diabetes. *Proceedings of the National Academy of Sciences of the United States of America, 104*(38), 15040–15044.
Sugiura, Y., Araki, K., Iemura, S., Natsume, T., Hoseki, J., & Nagata, K. (2010). Novel thioredoxin-related transmembrane protein TMX4 has reductase activity. *The Journal of Biological Chemistry, 285*(10), 7135–7142.
Swanton, E., & High, S. (2006). ER targeting signals: More than meets the eye? *Cell, 127*(5), 877–879.
Talmadge, K., Stahl, S., & Gilbert, W. (1980). Eukaryotic signal sequence transports insulin antigen in Escherichia coli. *Proceedings of the National Academy of Sciences of the United States of America,* 77(6), 3369–3373.
Tang, J. G., & Tsou, C. L. (1990). The insulin A and B chains contain structural information for the formation of the native molecule. Studies with protein disulphide-isomerase. *The Biochemical Journal, 268*(2), 429–435.
Tang, J. G., Wang, C. C., & Tsou, C. L. (1988). Formation of native insulin from the scrambled molecule by protein disulphide-isomerase. *The Biochemical Journal, 255*(2), 451–455.
Uchizono, Y., Alarcón, C., Wicksteed, B. L., Marsh, B. J., & Rhodes, C. J. (2007). The balance between proinsulin biosynthesis and insulin secretion: Where can imbalance lead? *Diabetes, Obesity and Metabolism, 9*, 56–66.
Varlamov, O., Fricker, L. D., Furukawa, H., Steiner, D. F., Langley, S. H., & Leiter, E. H. (1997). β-Cell lines derived from transgenic Cpefat/Cpefat mice are defective in carboxypeptidase e and proinsulin processing. *Endocrinology, 138*(11), 4883–4892.
von Heijne, G. (1986). Net N-C charge imbalance may be important for signal sequence function in bacteria. *Journal of Molecular Biology, 192*(2), 287–290.
von Heijne, G. (1998). Protein transport: Life and death of a signal peptide. *Nature, 396*(6707), 111–113.
Wahlberg, J. M., & Spiess, M. (1997). Multiple determinants direct the orientation of signal ‚äìanchor proteins: The topogenic role of the hydrophobic signal domain. *The Journal of Cell Biology, 137*(3), 555–562.
Walczak, C. P., Bernardi, K. M., & Tsai, B. (2012). Endoplasmic reticulum-dependent redox reactions control endoplasmic reticulum-associated degradation and pathogen entry. *Antioxidants & Redox Signaling, 16*(8), 809–818.

Walter, P., & Blobel, G. (1983). Subcellular distribution of signal recognition particle and 7SL-RNA determined with polypeptide-specific antibodies and complementary DNA probe. *The Journal of Cell Biology*, *97*(6), 1693–1699.

Wang, J., Chen, Y., Yuan, Q., Tang, W., Zhang, X., & Osei, K. (2011). Control of precursor maturation and disposal is an early regulative mechanism in the normal insulin production of pancreatic beta-cells. *PLoS One*, *6*(4), e19446.

Wang, J., & Osei, K. (2011). Proinsulin maturation disorder is a contributor to the defect of subsequent conversion to insulin in beta-cells. *Biochemical and Biophysical Research Communications*, *411*(1), 150–155.

Winter, J., Klappa, P., Freedman, R. B., Lilie, H., & Rudolph, R. (2002). Catalytic activity and chaperone function of human protein-disulfide isomerase are required for the efficient refolding of proinsulin. *The Journal of Biological Chemistry*, *277*(1), 310–317.

Wolin, S. L., & Walter, P. (1993). Discrete nascent chain lengths are required for the insertion of presecretory proteins into microsomal membranes. *The Journal of Cell Biology*, *121*(6), 1211–1219.

Zhang, B.-Y., Liu, M., & Arvan, P. (2003). Behavior in the eukaryotic secretory pathway of insulin-containing fusion proteins and single-chain insulins bearing various B-chain mutations. *The Journal of Biological Chemistry*, *278*(6), 3687–3693.

Zhang, X., Rashid, R., Wang, K., & Shan, S.-O. (2010). Sequential checkpoints govern substrate selection during cotranslational protein targeting. *Science*, *328*(5979), 757–760.

Zheng, N., & Gierasch, L. M. (1996). Signal sequences: The same yet different. *Cell*, *86*(6), 849–852.

Zhu, X., Orci, L., Carroll, R., Norrbom, C., Ravazzola, M., & Steiner, D. F. (2002). Severe block in processing of proinsulin to insulin accompanied by elevation of des-64,65 proinsulin intermediates in islets of mice lacking prohormone convertase 1/3. *Proceedings of the National Academy of Sciences of the United States of America*, *99*(16), 10299–10304.

Zimmermann, R., Eyrisch, S., Ahmad, M., & Helms, V. (2011). Protein translocation across the ER membrane. *Biochimica et Biophysica Acta (BBA)—Biomembranes*, *1808*(3), 912–924.

Zito, E., Chin, K. T., Blais, J., Harding, H. P., & Ron, D. (2010). ERO1-beta, a pancreas-specific disulfide oxidase, promotes insulin biogenesis and glucose homeostasis. *The Journal of Cell Biology*, *188*(6), 821–832.

CHAPTER THREE

Metabolism–Secretion Coupling and Mitochondrial Calcium Activities in Clonal Pancreatic β-Cells

Lukas N. Groschner, Muhammad Rizwan Alam, Wolfgang F. Graier[1]
Institute of Molecular Biology and Biochemistry, Center of Molecular Medicine, Medical University of Graz, Graz, Austria
[1]Corresponding author: e-mail address: wolfgang.graier@medunigraz.at

Contents

Abstract

Pancreatic β-cells are the only cells capable of lowering blood glucose by secreting insulin. The β-cell continuously adjusts its secretory activity to substrate availability in order to keep blood glucose levels within the physiological range—a process called metabolism–secretion coupling. Glucose is readily taken up by the β-cell and broken down into intermediates that fuel oxidative metabolism inside the mitochondria to generate ATP. The resulting increase in the ATP/ADP ratio causes closure of plasma membrane K_{ATP} channels, thereby depolarizing the cell and triggering the opening of voltage-gated Ca^{2+} channels. Consequential oscillations of cytosolic Ca^{2+} not only mediate the exocytosis of insulin granules but are also relayed to other subcellular compartments including the mitochondria, where Ca^{2+} is required to accelerate mitochondrial metabolism in response to nutrient stimulation. The mitochondrial Ca^{2+} uptake

Vitamins and Hormones, Volume 95
ISSN 0083-6729
http://dx.doi.org/10.1016/B978-0-12-800174-5.00003-X

machinery plays a fundamental role in this feed-forward mechanism that guarantees sustained insulin secretion and, thus, represents a promising therapeutic target for type 2 diabetes.

1. INTRODUCTION

The pancreatic β-cell is a particularly exciting type of cell, not only because its membrane harbors voltage-gated ion channels, which by definition make it an electrically excitable cell, but especially because of its unique way of adjusting secretory activity to substrate availability. There are not many cell types that are capable of accomplishing similar tasks and most certainly no other type of cell can secrete insulin, the one and only blood glucose-lowering hormone (Rorsman & Braun, 2013). Its importance is illustrated by the fact that depletion or dysfunction of β-cells is unavoidably linked to the development of diabetes mellitus, a disease currently affecting over 6.4% of adults worldwide (Shaw, Sicree, & Zimmet, 2010) and causing one death every 7 s (Ashcroft & Rorsman, 2012). Along with the prevalence of this disease, diabetes-associated healthcare costs are also increasing at an enormous speed, accounting already for 2–7% of national healthcare expanses in Western Europe (Zimmet, 2003), hence placing a growing burden on both individual patients and national economies.

In order to provide better insight into the pathophysiology of diabetes mellitus, a detailed understanding of the process of insulin secretion is of utmost importance and has thus turned the pancreatic β-cell into an attractive target for both basic and clinical research. In the 1960s, it was already found that metabolic substrates and intermediates other than glucose had a similar effect on insulin secretion and that inhibition of intracellular metabolism was sufficient to prevent insulin secretion even in the presence of glucose (Ashcroft, Hedeskov, & Randle, 1970). These observations have led to the idea that glucose elicits insulin release not through interaction with a specific receptor but through metabolism of the hexose within the β-cell, ruling out the concept of a surface bound "glucoreceptor."

Since then, the exceptional way of adjusting insulin secretion to the availability of metabolic substrates, a process also referred to as "metabolism–secretion coupling," has attracted a lot of attention. In essence, this is achieved by different K_{ATP} channel-dependent and -independent mechanisms (Henquin, 2000; Wiederkehr & Wollheim, 2008). The uptake of glucose by the β-cell through glucose transporter 1 in humans and 2 in rodents and its oxidative metabolism yields a rise in the cytosolic ATP/ADP ratio. This in turn decreases the K_{ATP} channel's open probability (Cook & Hales, 1984; Tarasov, Dusonchet, & Ashcroft, 2004), thus reducing the membrane potential and causing the opening of voltage-gated Ca^{2+} channels. Triggered by the influx of Ca^{2+}, insulin-filled vesicles subsequently release their cargo and thereby lower blood glucose levels (Eliasson et al., 2008).

The dependence of glucose-stimulated insulin secretion (GSIS) on cytosolic Ca^{2+} activity has been known for more than half a century. Over the past 30 years, however, more and more evidence has accumulated, supporting the notion that not only cytosolic Ca^{2+} activity but also its propagation to other cellular organelles are essential for the β-cell to adequately fulfill its function. Especially, the mitochondria as central hub connecting oxidative metabolism to insulin secretion have proven to hinge on Ca^{2+} in order to maintain and adjust their metabolic function (Wiederkehr & Wollheim, 2012). This chapter focuses on the role of mitochondrial Ca^{2+} handling in the function and dysfunction of clonal pancreatic β-cells.

2. THE IMPORTANCE OF MITOCHONDRIA TO β-CELL FUNCTION

Electron micrographs have shown that mitochondria are frequently found within close proximity to secretory granules of β-cells (Wollheim, 2000). This observation already points to an integral role of this organelle in the process of insulin secretion. However, the study of mitochondrial physiology in pancreatic β-cells is more or less limited to methods that allow the assessment of mitochondrial function in intact cells, since the quantity of β-cell mitochondria that can be isolated from primary islets is comparatively small and potentially contaminated with mitochondria from other islet cells. Yet, recent technical advancements in the field of fluorescent sensors have opened up new possibilities of studying mitochondrial function in one given cell on multiple levels in parallel (Tarasov, Griffiths, & Rutter, 2012; Waldeck-Weiermair et al., 2012). Such sensors can be used in primary cells, but are particularly applicable in β-cell lines in order to investigate basic concepts in β-cell physiology. Several widely used clonal cell lines have proven to be valuable in overcoming the shortage and limitations of primary β-cells (Hohmeier et al., 2000; Skelin, Rupnik, & Cencic, 2010) and have helped to study mitochondrial function in this very special type of cell.

The functional integrity of mitochondria is fundamental to β-cell physiology, which is highlighted by the finding that depletion of mitochondrial DNA (mtDNA) causes severe impairment of GSIS in β-cell lines such as MIN6 (Soejima et al., 1996; Tsuruzoe et al., 1998) and INS-1 (Kennedy, Maechler, & Wollheim, 1998). Certain types of diabetes are linked to mutations affecting mitochondrial function. Mutations in hepatic nuclear factor 1-α, for example, lead to uncoupling of mitochondrial oxidative phosphorylation (OXPHOS) in INS-1 cells and are associated with type 3 of maturity onset diabetes of the young (Pongratz et al., 2009). β-Cell-specific knockout of the mitochondrial transcription factor A also causes impaired insulin secretion and loss of β-cell mass resulting in a form of mitochondrial diabetes in mice (Silva et al., 2000). Mutations in mtDNA have been proposed to account for 0.5–1% of all cases of diabetes in humans (Kadowaki et al., 1994). Taking into consideration that the majority of all mitochondrial proteins are coded for by nuclear DNA, it can be assumed that the actual prevalence of mitochondrial diabetes is exceeding these estimates. Increasing evidence implicates not only mutations in mtDNA but also environmental factors such as a surfeit of metabolic substrates and a concomitant increase in reactive oxygen species in the pathogenesis of mitochondrial dysfunction, thus uncovering the mitochondrion as one of the major culprits in the development of impaired glucose tolerance and diabetes mellitus (Coughlan et al., 2011).

The general importance of mitochondrial metabolism to the process of GSIS is reflected by the fact that inhibition of the mitochondrial adenine nucleotide translocase, responsible for transporting ATP out of and ADP into the mitochondrial matrix, completely abolishes glucose-induced electrical activity of β-cells, indicating that glycolysis-derived ATP is not sufficient to maintain proper function (Kiranadi, Bangham, & Smith, 1991). Overexpression of the adenine nucleotide translocase in INS-1 cells, however, does not potentiate O_2 consumption rates, Ca^{2+} signals, or insulin secretion in response to glucose (unpublished observations), prompting the idea that the transport of ADP/ATP across mitochondrial membranes is not a rate-limiting factor. Inorganic phosphate, which is required by complex V of the electron transport chain to synthesize ATP, is transported into the mitochondria via a phosphate carrier. Silencing of this carrier decreases ATP production and insulin secretion in response to glucose (Nishi et al., 2011). Pharmacological dissipation of the mitochondrial inner membrane potential ($\Delta\Psi_{mito}$) using protonophores effectively inhibits β-cell secretory activity despite an increase in cytosolic Ca^{2+} (Rustenbeck, Herrmann, & Grimmsmann, 1997), emphasizing the relevance of the spatiotemporal coordination of metabolic and ionic signals. Similar to protonophores, also overexpression of mitochondrial uncoupling protein 1 (UCP1), which reduces the coupling of OXPHOS, results in decreased ATP production, increased K_{ATP} channel activity, hyperpolarized plasma membrane potential, and drastically impaired GSIS in a mouse β-cell line (Nakazaki et al., 2002). It is noteworthy, however, that a potentiation of insulin secretion, such as that evoked by glucagon-like peptide-1, is not necessarily associated with an increase in OXPHOS (Peyot et al., 2009) supporting the notion that mitochondrial energy metabolism is essential for insulin secretin, but stimulation of GSIS does not always involve changes in energy metabolism.

3. OXIDATIVE METABOLISM OF β-CELLS

The metabolism of the β-cell is quite distinctive as it is directly coupled to an important cellular function, exceeding the mere task of supplying the cell with energy-rich molecules. In addition, the β-cell has special preferences when it comes to metabolic substrates. So far, a number of substances have been shown to stimulate insulin secretion, the most relevant of these being D-glucose. The branched-chain amino acid leucine and—to a lesser extent—free fatty acids are also among the nutrients that evoke insulin secretion. Various hormones and neurotransmitters potentiate insulin secretion via interaction with specific receptors. The main nutrient secretagogues, in contrast, undergo metabolism within the β-cell—more precisely, within its mitochondria—to create second messengers, which then influence β-cell electrical activity and thereby give rise to insulin exocytosis (Jitrapakdee, Wutthisathapornchai, Wallace, & MacDonald, 2010).

Metabolic intermediates that serve as source of energy during physical exercise or catabolic states, such as pyruvate, lactate, and ketone bodies, need to be ignored by the β-cell in order to avoid hypoglycemic episodes (Wiederkehr & Wollheim, 2012). This apparent fuel selectivity requires the cell to express a very specific set of enzymes that make it possible to favor certain substrates, that is, glucose, over others. In this regard, the expression of specific genes has emerged to be just as important as the disallowance of others (Schuit et al., 2012; Sekine et al., 1994). Loss of the β-cells' ability to discriminate between different substrates has been linked to phenotypes associated with inadequate insulin secretion. In contrast to primary islet cells (Mertz, Worley, Spencer, Johnson, & Dukes, 1996), INS-1 insulinoma cell lines, for example, express significant amounts of the plasma membrane monocarboxylate transporter-1 (MCT1) and thus exhibit robust secretory response also after stimulation with pyruvate (Goehring et al., 2012). A similar phenomenon can be observed in patients manifesting exercise-induced hyperinsulinism, where a defect in the β-cell-specific silencing of MCT1 accounts for insulin secretion at times when it is least needed—in response to physical exercise (Otonkoski et al., 2007). Using a mouse model overexpressing MCT1 in β-cells, it was recently demonstrated that the transport of pyruvate across the plasma membrane is sufficient to induce this form of hyperinsulinism (Pullen et al., 2012).

Being the primary end-product of glycolysis, pyruvate represents a key metabolite in β-cells, and not only its oxidation within the mitochondria but also its exchange with tricarboxylic acid (TCA) cycle intermediates have been shown to correlate with glucose responsiveness in different INS-1 cell lines (Lu et al., 2002). It can hence be assumed that the recently identified mitochondrial pyruvate carrier (Bricker et al., 2012; Herzig et al., 2012) is essential for intact metabolism–secretion coupling in β-cells, but its exact role in this context is still awaiting clarification. Once pyruvate has entered the mitochondrial matrix, it can be converted to acetyl-CoA by the pyruvate dehydrogenase (PDH), a protein complex that indirectly depends on free Ca^{2+} in its activity, or it can be carboxylated to form oxaloacetate via the pyruvate carboxylase. Either way, pyruvate enters the TCA cycle and thereby fuels the mitochondrial electron transport chain. Lactate dehydrogenase (LDH) is an enzyme that prevents pyruvate from entering oxidative metabolism by converting it into lactate and regenerating NAD^+ needed during glycolysis. Correspondingly, INS-1 cell clones expressing high levels of LDH fail to accelerate O_2 consumption rates and insulin secretion in response to high glucose (Malmgren et al., 2009). Under normal conditions, NADH generated through glycolysis is efficiently shuttled into the mitochondria where it acts as another glycolysis-derived factor fueling mitochondrial metabolism (Eto et al., 1999).

Unlike most other cell lines, glucose-responsive INS-1 cells have the remarkable ability to further boost their respiratory rate in response to increasing levels of glucose. Strictly speaking, this phenomenon can be considered a reverse Crabtree effect: Under high-glucose conditions, most clonal (tumor) cell lines tend to reduce OXPHOS to a minimum and solely rely on anaerobic glycolysis in order to meet their energy demands (Koziel, Woyda-Ploszczyca, Kicinska, & Jarmuszkiewicz, 2012). To the β-cell, however, ATP is more than just an energy-rich molecule as its intracellular concentration is directly coupled to insulin secretion. In order to adjust granule exocytosis to glucose concentrations over a wide dynamic range, ATP synthesis is required to closely reflect glucose supply. If the β-cell would start generating only two molecules of ATP per molecule of glucose instead of the 30–32 that can be achieved through OXPHOS (Nelson & Cox, 2008), the moment glucose levels exceed a certain threshold, it could clearly not keep up with the increasing insulin demand. For this reason, β-cells need to increase their O_2 consumption rates even further under high-glucose conditions. Extracellular glucose concentration relates to the rate of glucose oxidation in a sigmoidal curve with the steepest slope between concentrations of 5.5 and 8 mM of glucose (Ashcroft et al., 1970), thereby corresponding very well to GSIS.

There are certain subclones of the INS-1 insulinoma cell line, which differ considerably in terms of their secretory response to high glucose. A study has linked these differences in metabolism–secretion coupling to the expression levels of genes related to OXPHOS. Any functional defects causing a Warburg-like shift from mitochondrial to anaerobic glycolytic metabolism were found to result in decreased glucose responsiveness of clonal β-cells and also correlate with the severity of a preexisting diabetic phenotype in humans (Malmgren et al., 2009). Taken together, these findings highlight the importance of mitochondrial oxidative metabolism in GSIS.

3.1. Mitochondrial coupling factors

Mitochondria represent the central hub of cellular bioenergetics and are also an organelle with crucial roles in cell signaling (Groschner, Waldeck-Weiermair, Malli, & Graier, 2012). In the pancreatic β-cell, these two functions overlap in many ways as the mitochondria are the main source not only of ATP but also of a multitude of other signaling molecules, which have been shown to regulate insulin secretion (Maechler & Wollheim, 2001).

The amino acid glutamate, for example, is formed from α-ketoglutarate in β-cell mitochondria during glucose stimulation and has been proposed to act as a mitochondrial signal driving the ATP-independent amplifying phase of insulin secretion (Maechler & Wollheim, 1999). Although this concept has been challenged by others using alternative means to increase cytosolic glutamate concentrations (Bertrand, Ishiyama, Nenquin, Ravier, & Henquin, 2002), measurements of membrane capacitance have revealed a direct effect of glutamate on insulin granule exocytosis (Hoy et al., 2002). Accordingly, disrupting either the generation of glutamate by knocking out glutamate dehydrogenase (Carobbio et al., 2009) or its transport out of the mitochondrial matrix by silencing the mitochondrial glutamate carrier (Casimir et al., 2009) impedes GSIS.

Mitochondrial GTP (mtGTP), another potent signaling molecule, forms within the mitochondrion as a product of the TCA cycle in the reaction of succinyl-CoA to succinate and is not exported to the cytosol. Two different isoforms of succinyl-CoA synthetase couple this reaction to the generation of one molecule of either ATP or GTP. Silencing of the ATP-producing isoform resulted in a pronounced increase in GSIS, while knockdown of the GTP-producing form had a negative effect on GSIS (Kibbey et al., 2007). Surprisingly, this shift from ATP to mtGTP synthesis was accompanied by a drop in $\Delta\Psi_{mito}$, an increase in O_2 consumption, and a potentiation of cytosolic Ca^{2+} activity despite a reduction in ATP. Given that mtGTP-depleted cells showed an increase in overall mitochondrial Ca^{2+} concentration ($[Ca^{2+}]_{mito}$) after stimulation with glucose, the authors argue that mtGTP might act to promote the extrusion of Ca^{2+} from the mitochondria, hence diverting the proton motive force from ATP production to the electrogenic Na^+/Ca^{2+} exchange. A more recent study implicates mtGTP in controlling mitochondrial production of phosphoenolpyruvate, another factor amplifying GSIS (Stark et al., 2009). Future work will be needed to elucidate the mechanisms behind mtGTP signaling.

Mitochondrial matrix pH, a parameter closely reflecting metabolic activity, naturally correlates very well with nutrient activation in INS-1E cells. Yet, matrix pH seems to affect metabolism–secretion coupling independent of its influence on the electrochemical gradient across the inner mitochondrial membrane (IMM) as proposed by a study using the unspecific K^+/H^+ ionophore nigericin to induce matrix acidification (Akhmedov et al., 2010). Further studies will be needed to identify the molecular mechanisms underlying this phenomenon.

Most of these coupling factors are likely to contribute to the feed-forward mechanism elicited by mitochondrial Ca^{2+} activity, which contributes mainly to the second phase of insulin secretion (unpublished observations).

3.2. Mitochondrial integrity and β-cell function

Mitochondria constitute an interconnected filamentous network of moving organelles continuously changing their shape through fission and fusion events (Groschner et al., 2012). Dynamics and ultrastructure of this organelle are inseparably linked to its bioenergetic function (Benard et al., 2007). Fis1, an integral component of the mitochondrial fission machinery, seems to be of particular importance to metabolism–secretion coupling. INS-1E cells overexpressing Fis1 exhibit fragmented mitochondria and fail to hyperpolarize $\Delta\Psi_{mito}$ when challenged with high glucose. Interestingly, also mitochondrial Ca^{2+} uptake and GSIS were significantly reduced under these conditions (Park et al., 2008). In the same study, overexpression of a dominant negative mutant of mitofusin 1 led to similar morphological changes but did not impede GSIS, indicating that changes in mitochondrial structure are not necessarily accompanied by changes on the functional level. These discrepancies might be explained by additional unknown functions of Fis1 or by differential effects on mitochondrial motility.

Knockdown of Fis1 resulted in decreased O_2 consumption and—just like its overexpression—in reduced GSIS (Twig et al., 2008).

We have recently described the fragmentation of mitochondrial networks in β-cells overexpressing proteins involved in Ca^{2+} sequestration such as mitochondrial Ca^{2+} uptake 1 (MICU1) (Alam et al., 2012), pointing out the bidirectional relationship between Ca^{2+} homeostasis, morphology, and motility of mitochondria. The Ca^{2+} sensitivity of mitochondrial dynamics is mediated by an EF-hand containing Miro GTPase, which causes mitochondria to halt at sites of high cytosolic Ca^{2+} concentrations ($[Ca^{2+}]_{cyto}$) (Saotome et al., 2008). It is tempting to speculate that this phenomenon contributes to the fact that β-cell mitochondria regularly localize at subplasmalemmal Ca^{2+} hot spots near the readily releasable pool of secretory granules (Wollheim, 2000) where they might have important functions in controlling local dynamics of Ca^{2+}, ATP, and other coupling factors (Kennedy et al., 1999).

4. MITOCHONDRIAL Ca^{2+} AND ENERGY METABOLISM

A rise of intracellular Ca^{2+} is generally associated with cell activation and, thus, with a concomitant increase in cellular energy expenditure. Under these conditions, a vast amount of ATP is utilized within the cell for specific functions such as contraction, ion transport, protein synthesis, motility, and exocytosis (Berridge, Lipp, & Bootman, 2000). In order to meet the increased energy demands, most cells are able to accelerate OXPHOS in dependence of cellular Ca^{2+} levels and so is the β-cell. Facing rapid, pulsatile changes of $[Ca^{2+}]_{cyto}$ during stimulation with glucose, the β-cell can boost its O_2 consumption rates up to four times compared to basal conditions (Wiederkehr et al., 2011). In the absence of extracellular Ca^{2+}, increases in response to glucose are comparatively modest, but still detectable, suggesting that the initial stimulation of mitochondrial metabolism by glucose does not necessarily require extracellular Ca^{2+}. The following acceleration of OXPHOS, in contrast, strictly depends on the presence of extracellular Ca^{2+}.

Yet, cytosolic Ca^{2+} has conflicting effects on mitochondrial metabolism. On the one hand, being a cation, its uptake into the mitochondrial matrix *per se* causes depolarization of $\Delta\Psi_{mito}$, thereby reducing the driving force for ATP synthesis. In β-cells, such transient depolarization occurs shortly after glucose-evoked cytosolic Ca^{2+} peaks and can be prevented by removal of extracellular Ca^{2+} (Kindmark et al., 2001). On the other hand, free Ca^{2+} acts as an activating signal for mitochondrial dehydrogenases, thus providing the electron transport chain with an increasing amount of reducing equivalents (McCormack, Halestrap, & Denton, 1990). Based on mathematical modeling of β-cell Ca^{2+} activity, Magnus and Keizer proposed in 1998 that the former would outweigh the latter effect. According to their β-cell model, the glucose-induced uptake of Ca^{2+} by mitochondria would cause a drop in $\Delta\Psi_{mito}$ in the range of 0.8 mV with slow temporal kinetics, but sufficient to suppress ATP synthesis to an extent that causes opening of K_{ATP} channels, thus implicating mitochondrial Ca^{2+} uptake in the termination of electrical bursting in the β-cell (Magnus & Keizer, 1998a, 1998b). This theoretical model, however, is not in line with experimental data from both cell lines and primary β-cells gathered since that time (Alam et al., 2012; Tarasov, Griffiths, et al., 2012; Wiederkehr et al., 2011).

Despite its pivotal role as a second messenger, Ca^{2+} can also be harmful to the cell when its concentration exceeds a threshold over a certain period of time. Apart from the deleterious effects of a persistent elevation of $[Ca^{2+}]_{mito}$ on mitochondrial permeability transition and the initiation of cell death (Bernardi & Rasola, 2007), prolonged intracellular Ca^{2+} signals observed under maximal stimulation with agonists accelerate mitochondrial metabolism only transiently, whereas oscillations of frequencies >0.5 min^{-1}, as typically seen in stimulated β-cells, provoke a sustained activation of Ca^{2+}-dependent mitochondrial dehydrogenases (Hajnoczky, Robb-Gaspers, Seitz, & Thomas, 1995). In this context, the kinetics of mitochondrial Ca^{2+} signals are of special interest; yet, in many cases, imaging techniques permit only limited inferences to be drawn about these. We recently developed a genetically encoded, FRET-based mitochondrial Ca^{2+} sensor, making it possible to record mitochondrial and cytosolic Ca^{2+} signals in parallel on the single cell level. This approach provides means to study subcellular Ca^{2+} handling with unprecedented temporal and spatial resolution while maintaining an excellent signal-to-noise ratio (Fig. 3.1) (Waldeck-Weiermair et al., 2012).

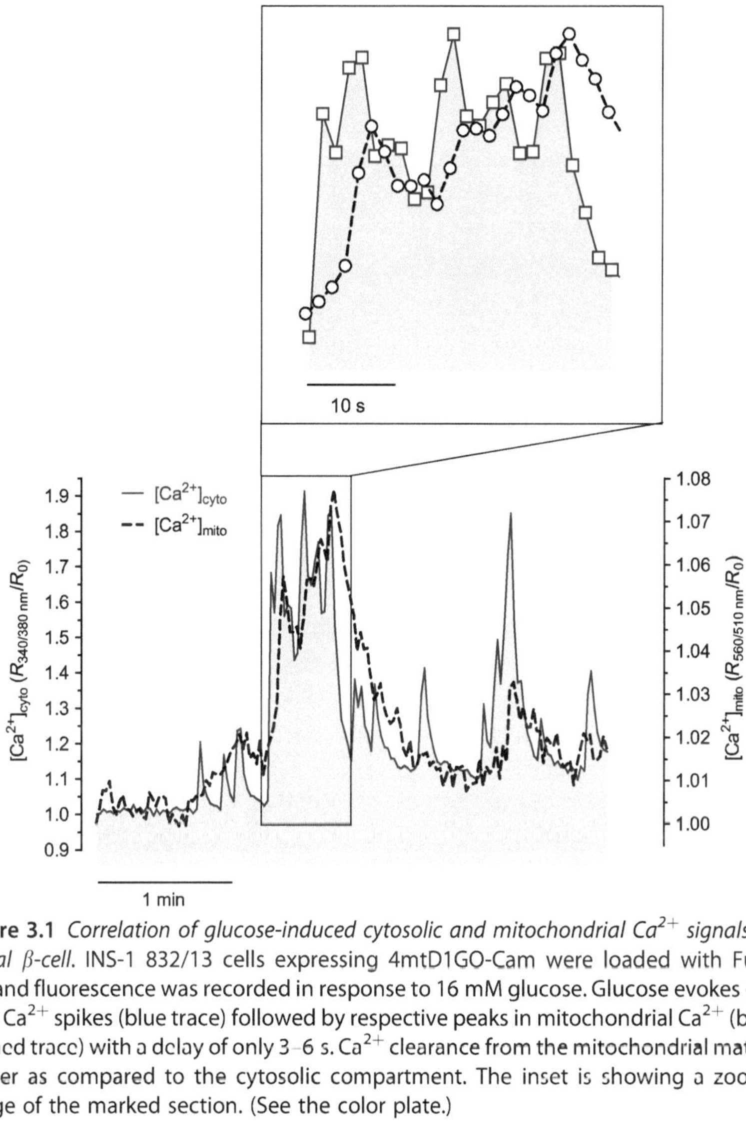

Figure 3.1 *Correlation of glucose-induced cytosolic and mitochondrial Ca^{2+} signals in a clonal β-cell.* INS-1 832/13 cells expressing 4mtD1GO-Cam were loaded with Fura-2 AM and fluorescence was recorded in response to 16 mM glucose. Glucose evokes cytosolic Ca^{2+} spikes (blue trace) followed by respective peaks in mitochondrial Ca^{2+} (black-dashed trace) with a delay of only 3–6 s. Ca^{2+} clearance from the mitochondrial matrix is slower as compared to the cytosolic compartment. The inset is showing a zoom in image of the marked section. (See the color plate.)

4.1. Ca^{2+}-dependent proteins within the mitochondria

A possible influence of Ca^{2+} ions on mitochondrial metabolism was first suggested in the late 1950s and was thereafter confirmed by Denton and McCormack who demonstrated that the activity of three key mitochondrial dehydrogenases is sensitive to Ca^{2+} (Denton & McCormack, 1986). PDH, one of the rate-limiting enzyme complexes of oxidative metabolism, is activated via dephosphorylation by PDH phosphatase, an enzyme highly dependent on the concentration of free Ca^{2+} (Denton, Randle, & Martin, 1972). Isocitrate dehydrogenase and α-ketoglutarate dehydrogenase, two TCA-cycle enzymes, in contrast, are regulated by direct binding of Ca^{2+} (Denton, Richards, & Chin, 1978; McCormack & Denton, 1979). In addition to these, a plethora of other mitochondrial metabolic enzymes have been reported to contain Ca^{2+}-binding domains and, thus, represent likely targets for the integration of cellular Ca^{2+} signals. The EF-hand protein S100A1, for instance, has been shown to activate the ATP synthase itself via Ca^{2+}-dependent interaction with its F1 portion (Boerries et al., 2007). The mitochondrial glycerophosphate dehydrogenase (mGDH) is another Ca^{2+}-regulated enzyme. As part of the glycerol phosphate shuttle, mGDH is localized to the outer part of the IMM allowing glycolysis-derived NADH to enter oxidative metabolism within the mitochondria (Wernette, Ochs, & Lardy, 1981). It was speculated that an islet-specific deficiency in mGDH activity might even contribute to the pathogenesis of type 2 diabetes (Ostenson et al., 1993). The mechanisms behind the Ca^{2+}-dependent increase of OXPHOS are manifold and involve both direct and indirect actions of Ca^{2+} on mitochondrial proteins. This increase of OXPHOS can be observed even beyond the immediate actions of Ca^{2+} (Jouaville, Pinton, Bastianutto, Rutter, & Rizzuto, 1999). After prestimulation with either high K^+ or a K_{ATP} channel blocker, MIN-6 cells exhibit an amplified response to glucose when compared to naive cells (Ainscow & Rutter, 2001).

Sound evidence for the activating role of mitochondrial Ca^{2+} in β-cells was provided by Wiederkehr and colleagues, who used a Ca^{2+}-buffering protein targeted to the mitochondrial matrix to modulate free matrix Ca^{2+} and found that buffering of $[Ca^{2+}]_{mito}$ resulted in reduced cellular respiration, ATP production, and a decrease in the amplifying phase of insulin secretion (Wiederkehr et al., 2011).

5. Ca^{2+} HANDLING IN β-CELLS

Glucose stimulates insulin secretion exclusively in the presence of Ca^{2+}, which is illustrated by the fact that hypocalcemic conditions can impair GSIS (Boucher, Mannan, Noonan, Hales, & Evans, 1995). Intracellular-free Ca^{2+} takes central stage in the process of GSIS by directly triggering exocytosis of insulin-filled large dense core vesicles. Several proteins encoded by the synaptotagmin gene family have been implicated in the Ca^{2+} dependency of vesicle membrane fusion (Gauthier & Wollheim, 2008) while others like syntaxin and synaptosomal protein of 25 kDa seem to be required for tight coupling between voltage-dependent Ca^{2+} channels and insulin granules (Vikman, Ma, Hockerman, Rorsman, & Eliasson, 2006). Close physical interaction between local sites of Ca^{2+} entry and the exocytotic apparatus is necessary to guarantee efficient utilization of cytosolic-free Ca^{2+}, which is limited even during electrical activity of the β-cell. This might be attributable to a comparatively low plasma membrane Ca^{2+} channel density (Rorsman, Braun, & Zhang, 2012). Under resting conditions, $[Ca^{2+}]_{cyto}$ is kept around 90 nM, and even during stimulation, overall cytosolic Ca^{2+} hardly exceeds concentrations of 400 nM (Rojas et al., 1994). Intracellular application of 10 mM of the Ca^{2+}-chelating agent EDTA does not prevent granule exocytosis (Hoppa et al., 2009), indicating that the β-cell has apparently developed a very efficient system of cellular Ca^{2+} handling to secure both insulin secretion and the transfer of Ca^{2+} signals from subplasmalemmal microdomains to cellular compartments such as the mitochondria (Rutter, Tsuboi, & Ravier, 2006).

5.1. Subcellular Ca^{2+} signals in clonal β-cells

Ca^{2+} enters the electrically excitable β-cell through different voltage-gated ion channels. The ATP-mediated increase in plasma membrane electrical resistance depolarizes the cell and thereby triggers electrical activity. L-type Ca^{2+} channels, which are rapidly activated during the upstroke of action potentials, account for bulk cytosolic Ca^{2+} signals, while Ca^{2+} influx via P/Q-type channels is required for exocytosis (Rorsman et al., 2012). A certain subpopulation of mitochondria are believed to be situated close to the inner mouth of L-type, possible also P/Q-type Ca^{2+} channels where they are confronted with oscillations of $[Ca^{2+}]_{cyto}$ at a high frequency. Therefore, the β-cell's mitochondria regulate their Ca^{2+} uptake differently as compared to other nonexcitable cell types such as endothelial and HeLa cells. We used INS-1 cells to characterize the spatiotemporal correlations of cytosolic and mitochondrial Ca^{2+} in parallel and found significant differences in the kinetics of subcellular Ca^{2+} handling. β-Cell mitochondria are able to take up Ca^{2+} at a higher speed than other cell types (Waldeck-Weiermair et al., 2012). In response to high glucose, the isolated transients of cytosolic Ca^{2+} seen in INS-1 cells are instantly transferred to the mitochondrial matrix, whereas Ca^{2+} spikes evoked by depolarizing concentrations of K^{+} were detected inside the matrix with a significant time lag. This phenomenon might be attributed to a glucose-induced increase in

$\Delta\Psi_{mito}$, which constitutes the driving force for a rapid mitochondrial Ca^{2+} uptake and is absent during stimulation with K^+. This hypothesis is in line with the observation that $\Delta\Psi_{mito}$ hyperpolarizes prior to Ca^{2+} influx into the cytosol (Duchen, Smith, & Ashcroft, 1993).

Ca^{2+} extrusion from β-cell mitochondria displays significantly slower kinetics compared to not only respective cytosolic peaks (Fig. 3.1) but also other cell types, hence allowing for maximal amplification of Ca^{2+} signals. Repetitive spiking of $[Ca^{2+}]_{cyto}$ consequently results in a long-lasting elevation of $[Ca^{2+}]_{mito}$. However, cytosolic Ca^{2+} peaks below a certain threshold are not detectable within the mitochondrial matrix (Waldeck-Weiermair et al., 2012). Differences in the Ca^{2+} affinities of Ca^{2+} channels themselves or of Ca^{2+}-sensing subunits such as MICU1 might explain that not every single cytosolic Ca^{2+} peak is relayed to the mitochondrial matrix. This could also account for the time-dependent desensitization of mitochondrial Ca^{2+} sequestration observed during persistent stimulation. Effectively, the mitochondria seem to be able to modify both their Ca^{2+} uptake and their Ca^{2+} buffering capacity according to the metabolic needs of the cell.

5.2. Mitochondrial Ca^{2+} uptake in β-cells

Since the early 1960s, it is known that respiring mitochondria are able to accumulate significant quantities of Ca^{2+} ions (Deluca & Engstrom, 1961), but today we are only beginning to understand the molecular basis of this intricate phenomenon. After entering the cytosol, Ca^{2+} ions have to permeate both the outer mitochondrial membrane and IMM before reaching the mitochondrial matrix. While the outer membrane constitutes less of a burden to ions and molecules smaller than 5 kDa, ion fluxes across the IMM are tightly regulated. So far a number of proteins, comprising ion channels, exchangers, and regulatory proteins, have been described to contribute to the shuttling of Ca^{2+} into and out of the mitochondrial matrix. Putative mitochondrial Ca^{2+} channels include the ryanodine receptor 1 (Beutner, Sharma, Giovannucci, Yule, & Sheu, 2001), uncoupling proteins 2 and 3 (UCP2/3) (Trenker, Malli, Fertschai, Levak-Frank, & Graier, 2007), and the mitochondrial Ca^{2+} uniporter (MCU). MCU is a two-transmembrane domain protein of the IMM representing the putative pore-forming subunit of what turns out to be a multiprotein MCU-complex (Baughman et al., 2011; De Stefani, Raffaello, Teardo, Szabo, & Rizzuto, 2011). Within this complex, MCU associates with multiple regulatory proteins, the first of which, MICU1, was discovered in 2010 by Mootha and colleagues screening a compendium of IMM proteins (Perocchi et al., 2010). MICU1 has one transmembrane domain and two EF-hand motifs that are crucial for its Ca^{2+}-sensing properties. More recent studies have suggested MICU1 as a negative regulator of the MCU, preventing mitochondrial Ca^{2+} overload under resting conditions (Mallilankaraman, Doonan, et al., 2012). MICU2 and MICU3, two additional paralogs of MICU1, have also been identified and might contribute to the tissue specificity of mitochondrial Ca^{2+} handling (Plovanich et al., 2013). Mitochondrial Ca^{2+} uniporter regulator 1 (MCUR1) is another novel regulatory protein that has been reported to act in concert with MCU (Mallilankaraman, Cardenas, et al., 2012). UCP2/3 have been found particularly important in adjusting mitochondrial Ca^{2+} uptake to differences in the concentration (Waldeck-Weiermair, Duan, et al., 2010) and the source (Waldeck-Weiermair, Malli, et al., 2010) of cytosolic Ca^{2+}. In contrast to UCP2/3, which preferentially localize at contact sites between the mitochondria and the ER, the mitochondrial Ca^{2+}/H^{+} antiporter leucine zipper EF-hand-containing protein 1 (LETM1) (Jiang, Zhao, & Clapham, 2009) seems to be responsible for the transfer of Ca^{2+} entering the cell through channels in the plasma membrane of endothelial cells (Waldeck-Weiermair et al., 2011). Similar differential Ca^{2+} uptake mechanisms might have important functions in β-cells, where the extracellular milieu rather than intracellular stores represents the main source of Ca^{2+}.

Single channel patch-clamp recordings in mitoplasts isolated from HeLa cells have so far revealed the presence of at least three inwardly rectifying Ca^{2+} currents of different amplitudes (Bondarenko, Jean-Quartier, Malli, & Graier, 2013; Jean-Quartier et al., 2012) pointing to the existence of multiple routes of mitochondrial Ca^{2+} uptake. To date, corresponding studies in β-cell mitoplasts are still to be carried out.

In order to assess the function of mitochondrial Ca^{2+} transport proteins in clonal pancreatic β-cells and their role in metabolism–secretion coupling, we recently employed a siRNA-based gene silencing strategy to selectively and efficiently suppress the expression of MICU1, MCU, UCP2, and LETM1 in INS-1 832/13 cells (Alam et al., 2012). Although the exact role of UCP2 in β-cells is debated, we demonstrated a source-specific involvement in mitochondrial Ca^{2+} uptake, which goes well in line with previous findings in other cell types where UCP2 is involved in the sequestration of intracellularly released Ca^{2+} (Waldeck-Weiermair et al., 2011; Waldeck-Weiermair, Malli, et al., 2010). LETM1 appeared to be involved in mitochondrial Ca^{2+} sequestration exclusively when Ca^{2+} is entering the cytosol from outside the cell. Knockdown of MCU and its regulatory subunit MICU1, in contrast, had a pronounced effect on mitochondrial Ca^{2+} sequestration irrespective of the source of mobilized Ca^{2+}. A combined knockdown of MICU1 and MCU did not result in any additional decrease in mitochondrial Ca^{2+} uptake, suggesting that these two proteins are indeed part of the same Ca^{2+} uptake pathway (Fig. 3.2).

Silencing of MICU1 and MCU effectively hampered mitochondrial Ca^{2+} signals in response to 16 mM glucose while leaving both frequency and amplitude of cytosolic Ca^{2+} oscillations unaffected. In addition, cells deficient of MICU1 or MCU showed a pronounced reduction in cytosolic ATP and insulin secretion in response to glucose. This discrepancy between the effect on GSIS despite a lack of effect on cytosolic Ca^{2+} might favor the idea of microdomains of high Ca^{2+} undetectable by the methods employed

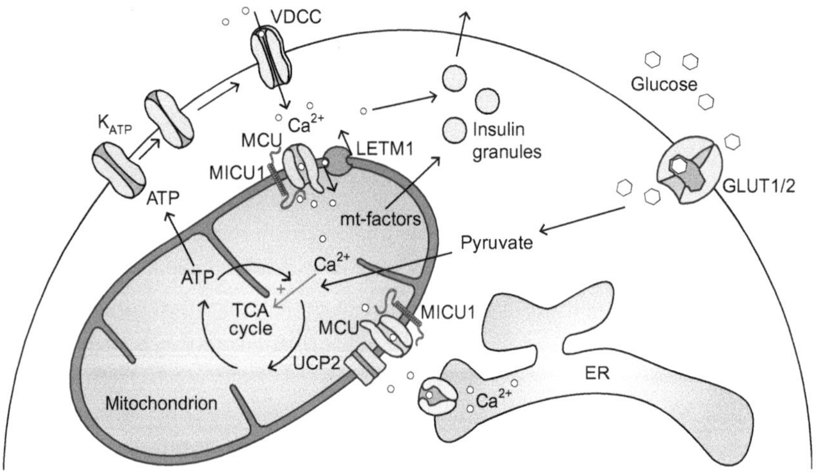

Figure 3.2 *Pathways of mitochondrial Ca^{2+} uptake in the pancreatic β-cell.* Glucose taken up by the β-cell via glucose transporter 1 or 2 (GLUT1/2) enters glycolysis to yield pyruvate. Pyruvate is transported into the mitochondrion where it fuels the TCA cycle and thereby oxidative metabolism to generate ATP and other mitochondrial coupling factors (mt-factors). ATP in turn causes K_{ATP} channels (K_{ATP}) to close triggering Ca^{2+} influx via voltage-dependent Ca^{2+} channels (VDCC). Ca^{2+} entering the cytosol does not only mediate insulin granule exocytosis, but is also transferred to the mitochondrial matrix. Proteins involved in this critical step are MICU1, MCU, and to some extent also LETM1, whereas Ca^{2+} released from the endoplasmic reticulum (ER) is taken up in a MICU1-, MCU-, and UCP2-dependent manner. Matrix-free Ca^{2+} activates mitochondrial dehydrogenases and thus acts as a feed-forward mechanism boosting the production of ATP and other factors required for a sustained amplifying phase of insulin secretion. (See the color plate.)

in this study. Expression of a Ca^{2+}-buffering protein targeted to the mitochondrial matrix also remained without effect on $[Ca^{2+}]_{cyto}$ (Wiederkehr et al., 2011). Again this could be explained by the existence of localized Ca^{2+} hot spots or by the fact that matrix Ca^{2+} modulates GSIS through additional mechanisms, which are not directly linked to $[Ca^{2+}]_{cyto}$. These mechanisms might also include the production of mitochondrial coupling factors other than ATP (Fig. 3.2) that are responsible for a sustained amplifying phase of GSIS. A recent report also supports the latter hypothesis by ruling out that subplasmalemmal Ca^{2+} contributes to the amplifying phase of insulin secretion (Ravier, Cheng-Xue, Palmer, Henquin, & Gilon, 2010). Tarasov and colleagues, however, confirmed the regulatory role of MCU in the glucose-induced generation of ATP (Tarasov, Semplici, Li, et al., 2012; Tarasov, Semplici, Ravier, et al., 2012).

5.3. Mitochondrial Ca^{2+} release in β-cells

Extrusion of Ca^{2+} from the mitochondrial matrix is accomplished by the mitochondrial $3Na^+/Ca^{2+}$ (Li^+) exchanger (NCLX), driven by the inwardly directed electrochemical gradient for Na^+ (Palty et al., 2010) and can be inhibited using the benzothiazepine CGP-37157 (Malli et al., 2003). The idea of blocking the NCLX in order to amplify mitochondrial Ca^{2+} signals and thereby also metabolic rates led to a series of experiments testing the effect of CGP-37157 on pancreatic β-cell function. An initial study performed in INS-1 cells and rats found that treatment with the compound had a positive effect on both ATP production and GSIS in a dose- and glucose-dependent manner (Lee et al., 2003). Similar to a study in human fibroblasts with mitochondrial complex I deficiency, where treatment with CGP-37157 could partly compensate for the lack in ATP synthesis (Visch et al., 2004), a more recent study showed that treatment with CGP-37157 could be beneficial in restoring GSIS in an *in vitro* model of mitochondrial diabetes (MODY4) (Gauthier et al., 2009). Conflicting research by Luciani et al. described a negative effect of CGP-37157 on GSIS despite the apparent activation of mitochondrial metabolism. This was proposed to be due to unspecific effects on VDCCs (Luciani, Ao, Hu, Warnock, & Johnson, 2007). According to a recent report, the changes in insulin secretion and overall ATP levels caused by silencing of NCLX are due to alterations in $[Ca^{2+}]_{cyto}$ provoked by defective mitochondrial Ca^{2+} shuttling (Nita et al., 2012). This idea still awaits confirmation by simultaneous measurement of cytosolic and mitochondrial Ca^{2+}.

The impact of proteins regulating mitochondrial Na^{+}/Ca^{2+} exchange, such as SLP-2 (Da Cruz et al., 2010), on β-cell function is still unknown. Modulating NCLX activity might, in any case, represent efficient therapeutic means of preserving metabolic function under conditions of mitochondrial deficiency not only in β-cells (Forbes et al., 2013).

5.4. Mitochondrial Ca^{2+} as potential therapeutic target for diabetes

In view of the observation that MCU is a highly conserved and ubiquitously expressed gene (Bick, Calvo, & Mootha, 2012), the MCU itself is far from being an ideal drug target. Yet, based on the assumption that mitochondrial Ca^{2+} handling is differentially regulated depending on cellular energy status, the source of Ca^{2+} (Alam et al., 2012) as well as the tissue-specific expression pattern of regulatory subunits (Plovanich et al., 2013), it might be possible to selectively manipulate mitochondrial Ca^{2+} channels and exchangers in β-cells and thereby potentiate GSIS. In order to make these proteins accessible to specific pharmacological interventions, it will be necessary to precisely characterize their molecular interactions and their contribution to metabolism–secretion coupling.

ACKNOWLEDGMENTS

The authors' work was supported by the Austrian Science Funds (FWF, P21857-B18 and P22553-B18). M. R. A. is funded by the FWF (P21857-B18) within the PhD program "Molecular Medicine" at the Medical University of Graz.

REFERENCES

Ainscow, E. K., & Rutter, G. A. (2001). Mitochondrial priming modifies Ca^{2+} oscillations and insulin secretion in pancreatic islets. *Biochemistry Journal*, *353*, 175–180.

Akhmedov, D., Braun, M., Mataki, C., Park, K. S., Pozzan, T., Schoonjans, K., et al. (2010). Mitochondrial matrix pH controls oxidative phosphorylation and metabolism-secretion coupling in INS-1E clonal beta cells. *FASEB Journal*, *24*, 4613–4626.

Alam, M. R., Groschner, L. N., Parichatikanond, W., Kuo, L., Bondarenko, A. I., Rost, R., et al. (2012). Mitochondrial Ca^{2+} uptake 1 (MICU1) and mitochondrial Ca^{2+} uniporter (MCU) contribute to metabolism-secretion coupling in clonal pancreatic beta-cells. *Journal of Biological Chemistry*, *287*, 34445–34454.

Ashcroft, S. J., Hedeskov, C. J., & Randle, P. J. (1970). Glucose metabolism in mouse pancreatic islets. *Biochemistry Journal*, *118*, 143–154.

Ashcroft, F. M., & Rorsman, P. (2012). Diabetes mellitus and the beta cell: The last ten years. *Cell*, *148*, 1160–1171.

Baughman, J. M., Perocchi, F., Girgis, H. S., Plovanich, M., Belcher-Timme, C. A., Sancak, Y., et al. (2011). Integrative genomics identifies MCU as an essential component of the mitochondrial calcium uniporter. *Nature*, *476*, 341–345.

Benard, G., Bellance, N., James, D., Parrone, P., Fernandez, H., Letellier, T., et al. (2007). Mitochondrial bioenergetics and structural network organization. *Journal of Cell Science, 120*, 838–848.
Bernardi, P., & Rasola, A. (2007). Calcium and cell death: The mitochondrial connection. *Subcellular Biochemistry, 45*, 481–506.
Berridge, M. J., Lipp, P., & Bootman, M. D. (2000). The versatility and universality of calcium signalling. *Nature Reviews Molecular Cell Biology, 1*, 11–21.
Bertrand, G., Ishiyama, N., Nenquin, M., Ravier, M. A., & Henquin, J. C. (2002). The elevation of glutamate content and the amplification of insulin secretion in glucose-stimulated pancreatic islets are not causally related. *Journal of Biological Chemistry, 277*, 32883–32891.
Beutner, G., Sharma, V. K., Giovannucci, D. R., Yule, D. I., & Sheu, S. S. (2001). Identification of a ryanodine receptor in rat heart mitochondria. *Journal of Biological Chemistry, 276*, 21482–21488.
Bick, A. G., Calvo, S. E., & Mootha, V. K. (2012). Evolutionary diversity of the mitochondrial calcium uniporter. *Science, 336*, 886.
Boerries, M., Most, P., Gledhill, J. R., Walker, J. E., Katus, H. A., Koch, W. J., et al. (2007). Ca2+-dependent interaction of S100A1 with F1-ATPase leads to an increased ATP content in cardiomyocytes. *Molecular and Cellular Biology, 27*, 4365–4373.
Bondarenko, A. I., Jean-Quartier, C., Malli, R., & Graier, W. F. (2013). Characterization of distinct single-channel properties of Ca^{2+} inward currents in mitochondria. *Pflügers Archiv, 465*, 997–1010.
Boucher, B. J., Mannan, N., Noonan, K., Hales, C. N., & Evans, S. J. (1995). Glucose intolerance and impairment of insulin secretion in relation to vitamin D deficiency in east London Asians. *Diabetologia, 38*, 1239–1245.
Bricker, D. K., Taylor, E. B., Schell, J. C., Orsak, T., Boutron, A., Chen, Y. C., et al. (2012). A mitochondrial pyruvate carrier required for pyruvate uptake in yeast, Drosophila, and humans. *Science, 337*, 96–100.
Carobbio, S., Frigerio, F., Rubi, B., Vetterli, L., Bloksgaard, M., Gjinovci, A., et al. (2009). Deletion of glutamate dehydrogenase in beta-cells abolishes part of the insulin secretory response not required for glucose homeostasis. *Journal of Biological Chemistry, 284*, 921–929.
Casimir, M., Lasorsa, F. M., Rubi, B., Caille, D., Palmieri, F., Meda, P., et al. (2009). Mitochondrial glutamate carrier GC1 as a newly identified player in the control of glucose-stimulated insulin secretion. *Journal of Biological Chemistry, 284*, 25004–25014.
Cook, D. L., & Hales, C. N. (1984). Intracellular ATP directly blocks K^+ channels in pancreatic B-cells. *Nature, 311*, 271–273.
Coughlan, M. T., Yap, F. Y., Tong, D. C., Andrikopoulos, S., Gasser, A., Thallas-Bonke, V., et al. (2011). Advanced glycation end products are direct modulators of beta-cell function. *Diabetes, 60*, 2523–2532.
Da Cruz, S., De Marchi, U., Frieden, M., Parone, P. A., Martinou, J. C., & Demaurex, N. (2010). SLP-2 negatively modulates mitochondrial sodium-calcium exchange. *Cell Calcium, 47*, 11–18.
Deluca, H. F., & Engstrom, G. W. (1961). Calcium uptake by rat kidney mitochondria. *Proceedings of the National Academy of Sciences of the United States of America, 47*, 1744–1750.
Denton, R. M., & McCormack, J. G. (1986). The calcium sensitive dehydrogenases of vertebrate mitochondria. *Cell Calcium, 7*, 377–386.
Denton, R. M., Randle, P. J., & Martin, B. R. (1972). Stimulation by calcium ions of pyruvate dehydrogenase phosphate phosphatase. *Biochemistry Journal, 128*, 161–163.
Denton, R. M., Richards, D. A., & Chin, J. G. (1978). Calcium ions and the regulation of NAD^+-linked isocitrate dehydrogenase from the mitochondria of rat heart and other tissues. *Biochemistry Journal, 176*, 899–906.

De Stefani, D., Raffaello, A., Teardo, E., Szabo, I., & Rizzuto, R. (2011). A forty-kilodalton protein of the inner membrane is the mitochondrial calcium uniporter. *Nature, 476*, 336–340.

Duchen, M. R., Smith, P. A., & Ashcroft, F. M. (1993). Substrate-dependent changes in mitochondrial function, intracellular free calcium concentration and membrane channels in pancreatic beta-cells. *Biochemistry Journal, 294*(Pt 1), 35–42.

Eliasson, L., Abdulkader, F., Braun, M., Galvanovskis, J., Hoppa, M. B., & Rorsman, P. (2008). Novel aspects of the molecular mechanisms controlling insulin secretion. *The Journal of Physiology, 586*, 3313–3324.

Eto, K., Tsubamoto, Y., Terauchi, Y., Sugiyama, T., Kishimoto, T., Takahashi, N., et al. (1999). Role of NADH shuttle system in glucose-induced activation of mitochondrial metabolism and insulin secretion. *Science, 283*, 981–985.

Forbes, J. M., Ke, B. X., Nguyen, T. V., Henstridge, D. C., Penfold, S. A., Laskowski, A., et al. (2013). Deficiency in mitochondrial complex I activity due to Ndufs6 gene trap insertion induces renal disease. *Antioxidants and Redox Signaling, 19*, 331–343.

Gauthier, B. R., Wiederkehr, A., Baquie, M., Dai, C., Powers, A. C., Kerr-Conte, J., et al. (2009). PDX1 deficiency causes mitochondrial dysfunction and defective insulin secretion through TFAM suppression. *Cell Metabolism, 10*, 110–118.

Gauthier, B. R., & Wollheim, C. B. (2008). Synaptotagmins bind calcium to release insulin. *American Journal of Physiology, Endocrinology and Metabolism, 295*, E1279–E1286.

Goehring, I., Gerencser, A. A., Schmidt, S., Brand, M. D., Mulder, H., & Nicholls, D. G. (2012). Plasma membrane potential oscillations in insulin secreting Ins-1 832/13 cells do not require glycolysis and are not initiated by fluctuations in mitochondrial bioenergetics. *Journal of Biological Chemistry, 287*, 15706–15717.

Groschner, L. N., Waldeck-Weiermair, M., Malli, R., & Graier, W. F. (2012). Endothelial mitochondria—Less respiration, more integration. *Pflügers Archiv, 464*, 63–76.

Hajnoczky, G., Robb-Gaspers, L. D., Seitz, M. B., & Thomas, A. P. (1995). Decoding of cytosolic calcium oscillations in the mitochondria. *Cell, 82*, 415–424.

Henquin, J. C. (2000). Triggering and amplifying pathways of regulation of insulin secretion by glucose. *Diabetes, 49*, 1751–1760.

Herzig, S., Raemy, E., Montessuit, S., Veuthey, J. L., Zamboni, N., Westermann, B., et al. (2012). Identification and functional expression of the mitochondrial pyruvate carrier. *Science, 337*, 93–96.

Hohmeier, H. E., Mulder, H., Chen, G., Henkel-Rieger, R., Prentki, M., & Newgard, C. B. (2000). Isolation of INS-1-derived cell lines with robust ATP-sensitive K^+ channel-dependent and -independent glucose-stimulated insulin secretion. *Diabetes, 49*, 424–430.

Hoppa, M. B., Collins, S., Ramracheya, R., Hodson, L., Amisten, S., Zhang, Q., et al. (2009). Chronic palmitate exposure inhibits insulin secretion by dissociation of Ca^{2+} channels from secretory granules. *Cell Metabolism, 10*, 455–465.

Hoy, M., Maechler, P., Efanov, A. M., Wollheim, C. B., Berggren, P. O., & Gromada, J. (2002). Increase in cellular glutamate levels stimulates exocytosis in pancreatic beta-cells. *FEBS Letters, 531*, 199–203.

Jean-Quartier, C., Bondarenko, A. I., Alam, M. R., Trenker, M., Waldeck-Weiermair, M., Malli, R., et al. (2012). Studying mitochondrial Ca^{2+} uptake—A revisit. *Molecular and Cellular Endocrinology, 353*, 114–127.

Jiang, D., Zhao, L., & Clapham, D. E. (2009). Genome-wide RNAi screen identifies Letm1 as a mitochondrial Ca^{2+}/H^+ antiporter. *Science, 326*, 144–147.

Jitrapakdee, S., Wutthisathapornchai, A., Wallace, J. C., & MacDonald, M. J. (2010). Regulation of insulin secretion: Role of mitochondrial signalling. *Diabetologia, 53*, 1019–1032.

Jouaville, L. S., Pinton, P., Bastianutto, C., Rutter, G. A., & Rizzuto, R. (1999). Regulation of mitochondrial ATP synthesis by calcium: Evidence for a long-term metabolic

priming. *Proceedings of the National Academy of Sciences of the United States of America, 96*, 13807–13812.
Kadowaki, T., Kadowaki, H., Mori, Y., Tobe, K., Sakuta, R., Suzuki, Y., et al. (1994). A subtype of diabetes mellitus associated with a mutation of mitochondrial DNA. *The New England Journal of Medicine, 330*, 962–968.
Kennedy, E. D., Maechler, P., & Wollheim, C. B. (1998). Effects of depletion of mitochondrial DNA in metabolism secretion coupling in INS-1 cells. *Diabetes, 47*, 374–380.
Kennedy, H. J., Pouli, A. E., Ainscow, E. K., Jouaville, L. S., Rizzuto, R., & Rutter, G. A. (1999). Glucose generates sub-plasma membrane ATP microdomains in single islet beta-cells. Potential role for strategically located mitochondria. *Journal of Biological Chemistry, 274*, 13281–13291.
Kibbey, R. G., Pongratz, R. L., Romanelli, A. J., Wollheim, C. B., Cline, G. W., & Shulman, G. I. (2007). Mitochondrial GTP regulates glucose-stimulated insulin secretion. *Cell Metabolism, 5*, 253–264.
Kindmark, H., Kohler, M., Brown, G., Branstrom, R., Larsson, O., & Berggren, P. O. (2001). Glucose-induced oscillations in cytoplasmic free Ca^{2+} concentration precede oscillations in mitochondrial membrane potential in the pancreatic beta-cell. *Journal of Biological Chemistry, 276*, 34530–34536.
Kiranadi, B., Bangham, J. A., & Smith, P. A. (1991). Inhibition of electrical activity in mouse pancreatic beta-cells by the ATP/ADP translocase inhibitor, bongkrekic acid. *FEBS Letters, 283*, 93–96.
Koziel, A., Woyda-Ploszczyca, A., Kicinska, A., & Jarmuszkiewicz, W. (2012). The influence of high glucose on the aerobic metabolism of endothelial EA.hy926 cells. *Pflügers Archiv, 464*, 657–669.
Lee, B., Miles, P. D., Vargas, L., Luan, P., Glasco, S., Kushnareva, Y., et al. (2003). Inhibition of mitochondrial Na^{+}-Ca^{2+} exchanger increases mitochondrial metabolism and potentiates glucose-stimulated insulin secretion in rat pancreatic islets. *Diabetes, 52*, 965–973.
Lu, D., Mulder, H., Zhao, P., Burgess, S. C., Jensen, M. V., Kamzolova, S., et al. (2002). 13C NMR isotopomer analysis reveals a connection between pyruvate cycling and glucose-stimulated insulin secretion (GSIS). *Proceedings of the National Academy of Sciences of the United States of America, 99*, 2708–2713.
Luciani, D. S., Ao, P., Hu, X., Warnock, G. L., & Johnson, J. D. (2007). Voltage-gated Ca^{2+} influx and insulin secretion in human and mouse beta-cells are impaired by the mitochondrial Na^{+}/Ca^{2+} exchange inhibitor CGP-37157. *European Journal of Pharmacology, 576*, 18–25.
Maechler, P., & Wollheim, C. B. (1999). Mitochondrial glutamate acts as a messenger in glucose-induced insulin exocytosis. *Nature, 402*, 685–689.
Maechler, P., & Wollheim, C. B. (2001). Mitochondrial function in normal and diabetic beta-cells. *Nature, 414*, 807–812.
Magnus, G., & Keizer, J. (1998a). Model of beta-cell mitochondrial calcium handling and electrical activity. I. Cytoplasmic variables. *The American Journal of Physiology, 274*, C1158–C1173.
Magnus, G., & Keizer, J. (1998b). Model of beta-cell mitochondrial calcium handling and electrical activity. II. Mitochondrial variables. *The American Journal of Physiology, 274*, C1174–C1184.
Malli, R., Frieden, M., Osibow, K., Zoratti, C., Mayer, M., Demaurex, N., et al. (2003). Sustained Ca^{2+} transfer across mitochondria is essential for mitochondrial Ca^{2+} buffering, sore-operated Ca^{2+} entry, and Ca^{2+} store refilling. *Journal of Biological Chemistry, 278*, 44769–44779.
Mallilankaraman, K., Cardenas, C., Doonan, P. J., Chandramoorthy, H. C., Irrinki, K. M., Golenar, T., et al. (2012). MCUR1 is an essential component of mitochondrial Ca^{2+} uptake that regulates cellular metabolism. *Nature Cell Biology, 14*, 1336–1343.

Mallilankaraman, K., Doonan, P., Cardenas, C., Chandramoorthy, H. C., Muller, M., Miller, R., et al. (2012). MICU1 is an essential gatekeeper for MCU-mediated mitochondrial Ca^{2+} uptake that regulates cell survival. *Cell, 151*, 630–644.

Malmgren, S., Nicholls, D. G., Taneera, J., Bacos, K., Koeck, T., Tamaddon, A., et al. (2009). Tight coupling between glucose and mitochondrial metabolism in clonal beta-cells is required for robust insulin secretion. *Journal of Biological Chemistry, 284*, 32395–32404.

McCormack, J. G., & Denton, R. M. (1979). The effects of calcium ions and adenine nucleotides on the activity of pig heart 2-oxoglutarate dehydrogenase complex. *Biochemistry Journal, 180*, 533–544.

McCormack, J. G., Halestrap, A. P., & Denton, R. M. (1990). Role of calcium ions in regulation of mammalian intramitochondrial metabolism. *Physiological Reviews, 70*, 391–425.

Mertz, R. J., Worley, J. F., Spencer, B., Johnson, J. H., & Dukes, I. D. (1996). Activation of stimulus-secretion coupling in pancreatic beta-cells by specific products of glucose metabolism. Evidence for privileged signaling by glycolysis. *Journal of Biological Chemistry, 271*, 4838–4845.

Nakazaki, M., Kakei, M., Ishihara, H., Koriyama, N., Hashiguchi, H., Aso, K., et al. (2002). Association of upregulated activity of K_{ATP} channels with impaired insulin secretion in UCP1-expressing insulinoma cells. *The Journal of Physiology, 540*, 781–789.

Nelson, D. L., & Cox, M. M. (2008). *Lehninger principles of biochemistry* (5th ed.). New York: W. H. Freeman and Company.

Nishi, Y., Fujimoto, S., Sasaki, M., Mukai, E., Sato, H., Sato, Y., et al. (2011). Role of mitochondrial phosphate carrier in metabolism-secretion coupling in rat insulinoma cell line INS-1. *Biochemistry Journal, 435*, 421–430.

Nita, I. I., Hershfinkel, M., Fishman, D., Ozeri, E., Rutter, G. A., Sensi, S. L., et al. (2012). The mitochondrial Na^{+}/Ca^{2+} exchanger upregulates glucose dependent Ca^{2+} signalling linked to insulin secretion. *PLoS One, 7*, e46649.

Ostenson, C. G., Abdel-Halim, S. M., Rasschaert, J., Malaisse-Lagae, F., Meuris, S., Sener, A., et al. (1993). Deficient activity of FAD-linked glycerophosphate dehydrogenase in islets of GK rats. *Diabetologia, 36*, 722–726.

Otonkoski, T., Jiao, H., Kaminen-Ahola, N., Tapia-Paez, I., Ullah, M. S., Parton, L. E., et al. (2007). Physical exercise-induced hypoglycemia caused by failed silencing of monocarboxylate transporter 1 in pancreatic beta cells. *American Journal of Human Genetics, 81*, 467–474.

Palty, R., Silverman, W. F., Hershfinkel, M., Caporale, T., Sensi, S. L., Parnis, J., et al. (2010). NCLX is an essential component of mitochondrial Na^{+}/Ca^{2+} exchange. *Proceedings of the National Academy of Sciences of the United States of America, 107*, 436–441.

Park, K. S., Wiederkehr, A., Kirkpatrick, C., Mattenberger, Y., Martinou, J. C., Marchetti, P., et al. (2008). Selective actions of mitochondrial fission/fusion genes on metabolism-secretion coupling in insulin-releasing cells. *Journal of Biological Chemistry, 283*, 33347–33356.

Perocchi, F., Gohil, V. M., Girgis, H. S., Bao, X. R., McCombs, J. E., Palmer, A. E., et al. (2010). MICU1 encodes a mitochondrial EF hand protein required for Ca^{2+} uptake. *Nature, 467*, 291–296.

Peyot, M. L., Gray, J. P., Lamontagne, J., Smith, P. J., Holz, G. G., Madiraju, S. R., et al. (2009). Glucagon-like peptide-1 induced signaling and insulin secretion do not drive fuel and energy metabolism in primary rodent pancreatic beta-cells. *PLoS One, 4*, e6221.

Plovanich, M., Bogorad, R. L., Sancak, Y., Kamer, K. J., Strittmatter, L., Li, A. A., et al. (2013). MICU2, a paralog of MICU1, resides within the mitochondrial uniporter complex to regulate calcium handling. *PLoS One, 8*, e55785.

Pongratz, R. L., Kibbey, R. G., Kirkpatrick, C. L., Zhao, X., Pontoglio, M., Yaniv, M., et al. (2009). Mitochondrial dysfunction contributes to impaired insulin secretion in INS-1

cells with dominant-negative mutations of HNF-1alpha and in HNF-1alpha-deficient islets. *Journal of Biological Chemistry*, *284*, 16808–16821.
Pullen, T. J., Sylow, L., Sun, G., Halestrap, A. P., Richter, E. A., & Rutter, G. A. (2012). Overexpression of monocarboxylate transporter-1 (SLC16A1) in mouse pancreatic beta-cells leads to relative hyperinsulinism during exercise. *Diabetes*, *61*, 1719–1725.
Ravier, M. A., Cheng-Xue, R., Palmer, A. E., Henquin, J. C., & Gilon, P. (2010). Sub-plasmalemmal Ca^{2+} measurements in mouse pancreatic beta cells support the existence of an amplifying effect of glucose on insulin secretion. *Diabetologia*, *53*, 1947–1957.
Rojas, E., Carroll, P. B., Ricordi, C., Boschero, A. C., Stojilkovic, S. S., & Atwater, I. (1994). Control of cytosolic free calcium in cultured human pancreatic beta-cells occurs by external calcium-dependent and independent mechanisms. *Endocrinology*, *134*, 1771–1781.
Rorsman, P., & Braun, M. (2013). Regulation of insulin secretion in human pancreatic islets. *Annual Review of Physiology*, *75*, 155–179.
Rorsman, P., Braun, M., & Zhang, Q. (2012). Regulation of calcium in pancreatic alpha- and beta-cells in health and disease. *Cell Calcium*, *51*, 300–308.
Rustenbeck, I., Herrmann, C., & Grimmsmann, T. (1997). Energetic requirement of insulin secretion distal to calcium influx. *Diabetes*, *46*, 1305–1311.
Rutter, G. A., Tsuboi, T., & Ravier, M. A. (2006). Ca^{2+} microdomains and the control of insulin secretion. *Cell Calcium*, *40*, 539–551.
Saotome, M., Safiulina, D., Szabadkai, G., Das, S., Fransson, A., Aspenstrom, P., et al. (2008). Bidirectional Ca^{2+}-dependent control of mitochondrial dynamics by the Miro GTPase. *Proceedings of the National Academy of Sciences of the United States of America*, *105*, 20728–20733.
Schuit, F., Van Lommel, L., Granvik, M., Goyvaerts, L., de Faudeur, G., Schraenen, A., et al. (2012). Beta-cell-specific gene repression: A mechanism to protect against inappropriate or maladjusted insulin secretion? *Diabetes*, *61*, 969–975.
Sekine, N., Cirulli, V., Regazzi, R., Brown, L. J., Gine, E., Tamarit-Rodriguez, J., et al. (1994). Low lactate dehydrogenase and high mitochondrial glycerol phosphate dehydrogenase in pancreatic beta-cells. Potential role in nutrient sensing. *Journal of Biological Chemistry*, *269*, 4895–4902.
Shaw, J. E., Sicree, R. A., & Zimmet, P. Z. (2010). Global estimates of the prevalence of diabetes for 2010 and 2030. *Diabetes Research and Clinical Practice*, *87*, 4–14.
Silva, J. P., Kohler, M., Graff, C., Oldfors, A., Magnuson, M. A., Berggren, P. O., et al. (2000). Impaired insulin secretion and beta-cell loss in tissue-specific knockout mice with mitochondrial diabetes. *Nature Genetics*, *26*, 336–340.
Skelin, M., Rupnik, M., & Cencic, A. (2010). Pancreatic beta cell lines and their applications in diabetes mellitus research. *ALTEX*, *27*, 105–113.
Soejima, A., Inoue, K., Takai, D., Kaneko, M., Ishihara, H., Oka, Y., et al. (1996). Mitochondrial DNA is required for regulation of glucose-stimulated insulin secretion in a mouse pancreatic beta cell line, MIN6. *Journal of Biological Chemistry*, *271*, 26194–26199.
Stark, R., Pasquel, F., Turcu, A., Pongratz, R. L., Roden, M., Cline, G. W., et al. (2009). Phosphoenolpyruvate cycling via mitochondrial phosphoenolpyruvate carboxykinase links anaplerosis and mitochondrial GTP with insulin secretion. *Journal of Biological Chemistry*, *284*, 26578–26590.
Tarasov, A., Dusonchet, J., & Ashcroft, F. (2004). Metabolic regulation of the pancreatic beta-cell ATP-sensitive K^{+} channel: A pas de deux. *Diabetes*, *53*(Suppl. 3), S113–S122.
Tarasov, A. I., Griffiths, E. J., & Rutter, G. A. (2012). Regulation of ATP production by mitochondrial Ca^{2+}. *Cell Calcium*, *52*, 28–35.
Tarasov, A. I., Semplici, F., Li, D., Rizzuto, R., Ravier, M. A., Gilon, P., et al. (2012). Frequency-dependent mitochondrial Ca2+ accumulation regulates ATP synthesis in pancreatic beta cells. *Pflügers Archiv*, *465*, 543–554.

Tarasov, A. I., Semplici, F., Ravier, M. A., Bellomo, E. A., Pullen, T. J., Gilon, P., et al. (2012). The mitochondrial Ca^{2+} uniporter MCU is essential for glucose-induced ATP increases in pancreatic beta-cells. *PLoS One*, 7, e39722.

Trenker, M., Malli, R., Fertschai, I., Levak-Frank, S., & Graier, W. F. (2007). Uncoupling proteins 2 and 3 are fundamental for mitochondrial Ca^{2+} uniport. *Nature Cell Biology*, *9*, 445–452.

Tsuruzoe, K., Araki, E., Furukawa, N., Shirotani, T., Matsumoto, K., Kaneko, K., et al. (1998). Creation and characterization of a mitochondrial DNA-depleted pancreatic beta-cell line: Impaired insulin secretion induced by glucose, leucine, and sulfonylureas. *Diabetes*, *47*, 621–631.

Twig, G., Elorza, A., Molina, A. J., Mohamed, H., Wikstrom, J. D., Walzer, G., et al. (2008). Fission and selective fusion govern mitochondrial segregation and elimination by autophagy. *EMBO Journal*, *27*, 433–446.

Vikman, J., Ma, X., Hockerman, G. H., Rorsman, P., & Eliasson, L. (2006). Antibody inhibition of synaptosomal protein of 25 kDa (SNAP-25) and syntaxin 1 reduces rapid exocytosis in insulin-secreting cells. *Journal of Molecular Endocrinology*, *36*, 503–515.

Visch, H. J., Rutter, G. A., Koopman, W. J., Koenderink, J. B., Verkaart, S., de Groot, T., et al. (2004). Inhibition of mitochondrial Na^{+}-Ca^{2+} exchange restores agonist-induced ATP production and Ca^{2+} handling in human complex I deficiency. *Journal of Biological Chemistry*, *279*, 40328–40336.

Waldeck-Weiermair, M., Alam, M. R., Khan, M. J., Deak, A. T., Vishnu, N., Karsten, F., et al. (2012). Spatiotemporal correlations between cytosolic and mitochondrial Ca^{2+} signals using a novel red-shifted mitochondrial targeted cameleon. *PLoS One*, 7, e45917.

Waldeck-Weiermair, M., Duan, X., Naghdi, S., Khan, M. J., Trenker, M., Malli, R., et al. (2010). Uncoupling protein 3 adjusts mitochondrial Ca^{2+} uptake to high and low Ca^{2+} signals. *Cell Calcium*, *48*, 288–301.

Waldeck-Weiermair, M., Jean-Quartier, C., Rost, R., Khan, M. J., Vishnu, N., Bondarenko, A. I., et al. (2011). Leucine zipper EF hand-containing transmembrane protein 1 (Letm1) and uncoupling proteins 2 and 3 (UCP2/3) contribute to two distinct mitochondrial Ca^{2+} uptake pathways. *Journal of Biological Chemistry*, *286*, 28444–28455.

Waldeck-Weiermair, M., Malli, R., Naghdi, S., Trenker, M., Kahn, M. J., & Graier, W. F. (2010). The contribution of UCP2 and UCP3 to mitochondrial Ca^{2+} uptake is differentially determined by the source of supplied Ca^{2+}. *Cell Calcium*, *47*, 433–440.

Wernette, M. E., Ochs, R. S., & Lardy, H. A. (1981). Ca^{2+} stimulation of rat liver mitochondrial glycerophosphate dehydrogenase. *Journal of Biological Chemistry*, *256*, 12767–12771.

Wiederkehr, A., Szanda, G., Akhmedov, D., Mataki, C., Heizmann, C. W., Schoonjans, K., et al. (2011). Mitochondrial matrix calcium is an activating signal for hormone secretion. *Cell Metabolism*, *13*, 601–611.

Wiederkehr, A., & Wollheim, C. B. (2008). Impact of mitochondrial calcium on the coupling of metabolism to insulin secretion in the pancreatic beta-cell. *Cell Calcium*, *44*, 64–76.

Wiederkehr, A., & Wollheim, C. B. (2012). Mitochondrial signals drive insulin secretion in the pancreatic beta-cell. *Molecular and Cellular Endocrinology*, *353*, 128–137.

Wollheim, C. B. (2000). Beta-cell mitochondria in the regulation of insulin secretion: A new culprit in type II diabetes. *Diabetologia*, *43*, 265–277.

Zimmet, P. (2003). The burden of type 2 diabetes: Are we doing enough? *Diabetes & Metabolism*, *29*, 6S9–6S18.

CHAPTER FOUR

Metabolic Syndrome and Ionic Channels in Pancreatic Beta Cells

Marcia Hiriart[1], Myrian Velasco, Carlos Larqué, Carlos Manlio Diaz-Garcia

Department of Neural Development and Physiology, Neuroscience Division, Instituto de Fisiología Celular, Universidad Nacional Autónoma de México, Mexico, Mexico

[1]Corresponding author: e-mail address: mhiriart@ifc.unam.mx

Contents

Abstract

Worldwide increase in the prevalence of metabolic syndrome and diabetes mellitus type 2 (DM2) during the past decades has converted them into a global epidemic disease. It is not well understood how these metabolic disorders initiate, but an increase in food consumption associated to low physical activity leads to increase in body weight and obesity. This in turn, elevates circulating lipids and cytokines release by adipose tissue, give the organism a chronic inflammation and potentiate insulin secretion, causing insulin resistance. Depending on genetics and probably other environmental factors, after a long period of hyperactivity, pancreatic beta cells become exhausted and DM2 overcomes.

Pancreatic beta cells are the only source of insulin known in mammals. They are unique because of their ability to sense and transform fuels into a chemical signal, which

Vitamins and Hormones, Volume 95
ISSN 0083-6729
http://dx.doi.org/10.1016/B978-0-12-800174-5.00004-1

affects mainly all the cells in the organism. Many other factors affect insulin secretion. We will focus on the alterations of glucose-induced insulin secretion coupling, particularly in ionic channels that have crucial importance in this process.

Different channel types can be affected by metabolic syndrome. The most studied are K_{ATP} and other potassium channels, calcium, sodium, and TRP channels. Much information comes from rodents that do not express exactly the same proportion and type of channels than humans. However, getting insight of how do they participate in insulin secretion and how to modulate them is important to completely understand beta-cell physiology and pathophysiological reactions to metabolic syndrome and diabetes, in order to stop the epidemic of these metabolic disorders.

ABBREVIATIONS

DM2 type 2 diabetes mellitus
FFAs free fatty acids
GLP-1 glucagon-like peptide 1
GLUT2 glucose transporter type-2
GLUT4 glucose transporter type-4
GSIS glucose-stimulated insulin secretion
HDL high-density lipoproteins
IL-6 interleukin-6
IR insulin receptor
IRS insulin receptor substrate
K_{ATP} channels ATP-sensitive potassium channels
KCa channel Ca^{2+}-sensitive voltage-dependent potassium channel
Kir channel inward rectifier potassium channel
Kv channel voltage-dependent potassium channel
MS metabolic syndrome
NDM neonatal diabetes mellitus
ROS reactive oxygen species
STZ streptozotocin
SUR sulfonylurea receptor
TNF-alpha tumor necrosis factor alpha
TRP channels transient receptor potential family
VDCCs voltage-dependent calcium channels
VLDLs low-density lipoproteins

1. INTRODUCTION

Glucose homeostasis is critical to maintain life in mammals. The mechanisms that participate in this process are finely tuned and not entirely understood to date. After feeding, glucose is absorbed and its plasma levels rise. This is a potent stimulus for pancreatic beta cells to secrete insulin.

This hormone increases glucose disposal by peripheral tissues, glycogen synthesis, and lipogenesis in the liver, and promotes the uptake of glucose and conversion to glycogen or triglycerides by muscle and adipocytes, respectively. All these processes lead to the reduction in glucose levels and stop the stimulus for secreting insulin. In contrast, during fasting state glucose remains between 4 and 5 mM, and insulin levels are low. In this condition, the liver is the main source of plasma glucose, because this organ controls glycogen breakdown and gluconeogenesis, which are mainly regulated by the counter-regulatory hormones of insulin.

Glucose homeostasis is disrupted in the metabolic syndrome (MS) and beta cells get exhausted under constant pressure, leading to type 2 diabetes mellitus (DM2). This process is not fully understood. In this chapter, we will analyze what is known on insulin secretion and ionic channels behavior in the MS.

2. A RAPID FLY ON METABOLIC SYNDROME

The term "metabolic syndrome" (MS) has been used for a long time to describe a group of alterations that increases the risk to develop DM2 and cardiovascular diseases (Eckel, Grundy, & Zimmet, 2005; Gallagher, Leroith, & Karnieli, 2010). The cardinal signs of MS include central obesity, hypertension, dyslipidemia, hyperinsulinemia, insulin resistance, impaired fasting glucose, and impaired glucose tolerance. A worldwide increase in its prevalence during the last three decades has converted MS into a global epidemic disease (Fig. 4.1).

Genetic and environmental factors contribute to the development of MS. The last includes high-carbohydrate, high-fat diets, and the lack of physical activity, and energy expenditure. The influence of these factors results in visceral obesity, insulin resistance, impaired glucose and lipid metabolism, and a chronic mild inflammatory state (Larqué et al., 2011). Free fatty acids (FFAs) constitute a link between insulin secretion and insulin resistance. Generation of lipid metabolites, reactive oxygen species (ROS), and inflammatory cytokines could be important mechanisms to generate insulin resistance (Corkey, 2012).

2.1. Obesity and dyslipidemia

Central obesity is a major risk factor to develop MS, and it is established by hypertrophy and hyperplasia of visceral adipocytes. Therefore, abdominal

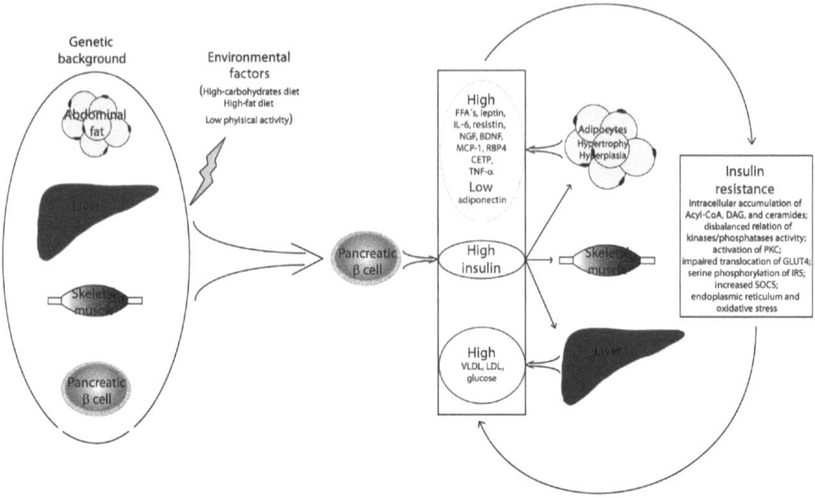

Figure 4.1 Pathophysiologic processes involved in metabolic syndrome (MS). Although the genetic background confers susceptibility, it is an unhealthy environment, which triggers obesity and MS. High-carbohydrate or high-fat diets produce increased insulin secretion by pancreatic B cells, hyperplasia and hypertrophy of adipocytes, altered secretion of adipokines and other inflammatory cytokines; and increased secretion of VLDL and LDL by the liver. Hyperinsulinemia and the mild inflammatory milieu impair insulin sensitivity in its target tissues by several mechanisms. Insulin resistance favors insulin hypersecretion, increased hepatic secretion of VLDL, LDL, and glucose, and adipokine secretion. (For color version of this figure, the reader is referred to the online version of this chapter.)

circumference, rather than body mass index (BMI), has become the most important parameter to identify central obesity (Alberti et al., 2009).

Adipose tissue is not only metabolically active and plays an important role in glucose and lipid metabolism but also secretes hormones known as adipokines, such as leptin, adiponectin, resistin, nerve growth factor (NGF), brain-derived neurotrophic factor (BDNF), interleukin-6 (IL-6), monocyte chemoattractant protein-1 (MCP-1), and retinol-binding protein-4 (RBP4) that could be related to the development of various pathologic processes including the MS (Hotamisligil, 2006). In addition, active adipose-infiltrated macrophages are the main source of inflammatory cytokines, such as tumor necrosis factor alpha (TNF-α) and IL-6 during obesity (Galic, Oakhill, & Steinberg, 2010).

Normally, fatty acids represent a very important energy source. They circulate free in the blood or as triglycerides within lipoproteins. FFAs are produced in adipocytes by the hydrolysis of triglycerides mediated by the hormone-sensitive lipase. This last process is inhibited by insulin.

Although lipolysis varies among the different visceral fat depots (Smith, Hammersten, Bjorntorp, & Kral, 1979), plasma FFA levels are increased in MS, reflecting an impaired insulin action in this tissue. Furthermore, increased plasma FFA impairs insulin signaling in its target tissues, causing FFA uptake to exceed its oxidation. This produces an intracellular accumulation of lipid derivates including acyl-coenzyme A (acyl-CoA), diacylglycerol (DAG), and ceramides, as well as a further disruption of insulin signaling. Finally, increased FFA supply enables the liver production and release of very low-density lipoproteins (VLDL). Additionally, during obesity, adipose tissue produces high amounts of cholesterol ester transferase protein (CETP) that facilitates the transfer of cholesteryl esters from high-density lipoproteins (HDLs) to VLDL, contributing to low HDL plasma levels (Gallagher et al., 2010).

2.2. Insulin resistance

The term "insulin resistance" can be explained as a defect in insulin ability to decrease plasma glucose levels, due to impaired signaling on sensitive tissues, resulting in fasting and postprandial hyperinsulinemia and increased glucose levels. Normal insulin signaling and its effects have been reviewed in several studies (Saltiel & Kahn, 2001; Taniguchi, Emanuelli, & Kahn, 2006). Insulin signaling pathway includes the insulin receptor (IR), which is a prototype of integral membrane proteins with tyrosine kinase activity, and is formed by two alpha-beta dimers. Insulin binding to alpha subunits in the extracellular domain of the receptor increases the beta subunit tyrosine kinase activity. When insulin binds to IR, it induces conformational changes that lead to the transphosphorylation of the beta subunits of IR and a cascade of phosphorylation of other IR-recruited proteins. Proteins recruited by the activated IR include insulin receptor substrate (IRS) proteins that mediate most of the insulin intracellular signaling and other scaffold proteins. These proteins contain an NH2-terminal pleckstrin homology domain and a phosphotyrosine-binding (PTB) domain that allows the coupling of IRS proteins to IR and other activated receptors such as growth hormone (GH) receptor, some IL receptors, and integrins. In addition, IRSs contain other tyrosine and serine phosphorylation sites capable to bind to numerous effectors or adapter proteins (White, 2003).

Phosphorylated IRS proteins activate three main intracellular signaling pathways. The first is the phosphoinositide 3-kinase (PI3K)–protein kinase C (PKC)–phosphoinositide-dependent kinase (PDK)–PKB/Akt pathway, which is related to most of the metabolic actions of insulin. These responses include modulation of glucose and lipid metabolic enzymes, regulation of mammalian target of rapamycin (mTOR)-related protein synthesis, activation of transcription factors that regulate metabolism such as forkhead box O1 (FOXO1) and sterol regulatory element-binding protein (SREBP), and partially in translocation of glucose transporter type-4 (GLUT4)-containing vesicles to the cell membrane (Taniguchi et al., 2006). The second pathway is the Ras–mitogen-activated protein kinase (MAPK) pathway, which regulates expression of genes related to cell growth and differentiation (Taniguchi et al., 2006). The third pathway involves the proto-oncogene Cbl, and the Cbl-associated protein, which are released from the IR complex after their activation and are accumulated in discrete plasma membrane regions due to interaction with a caveolar protein, flotilin. It has been suggested that this complex partially mediates translocation of the GLUT4-containing vesicles to the membrane (Vollenweider, 2003).

Interaction of insulin pathway proteins with noncanonical insulin pathway proteins such as SOCS has been suggested as an important mechanism of insulin resistance. TNF-α, IL-6, and even insulin signaling enhance the transcription of *SOCS* genes. These proteins are suggested to play different roles in insulin resistance (Howard & Flier, 2006).

Chronic or increased production of ROS or a reduced capacity for their elimination could lead to impairment of intracellular signaling and result either in inflammation or in insulin resistance. The activation of oxidative stress-sensitive kinases could lead to serine/threonine phosphorylation of proteins like IR and IRS (Evans, Maddux, & Goldfine, 2005).

2.3. MS can be induced by changes in diet

Changing the amount of fat or sugar in the diet provides the possibility of developing MS in animal models. MS development in response to different diets is remarkable in rodents. Mice develop MS faster with a high-fat diet, while rats are more susceptible to the increase in carbohydrates.

We developed a MS rat model using normal young adult Wistar rats, which do not show a particular genetic susceptibility to develop obesity and diabetes. We used 20% sucrose in drinking water and normal rat chow during 8 and 24 weeks. After 2 months, this model shows obesity and increased abdominal fat, hyperinsulinemia, hypertriglyceridemia, increased systolic blood pressure, impaired glucose tolerance in IPGTT, and insulin resistance (Larqué et al., 2011; Velasco et al., 2012). We will refer later to this model to discuss changes in pancreatic beta cells due to MS.

3. PHYSIOLOGY OF PANCREATIC ISLETS IN GLUCOSE HOMEOSTASIS

Pancreas in mammals is a mixed gland, composed of 97% of acinar exocrine tissue and only nearly 1–2% of endocrine pancreatic islets. Pancreas derives from evaginations of the posterior foregut endoderm. Endocrine progenitor cells express the transcription factor neurogenin 3 (Ngn3), they differentiates into the endocrine cells and proliferates (Guney et al., 2011). Several other transcription factors are needed for the normal development of islets and pancreatic beta cells, among them, MafA (v-maf musculoaponeurotic fibrosarcoma oncogene homolog A) and Pdx-1 (Pancreatic and duodenal homeobox 1), the last is necessary during organogenesis of islets, differentiation of cells, and maintenance of beta-cell functions (Cerf, 2011).

At least four different types of cells form pancreatic islets, beta, alpha, delta, and pp cells that secrete, respectively, insulin, glucagon, somatostatin, and pancreatic polypeptide. The diameter of islets goes from 50 to 500 μm and each one contains from 50 to 300 endocrine cells (Taborsky, Ahren, Mundinger, Mei, & Havel, 2002). The complete function of pancreatic islets depends on the correct angiogenesis and innervation (Cerf, 2011).

Pancreatic beta cells' sensing of extracellular glucose and insulin secretion are finely regulated by the nervous and endocrine systems. When glucose passes through the proximal portions of the intestine, hormones-denominated incretins (i.e., glucagon-like peptide 1 (GLP-1) and glucose-dependent insulinotropic polypeptide (GIP)) are secreted and potentiate nutrient-induced insulin secretion. Incretins also increase beta-cell proliferation and decrease apoptosis. Incretin-based therapies are now used to treat DM2 (Phillips & Prins, 2011).

Insulin and glucagon secretions are regulated by parasympathetic and sympathetic innervation of islets. The classical view is that neurotransmitters released from these nerves may directly regulate insulin and glucagon secretion. Sympathetic innervation acting through adrenoceptors alpha2 and beta, respectively, decreases insulin and increases glucagon secretion, for example, in response to hypoglycemia and fly or fight stressors. Sympathetic fibers are also related to arterioles that supply the islets, indicating that they control blood flow to the islets. This innervation is remodeled in cases of injury, such as STZ treatment and insulinitis (Chiu, Hua, Fu, Pasricha, & Tang, 2012).

On the other hand, parasympathetic innervation, through vague release of acetylcholine acting on muscarinic receptors, is a major regulatory pathway for insulin secretion; for example, increasing insulin secretion during the cephalic phase of digestion, anticipating feeding (Ahren, 2012).

Pancreatic beta cells are electrically excitable and are capable of transducing variations in fuels into secretory signals through changes in their metabolism. The best analyzed coupling of insulin secretion is that induced by glucose (Henquin et al., 2009).

3.1. Glucose stimulation–insulin secretion coupling in pancreatic beta cells

During fasting, at glucose concentration nearly 5 mM, beta cells are electrically inactive and have a resting potential from −70 to −80 mV. This potential is due to the activity of ATP-sensitive potassium channels (K_{ATP}); when these channels are opened, potassium outflows. Moreover, in many beta cells, a cationic background current through transient receptor potential family (TRP)-type channels that are constantly opened counteracts the K^+ outward flow and electrogenic Na^+/K^+-ATPase pump preserves the cationic gradient.

The increase in glucose concentration above 7 mM leads to membrane depolarization; when a threshold potential is reached, beta cells start firing action potentials. This electrical activity is oscillatory and consists of groups of action potential superimposed on depolarized plateau that are separated by the repolarized intervals, as shown in Fig. 4.2.

Insulin secretion stimulated by glucose is a complex process of signal transduction in beta cells, comprised of proximal events which include glucose internalization through glucose transporters (GLUT) and its catabolism through glycolysis, Krebs cycle, and oxidative phosphorylation, leading to a rise in ATP/ADP ratio, and by distal events, which include the activation of different ionic channels (Velasco et al., 2012).

In the rat, the closure of K_{ATP} channels initiates a slow depolarization of membrane potential, due in part to cationic nonselective TRP channels, to nearly −40 mV. At this potential, the open probability of Na^+ and T-type calcium voltage-dependent channels increases, and Na^+ and Ca^{2+} enter the cells, causing a rapid depolarization. Finally around −20 mV, larger conductance L-type calcium channels activate, resulting in an increase of intracellular calcium and insulin exocytosis (Hiriart & Aguilar-Bryan, 2008).

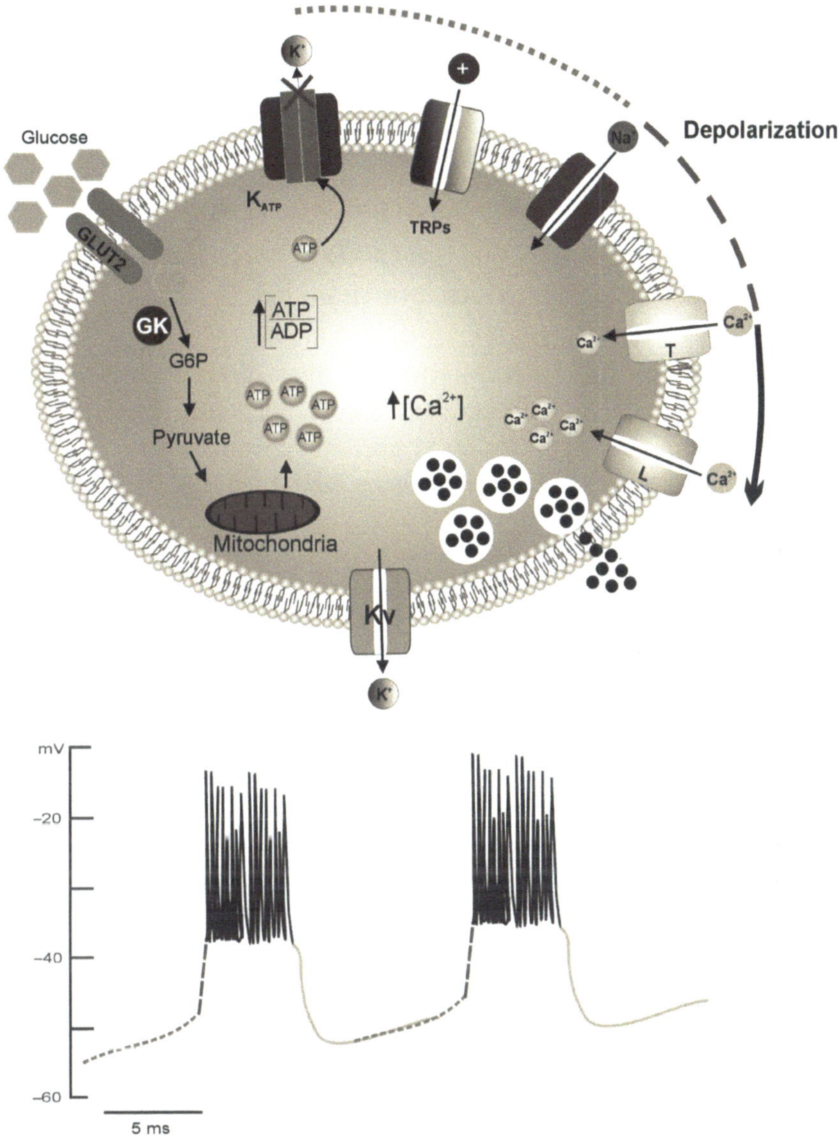

Figure 4.2 Ion channels that participate in glucose-stimulated insulin secretion (GSIS). When extracellular glucose concentration increases, it is internalized into the beta cell by GLUT2 (rodents) and metabolized. The ATP/ADP ratio raises and promotes closure of KATP channels, simultaneously Na^+ and Ca^{2+} entry trough TRP channels depolarize the membrane potential (blue line). This depolarization reaches a threshold, which increases the open probability of voltage-dependent T-type Ca^{2+} and Na^+ channels (pink line). Further depolarization provokes the opening of L-type Ca^{2+} channels and increases intracellular calcium, triggering insulin exocytosis. Lower part, scheme of electrical activity of beta cell, the color corresponds to the participation of each type of channels. (For interpretation of the references to color in this figure legend, the reader is referred to the online version of this chapter.)

Then electrical activity of beta cells is due to the activity of different ionic channels, which may vary among species, but play an important role in insulin secretion. We will review some properties of the most important channels to understand their dysfunction in MS.

4. PHYSIOLOGY AND PATHOPHYSIOLOGY OF IONIC CHANNELS

4.1. ATP-sensitive potassium channels

K_{ATP} channels link the metabolic status with the electrical activity and are named to describe their blockage when the intracellular ATP/ADP ratio increases. They are present in many tissues including, heart (Noma, 1983), skeletal muscle (Spruce, Standen, & Stanfield, 1987), brain (Ashford, Sturgess, Trout, Gardner, & Hales, 1988), and pancreatic beta cells (Cook & Hales, 1984).

The K_{ATP} channels are heteroctameric complexes formed by two different subunits, an inward rectifying potassium channel (Kir6.X) and a sulfonylurea receptor SURx (see Fig. 4.3). To form a functional K_{ATP} channel, four monomers of each subunit are necessary (Clement et al., 1997). "Inwardly rectifying" refers to the property of these channels to allow K^+ flow to move more easily into (negative voltage) rather than out (positive voltage) of the cell (Hibino et al., 2010).

The Kir6.1 or Kir6.2 channels determine biophysical properties of K_{ATP} channels, which are encoded by two genes *KCNJ8* and *KCNJ11*, respectively. Both types are formed by two transmembranal domains linked by highly conserved amino acids that form the ion-selectivity filter (glycine-phenylalanine-glycine) and have cytoplasmic amino NH2 and carboxy COOH terminal domains which bind ATP.

Sulfonylurea receptor is a member of ABC family (from the ATP-binding cassette). Two different genes, *ABCC8* and *ABCC9*, encode for SUR1 and SUR2, respectively. The last one also presents two splice variants SUR2A and SUR2B. SUR1 or SUR2 has a topology of 17 transmembranal domains, grouped in three segments TD0, TD1 and TD2 (reviewed in Hiriart & Aguilar-Bryan, 2008). All SUR proteins have two nucleotide-binding folds (NBF1 and NBF2); NBF1 is located between 11th and 12th transmembranal domains, while NBF2 locates in carboxyl terminal domains. NBF1 has high-affinity ATP-binding, while NBF2 binds ATPMg or ADPMg, causing opening of the channels (reviewed in Hiriart & Aguilar-Bryan, 2008).

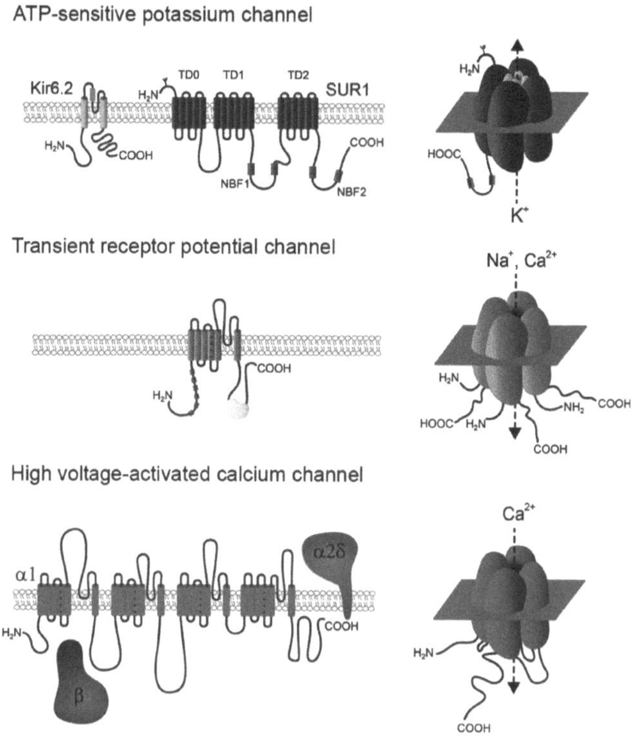

Figure 4.3 Structural properties of ionic channels involved in insulin secretion. General structures of three ion channels are depicted in this cartoon: ATP-sensitive potassium channel (K_{ATP}), transient receptor potential channel (TRP), and high-voltage-activated calcium channel (HVA-CC). Left panels show the topology of ion channel in plasma membrane and right panels represent how they aggregate and form hydrophilic pathways for ions. KATP channels are formed by two subunits, the pore-forming Kir6.2 subunits and the regulatory SUR1. This protein is glycosylated at the N-terminal domain and presents several membrane-spanning segments, grouped in three transmembranal domains (TD0, TD1, and TD2). SUR1 also presents two intracellular nucleotide-binding foldings (NBF1 and NBF2). As depicted in the right panel, KATP channels are heteroctamers, which form K^+ permeable ionic channels. TRP channels are formed by six transmembranal segments that form homotetramers. The fifth and sixth alpha helices and the loop connecting them form the pore and the selectivity filter. They are selectively permeable to cations (mainly Na^+ and Ca^{2+} in physiologic conditions) and present large N- and C-terminal domains that can present several ankyrin repeat domains (i.e., TRPA1 and TRPV1) or enzymatic activities (i.e., TRPM2), respectively. HVA-CC is responsible for Ca^{2+} entry in beta cells and triggering insulin exocytosis. The α1 pore-forming subunits, and consequently L-type currents, predominate in insulin-secreting cells. These subunits are composed by a single polypeptide chain; with four domains of six transmembranal segments each (similar to a TRP subunit). Segment 4 (S4) in each domain is positively charged and determines the activation gating, while S5–S6 form the pore and selectivity filter as in TRP channels. Native ion channel is composed by additional accessory subunits (β and α2δ). (For color version of this figure, the reader is referred to the online version of this chapter.)

The combinations of Kir channel and the sulfonylurea receptor isoforms form different K_{ATP} channels. For example, cardiac and skeletal muscles have K_{ATP} channels isoform Kir6.1/SUR2A, while neuronal and pancreatic beta cells, Kir6.2/SUR1. The biophysical and pharmacological properties depend on these isoforms.

K_{ATP} channels in pancreatic beta cells have a conductance between 50 to 80 pS, and they are weak inward rectifiers (reviewed in Aguilar-Bryan & Bryan, 1999; Quan, Barszczyk, Feng, & Sun, 2011). Pancreatic K_{ATP} channels are the targets of oral hypoglycemic agents like sulfonylureas, which had been used to treat DM2 because they increase insulin secretion. The most important are tolbutamide and glibenclamide, which bind to SUR and close the channels. Other drug group is named KCOs (potassium channels openers) that open the K_{ATP} channels in beta cells. The most potent is diazoxide, which is used to decrease insulin secretion in the congenital hyperinsulinism (CHI) (reviewed in Hibino et al., 2010).

4.1.1 K_{ATP} channels mutation

The most common pathologies due to pancreatic K_{ATP} channels dysfunction are neonatal diabetes mellitus (NDM) (Gloyn et al., 2004) and CHI (Tornovsky et al., 2004).

NDM is defined as the insulin-requiring monogenic diabetes that presents during the first 6 months of life and can be transient or permanent. Extensive clinical and molecular studies have demonstrated that mutations in the genes encoding for Kir6.2 (KCNJ11) and the sulfonylurea receptor SUR1 (ABCC8) produce neonatal diabetes (reviewed in Quan et al., 2011). In NDM, all the mutations on Kir6.2 decrease the channel sensitivity to ATP, while mutations in SUR1 increases the Mg-nucleotide-mediated activation of the channels, or changes their intrinsic gating properties (reviewed by Hibino et al., 2010).

CHI is a genetic heterogeneous disease characterized by dysregulation of insulin secretion resulting in severe hypoglycemia. About 50% of patients have mutations in one of the two subunits of the K_{ATP} channels (Nichols et al., 1996). The functional consequences of these mutations are classified in two groups; one of them comprises a total loss of K_{ATP} channels in the plasma membrane and no K_{ATP} currents. In the other group, the K_{ATP} channels are present but show a reduced sensitivity to Mg-nucleotide activation or to the intrinsic channel-open probability (reviewed by Dunne, Cosgrove, Shepherd, Aynsley-Green, & Lindley, 2004).

4.1.2 K_{ATP} in metabolic syndrome

Since the discovery of adipokines, it has been proposed that they could be related to glucose and lipid homeostasis (Hotamisligil, 2006). For example, leptin decreases insulin secretion and protects beta cells from overnutrition (Morioka et al., 2007), probably by increasing K_{ATP} channels activation (Wagoner, Chen, Worley, Dukes, & Oxford, 1993).

We recently reported that adult male Wistar rats treated with 20% sucrose in the drinking water develop MS. Pancreatic beta cells from MS rats secrete more insulin, compared to controls. After 2 months of treatment, we observed an increase in the total amount of glucose transporter type-2 (GLUT2) protein, located in the membrane (Larqué et al., 2011).

After a 6-month treatment, electrophysiological studies of K_{ATP} single-channel activity demonstrated that the conductance of the channels was not modified by the treatment. However, the sensitivity of K_{ATP} channels to ATP in MS rats, studied in isolated patches of membrane, increased with respect to control rats. The change in the K_d for ATP indicates that the channel closes at lower ATP concentrations in the MS beta cells due to an increased sensitivity to this metabolic signal (Velasco et al., 2012).

4.2. Transient receptor potential channels

The recent identification of the channels underlying the cationic nonselective currents of pancreatic beta cells has been associated to some members of the TRP family (Islam, 2011). In mammals, these ionic channels are grouped in six subfamilies known as canonical (C), vanilloid (V), ankyrin (A), melastatin (M), polycistin (PP), and mucolipin (ML) (Venkatachalam & Montell, 2007). They share a common tetrameric structure with six putative transmembrane segments in each subunit (Li, Yu, & Yang, 2011), which is similar to voltage-gated K^+ channels (Fig. 4.3).

The expression of several members of TRP family has been reported in insulin-secreting cells, although their exact roles are not yet fully elucidated. The observations from knock-out mice points out to TRPM2 and TRPM5 as key regulators of glucose-stimulated insulin secretion (GSIS) (Colsoul, Vennekens, & Nilius, 2011). For example, TRPM2 can be activated by ROS such as H_2O_2, linking the cellular redox state to membrane depolarization, Ca^{2+} mobilization from intracellular stores, and beta-cell viability (Ishii et al., 2006). Interestingly, beta cells are particularly susceptible to oxidative stress in MS (Guichard, Moreau, Pessayre, Epperson, & Krause, 2008). Moreover, TRPM2 channel is a downstream effector in GLP-1 signaling. This incretin protects obese mice from MS (Tomas, Wood, Stanojevic, & Habener, 2011), and it has been described in beta cells as an inductor of GSIS after protein kinase A activation and Ca^{2+} entry through TRPM2 channels (Uchida et al., 2011; Uchida & Tominaga, 2011b).

In humans, three single-nucleotide polymorphisms of TRPM2 have been negatively associated with the homeostatic model assessment of beta-cell function but not with insulin resistance or DM2, raising many questions on how these gene variants affect beta-cell physiology (Romero et al., 2010). Moreover, it is known that TRPM2 null mice present increased energy expenditure and ameliorated high-fat diet-induced insulin resistance and obesity, which confer a better glucose homeostasis despite a reduced insulin secretion (Zhang et al., 2012).

On the other hand, TRPM5 has been reported as an important determinant of Ca^{2+} oscillations in mouse beta cells (Colsoul et al., 2010). Absence of this channel causes a significant glucose intolerance in adult animals, which has been associated with an impaired GSIS (Brixel et al., 2010; Colsoul et al., 2010). TRPM5 connects insulin release to circulating fructose levels through the gustducin receptor in beta cells (Kyriazis, Soundarapandian, & Tyrberg, 2012) and a possible modulation of GLP-1 secretion in the gut has been suggested (Colsoul et al., 2011). The complexity of TRPM5 roles in the overall metabolic state has also been studied in humans, where single-nucleotide polymorphisms of *TRPM5* gene are associated with prediabetic phenotypes, including insulin resistance (Ketterer et al., 2011).

The close-related TRPM4 channel does not seem to be as relevant as TRPM5 in mice, since knock-out animals show no differences in glucose tolerance with respect to wild-type mice (Vennekens et al., 2007). However, there is a great amount of evidence regarding the presence of TRPM4-like currents and channel expression in rat insulinomas and native cells (Marigo, Courville, Hsu, Feng, & Cheng, 2009). Furthermore, arginine-vasopressin, a hormone that correlates with MS (Enhorning et al., 2012; Enhorning et al., 2011), cannot exert a stimulating effect on insulin secretion when a dominant negative TRPM4 construct is expressed (Cheng et al., 2007).

The melastatin family member 3, which acts as a steroid receptor, has been observed in beta cells where it can be activated by pregnenolone sulphate (Wagner et al., 2008) and participates in Zn^{2+} influx (Wagner et al., 2010). Moreover, this channel can also be activated by sphingolipids (Grimm, Kraft, Schultz, & Harteneck, 2005), which are increased in obesity, inflammation, and MS (Brozinick et al., 2012; Majumdar & Mastrandrea, 2012; Othman et al., 2012).

The TRPA1 channel has been detected in the insulin-secreting cell line RINm5F and freshly isolated rat beta cells, and involved in insulin secretion (Cao et al., 2012). This study demonstrated that TRPA1 also links insulin release to oxidative stress through intracellular Ca^{2+} elevation in the insulinoma cell line. This indicates that more TRP channels, other than TRPM2, can modulate beta-cell excitability as a function of ROS. Moreover, this channel has also been highlighted as a polyunsaturated fatty acid sensor, whose activation is proportional to fatty acid chain length and its number of double bonds (Motter & Ahern, 2012). Interestingly, some of these polyunsaturated fatty acids are diminished in patients with MS (Shin et al., 2009), while their dietary intake is associated with lower prevalence of this condition (Mirmiran et al., 2012).

Expression of canonical TRP channels has also been reported in insulin-secreting cells (Li & Zhang, 2009; Sakura & Ashcroft, 1997; Qian et al., 2002), and though their exact roles are not fully unraveled in insulin release, their activities in other tissues are associated with many symptoms of MS (such as obesity, hypertension, and dyslipidemia), and even diabetes (Graham, Yuan, & Ma, 2012; Zhu, Luo, Ma, & Liu, 2011).

Amylin is a determinant of islet dysfunction (Hayden, 2002), and it has been associated with MS in humans (Hou et al., 2011). TRPV4 has been detected in MIN6 and mouse pancreas, and its activation by human islet amyloid polypeptide (amylin) has been linked to beta-cell cytotoxicity due to an exacerbated Ca^{2+} influx and endoplasmic reticulum stress (Casas, Novials, Reimann, Gomis, & Gribble, 2008). Moreover, TRPV4 inhibition in mice through pharmacological blockade or loss of function mutations ameliorates high-fat diet-induced obesity, adipose inflammation, and insulin resistance (Ye et al., 2012).

In summary, the participation of TRP channels in the overall metabolic status of mammals and particularly in the pathophysiology of pancreatic beta cells has been increasingly studied. There is no doubt about their roles not only in controlling insulin release in response to many neurotransmitters, hormones, and autocrine signals (Diaz-Garcia, Sanchez-Soto, & Hiriart, 2013; Uchida & Tominaga, 2011a) but also in regulating metabolism in many other tissues and thus their suceptibility to MS (Liu, Zhu, & Tepel, 2008).

4.3. Voltage-gated Na^+ channels

Voltage-dependent Na^+ channels are functionally expressed in murine, canine, and human beta cells and participate in GSIS (Braun et al., 2008;

Hiriart & Matteson, 1988; Pressel & Misler, 1990). Consequently, the dysfunction of this channel as observed in a beta 1 subunit deficiency model, the Scn1b null mice, causes a reduction of both *in vitro* and *in vivo* insulin secretion, as well as glucose intolerance compared to wild-type animals (Ernst, Aguilar-Bryan, & Noebels, 2009).

Voltage-gated Na^+ channels are heteromeric proteins composed of a glycosylated pore-forming alpha subunit and two auxiliary beta subunits (Catterall, 2000a). Four homologous domains (I–IV), with six transmembrane segments (S1–S6) each, form the alpha subunit, which structurally resembles a voltage-gated K^+ channel subunit. Other important regions of the channel are the pore loop, located between S5 and S6, which contributes to permeation and selectivity; the positively charged S4 segment, which participates in depolarization-induced activation; and the linker region between domains III and IV that works as an inactivation gate (Catterall, Goldin, & Waxman, 2005).

Nine isoforms with a significant sequence homology have been described in the family of voltage-sensitive Na^+ channels (Nav1.1–Nav1.9), which share similar biophysical and pharmacological properties (Catterall et al., 2005). The member Nav1.7 is ubiquitously expressed in insulin-secreting cells, and also the Nav1.3 and Nav1.6 isoforms have been reported in murine and human pancreatic beta cells, respectively (Braun et al., 2008; Philipson, Kusnetsov, Larson, Zeng, & Westermark, 1993).

The role of VGSC in GSIS coupling is far from being a single-intermediate step between K_{ATP} inhibition and Ca^{2+} entry, as suggested by a recent work of Zou and coworkers. Their results showed that cytosolic ATP exerts a dynamic regulation of Na^+ channel activity, increasing the recovery from inactivation and causing a rightward shift of both the current to voltage curve and the voltage-dependent inactivation (Zou et al., 2013). Sodium channels mediate in part, the potentiating effect of neural growth factor on insulin secretion by increasing channel expression and beta-cell excitability (Vidaltamayo, Sanchez-Soto, & Hiriart, 2002).

Interestingly, in obesity and early stages of MS, it has been observed that neurotrophin levels increase, along with higher insulin levels, insulin resistance and other inflammatory mediators (Bullo, Peeraully, Trayhurn, Folch, & Salas-Salvado, 2007; Hristova & Aloe, 2006). Indeed, further research is needed about the mechanisms leading to hyperinsulinemia in MS and specifically in the modulation of ion channels participating in insulin secretion.

4.4. Voltage-dependent calcium channels

Voltage-dependent calcium channels (VDCCs) play a key role in GSIS (Yang & Berggren, 2006). Native pancreatic beta cells and cell lines have different types of VDCC (reviewed in Hiriart & Aguilar-Bryan, 2008) and the dysfunctions of these channels alter insulin secretion. The activity and density of calcium channels are regulated by several mechanisms such as protein phosphorylation, calmodulin, etc. When Ca^{2+} channels expression in human beta cells decrease, patients show impaired insulin secretion, glucose intolerance, and type 2 diabetes mellitus (reviewed in Yang & Berggren, 2006).

VDCCs were first classified according to their voltage activation in low-voltage-activated type T channels (approximately −60 mV) or high-voltage-activated (HVA, approximately −30 mV) that included types L (long lasting), N (neuron), P/Q (first recorded in Purkinje neurons), and R channels (Fig. 4.3). The initial purification studies revealed alpha1, beta, and gamma subunits (Catterall, 2000b) and later biochemical analyses revealed an additional alpha2-delta subunit that comigrated with alpha1 (Hosey et al., 1987).

Calcium channels are heteromeric complexes composed of alpha1, beta, alpha2-delta, and gamma subunits. Alpha1 is the pore-forming subunit, while the other (beta, alpha2-delta, and gamma) act like auxiliary subunits (Hiriart & Aguilar-Bryan, 2008). To date, ten alpha1 subunit genes have been described and the putative channels have been classified according to pharmacological and electrophysiological criteria (Yang & Berggren, 2006).

The pore-forming alpha1 subunit is organized in four repeated domains and each of them contains six transmembranal segments (S1–S6); the S4 segment contains the voltage sensor, similar to voltage-dependent sodium channels. Beta subunit is intracellular, while the gamma subunit is formed by four transmembranal segments and the alpha2 subunit is extracellular and attached to the membrane through a disulfide linkage to the transmembranal delta subunit (Catterall, 2000b).

The rodent beta cells express type L, P/Q, R, and T calcium channels (Mears, 2004); of these channels, type T and L are the most important in insulin secretion (Satin, 2000). In rat beta cells, T-type channels are activated at approximately −40 mV and exhibit slow deactivation and rapid inactivation (Hiriart & Matteson, 1988). The T-type channel opening could contribute to the membrane potential depolarization.

L-type channels are the best characterized in beta cells and Ca^{2+} currents through them represent the largest contribution to the increases in calcium during insulin secretion. Type L channels conduct barium better than calcium, and the unitary conductance changes from 2 pS with calcium to 20–25 pS with barium as current carrier (Rorsman, Ashcroft, & Trube, 1988). L-type channels are activated by strong depolarization and are not inactivated by long-lasting voltage pulses. According to the alpha subunit expressed, the rat shows two different L-type channels, alpha1D (Cav1.3) and alpha1C (Cav1.2). In the rat, mRNA levels of the alpha1D subunit is 2.5 times higher than alpha1C subunit (Iwashima et al., 1993), and this channel type is the most important for the insulin secretion process (Scholze, Plant, Dolphin, & Nurnberg, 2001). On the other hand, mice express higher amounts of alpha1C subunit (Yang et al., 1999). The contributions of the different channel types have not been thoroughly studied in different species and remain controversial. It has been recently described in human beta cells from human cadaver donors that mRNA for Cav1.3 channels and protein predominate over Cav1.2 type. Moreover, a variant SNP in the gene *CACNA1D*, encoding for Cav1.3 was described. This change was associated with a reduction in the expression of Cav1.3 channel mRNA and DM2 (Reinbothe et al., 2013).

A point mutation of human Cav1.2 channels makes the beta cell secrete insulin excessively, causing hypoglycemic episodes in children with this mutation (Splawski et al., 2004).

R-type channels, that inactivate faster than other HVA, are also present in rodent beta cells. These channels may play a role in the supply of new secretory granules to the release sites. Interestingly, these channels are not expressed in human islets, which express P/Q calcium channels that play an important role in insulin exocytosis (Rorsman, Eliasson, Kanno, Zhang, & Gopel, 2011).

The sensitivity to drugs is being used to further classify the channels, L-type channels are sensitive to dihydropyridines, N-type are blocked by omega-conotoxin GVIA (w-CgTx) (Snutch & Reiner, 1992), P/Q type are blocked by omega-agatoxine (Catterall, 2011), while it has been proposed that mibefradil is a potent blocker for T-type channels in several cell types including pancreatic beta cells (Wu et al., 2000). Pharmacological experiments have shown that 60–80% of glucose-induced insulin secretion from mouse, rat, and human, can be attributed to calcium influx through the L-type calcium channel (Davalli et al., 1996).

It is clear that calcium channels play an important role in insulin secretion; however, the pathophysiological changes during hyperinsulinemia in the MS are not entirely clear. MS may precede diabetes mellitus and constitutes a model to study beta-cell dysfunction.

We used an MS model in rat fed for 24 weeks with 20% sucrose to study the calcium currents, and we found three subpopulations of cells regarding calcium currents. One half of the cells had low-current density (we named them MS1), 35% of the cells showed large currents (MS2), and 15% of them showed no IBa^{2+} at all (Fig. 4.4). We propose that during MS, the MS2 cells increase by 92% the maximum peak of barium current density, explaining in part, the hyperinsulinemia observed in our model. However, with the chronic treatment, cells begin to get exhausted by showing less current and probably less insulin secretion, probably running to exhaustion.

4.5. Returning to resting potential

The depolarization of the membrane potential is caused by the different ionic channels above described. In the repolarization to resting potential, several types of potassium channels participate, among them being voltage-dependent potassium channels (Kv) and Ca^{2+}-sensitive voltage-dependent potassium channels (KCa) (Braun et al., 2008). These channels are described in all beta cells and in several cell lines studied to date (reviewed in MacDonald & Wheeler, 2003).

The pore-forming subunits (alpha1) of Kv and KCa channels are formed by six and seven transmembrane domains (TMD), respectively, and like other voltage-dependent channels, the Kv channels have a voltage sensor in the fourth TMD, while KCa channels in the fifth TMD (reviewed in MacDonald & Wheeler, 2003).

Voltage-dependent currents are classified based on their biophysical and pharmacological properties, that is, the KA-type current (Kv1.4), which is blocked by 4-aminopyridine and insensitive to tetraethylammonium (TEA), and the delayed-rectifier potassium current (Kv2.1), which is TEA-sensitive. The first direct evidence that suggested that repolarizing outward potassium currents are involved in insulin secretion arose from studies that showed that TEA prolongs mouse beta-cell action potentials and increases insulin secretion. KA currents activate and inactivate rapidly, while delayed-rectifier currents activate more slowly and do not inactivate, or inactivate

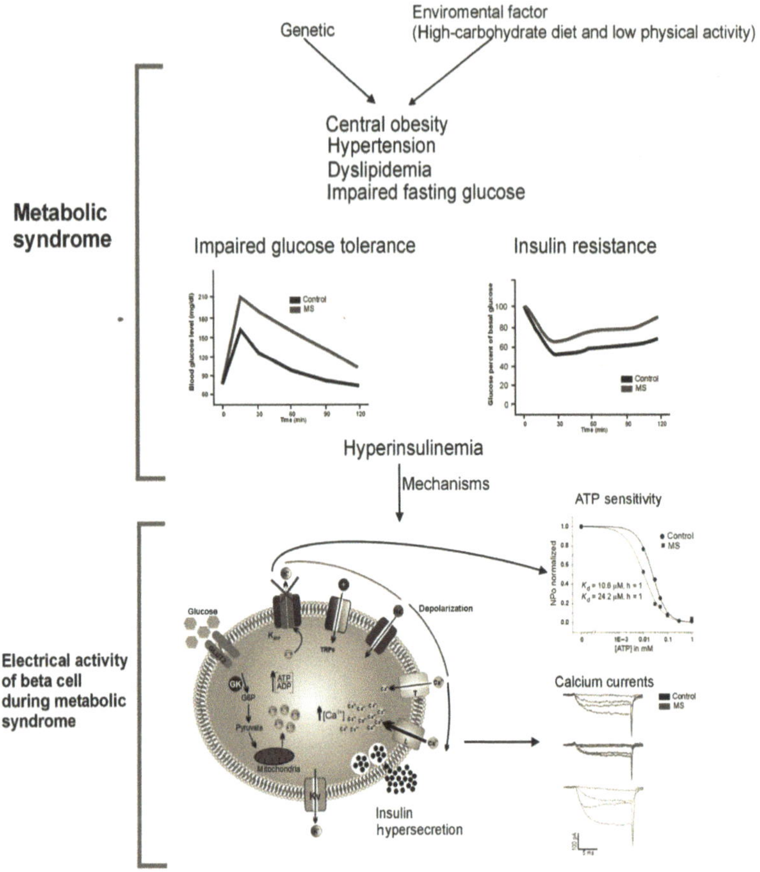

Figure 4.4 Model of the mechanisms of beta-cell dysfunction during metabolic syndrome. Genetic and environmental factors contribute to the development of metabolic syndrome. Metabolic syndrome included signs such as insulin resistance and hyperinsulinemia. During MS, the KATP channels change their ATP-sensitivity and beta-cell calcium currents show two behavior modes. (For color version of this figure, the reader is referred to the online version of this chapter.)

slowly over seconds. A recently described toxin Conkunitzin-S1 that preferentially blocks the delayed rectifiers Kv1.7 channels increases glucose-stimulated insulin release, by increasing action potential firing, without effects on basal glucose (Finol-Urdaneta et al., 2012).

KCa currents are Ca^{2+} sensitive and are classified according to their conductance in SK (small) and BK (big) (reviewed in Hiriart & Aguilar-Bryan, 2008). It has been proposed that Kv2.1 (Jacobson et al., 2007) and BK could also participate in repolarizing the plateau or the fast spikes.

4.6. Calcium release from intracellular reservoirs

Calcium elevation may also originates from internal stores. Cytosolic Ca^{2+} oscillations have been observed in all beta cells studied that are associated to filling and emptying of Ca^{2+} stores, mainly the endoplasmic reticulum (Gilon, Arredouani, Gailly, Gromada, & Henquin, 1999). The increment of intracellular Ca^{2+} levels could be further enhanced by Ca^{2+}-induced Ca^{2+}-release through ryanodine receptors (Islam, 2002) and inositol triphosphate receptors (Joseph, Williams, Corkey, Matschinsky, & Williamson, 1984). The expression of the later is regulated by glucose (Lee, Jonas, Weir, & Laychock, 1999) and is increased in islets from diabetic mice (Takasawa et al., 1998).

The interaction between surface voltage-independent ion channels and receptors located at intracellular Ca^{2+} pools is responsible for slow Ca^{2+} oscillations in beta cells (Leech, Holz, & Habener, 1994). This relationship is manifested in the activation of cationic nonselective currents after emptying of intracellular reservoirs (Cruz-Cruz, Salgado, Sanchez-Soto, Vaca, & Hiriart, 2005). Moreover, one of these channels, TRPM2, is located in lysosomes and participates in Ca^{2+} release in response to oxidative stress (Lange et al., 2009).

It is worth to mention that impairment of mitochondrial function affects Ca^{2+} homeostasis in beta cells (Dufer, Krippeit-Drews, & Drews, 2002). Recently, mitochondria have been suggested as a nonendoplasmic reticulum store that contributes to Ca^{2+} release after K_{ATP} silencing (Dufer et al., 2007). Taking together the evidence, several organelles and receptors are implicated in Ca^{2+} dynamics, and some of them could be implicated in beta-cell dysfunction during the MS, as observed in cardiomyocytes (Dincer et al., 2006).

5. CONCLUDING REMARKS

It has come a long way to describe the activity of ion channels in coupling insulin secretion stimulated by glucose. Understanding how are they altered by MS medium could lead us to develop new strategies to prevent beta-cell hyperfunction and exhaustion and also treating type 2 diabetes mellitus epidemics.

REFERENCES

Aguilar-Bryan, L., & Bryan, J. (1999). Molecular biology of adenosine triphosphate-sensitive potassium channels. *Endocrine Reviews, 20*, 101–135.

Ahren, B. (2012). Islet nerves in focus—Defining their neurobiological and clinical role. *Diabetologia, 55*, 3152–3154.

Alberti, K. G., Eckel, R. H., Grundy, S. M., Zimmet, P. Z., Cleeman, J. I., Donato, K. A., et al. (2009). Harmonizing the metabolic syndrome: A joint interim statement of the International Diabetes Federation Task Force on Epidemiology and Prevention; National Heart, Lung, and Blood Institute; American Heart Association; World Heart Federation; International Atherosclerosis Society; and International Association for the Study of Obesity. *Circulation, 120*, 1640–1645.

Ashford, M. L., Sturgess, N. C., Trout, N. J., Gardner, N. J., & Hales, C. N. (1988). Adenosine-5′-triphosphate-sensitive ion channels in neonatal rat cultured central neurones. *Pflügers Archiv, 412*, 297–304.

Braun, M., Ramracheya, R., Bengtsson, M., Zhang, Q., Karanauskaite, J., Partridge, C., et al. (2008). Voltage-gated ion channels in human pancreatic beta-cells: Electrophysiological characterization and role in insulin secretion. *Diabetes, 57*, 1618–1628.

Brixel, L. R., Monteilh-Zoller, M. K., Ingenbrandt, C. S., Fleig, A., Penner, R., Enklaar, T., et al. (2010). TRPM5 regulates glucose-stimulated insulin secretion. *Pflügers Archiv, 460*, 69–76.

Brozinick, J. T., Hawkins, E., Hoang Bui, H., Kuo, M. S., Tan, B., Kievit, P., et al. (2012). Plasma sphingolipids are biomarkers of metabolic syndrome in non-human primates maintained on a Western-style diet. *International Journal of Obesity, 37*, 1064–1070.

Bullo, M., Peeraully, M. R., Trayhurn, P., Folch, J., & Salas-Salvado, J. (2007). Circulating nerve growth factor levels in relation to obesity and the metabolic syndrome in women. *European Journal of Endocrinology, 157*, 303–310.

Cao, D. S., Zhong, L., Hsieh, T. H., Abooj, M., Bishnoi, M., Hughes, L., et al. (2012). Expression of transient receptor potential ankyrin 1 (TRPA1) and its role in insulin release from rat pancreatic beta cells. *PLoS One*, 7, e38005.

Casas, S., Novials, A., Reimann, F., Gomis, R., & Gribble, F. M. (2008). Calcium elevation in mouse pancreatic beta cells evoked by extracellular human islet amyloid polypeptide involves activation of the mechanosensitive ion channel TRPV4. *Diabetologia, 51*, 2252–2262.

Catterall, W. A. (2000a). From ionic currents to molecular mechanisms: The structure and function of voltage-gated sodium channels. *Neuron, 26*, 13–25.

Catterall, W. A. (2000b). Structure and regulation of voltage-gated Ca^{2+} channels. *Annual Review of Cell and Developmental Biology, 16*, 521–555.

Catterall, W. A. (2011). Voltage-gated calcium channels. *Cold Spring Harbor Perspectives in Biology, 3*, a003947.

Catterall, W. A., Goldin, A. L., & Waxman, S. G. (2005). International Union of Pharmacology. XLVII. Nomenclature and structure-function relationships of voltage-gated sodium channels. *Pharmacological Reviews, 57*, 397–409.

Cerf, M. E. (2011). Islet organogenesis, angiogenesis and innervation. *Cell Biology International, 35*, 1065–1078.

Cheng, H., Beck, A., Launay, P., Gross, S. A., Stokes, A. J., Kinet, J. P., et al. (2007). TRPM4 controls insulin secretion in pancreatic beta-cells. *Cell Calcium, 41*, 51–61.

Chiu, Y. C., Hua, T. E., Fu, Y. Y., Pasricha, P. J., & Tang, S. C. (2012). 3-D imaging and illustration of the perfusive mouse islet sympathetic innervation and its remodelling in injury. *Diabetologia, 55*, 3252–3261.

Clement, J. P., 4th., Kunjilwar, K., Gonzalez, G., Schwanstecher, M., Panten, U., Aguilar-Bryan, L., et al. (1997). Association and stoichiometry of K(ATP) channel subunits. *Neuron, 18*, 827–838.

Colsoul, B., Schraenen, A., Lemaire, K., Quintens, R., Van Lommel, L., Segal, A., et al. (2010). Loss of high-frequency glucose-induced Ca^{2+} oscillations in pancreatic islets correlates with impaired glucose tolerance in Trpm5 −/− mice. *Proceedings of the National Academy of Sciences of the United States of America, 107*, 5208–5213.

Colsoul, B., Vennekens, R., & Nilius, B. (2011). Transient receptor potential cation channels in pancreatic beta cells. *Reviews of Physiology Biochemistry and Pharmacology*, *161*, 87–110.

Cook, D. L., & Hales, C. N. (1984). Intracellular ATP directly blocks K+ channels in pancreatic B-cells. *Nature*, *311*, 271–273.

Corkey, B. E. (2012). Diabetes: Have we got it all wrong? Insulin hypersecretion and food additives: Cause of obesity and diabetes? *Diabetes Care*, *35*, 2432–2437.

Cruz-Cruz, R., Salgado, A., Sanchez-Soto, C., Vaca, L., & Hiriart, M. (2005). Thapsigargin-sensitive cationic current leads to membrane depolarization, calcium entry, and insulin secretion in rat pancreatic beta-cells. *American Journal of Physiology, Endocrinology and Metabolism*, *289*, E439–E445.

Davalli, A. M., Biancardi, E., Pollo, A., Socci, C., Pontiroli, A. E., Pozza, G., et al. (1996). Dihydropyridine-sensitive and -insensitive voltage-operated calcium channels participate in the control of glucose-induced insulin release from human pancreatic beta cells. *The Journal of Endocrinology*, *150*, 195–203.

Diaz-Garcia, C. M., Sanchez-Soto, C., & Hiriart, M. (2013). TRPM channels phosphorylation as a potential bridge between old signals and novel regulatory mechanisms of insulin secretion. *Current Diabetes Reviews*, *9*, 117–125.

Dincer, U. D., Araiza, A., Knudson, J. D., Shao, C. H., Bidasee, K. R., & Tune, J. D. (2006). Dysfunction of cardiac ryanodine receptors in the metabolic syndrome. *Journal of Molecular and Cellular Cardiology*, *41*, 108–114.

Dufer, M., Haspel, D., Krippeit-Drews, P., Kelm, M., Ranta, F., Nitschke, R., et al. (2007). The KATP channel is critical for calcium sequestration into non-ER compartments in mouse pancreatic beta cells. *Cellular Physiology and Biochemistry*, *20*, 65–74.

Dufer, M., Krippeit-Drews, P., & Drews, G. (2002). Inhibition of mitochondrial function affects cellular Ca2+ handling in pancreatic B-cells. *Pflügers Archiv*, *444*, 236–243.

Dunne, M. J., Cosgrove, K. E., Shepherd, R. M., Aynsley-Green, A., & Lindley, K. J. (2004). Hyperinsulinism in infancy: From basic science to clinical disease. *Physiological Reviews*, *84*, 239–275.

Eckel, R. H., Grundy, S. M., & Zimmet, P. Z. (2005). The metabolic syndrome. *Lancet*, *365*, 1415–1428.

Enhorning, S., Bankir, L., Bouby, N., Struck, J., Hedblad, B., Persson, M., et al. (2012). Copeptin, a marker of vasopressin, in abdominal obesity, diabetes and microalbuminuria: The prospective Malmo Diet and Cancer Study cardiovascular cohort. *International Journal of Obesity*, *37*, 598–603.

Enhorning, S., Struck, J., Wirfalt, E., Hedblad, B., Morgenthaler, N. G., & Melander, O. (2011). Plasma copeptin, a unifying factor behind the metabolic syndrome. *The Journal of Clinical Endocrinology and Metabolism*, *96*, E1065–E1072.

Ernst, S. J., Aguilar-Bryan, L., & Noebels, J. L. (2009). Sodium channel beta1 regulatory subunit deficiency reduces pancreatic islet glucose-stimulated insulin and glucagon secretion. *Endocrinology*, *150*, 1132–1139.

Evans, J. L., Maddux, B. A., & Goldfine, I. D. (2005). The molecular basis for oxidative stress-induced insulin resistance. *Antioxidants and Redox Signaling*, *7*, 1040–1052.

Finol-Urdaneta, R. K., Remedi, M. S., Raasch, W., Becker, S., Clark, R. B., Struver, N., et al. (2012). Block of Kv1.7 potassium currents increases glucose-stimulated insulin secretion. *EMBO Molecular Medicine*, *4*, 424–434.

Galic, S., Oakhill, J. S., & Steinberg, G. R. (2010). Adipose tissue as an endocrine organ. *Molecular and Cellular Endocrinology*, *316*, 129–139.

Gallagher, E. J., Leroith, D., & Karnieli, E. (2010). Insulin resistance in obesity as the underlying cause for the metabolic syndrome. *The Mount Sinai Journal of Medicine*, *77*, 511–523.

Gilon, P., Arredouani, A., Gailly, P., Gromada, J., & Henquin, J. C. (1999). Uptake and release of Ca2+ by the endoplasmic reticulum contribute to the oscillations of the cytosolic Ca2+ concentration triggered by Ca2+ influx in the electrically excitable pancreatic B-cell. *The Journal of Biological Chemistry, 274*, 20197–20205.

Gloyn, A. L., Pearson, E. R., Antcliff, J. F., Proks, P., Bruining, G. J., Slingerland, A. S., et al. (2004). Activating mutations in the gene encoding the ATP-sensitive potassium-channel subunit Kir6.2 and permanent neonatal diabetes. *The New England Journal of Medicine, 350*, 1838–1849.

Graham, S., Yuan, J. P., & Ma, R. (2012). Canonical transient receptor potential channels in diabetes. *Experimental Biology and Medicine (Maywood, NJ), 237*, 111–118.

Grimm, C., Kraft, R., Schultz, G., & Harteneck, C. (2005). Activation of the melastatin-related cation channel TRPM3 by D-erythro-sphingosine [corrected]. *Molecular Pharmacology, 67*, 798–805.

Guichard, C., Moreau, R., Pessayre, D., Epperson, T. K., & Krause, K. H. (2008). NOX family NADPH oxidases in liver and in pancreatic islets: A role in the metabolic syndrome and diabetes? *Biochemical Society Transactions, 36*, 920–929.

Guney, M. A., Petersen, C. P., Boustani, A., Duncan, M. R., Gunasekaran, U., Menon, R., et al. (2011). Connective tissue growth factor acts within both endothelial cells and beta cells to promote proliferation of developing beta cells. *Proceedings of the National Academy of Sciences of the United States of America, 108*, 15242–15247.

Hayden, M. R. (2002). Islet amyloid, metabolic syndrome, and the natural progressive history of type 2 diabetes mellitus. *Journal of the Pancreas, 3*, 126–138.

Henquin, J. C., Nenquin, M., Ravier, M. A., & Szollosi, A. (2009). Shortcomings of current models of glucose-induced insulin secretion. *Diabetes, Obesity and Metabolism, 11*(Suppl. 4), 168–179.

Hibino, H., Inanobe, A., Furutani, K., Murakami, S., Findlay, I., & Kurachi, Y. (2010). Inwardly rectifying potassium channels: Their structure, function, and physiological roles. *Physiological Reviews, 90*, 291–366.

Hiriart, M., & Aguilar-Bryan, L. (2008). Channel regulation of glucose sensing in the pancreatic beta-cell. *American Journal of Physiology, Endocrinology and Metabolism, 295*, E1298–E1306.

Hiriart, M., & Matteson, D. R. (1988). Na channels and two types of Ca channels in rat pancreatic B cells identified with the reverse hemolytic plaque assay. *The Journal of General Physiology, 91*, 617–639.

Hosey, M. M., Barhanin, J., Schmid, A., Vandaele, S., Ptasienski, J., O'Callahan, C., et al. (1987). Photoaffinity labelling and phosphorylation of a 165 kilodalton peptide associated with dihydropyridine and phenylalkylamine-sensitive calcium channels. *Biochemical and Biophysical Research Communications, 147*, 1137–1145.

Hotamisligil, G. S. (2006). Inflammation and metabolic disorders. *Nature, 444*, 860–867.

Hou, X., Sun, L., Li, Z., Mou, H., Yu, Z., Li, H., et al. (2011). Associations of amylin with inflammatory markers and metabolic syndrome in apparently healthy Chinese. *PLoS One, 6*, e24815.

Howard, J. K., & Flier, J. S. (2006). Attenuation of leptin and insulin signaling by SOCS proteins. *Trends in Endocrinology and Metabolism, 17*, 365–371.

Hristova, M., & Aloe, L. (2006). Metabolic syndrome—Neurotrophic hypothesis. *Medical Hypotheses, 66*, 545–549.

Ishii, M., Shimizu, S., Hara, Y., Hagiwara, T., Miyazaki, A., Mori, Y., et al. (2006). Intracellular-produced hydroxyl radical mediates H2O2-induced Ca2+ influx and cell death in rat beta-cell line RIN-5F. *Cell Calcium, 39*, 487–494.

Islam, M. S. (2002). The ryanodine receptor calcium channel of beta-cells: Molecular regulation and physiological significance. *Diabetes, 51*, 1299–1309.

Islam, M. S. (2011). TRP channels of islets. *Advances in Experimental Medicine and Biology, 704*, 811–830.

Iwashima, Y., Pugh, W., Depaoli, A. M., Takeda, J., Seino, S., Bell, G. I., et al. (1993). Expression of calcium channel mRNAs in rat pancreatic islets and downregulation after glucose infusion. *Diabetes, 42*, 948–955.

Jacobson, D. A., Kuznetsov, A., Lopez, J. P., Kash, S., Ammala, C. E., & Philipson, L. H. (2007). Kv2.1 ablation alters glucose-induced islet electrical activity, enhancing insulin secretion. *Cell Metabolism, 6*, 229–235.

Joseph, S. K., Williams, R. J., Corkey, B. E., Matschinsky, F. M., & Williamson, J. R. (1984). The effect of inositol trisphosphate on Ca2+ fluxes in insulin-secreting tumor cells. *The Journal of Biological Chemistry, 259*, 12952–12955.

Ketterer, C., Mussig, K., Heni, M., Dudziak, K., Randrianarisoa, E., Wagner, R., et al. (2011). Genetic variation within the TRPM5 locus associates with prediabetic phenotypes in subjects at increased risk for type 2 diabetes. *Metabolism, 60*, 1325–1333.

Kyriazis, G. A., Soundarapandian, M. M., & Tyrberg, B. (2012). Sweet taste receptor signaling in beta cells mediates fructose-induced potentiation of glucose-stimulated insulin secretion. *Proceedings of the National Academy of Sciences of the United States of America, 109*, E524–E532.

Lange, I., Yamamoto, S., Partida-Sanchez, S., Mori, Y., Fleig, A., & Penner, R. (2009). TRPM2 functions as a lysosomal Ca^{2+} – release channel in beta cells. *Science Signaling, 2*, ra23.

Larqué, C., Velasco, M., Navarro-Tableros, V., Duhne, M., Aguirre, J., Gutierrez-Reyes, G., et al. (2011). Early endocrine and molecular changes in metabolic syndrome models. *IUBMB Life, 63*, 831–839.

Lee, B., Jonas, J. C., Weir, G. C., & Laychock, S. G. (1999). Glucose regulates expression of inositol 1,4,5-trisphosphate receptor isoforms in isolated rat pancreatic islets. *Endocrinology, 140*, 2173–2182.

Leech, C. A., Holz, G. G., 4th., & Habener, J. F. (1994). Voltage-independent calcium channels mediate slow oscillations of cytosolic calcium that are glucose dependent in pancreatic beta-cells. *Endocrinology, 135*, 365–372.

Li, M., Yu, Y., & Yang, J. (2011). Structural biology of TRP channels. *Advances in Experimental Medicine and Biology, 704*, 1–23.

Li, F., & Zhang, Z. M. (2009). Comparative identification of Ca2+ channel expression in INS-1 and rat pancreatic beta cells. *World Journal of Gastroenterology, 15*, 3046–3050.

Liu, D., Zhu, Z., & Tepel, M. (2008). The role of transient receptor potential channels in metabolic syndrome. *Hypertension Research, 31*, 1989–1995.

MacDonald, P. E., & Wheeler, M. B. (2003). Voltage-dependent K(+) channels in pancreatic beta cells: Role, regulation and potential as therapeutic targets. *Diabetologia, 46*, 1046–1062.

Majumdar, I., & Mastrandrea, L. D. (2012). Serum sphingolipids and inflammatory mediators in adolescents at risk for metabolic syndrome. *Endocrine, 41*, 442–449.

Marigo, V., Courville, K., Hsu, W. H., Feng, J. M., & Cheng, H. (2009). TRPM4 impacts on Ca2+ signals during agonist-induced insulin secretion in pancreatic beta-cells. *Molecular and Cellular Endocrinology, 299*, 194–203.

Mears, D. (2004). Regulation of insulin secretion in islets of Langerhans by Ca(2+)channels. *The Journal of Membrane Biology, 200*, 57–66.

Mirmiran, P., Hosseinpour-Niazi, S., Naderi, Z., Bahadoran, Z., Sadeghi, M., & Azizi, F. (2012). Association between interaction and ratio of omega-3 and omega-6 polyunsaturated fatty acid and the metabolic syndrome in adults. *Nutrition, 28*, 856–863.

Morioka, T., Asilmaz, E., Hu, J., Dishinger, J. F., Kurpad, A. J., Elias, C. F., et al. (2007). Disruption of leptin receptor expression in the pancreas directly affects beta cell growth and function in mice. *The Journal of Clinical Investigation, 117*, 2860–2868.

Motter, A. L., & Ahern, G. P. (2012). TRPA1 is a polyunsaturated fatty acid sensor in mammals. *PLoS One*, 7, e38439.

Nichols, C. G., Shyng, S. L., Nestorowicz, A., Glaser, B., Clement, J. P., 4th., Gonzalez, G., et al. (1996). Adenosine diphosphate as an intracellular regulator of insulin secretion. *Science*, *272*, 1785–1787.

Noma, A. (1983). ATP-regulated K+ channels in cardiac muscle. *Nature*, *305*, 147–148.

Othman, A., Rutti, M. F., Ernst, D., Saely, C. H., Rein, P., Drexel, H., et al. (2012). Plasma deoxysphingolipids: A novel class of biomarkers for the metabolic syndrome? *Diabetologia*, *55*, 421–431.

Philipson, L. H., Kusnetsov, A., Larson, T., Zeng, Y., & Westermark, G. (1993). Human, rodent, and canine pancreatic beta-cells express a sodium channel alpha 1-subunit related to a fetal brain isoform. *Diabetes*, *42*, 1372–1377.

Phillips, L. K., & Prins, J. B. (2011). Update on incretin hormones. *Annals of the New York Academy of Sciences*, *1243*, E55–E74.

Pressel, D. M., & Misler, S. (1990). Sodium channels contribute to action potential generation in canine and human pancreatic islet B cells. *The Journal of Membrane Biology*, *116*, 273–280.

Qian, F., Huang, P., Ma, L., Kuznetsov, A., Tamarina, N., & Philipson, L. H. (2002). TRP genes: Candidates for nonselective cation channels and store-operated channels in insulin-secreting cells. *Diabetes*, *51*(Suppl. 1), S183–S189.

Quan, Y., Barszczyk, A., Feng, Z. P., & Sun, H. S. (2011). Current understanding of K ATP channels in neonatal diseases: Focus on insulin secretion disorders. *Acta Pharmacologica Sinica*, *32*, 765–780.

Reinbothe, T. M., Alkayyali, S., Ahlqvist, E., Tuomi, T., Isomaa, B., Lyssenko, V., et al. (2013). The human L-type calcium channel Ca(v)1.3 regulates insulin release and polymorphisms in CACNA1D associate with type 2 diabetes. *Diabetologia*, *56*, 340–349.

Romero, J. R., Germer, S., Castonguay, A. J., Barton, N. S., Martin, M., & Zee, R. Y. (2010). Gene variation of the transient receptor potential cation channel, subfamily M, member 2 (TRPM2) and type 2 diabetes mellitus: A case-control study. *Clinica Chimica Acta*, *411*, 1437–1440.

Rorsman, P., Ashcroft, F. M., & Trube, G. (1988). Single Ca channel currents in mouse pancreatic B-cells. *Pflügers Archiv*, *412*, 597–603.

Rorsman, P., Eliasson, L., Kanno, T., Zhang, Q., & Gopel, S. (2011). Electrophysiology of pancreatic beta-cells in intact mouse islets of Langerhans. *Progress in Biophysics and Molecular Biology*, *107*, 224–235.

Sakura, H., & Ashcroft, F. M. (1997). Identification of four trp1 gene variants murine pancreatic beta-cells. *Diabetologia*, *40*, 528–532.

Saltiel, A. R., & Kahn, C. R. (2001). Insulin signalling and the regulation of glucose and lipid metabolism. *Nature*, *414*, 799–806.

Satin, L. S. (2000). Localized calcium influx in pancreatic beta-cells: Its significance for Ca2+ − dependent insulin secretion from the islets of Langerhans. *Endocrine*, *13*, 251–262.

Scholze, A., Plant, T. D., Dolphin, A. C., & Nurnberg, B. (2001). Functional expression and characterization of a voltage-gated CaV1.3 (alpha1D) calcium channel subunit from an insulin-secreting cell line. *Molecular Endocrinology*, *15*, 1211–1221.

Shin, M. J., Shim, E., Kang, B., Park, S., Lee, S. H., Shim, C. Y., et al. (2009). Increased inflammation, reduced plasma phospholipid eicosapentaenoic acid and reduced antioxidant potential of treated hypertensive patients with metabolic syndrome. *Yonsei Medical Journal*, *50*, 757–763.

Smith, U., Hammersten, J., Bjorntorp, P., & Kral, J. G. (1979). Regional differences and effect of weight reduction on human fat cell metabolism. *European Journal of Clinical Investigation*, *9*, 327–332.

Snutch, T. P., & Reiner, P. B. (1992). Ca2+ channels: Diversity of form and function. *Current Opinion in Neurobiology*, *2*, 247–253.

Splawski, I., Timothy, K. W., Sharpe, L. M., Decher, N., Kumar, P., Bloise, R., et al. (2004). Ca(V)1.2 calcium channel dysfunction causes a multisystem disorder including arrhythmia and autism. *Cell, 119*, 19–31.

Spruce, A. E., Standen, N. B., & Stanfield, P. R. (1987). Studies of the unitary properties of adenosine-5′-triphosphate-regulated potassium channels of frog skeletal muscle. *The Journal of Physiology, 382*, 213–236.

Taborsky, G. J., Jr., Ahren, B., Mundinger, T. O., Mei, Q., & Havel, P. J. (2002). Autonomic mechanism and defects in the glucagon response to insulin-induced hypoglycaemia. *Diabetes, Nutrition and Metabolism, 15*, 318–322, discussion 322–313.

Takasawa, S., Akiyama, T., Nata, K., Kuroki, M., Tohgo, A., Noguchi, N., et al. (1998). Cyclic ADP-ribose and inositol 1,4,5-trisphosphate as alternate second messengers for intracellular Ca^{2+} mobilization in normal and diabetic beta-cells. *The Journal of Biological Chemistry, 273*, 2497–2500.

Taniguchi, C. M., Emanuelli, B., & Kahn, C. R. (2006). Critical nodes in signalling pathways: Insights into insulin action. *Nature Reviews Molecular Cell Biology, 7*, 85–96.

Tomas, E., Wood, J. A., Stanojevic, V., & Habener, J. F. (2011). Glucagon-like peptide-1 (9–36)amide metabolite inhibits weight gain and attenuates diabetes and hepatic steatosis in diet-induced obese mice. *Diabetes, Obesity and Metabolism, 13*, 26–33.

Tornovsky, S., Crane, A., Cosgrove, K. E., Hussain, K., Lavie, J., Heyman, M., et al. (2004). Hyperinsulinism of infancy: Novel ABCC8 and KCNJ11 mutations and evidence for additional locus heterogeneity. *The Journal of Clinical Endocrinology and Metabolism, 89*, 6224–6234.

Uchida, K., Dezaki, K., Damdindorj, B., Inada, H., Shiuchi, T., Mori, Y., et al. (2011). Lack of TRPM2 impaired insulin secretion and glucose metabolisms in mice. *Diabetes, 60*, 119–126.

Uchida, K., & Tominaga, M. (2011a). The role of thermosensitive TRP (transient receptor potential) channels in insulin secretion. *Endocrine Journal, 58*, 1021–1028.

Uchida, K., & Tominaga, M. (2011b). TRPM2 modulates insulin secretion in pancreatic beta-cells. *Islets, 3*, 209–211.

Velasco, M., Larqué, C., Gutierrez-Reyes, G., Arredondo, R., Sanchez-Soto, C., & Hiriart, M. (2012). Metabolic syndrome induces changes in KATP-channels and calcium currents in pancreatic beta-cells. *Islets, 4*, 302–311.

Venkatachalam, K., & Montell, C. (2007). TRP channels. *Annual Review of Biochemistry, 76*, 387–417.

Vennekens, R., Olausson, J., Meissner, M., Bloch, W., Mathar, I., Philipp, S. E., et al. (2007). Increased IgE-dependent mast cell activation and anaphylactic responses in mice lacking the calcium-activated nonselective cation channel TRPM4. *Nature Immunology, 8*, 312–320.

Vidaltamayo, R., Sanchez-Soto, M. C., & Hiriart, M. (2002). Nerve growth factor increases sodium channel expression in pancreatic beta cells: Implications for insulin secretion. *The FASEB Journal, 16*, 891 892.

Vollenweider, P. (2003). Insulin resistant states and insulin signaling. *Clinical Chemistry and Laboratory Medicine, 41*, 1107–1119.

Wagner, T. F., Drews, A., Loch, S., Mohr, F., Philipp, S. E., Lambert, S., et al. (2010). TRPM3 channels provide a regulated influx pathway for zinc in pancreatic beta cells. *Pflügers Archiv, 460*, 755–765.

Wagner, T. F., Loch, S., Lambert, S., Straub, I., Mannebach, S., Mathar, I., et al. (2008). Transient receptor potential M3 channels are ionotropic steroid receptors in pancreatic beta cells. *Nature Cell Biology, 10*, 1421–1430.

Wagoner, P. K., Chen, C., Worley, J. F., Dukes, I. D., & Oxford, G. S. (1993). Amylin modulates beta-cell glucose sensing via effects on stimulus-secretion coupling. *Proceedings of the National Academy of Sciences of the United States of America, 90*, 9145–9149.

White, M. F. (2003). Insulin signaling in health and disease. *Science, 302*, 1710–1711.
Wu, S., Zhang, M., Vest, P. A., Bhattacharjee, A., Liu, L., & Li, M. (2000). A mibefradil metabolite is a potent intracellular blocker of L-type Ca(2+) currents in pancreatic beta-cells. *The Journal of Pharmacology and Experimental Therapeutics, 292*, 939–943.
Yang, S. N., & Berggren, P. O. (2006). The role of voltage-gated calcium channels in pancreatic beta-cell physiology and pathophysiology. *Endocrine Reviews, 27*, 621–676.
Yang, S. N., Larsson, O., Branstrom, R., Bertorello, A. M., Leibiger, B., Leibiger, I. B., et al. (1999). Syntaxin 1 interacts with the L(D) subtype of voltage-gated Ca(2+) channels in pancreatic beta cells. *Proceedings of the National Academy of Sciences of the United States of America, 96*, 10164–10169.
Ye, L., Kleiner, S., Wu, J., Sah, R., Gupta, R. K., Banks, A. S., et al. (2012). TRPV4 is a regulator of adipose oxidative metabolism, inflammation, and energy homeostasis. *Cell, 151*, 96–110.
Zhang, Z., Zhang, W., Jung, D. Y., Ko, H. J., Lee, Y., Friedline, R. H., et al. (2012). TRPM2 Ca2+ channel regulates energy balance and glucose metabolism. *American Journal of Physiology, Endocrinology and Metabolism, 302*, E807–E816.
Zhu, Z., Luo, Z., Ma, S., & Liu, D. (2011). TRP channels and their implications in metabolic diseases. *Pflügers Archiv, 461*, 211–223.
Zou, N., Wu, X., Jin, Y. Y., He, M. Z., Wang, X. X., Su, L. D., et al. (2013). ATP regulates sodium channel kinetics in pancreatic islet beta cells. *The Journal of Membrane Biology, 246*, 101–107.

CHAPTER FIVE

The Beta Cell Immunopeptidome

Nadine L. Dudek[1], Anthony W. Purcell
Department of Biochemistry and Molecular Biology, Monash University, Clayton, Victoria, Australia
[1]Corresponding author: e-mail address: nadine.dudek@monash.edu

Contents

Abstract

Type 1 diabetes results from the autoimmune-mediated destruction of insulin-secreting beta cells, leading to beta cell loss and insulin deficiency. Presentation of peptides derived from beta cell proteins to autoreactive lymphocytes is critical for the development of disease, and the list of antigens recognized is increasing. A number of these proteins are found within the beta cell secretory granules, which are transiently exposed to the immune system during normal cellular function. How the interplay of environmental and genetic determinants culminates in destructive autoimmunity remains to be clearly defined. Nonconventional presentation of peptide ligands, posttranslational modification of peptides, and the role of the gut microbiome in the development of the immune system are all considered central topics in disease pathogenesis. Each of these may provide a mechanism by which presentation of antigenic peptides in the target tissue differs from presentation in the thymus, allowing autoreactive cells to escape tolerance induction. The high metabolic demand on pancreatic islets, the high concentration of granule proteins, and the susceptibility of islets to cellular stress may all contribute to the presentation of abnormal ligands in the pancreas. Moreover, the finding that small molecules can alter the repertoire of peptides presented by major histocompatibility complex molecules provides a tantalizing hypothesis for the presentation

Vitamins and Hormones, Volume 95
ISSN 0083-6729
http://dx.doi.org/10.1016/B978-0-12-800174-5.00005-3

of autoantigenic peptides in the presence of microbial or endogenous metabolites. In this chapter, we provide an overview of the immunopeptidome of beta cells and the key factors that may influence presentation of beta cell antigens to the immune system.

1. INTRODUCTION

The cellular immune response depends upon recognition of peptides presented on the cell surface by human leukocyte antigen (HLA) molecules encoded by the major histocompatibility complex (MHC). These peptides are derived from the degradation of intracellular or extracellular proteins with hundreds of thousands of different HLA-bound peptides (the immunopeptidome) displayed simultaneously on the cell surface for scrutiny by passing T cells. Because of pathogen-driven genetic diversification of the MHC region, HLA alleles and their gene products are frequently associated with resistance to disease. However, the very polymorphism that drives antigen specificity is also linked to selective presentation of self-peptides, leading to autoimmune diseases such as type 1 diabetes (T1D), rheumatoid arthritis, and multiple sclerosis. Over 40 susceptibility loci have been identified in genetic studies of T1D (Pociot et al., 2010). However, of the genes that predispose to this disease in humans, the strongest contributing factor is the genotype of an individual's MHC molecules. Between 50% and 60% of the familial clustering seen in T1D can be attributed to allelic variation in the HLA genes encoding classical class I and II MHC proteins (Concannon et al., 2005; Noble & Erlich, 2012). In Caucasian populations, the most commonly associated HLA class II haplotypes are HLA-DR3/DQ2 and HLA-DR4/DQ8, with approximately 30–50% of patients carrying both haplotypes. Indeed, heterozygosity for both haplotypes confers the greatest risk for developing T1D, potentially through the formation of an additional *trans*-encoded HLA-DQ molecule (Kooy-Winkelaar et al., 2011; van Lummel et al., 2012). In the nonobese diabetic (NOD) mouse, a widely used murine model of spontaneous diabetes, genetic susceptibility is linked to the MHC class II allele IA^{g7}. IA^{g7} is highly homologous to the human HLA-DQ8 molecule and shares a common peptide-binding specificity during selection of natural ligands (Suri, Walters, Gross, & Unanue, 2005). Although not as striking as class II associations, a number of class I alleles are also linked to the development of T1D. The most commonly associated alleles include HLA-A2, HLA-A24, HLA-B39, and HLA-A11 (Nejentsev et al., 2007). These HLA associations, taken together with findings in murine models that the interaction of autoreactive lymphocytes with both class I and II molecules is required for the initiation and progression of T1D (Eisenbarth, 2007), have led to the hypothesis that islet-derived peptides are presented differentially by disease-associated and nonassociated alleles. Although this is a simple postulate, the complexity of the immunopeptidome and the multitude of other environmental and genetic influences involved in rendering an individual susceptible to developing T1D have made this difficult to assess.

2. AUTOANTIGENS IN T1D

T1D results from the immune-mediated destruction of insulin-secreting beta cells, leading to insulin deficiency and hyperglycemia. This damage occurs slowly over months to years, eventually resulting in the near complete loss of insulin-secreting cells. Both humoral and cellular immune responses can be detected prior to and at diagnosis of disease (Roep & Peakman, 2011; Vehik et al., 2011). Serological screening for serum autoantibodies against (pro)insulin, glutamic acid decarboxylase (GAD65), and the islet tyrosine phosphatase (IA-2) has long been used to confirm diagnosis in patients with T1D (Bingley, 2010), and at least one of these specificities can generally detected during the preclinical phase. More recently, the islet-specific zinc transporter isoform 8 has been added to the list of antigens used for routine screening as a high fraction of new-onset T1D patients have circulating autoantibodies against this zinc transporter (Wenzlau et al., 2008). Autoantibody testing for diagnostic purposes shows that up to 2–5% of patients with clinically diagnosed T1D are negative for known antibodies, suggesting that T1D autoantigen panel is incomplete.

Although autoantibodies may be readily detected in serum, there is no experimental evidence to suggest that they are themselves pathogenic. While in murine models of diabetes, B cells have been shown to be important antigen-presenting cells, it is autoreactive T lymphocytes that are implicated as the prime effectors of disease. The lag between initiation of immune reactivity against self and the development of clinical symptoms has made it difficult to determine whether there is a common antigen that initiates diabetes or whether immunity to multiple proteins occurs simultaneously. Moreover, the list of proteins targeted during the development of diabetes in murine models and in humans is still increasing (Table 5.1, reviewed in Roep & Peakman, 2012). Some of these islet autoantigens are expressed primarily in pancreatic beta cells; however, others show wider patterns of

Table 5.1 Targets of autoimmunity in T1D

Autoantigen	Mouse	Human	Tissue distribution
Carboxypeptidase H/E[a]		autoAbs	Neuroendocrine, adrenal
Chromogranin A[a]	CD4		Neuroendocrine
DNA TopII		autoAbs	Wide tissue distribution
GAD65	CD4	CD8, CD4 autoAbs	Islet cells, CNS, testis, ovary, adrenal gland, neurons
GAD67	CD4	CD4, autoAbs	Islet cells, neurons
Ganglioside GM2-1[a]		autoAbs	Neuroendocrine
Ganglioside GT3		autoAbs	Neuroendocrine
Glima38[a]		autoAbs	Neuroendocrine
Glial fibrillary acidic protein	CD4	CD8, CD4	Neuroendocrine
GLUT2		autoAbs	Wide tissue distribution
Imogen38		CD4	Wide tissue distribution
HIP/PAP[a]	CD4		Islets
Hsp60	CD4	CD4	Wide tissue distribution
Hsp70		CD4, autoAbs	Wide tissue distribution
Hsp90		autoAbs	Wide tissue distribution
IAPP[a]	CD4	CD8	Islets
IA-2 (ICA512)[a]	CD4, autoAbs	CD4, CD8, autoAbs	Neuroendocrine
IA-2β (phogrin)[a]	CD4	CD4, autoAbs	Neuroendocrine
ICA69		CD4, autoAbs	Pancreas, heart, brain
IGRP	CD8	CD8	Islets
JunB		CD4, autoAbs	Wide tissue distribution
Peripherin	CD4, autoAbs		Neuroendocrine

Table 5.1 Targets of autoimmunity in T1D—cont'd

Autoantigen	Mouse	Human	Tissue distribution
Preproinsulin[a]	CD8, CD4, autoAbs	CD8, CD4, autoAbs	Beta cells, thymus
SOX13 (IAC12)		autoAbs	Wide tissue distribution
Sulfatide[a]		autoAbs	Wide tissue distribution
S100β	CD4	CD4	Neuroendocrine
ZnT8[a]		CD4, CD8, autoAbs	Beta cells

autoAbs, autoantibodies; GAD, glutamic acid decarboxylase; Hsp, heat-shock protein; IGRP, islet-specific glucose-6-phosphatase catalytic subunit-related protein; IA-2, tyrosine phosphatase-like antigen-2; IA-2β, tyrosine phosphatase-like antigen-2β; ICA69, islet cell antigen 69; IAPP, islet amyloid polypeptide; ZnT8, islet-specific zinc transporter isoform 8.
[a]Expressed in secretory granules.
Based on Roep and Peakman (2012).

expression in the neuroendocrine system. It is more than likely that as the cellular immune response evolves, many of these proteins become targets through a mechanism known as epitope spreading and are not the initial targets of disease. In T1D, it is hypothesized that once autoimmunity is initiated, beta cell injury or activation results in the exposure of more antigens, increasing the number of targeted islet proteins. Typically, epitope spreading is thought to occur when antigens interact or colocalize and are taken up simultaneously by B cells with surface immunoglobulin specific for the new antigen. These B cells receive T cell help by virtue of an existing response to the primary antigen, leading to maturation of the B cells and secretion of autoantibodies to the secondary target. Colocalization of antigens within secretory granules may fuel such a mechanism of B and T cell epitope spreading in the face of increasing inflammation during the development of T1D.

There is substantial evidence in both mice and humans to implicate proinsulin as a dominant triggering antigen. Proinsulin is produced by beta cells as a 110 amino acid precursor (pre-proinsulin). Successive cleavages result in the removal of the leader sequence and the intervening C-peptide to generate mature insulin, consisting of a disulfide-linked dimer of A and B chains. As changes in metabolic demand may exceed the rate at which new insulin molecules can be synthesized, the beta cell stores insulin within cytoplasmic secretory granules ready for release. In humans, autoantibodies against insulin are a major risk factor for the development of T1D and are the earliest markers of islet autoimmunity in at-risk children (Bingley, 1996; Ziegler, Hummel, Schenker, & Bonifacio, 1999). Resistance to the development of diabetes is associated with the level of insulin mRNA transcripts expressed in the thymus by way of a variable number of tandem repeats (VNTR) upstream of the human proinsulin gene. The short and long class I and III VNTR alleles are associated with low and high thymic proinsulin mRNA expression, respectively. Homozygosity for the class I VNTR alleles is associated with increased risk, while the class III VNTR alleles are dominantly protective (Bennett et al., 1995; Pugliese et al., 1997; Vafiadis et al., 2001). It is hypothesized that lower thymic expression of proinsulin allows autoreactive T cells to escape thymic deletion and move to the periphery. This is supported by studies in the NOD mouse in which thymic overexpression of proinsulin protects from disease (French et al., 1997). Moreover, graded expression of proinsulin in the thymus of NOD mice shows a dose-dependent, inverse correlation with peripheral T cell responses to proinsulin (Chentoufi & Polychronakos, 2002).

In NOD mice, insulin-specific T cells are among the earliest to appear within the infiltrated islets. Many of these recognize peptides derived from amino acids 9–23 of the insulin B chain (Wegmann, Norbury-Glaser, & Daniel, 1994) and both $CD8^+$ and $CD4^+$ T cells recognizing this region can transfer disease to susceptible mice (Daniel, Gill, Schloot, & Wegmann, 1995; Wong et al., 2009). Nakayama et al. (2005) demonstrated the key role of insulin B_{9-23} in NOD mice by combining insulin 1 and 2 knockout mice with a mutated proinsulin gene. These mice, in which the insulin produced was metabolically active but contained a single amino acid change in the B_{9-23} region, were completely protected from the development of diabetes. Deletion of other known autoantigens such as IA-2 (Kubosaki, Miura, & Notkins, 2004; Kubosaki, Nakamura, & Notkins, 2005), IA2β (Kubosaki et al., 2004, 2005), ICA69 (Winer et al., 2002), and GAD65 (Kash, Condie, & Baekkeskov, 1999; Yamamoto et al., 2004) does not protect NOD mice from diabetes, suggesting that these proteins are dispensable at least for the initiation of disease.

Islet-specific glucose 6 phosphatase catalytic subunit-related protein (IGRP) is another important T cell target in NOD mice. A high percentage of islet-infiltrating $CD8^+$ T cells recognize IGRP, and T cells specific for $IGRP_{206-214}$ are able to transfer diabetes. Furthermore, transgenic mice expressing a T cell receptor specific for $IGRP_{206-214}$ develop accelerated disease (Verdaguer et al., 1997). IGRP-specific T cells undergo a process of avidity maturation during progression toward diabetes, and strikingly, tracking of these T cells in the peripheral blood can be used to predict which animals will go on to become diabetic (Trudeau et al., 2003). However, unlike proinsulin, mice made tolerant to IGRP through thymic expression of the protein still develop diabetes, suggesting that proinsulin precedes IGRP in the hierarchy of responses to islet antigens (Krishnamurthy et al., 2006). Both $CD8^+$ and $CD4^+$ T cells recognizing IGRP have also been identified in humans and IGRP-specific $CD8^+$ T cells have been detected in insulitis lesions of human T1D patients (Unger et al., 2012). Recently, an IGRP-specific HLA-A2-restricted T cell clone isolated from a patient with T1D was demonstrated to cause beta cell destruction in susceptible HLA-A2 transgenic NOD mice (Unger et al., 2012). The use of these "humanized" mice for testing of pathogenic potential of islet-specific T cells from humans provides a valuable tool for assessing cytotoxic potential *in vivo*. This is an important consideration as one of the main criteria for selecting whether a given epitope is relevant to disease is whether epitope-specific T cells are able to transfer insulitis or diabetes, something that is not possible in human subjects. Irrespective of whether any of these candidate autoantigens are involved in the initiation of disease or the effector phase of disease, or whether they are simply along for the ride, each epitope must be generated by antigen processing and presented to the immune system in complex with an MHC molecule.

3. ANTIGEN PROCESSING

3.1. Class I presentation

A large number of factors influence the processing and presentation of peptides by MHC molecules. These include protein turnover, protein accessibility, protease specificity, and the ability to bind to specific MHC molecules. Cytokine-induced expression of proteasome subunits and the action of signal peptidases together with cytoplasmic and endoplasmic reticulum (ER)-associated aminopeptidases all contribute to the complexity and plasticity of peptide generation. Tissue-specific differences in antigen processing or, indeed, differences in the milieu of inflammatory mediators at the site of antigen presentation may facilitate the development of autoimmunity. Both MHC class I and II molecules are critical for the development of T1D. NOD mice deficient in MHC class I do not develop diabetes, and studies aimed at specifically reducing class I expression on beta cells show an inverse correlation between the level of cell surface class I molecules and protection from disease (Gianani et al., 2010; Kay, Parker, Stephens, Thomas, & Allison, 1996; Yamanouchi et al., 2003). In humans, increased expression of MHC class I molecules on beta cells is observed in biopsies of patients with T1D reflecting the inflammatory nature of the lesion (Imagawa et al., 1999; Itoh et al., 1993). This also implies that with this increase in MHC class I expression, there are alterations in the nature of the bound peptide cargo of these molecules presented under these inflammatory conditions.

The major source of peptides for class I MHC molecules is protein degradation within the proteasome, a multisubunit cytosolic structure whose specificity can be altered depending on the expression of constitutive or inducible subunits. Peptides released from the proteasome are translocated into the ER by the transporter associated with antigen-processing (TAP) molecules (Fig. 5.1). The TAP heterodimer associates with a number of other proteins including tapasin, calreticulin, and ERp57 to form the peptide-loading complex (PLC). Within the PLC, the class I heavy chain is assembled with beta-2 microglobulin and peptide (reviewed in Blum, Wearsch, & Cresswell, 2013), and correctly folded complexes are trafficked to the cell surface for recognition by circulating $CD8^+$ T cells. MHC class I molecules generally bind peptides of 8–10 amino acids in length, constrained by the closed nature of the peptide-binding cleft. However, much longer peptides can be transported in the ER by the TAP molecules. These are usually further trimmed by ER aminopeptidase 1 (Saric et al., 2002; Serwold, Gonzalez, Kim, Jacob, & Shastri, 2002); however, peptides up to 16 amino acids in length have been observed to bind to some HLA molecules (Bade-Doding et al., 2011). MHC class I molecules are also able to bind peptides from exogenous proteins internalized by the cells in a process termed cross-presentation. This occurs largely in specialized subsets of dendritic cells and is crucial in priming $CD8^+$ T lymphocytes.

3.2. Class II presentation

Primary beta cells do not express MHC class II molecules. The capture and presentation of beta cell-derived peptides for presentation to $CD4^+$ T cells is performed by antigen-presenting cells within the islet itself or the draining pancreatic lymph nodes. Following capture and internalization, antigens destined for presentation by class II molecules are generated though proteolysis in the lysosomal or late endocytic compartments (Fig. 5.1;

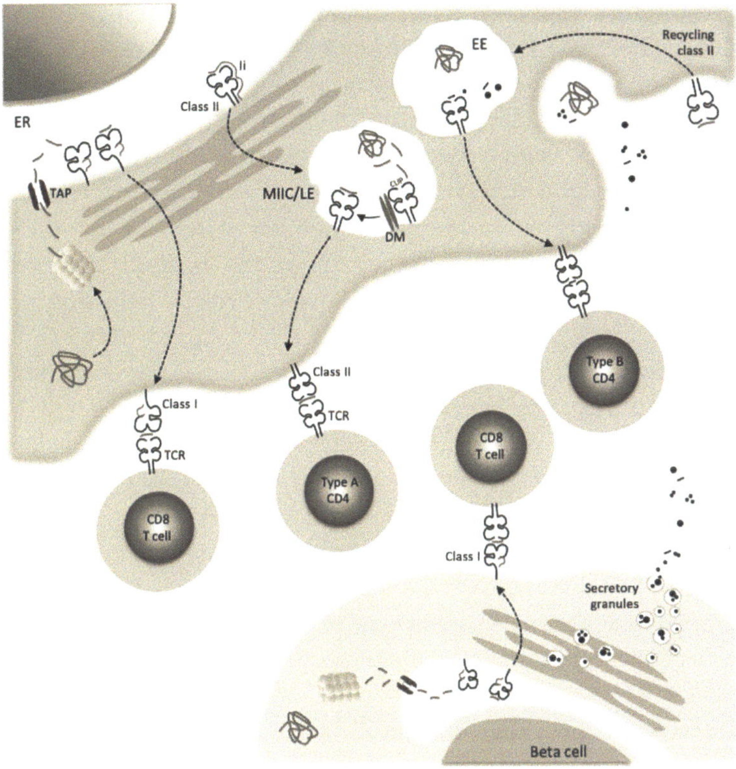

Figure 5.1 Antigen-processing pathways for the delivery of peptides to MHC class I and II molecules. Cytosolic proteins are processed primarily through the proteasome, leading to the generation of short peptides. These are transported into the ER via the TAP for assembly with class I MHC molecules. In some cell types such as dendritic cells, exogenous antigens can enter the class I pathway in a process termed cross-presentation. Exogenous proteins acquired through phagocytosis, macropinocytosis, and endocytosis traffic to the late endosomes (MHC-II compartment, MIIC) for processing and loading onto class II molecules. Class II MHC molecules are assembled with invariant chain (Ii) in the endoplasmic reticulum (ER) where the CLIP peptide protects the binding cleft from premature peptide binding. After egress to the late endosomes, Ii chain is removed and CLIP is exchanged for antigenic peptide through the action of HLA–DM. These stable MHC–peptide complexes are displayed on the cell surface for recognition by $CD4^+$ T cells. T cells recognizing these types of class II MHC molecules represent "Type A" $CD4^+$ T cells. Peptides may also be loaded directly at the cell surface or in early endosomes in the absence of HLA–DM. These complexes may be less stable and are proposed to be the targets of "Type B" $CD4^+$ T cells. Pancreatic beta cells only express MHC class I and process antigens for recognition by $CD8^+$ T cells. APC, antigen-presenting cell; EE, early endosome; LE, late endosome; TCR, T cell receptor.

Neefjes, Jongsma, Paul, & Bakke, 2011). Nascent MHC class II molecules assemble in the ER, a process facilitated by the invariant chain chaperone, which protects the antigen-binding cleft and traffics the molecules to the late endosomal compartments via the trans-Golgi network. Progressive proteolysis of the invariant chain leaves only the class II-associated invariant chain peptide (CLIP) segment within the binding cleft. CLIP is released and exchanged for antigenic peptides through the action of HLA-DM or H2-DM in mice. HLA-DM molecules favor the creation of stable peptide–MHC complexes, thereby acting as a peptide editor, removing peptides that form unstable complexes or have bound in registers with weak affinity (van den Hoorn, Paul, Jongsma, & Neefjes, 2011). The importance of DM-mediated peptide selection was recently highlighted using H2-DM-deficient NOD mice which were protected from the development of disease (Morgan et al., 2013). Another chaperone HLA-DO (H2-DO in mice) is believed to modulate the function of HLA-DM, potentially as a negative regulator (Denzin, Sant'Angelo, Hammond, Surman, & Cresswell, 1997; Liljedahl et al., 1998). Overexpression of H2-DO in NOD mice reduces the incidence of diabetes, most likely through the impairment of acquisition of antigenic peptides by MHC class II (Fallas et al., 2004; Yi et al., 2010).

Processing of class II ligands typically generates large sets of nested peptides with varying N- and C-terminal extensions flanking the same central core sequence (Chicz et al., 1992). These peptides can be accommodated by class II molecules due to the open conformation of the peptide-binding cleft, allowing greater flexibility in the length of bound peptides compared to MHC class I molecules. As a result, peptides typically between 14 and 20 amino acids are found naturally bound to MHC class II molecules. The segment of the peptide that binds to the class II molecule contains a nine amino acid core, which determines the binding register. The remaining peptide residues are outside the groove. These flanking residues can have a major impact on both binding potential and capacity to stimulate $CD4^+$ T cell cells (Bartnes, Leon, Briand, Travers, & Hannestad, 1999; Carson, Desai, Vignali, & Vignali, 1999; Carson, Vignali, Woodland, & Vignali, 1997). Following assembly, stable peptide–MHC complexes traffic to the plasma membrane for recognition by $CD4^+$ T lymphocytes. It is normally the case that T cells recognizing class II MHC–peptide complexes generated by processing of whole antigen can also recognize the same peptide when loaded exogenously onto the cell surface. That is to say that T cells will recognize the peptide–MHC complex irrespective of whether the complex has been generated internally from antigen processing or delivered exogenously. However, binding of synthetic peptides or sequences from denatured proteins bypasses the normal processing pathways. MHC class II–peptide complexes may result through direct binding at the cell surface or in recycling cellular compartments through peptide exchange (Lovitch & Unanue, 2005). The stability of these complexes may vary, given that they are not facilitated by HLA–DM interactions. Such non-conventional acquisition of peptide may have significant implications for the development of autoimmunity, which will be discussed later.

4. IDENTIFYING T CELL EPITOPES IN T1D

The inaccessibility of the target tissue in humans and the limited amount of islet material in NOD mice makes identifying the peptides presented by beta cells or antigen-presenting cells in the surrounding tissues difficult. In NOD mice, it has often been the case that a diabetogenic T cell clone has been used for many years to study the mechanisms of disease without knowing the precise specificity of the clone. This is true for two of the best-studied T cell clones in NOD mice, the $CD8^+$ NY8.3 and the $CD4^+$ BDC2.5. These clones, isolated in the mid 1990s, were used to generate a wealth of information about the disease in NOD mice long before they were found to recognize peptides from IGRP and chromogranin A, respectively. Mapping T cell epitopes is most commonly achieved using libraries of synthetic peptides, spanning the antigen of interest. This approach has been used successfully for the identification of autoantigenic peptides in many autoimmune diseases, including T1D. For example, Pinkse et al. (2005) identified a HLA-A2 restricted epitope from the B chain of insulin (B_{10-18}) by testing synthetic peptides predicted to bind to HLA-A2 using binding algorithms. Increasing numbers of insulin B_{10-18}-specific T cells were found to correlate with islet destruction in T1D islet allograft recipients undergoing graft rejection. This highlights the potential for using T cell epitopes to monitor disease status and graft function. The caveat is that knowledge of the target antigen is required in order to generate suitable synthetic peptides. Furthermore, this approach does not take into account whether a peptide is naturally processed and presented. It may be possible to isolate T cell clones specific for an autoantigenic peptide that is never generated and presented *in vivo* and therefore may have little relevance to disease. A number of groups have turned instead to using naturally processed peptides for T cell screening studies. For example, Hassainya et al. (2005) utilized purified proteasome complexes to digest recombinant human proinsulin, generating a series of potential HLA-A2 epitopes. Of 10 selected candidates, based on predicted HLA binding efficiency, 6 were immunogenic in HLA-A2 transgenic mice, and importantly 3 were processed and presented by cells expressing proinsulin. Toma et al. (2005) used a similar approach in which they selected proinsulin peptides by combining analysis of proteasome cleavage and binding to purified class I molecules commonly associated with T1D. The epitopes selected within proinsulin region 28–64 were recognized by PBMCs from diabetic patients but not healthy controls, highlighting the usefulness of this approach. Other groups have relied on direct isolation and characterization of peptides bound to HLA molecules on the surface of antigen-presenting cells, a method frequently referred to as peptide elution. A series of naturally processed and presented epitopes from IA-2 presented by HLA-DR4 were identified using affinity-purified MHC molecules from cells fed with the autoantigen (Peakman et al., 1999). In this elegant approach, biotinylated antigen was targeted onto antigen-presenting cells using a lectin-based delivery system. The elution of peptides from these cells identified naturally presented IA-2 ligands that could stimulate T cell proliferation from HLA-DR4-positive T1D patients but not HLA-matched nondiabetic controls. More recently, this group has identified a HLA-A2-restricted peptide from proinsulin by overexpressing proinsulin and HLA-A2 in K562 cells and sequencing the HLA-bound peptides (Skowera et al., 2008). $CD8^+$ T cells specific for this epitope were found to kill beta cells *in vitro* in a glucose concentration-dependent fashion. The same parental K562 line transfected instead with HLA-A24 and proinsulin was also used to identify a peptide from the signal peptide of proinsulin (amino acids 3–11) (Kronenberg et al., 2012). Tetramer staining of peripheral blood demonstrated a higher frequency of these cells in HLA-A24-positive individuals with recent onset disease compared with HLA-matched controls.

Despite their success, these types of studies still require prior knowledge of the target antigen. Different approaches are required when looking for the target of a T cell clone with unknown antigen specificity. Identification of $IGRP_{206-214}$ and chromogranin WE14 as the targets of the NY8.3 and BDC2.5 T cell clones, respectively, relied on fractionation of islet material derived from NOD mice. For BDC2.5, the target antigen was identified by using mass spectrometric analysis of antigenic material produced from an islet beta cell tumor in transgenic NOD mice (Stadinski et al., 2010). Partially purified membrane preparations taken from the murine adenomas were further fractionated by size exclusion and ion exchange chromatography. Proteins contained within fractions able to stimulate diabetogenic $CD4^+$ T cell clones were identified by mass spectrometry, ultimately leading to the identification of chromogranin A as the target autoantigen. In the case of IGRP, the NOD-derived cell line NIT-1 was used for peptide elution and screening for active fractions. NIT-1 cells, like primary pancreatic beta cells, express relatively modest levels of MHC class I ($H\text{-}2K^d$ and $H\text{-}2D^b$) under noninflammatory conditions compared with hematopoietic cells. Class I levels can be significantly increased following treatment with IFNγ. Lieberman et al. (2003) utilized over 10^{10} IFNγ-treated NIT-1 cells to identify $IGRP_{206-214}$ as the target of one of the most dominant $CD8^+$ T cell specificities in NOD mice. These types of studies highlight the need for large amounts of material to facilitate the identification of novel diabetogenic antigens. However, systematic and comprehensive analysis of both the proteome and immunoproteome of pancreatic beta cells to facilitate the identification of potential T cell epitopes is becoming a more realistic goal with increasing accessibility to human material and the steadily increasing sensitivity and coverage of proteomes achieved using modern mass spectrometers. Indeed, Matthias Mann's group reported quantitative proteomic analysis of single pancreatic islets in 2009 using high-end mass spectrometry. This study achieved the identification of around 7000 proteins and identified a subset of these proteins (77 up- and 65 down-regulated) that significantly changed in their expression under hyperglycemic conditions. Mapping of the beta cell immunopeptidome is somewhat more challenging, given the requirement to isolate and sequence peptides generated not through tryptic digestion, but through endogenous cellular processing and bound to MHC molecules. Indeed, in our experience, generally 100-fold more material is required for immunopeptidome studies indicating the relative low abundance of peptides displayed on the cell surface compared to the levels of native antigen available for shotgun proteomics-type experiments. These studies may be greatly facilitated by the development of cell lines such as 1.1B4, a human insulin-secreting cell line generated by electrofusion of normal human islet cells with immortal human PANC-1 cells (McCluskey et al., 2011), which can be expanded to large numbers in high-density cell culture.

4.1. The beta cell immunopeptidome

Few studies have examined in detail the peptides presented by MHC class I molecules on beta cells. We hypothesized that identification of peptides presented by beta cells under basal and inflammatory conditions may provide insight into the mechanisms by which beta cells become targeted by autoreactive T cells. In particular, changes in the peptides presented by beta cells under inflammatory conditions may dictate the transition from benign to destructive insulitis. We examined the repertoire of peptides presented by K^d and D^b class I molecules expressed by NIT-1 cells with and without IFNγ stimulation (Dudek et al., 2012). We sequenced over 2000 class I peptides from these cells under basal conditions or following treatment with IFNγ by LC-MS/MS. The majority of peptides were derived from ubiquitously expressed proteins, were common to NIT-1 cells and NOD tissues such as spleen and thymus, and were detected in the presence or absence of cytokine stimulation. Peptides from neuroendocrine or neuronal origin were identified along with sequences from a number of proteins involved in secretory processes in both K^d and D^b datasets. Although peptides derived from known autoantigens such as insulin, IGRP, chromogranin A, and islet amyloid polypeptide could be identified among the MHC-bound peptides isolated from the surface of beta cells, these did not include previously identified T cell epitopes from NOD mice. NIT-1 cells are able to stimulate diabetogenic $CD8^+$ T cells when they are cultured under normal conditions or following cytokine treatment; this suggested that the antigenic peptides were of lower abundance since LC-MS/MS analysis tends to lead to the preferential sequencing of the most highly abundant peptides. In order to detect and quantitate known T cell epitopes from these autoantigens, we therefore utilized a targeted mass spectrometry approach known as multiple reaction monitoring (MRM). In particular, MRM was used to specifically examine the presentation of the immunodominant peptide $IGRP_{206-214}$. This targeted method also allows for the absolute quantitation of peptide epitopes through the inclusion of an isotopically labeled peptide standard added to the MHC–peptide extraction step at a known concentration. We observed that under basal conditions, NIT-1 cells express as little as one $IGRP_{206-214}$ complex per cell. Even after IFNγ treatment, the increase is minimal with only 25 complexes of $IGRP_{206-214}$-H2-K^d per cell detected by this LC-MRM-MS approach. This is in sharp contrast with other endogenous peptides, which may be presented in excess of 15,000 copies per cell, as we observed for the JAK-1-derived peptide SYFPEITHI (Dudek et al., 2012). This speaks to the exquisite sensitively of $CD8^+$ T cells that may require only a few MHC–peptide complexes to trigger full cytotoxic potential and suggests that those autoantigen-derived peptides identified by normal LC-MS/MS are relatively abundant and likely to be tolerogenic. This conclusion is supported by the observation that the IGRP peptide we did identify from LC-MS/MS analysis does not elicit a T cell response in NOD mice (Han et al., 2005).

Although beta cells do not express class II MHC, Suri, Walters, Rohrs, Gross, and Unanue (2008) engineered NIT-1 cells to express IA^{g7} to facilitate the identification of beta cell-derived class II ligands. This was done by transfection of the class II transactivator CIITA into NIT-1 cells and resulted in high cell surface expression of the class II molecules. Importantly, these NIT-1 CIITA cells were able to stimulate diabetogenic $CD4^+$ T cells. Notably, the introduction of IA^{g7} alone was unable to stimulate the same T cells, highlighting the requirement of other members of the class II pathway for the production of antigenic ligands. Immunoaffinity purification of the class II molecules from these cells and sequencing of the associated peptides by tandem mass spectrometry yielded over 300 peptide identifications. Although most were derived from ubiquitous proteins, approximately 10% of the peptides were derived from proteins with restricted tissue expression. Among these included components of the secretory granule such as chromogranin A and secretogranin. Three peptides identified in this study were able to induce proliferation of $CD4^+$ T cells isolated from the draining pancreatic lymph node of NOD mice. However, known peptides from autoantigens such as insulin were not identified. Moreover, although the NIT-CIITA cells were able to stimulate BDC2.5 T cells, the chromogranin A peptide that was subsequently shown to be the target of these cells (Stadinski et al., 2010) was not among the chromogranin peptides identified in the NIT-1 CIITA cell immunopeptidome. This again highlights the probability that disease-relevant epitopes may well be presented at low levels and cannot be readily seen by standard LC-MS/MS analysis.

4.2. The secretory granule as a source of autoantigens

Although beta cells express a large number of proteins, only a small number of these become major targets of autoimmunity. It has been suggested that this selectivity is due to their association with secretory granules. Many of the proteins targeted by autoreactive lymphocytes are located within the secretory pathway or the insulin granule itself (Table 5.1). Granular membrane proteins are highly accessible to the immune system as they are transiently exposed on the cell surface during the normal secretory function of beta cell exocytosis. The high abundance of the major proteins involved in the secretory pathway makes them prime candidates as autoantigens.

Moreover, antigen-presenting cells within the islets constitutively capture insulin granules released from beta cells irrespective of the level of inflammation or cell death (Calderon, Suri, Miller, & Unanue, 2008; Mohan et al., 2010). Evidence from two granule proteins, insulin and chromogranin A, suggest a role for nonconventional peptide–MHC interactions, similar to that reported for immunodominant $CD4^+$ T cells involved in murine models of multiple sclerosis (He et al., 2002). Stadinski et al. (2010) demonstrated that the chromogranin A peptide WE14, a natural cleavage product of the protein, was recognized by BDC2.5 cells in an unusual manner. The carboxyl terminus of the WE14 peptide appears to interact with $I\text{-}A^{g7}$ outside the normal binding groove and lacks the N-terminal amino acids that would occupy positions 1 and 4 of the cleft, anchors which are usually important for stable MHC binding. Truncation of C-terminal amino acids of the WE14 peptide reduced MHC binding and T cell stimulatory capacity, highlighting the importance of the flanking residues lying outside the binding groove.

Nonconventional interactions have also been demonstrated in the recognition of the insulin B_{9-23} epitope. Mohan et al. (2010) identified two sets of islet-infiltrating $CD4^+$ T cells, designated Type A and B, that recognize amino acids 9–23 of the insulin B chain. These cells display differential recognition of peptide–MHC complexes generated by interaction with free peptides or denatured protein versus processing of whole native protein. Type A cells were shown to recognize insulin presented by antigen-presenting cells with the B_{9-23} peptides presented in a standard peptide-binding register. In contrast, Type B cells were shown to react only with antigen-presenting cells fed with soluble B chain peptide and not with native insulin protein. In the case of Type B cells, the peptide is recognized in a binding register that is shifted by a single amino acid. The recognition of insulin presented in this nonconventional manner by Type B T cells is thought to result from the uptake of secretory granules containing degradation products of insulin by antigen-presenting cells tightly associated with blood vessels in the islets. Loading of soluble peptides (in this case, insulin degradation products) onto class II molecules at the cell surface or on recycling molecules occurs in the absence of HLA–DM. The loss of HLA–DM-mediated quality control allows presentation of multiple conformations and binding registers that are not normally permitted in the presence of the chaperone. These nonconventional peptide–MHC complexes are only presented in the target tissue and not in the thymus, allowing Type B insulin reactive cells to escape thymic deletion and become activated in the periphery. The first evidence supporting the existence of Type B cells came from elegant studies of responses to the model protein hen egg lysozyme (Pu, Carrero, & Unanue, 2002; Viner, Nelson, Deck, & Unanue, 1996; Viner, Nelson, & Unanue, 1995) and have also been demonstrated with responses to peptides derived from MHC class II molecules themselves (Barlow, He, & Janeway, 1998; Gyotoku, Fukui, & Sasazuki, 1998; Lovitch, Walters, Gross, & Unanue, 2003). In human autoimmune disease, T cells responding to exogenous peptides but not to cells presenting peptides derived from processing of full-length protein have been described in myasthenia gravis (Bellone, Ostlie, Karachunski, Manfredi, & Conti-Tronconi, 1993; Matsuo et al., 1995), multiple sclerosis (Markovic-Plese et al., 1995), and T1D (Semana, Gausling, Jackson, & Hafler, 1999). These may represent the Type B cells that have been described in murine models.

4.3. Posttranslational modification in T1D

In the case of Type A and Type B cells, conformational isomers of peptide–MHC complexes or complexes in which the peptide is bound in a different register within the binding groove provide the basis of differential recognition (Lovitch & Unanue, 2005; Mohan et al., 2010; Mohan, Petzold, & Unanue, 2011). Another emerging theme in the development of autoimmunity is posttranslational modification. The hypothesis that T cells become activated in the islets due to high local concentrations of antigen and tissue-specific differences in antigen processing and posttranslational modification is highly plausible, given the high metabolic demand on the pancreatic islets and the susceptibility of beta cells to ER and oxidative stress during inflammation. These conditions are likely to lead to changes in posttranslational modifications, protein misfolding, translational infidelity, and alternative splicing and may alter the way peptides are processed and presented in the target tissue (Dunne, Overbergh, Purcell, & Mathieu, 2012). In this scenario, autoreactive T cells escape negative selection because the antigenic form of a protein is not presented in the thymus and is thus able to be activated in the periphery through the presentation of novel posttranslationally modified epitopes. Evidence of posttranslational modification of diabetogenic epitopes includes the identification of modified peptides of proinsulin and chromogranin A. Mannering et al. (2005) demonstrated that a spontaneous modification of adjacent cysteine residues in the insulin A chain is essential for T cell recognition. The formation of a vicinal disulfide bond in this A chain epitope is not in a native disulfide configuration, suggesting that it may form from misfolded insulin or during antigen processing. Post-translational modification of the chromogranin A peptide recognized by BDC2.5 T cell clone has also been reported (Delong et al., 2012). The immunogenicity of the target peptide WE14 is greatly increased by treatment with tissue transglutaminase, an enzyme that is involved in tissue remodeling and implicated in the development of celiac disease. This enzyme catalyzes the deamidation of glutamine and asparagine residues, in addition to forming isopeptide bonds between the side chain amine of lysine and the side chain carboxyl groups of either glutamate or aspartate residues. Post-translational modification may have a number of influences on antigen presentation and not only generate novel immunogenic peptides but also affect the specificity of proteolytic cleavage and change the affinity of the peptide for binding to MHC. There is also mounting evidence for splice variation in the generation of novel epitopes within the islets. For example, IGRP has at least eight splice products, six of which are expressed exclusively in beta cells (Dogra et al., 2006). Diez et al. (2001) demonstrated differential expression of IA-2 in the islets compared with the thymus and spleens. While the full-length mRNA transcript was expressed in the islets along with two alternative transcripts, the spleen and thymus expressed a splice variant lacking an exon encoding membrane regions that are targeted in T1D.

5. PEPTIDE-BASED INTERVENTION AND THE ROLE OF SMALL MOLECULES

One of the aims of mapping T cell responses in T1D is to provide avenues for immunotherapeutic intervention, prior to the initiation of disease in at-risk individuals, during the long progression to clinical diabetes, or after diagnosis. In some patients, residual beta cell function remains, giving impetus to studies aimed at beta cell regeneration or replacement. Strategies aimed at replacement also require immunomodulation to prevent recurrent autoimmunity. While this may be achieved by broad immunosuppression, antigen-specific therapy may potentially offer fewer side effects. To date, disease modulation using antigen-specific therapy has been successfully achieved in murine models. In humans, only limited success has been demonstrated thus far although a large number of clinical trials are still in progress (Rewers & Gottlieb, 2009). One of the most promising murine studies came from Tsai et al. (2010) who prevented disease in NOD mice by expanding IGRP-specific cells with suppressor function. This was achieved by immunization with nanoparticles coated with specific peptide–MHC complexes.

Remarkably, this strategy was able to reverse diabetes in overtly diabetic mice. This particular study is of note as antigen-specific therapies in mice are generally effective when used prior to the onset of disease and are not as effective in animals with established disease. Another approach to modulating the insulin response has been to use small molecules to alter the presentation of diabetogenic peptides. Michels et al. (2011) identified a number of small molecules able to occupy different pockets along the IA^{g7} antigen-binding cleft. By using the insulin B_{9-23} peptide, the authors were able to demonstrate either inhibition or enhancement of T cell stimulatory capacity based on the small molecule used and the peptide-binding pocket that was subsequently targeted. In particular, glyphosine, which occupies pocket 9 of the binding groove, was able to enhance peptide presentation, leading to IL-10 secretion and protection from diabetes in NOD mice. The use of small molecules to alter the binding of a peptide and thereby either stimulating or inhibiting T cell responses provides an interesting avenue for therapeutic intervention. However, small molecule interference in the antigen-binding cleft can have devastating consequences as recently demonstrated for Abacavir hypersensitivity (Illing et al., 2012). Abacavir is an antiretroviral drug used to treat HIV-I infection, which in some cases induces severe cutaneous hypersensitivity reactions. In 2002, two studies demonstrated that 100% of individuals experiencing abacavir hypersensitivity syndrome possessed HLA-B*57:01, and predisposition to this hypersensitivity was associated with an odds ratio greater than 500 if the individual was HLA-B*57:01 positive (Hetherington et al., 2002; Mallal et al., 2002). $CD8^+$ infiltrates are present in the abacavir-associated rash, and drug-specific $CD8^+$ T cell responses can be elicited from peripheral blood mononuclear cells. We recently demonstrated perturbation of the HLA-B*57:01 peptide repertoire in the presence of abacavir using mass spectrometric analysis of HLA-bound peptides (Illing et al., 2012). The alteration in the repertoire was due to the specific and noncovalent interaction of abacavir with HLA-B*57:01, binding in a region that surrounded the F pocket of the antigen-binding cleft. The dramatic change in the repertoire of peptides selected and presented in the presence of abacavir facilitates the robust activation of a broad range of T cell clonotypes against "altered self." The immune response to abacavir-exposed antigen-presenting cells resembles allograft rejection in magnitude and severity, highlighting potential risks associated with using small molecule modulators of peptide binding to treat autoimmune disorders.

That the interaction of a small molecule with a single pocket of the antigen-binding cleft can have such a dramatic impact on peptide presentation and T cell activation raises the possibility that this is an important mechanism in the development of autoimmunity. The last few decades have seen a reduction in the number of patients carrying the high-risk HLA-DR3/DQ2 and HLA-DR4/DQ8 haplotypes accompanied by an increase in the number of patients carrying moderately associated HLA types. This suggests that HLA-associated predisposition is being influenced by increasing environmental pressures. Biological environmental influences may include viral infections, parasitic infections, dietary challenges, and colonization with microbes, either commensal or pathogenic. There is currently great interest in the role of commensal intestinal microbiota and microbial infections in genetically susceptible individuals. Studies in mice have demonstrated the importance of the gastrointestinal flora as mice bred in germ-free conditions have reduced intestinal lymphatic tissue and underdeveloped lymphoid organs. Most of the immune functions in these mice can, however, be restored by reconstitution of germ-free animals with a normal microbiota. In T1D, the composition of the gut microbiota may stay neutral or attenuate the disease in murine models, although in these settings of conventional microbiota, modulation does not normally accelerate diabetes. King et al. found that a spontaneous contamination with a monoculture of gram-positive aerobic spore-forming bacteria in their "germ-free" colony delayed the onset and reduced the incidence of diabetes NOD mice (King & Sarvetnick, 2011). In the same year, Kriegel et al. (2011) published results showing that a naturally transmitted segmented filamentous bacterium was associated with protection of NOD mice from developing diabetes. This bacterium has been shown to induce a strong T-helper cell-type 17 population in the small-intestinal lamina propria of the mouse gut. The same bacterium had also been shown to contribute to inflammation in a murine model of arthritis (Wu et al., 2010), demonstrating a dichotomous role in the development of autoimmunity. It is a reasonable assumption that some microbial lineages will be better suited to the induction or the prevention of disease than others. Recently, differences in the gut microbiota of children with T1D and healthy children were also reported (Murri et al., 2013). Although these observations cannot address whether these differences in gut microbiota have any bearing on disease pathogenesis or whether they are the end result of differences in glycemic index, they provide an interesting baseline for more comprehensive studies of changes in the resident intestinal microbiota and comparison with metabolism and immune reactivity in patients with established disease and at-risk individuals. The normal commensals within an organism provide essential nutrients, such as vitamins, to the host. The reverse is also true where some microbes rely on products produced only by the host organism. It follows that changes in the microbiome will change the types and/or quantities of circulating metabolites. A tantalizing possibility combines the observations that small molecules can modulate determinant selection of MHC molecules and the potential of circulating metabolites derived from certain gut microbes to also demonstrate this functionality. Although no microbial metabolite has been observed to bind to conventional MHC class I or class II molecules and alter peptide binding, we have recently shown that MAIT cells, a dominant T cell population in the gut, recognize bacterial Vitamin B metabolites in complex with the nonclassical HLA molecule MR1 (Kjer-Nielsen et al., 2012).

6. ADVANCES IN MASS SPECTROMETRY FOR THE IDENTIFICATION OF PTMs

The identification of peptide ligands of disease relevance in T1D presents some major technical hurdles, given the complexity of the immunopeptidome and the compounding factors of register shifting, noncanonical acquisition of peptides, posttranslational modification, and low ligand abundance. While one strategy alone will not be sufficient to identify and assess the importance of candidate peptides, several advances in mass spectrometry make identifying relevant peptides from primary beta cells or beta cell lines a more achievable goal (Fig. 5.2). The first of these is the application of MRM for the detection and quantitation of MHC-bound peptides (Tan, Croft, Dudek, Williamson, & Purcell, 2011). MRM combines knowledge of the mass of the targeted peptide with diagnostic fragmentation information to provide highly sensitive and specific detection and quantitation of peptides of interest. In essence, it searches for the mass spectral fingerprint of the peptide(s) being monitored for and, when combined with an isotopically labeled internal peptide standard, allows absolute quantitation in the same experiment. In our hands, MRM analysis provides a 500-fold increase in the sensitivity of detection over standard LC-MS/MS experiments. One of the most important applications of MRM analysis of MHC peptide epitopes lies in the ability to examine hundreds of peptides in a single analysis. Not only does this allow changes in the presentation of known autoantigenic peptides to be determined, but this also enables changes in the presentation of peptides generated from a single antigen to be assessed. Comparing the absolute levels of peptide–MHC complexes

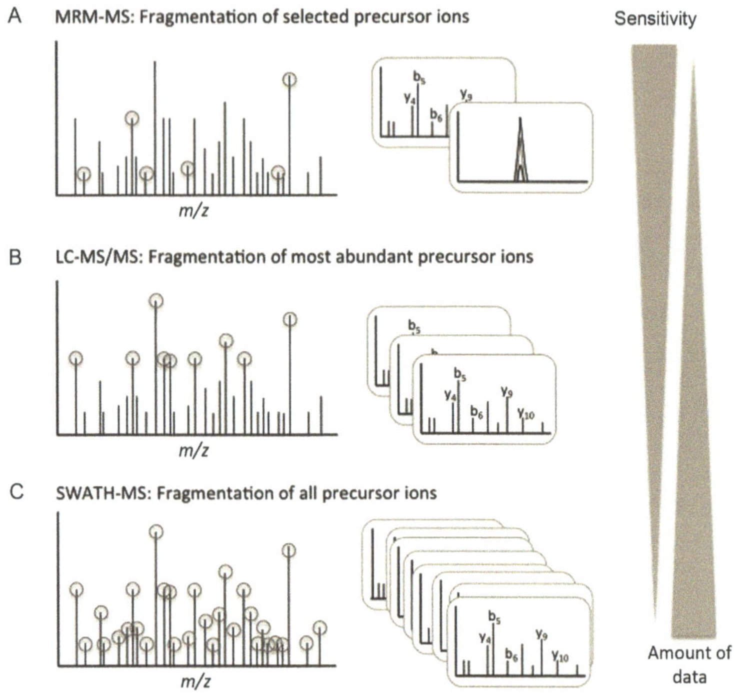

Figure 5.2 Mass spectrometry approaches for the identification and quantitation of MHC-bound peptides. (A) Multiple reaction monitoring (MRM): During MRM-LC-MS, a known peptide(s) of interest is detected based on its precursor mass and characteristic daughter ions generated upon fragmentation. Incorporation of an isotopically labeled internal peptide standard allows absolute quantitation in the same experiment. (B) LC-MS/MS analysis: Only the most abundant precursor ions are selected for fragmentation. Although this technique is not as sensitive as MRM analysis, it does not require any prior knowledge of the peptide of interest, providing a tool for the identification of novel sequences. (C) SWATH-MS: All analytes entering the mass spectrometer are subjected to MS/MS-based fragmentation, even those present in low abundance. Postacquisition extraction of peptide precursor mass and fragmentation information allow the detection of peptides of interest. *Modified from Dudek, Giam, and Purcell (2013).*

from the same autoantigens presented by the same cell may provide a rationale for selecting peptides that may be poorly tolerogenic. Moreover, the ability to detect hundreds of peptides in a single sample provides scope for incorporating potential PTMs and peptide variations within the analysis. For example, MRMs can be designed *in silico* for potential modifications of a target peptide such as deamidation, pyroglutamation, glutathionylation, oxidation, and phosphorylation. It is also possible to design MRMs to cover the peptide core and flanking sequences. This is especially important when synthetic peptides have been used to map both MHC class I and class II epitopes as the naturally processed ligand may differ from the mapped sequence. This is particularly true for class II epitopes since naturally processed forms of these peptides exhibit substantial N- and C-terminal heterogeneity. Recently, we have also reported the parallel detection and quantitation of both the native antigen- and MHC-bound peptides formed from the degradation of this antigen (Croft et al., 2013). This study highlights the ability to multiplex analysis to detect multiple MHC-bound peptides and in parallel to sample antigen expression levels, providing a definitive picture of the dynamics of antigen expression and epitope generation.

The only caveat of MRM analysis is that data are collected for a set number of peptides of known sequence; other analytes entering the mass spectrometer are not selected for fragmentation. While this is the very attribute that makes MRM analysis so sensitive, it limits the use of MRM as a discovery tool. This may be overcome by the most recent addition in the arsenal of mass spectrometric techniques involving data-independent acquisition strategies such as SWATH-MS (Gillet et al., 2012). Data-independent acquisition changes the paradigm of how specific peptides are detected and quantitated in mass spectrometry. This technique allows all analytes entering the mass spectrometer to be subjected to MS/MS-based fragmentation. This is achieved by taking a small packet of analytes contained within a defined mass window and subjecting everything to MS/MS. By systematically moving through an entire mass range taking individual and consecutive mass windows or SWATHs, a comprehensive data set of MS/MS data can be obtained. Postacquisition data interrogation allows MS/MS spectral information to be extracted from each SWATH and for the detection and quantitation of peptides of interest. Thus, unlike MRM analysis, the identity of the peptide of interest need not be known prior to data acquisition.

The major point of differentiation between SWATH and standard LC-MS/MS analysis is that the later collects fragmentation information only for the most abundant ions entering the mass spectrometer. Typically, this means that MS/MS spectra are collected for the top 20–30 precursor ions per second, irrespective of how many other ions are present. With SWATH-MS, fragmentation data are collected for all ions, even low abundance species, allowing data to be interrogated for fragment ions characteristic of a peptide of interest. One of the most exciting aspects of SWATH-MS is that once collected, the data can be analyzed retrospectively for any newly emerging antigen of interest making it an excellent tool for the identification of novel epitopes. This is particularly relevant when analyzing precious samples such as human islets that are difficult to obtain. The wealth of information that can be obtained from a single experiment is vastly expanded through the use of SWATH analysis.

7. CONCLUSIONS

Identifying the peptides presented by pancreatic beta cells and by the antigen-presenting cells within and around the target tissue remains an important goal in T1D research. Many factors impact on the generation of peptide ligands during antigen processing. Protein turnover, protein accessibility, protease specificity, and the affinity for MHC molecules all come into play before a peptide can be presented at the cell surface. The site of presentation, the type of cell type displaying the peptide–MHC complex, and the inflammatory and redox state under which the peptide is presented will all influence the outcome of T cell engagement and determine whether the balance between tolerance and autoimmunity is tipped. Posttranslational modification, peptide-binding register shifts, tissue-specific presentation, and low abundance make the identification of disease-relevant epitopes particularly challenging. It is clear that a combinatorial approach utilizing predictive tools, elution of natural sequences, and functional readouts are all required to delineate the complexity of this disease. Using mice susceptible to disease, it is likely that those peptides recognized by islet-infiltrating T cells are most relevant. In humans, comparison of T cell response between healthy individuals, at-risk individuals, patients with recent onset or established disease, and islet/pancreas transplant recipients may indicate which peptides are most relevant. This is complicated by the possibility that both healthy and diabetic samples may respond to the same peptide, but with a functionally distinct outcome. Mapping responses to islet antigens will, however, allow better evaluation of self-reactive T cells and their role in the onset and progression of disease and may also provide valuable candidates for disease prediction and monitoring of patients following therapeutic intervention.

REFERENCES

Bade-Doding, C., Theodossis, A., Gras, S., Kjer-Nielsen, L., Eiz-Vesper, B., Seltsam, A., et al. (2011). The impact of human leukocyte antigen (HLA) micropolymorphism on ligand specificity within the HLA-B*41 allotypic family. *Haematologica*, *96*(1), 110–118.

Barlow, A. K., He, X., & Janeway, C., Jr. (1998). Exogenously provided peptides of a self-antigen can be processed into forms that are recognized by self-T cells. *The Journal of Experimental Medicine*, *187*(9), 1403–1415.

Bartnes, K., Leon, F., Briand, J. P., Travers, P. J., & Hannestad, K. (1999). N-terminal elongation of a peptide determinant beyond the first primary anchor improves binding to H-2 I-Ad and HLA-DR1 by backbone-dependent and aromatic side chain-dependent interactions, respectively. *European Journal of Immunology*, *29*(1), 189–195.

Bellone, M., Ostlie, N., Karachunski, P., Manfredi, A. A., & Conti-Tronconi, B. M. (1993). Cryptic epitopes on the nicotinic acetylcholine receptor are recognized by autoreactive $CD4^+$ cells. *Journal of Immunology*, *151*(2), 1025–1038.

Bennett, S. T., Lucassen, A. M., Gough, S. C., Powell, E. E., Undlien, D. E., Pritchard, L. E., et al. (1995). Susceptibility to human type 1 diabetes at IDDM2 is determined by tandem repeat variation at the insulin gene minisatellite locus. *Nature Genetics*, *9*(3), 284–292.

Bingley, P. J. (1996). Interactions of age, islet cell antibodies, insulin autoantibodies, and first-phase insulin response in predicting risk of progression to IDDM in ICA+relatives: The ICARUS data set. Islet Cell Antibody Register Users Study. *Diabetes*, *45*(12), 1720–1728.

Bingley, P. J. (2010). Clinical applications of diabetes antibody testing. *The Journal of Clinical Endocrinology and Metabolism*, *95*(1), 25–33.

Blum, J. S., Wearsch, P. A., & Cresswell, P. (2013). Pathways of antigen processing. *Annual Review of Immunology*, *31*, 443–473.

Calderon, B., Suri, A., Miller, M. J., & Unanue, E. R. (2008). Dendritic cells in islets of Langerhans constitutively present beta cell-derived peptides bound to their class II MHC molecules. *Proceedings of the National Academy of Sciences of the United States of America*, *105*(16), 6121–6126.

Carson, R. T., Desai, D. D., Vignali, K. M., & Vignali, D. A. (1999). Immunoregulation of Th cells by naturally processed peptide antagonists. *Journal of Immunology*, *162*(1), 1–4.

Carson, R. T., Vignali, K. M., Woodland, D. L., & Vignali, D. A. (1997). T cell receptor recognition of MHC class II-bound peptide flanking residues enhances immunogenicity and results in altered TCR V region usage. *Immunity*, *7*(3), 387–399.

Chentoufi, A. A., & Polychronakos, C. (2002). Insulin expression levels in the thymus modulate insulin-specific autoreactive T-cell tolerance: The mechanism by which the IDDM2 locus may predispose to diabetes. *Diabetes*, *51*(5), 1383–1390.

Chicz, R. M., Urban, R. G., Lane, W. S., Gorga, J. C., Stern, L. J., Vignali, D. A., et al. (1992). Predominant naturally processed peptides bound to HLA-DR1 are derived from MHC-related molecules and are heterogeneous in size. *Nature*, *358*(6389), 764–768.

Concannon, P., Erlich, H. A., Julier, C., Morahan, G., Nerup, J., Pociot, F., et al. (2005). Type 1 diabetes: Evidence for susceptibility loci from four genome-wide linkage scans in 1,435 multiplex families. *Diabetes*, *54*(10), 2995–3001.

Croft, N. P., Smith, S. A., Wong, Y. C., Tan, C. T., Dudek, N. L., Flesch, I. E., et al. (2013). Kinetics of antigen expression and epitope presentation during virus infection. *PLoS Pathogens*, *9*(1), e1003129.

Daniel, D., Gill, R. G., Schloot, N., & Wegmann, D. (1995). Epitope specificity, cytokine production profile and diabetogenic activity of insulin-specific T cell clones isolated from NOD mice. *European Journal of Immunology*, *25*(4), 1056–1062.

Delong, T., Baker, R. L., He, J., Barbour, G., Bradley, B., & Haskins, K. (2012). Diabetogenic T-cell clones recognize an altered peptide of chromogranin A. *Diabetes*, *61*(12), 3239–3246.

Denzin, L. K., Sant'Angelo, D. B., Hammond, C., Surman, M. J., & Cresswell, P. (1997). Negative regulation by HLA-DO of MHC class II-restricted antigen processing. *Science, 278*(5335), 106–109.

Diez, J., Park, Y., Zeller, M., Brown, D., Garza, D., Ricordi, C., et al. (2001). Differential splicing of the IA-2 mRNA in pancreas and lymphoid organs as a permissive genetic mechanism for autoimmunity against the IA-2 type 1 diabetes autoantigen. *Diabetes, 50*(4), 895–900.

Dogra, R. S., Vaidyanathan, P., Prabakar, K. R., Marshall, K. E., Hutton, J. C., & Pugliese, A. (2006). Alternative splicing of G6PC2, the gene coding for the islet-specific glucose-6-phosphatase catalytic subunit-related protein (IGRP), results in differential expression in human thymus and spleen compared with pancreas. *Diabetologia, 49*(5), 953–957.

Dudek, N. L., Giam, K., & Purcell, A. W. (2013). The use of proteomics to dissect the molecular specificities of T cells in type 1 diabetes. *Journal of Diabetes & Metabolism, S12*, 006.

Dudek, N. L., Tan, C. T., Gorasia, D. G., Croft, N. P., Illing, P. T., & Purcell, A. W. (2012). Constitutive and inflammatory immunopeptidome of pancreatic beta-cells. *Diabetes, 61*(11), 3018–3025.

Dunne, J. L., Overbergh, L., Purcell, A. W., & Mathieu, C. (2012). Posttranslational modifications of proteins in type 1 diabetes: The next step in finding the cure? *Diabetes, 61*(8), 1907–1914.

Eisenbarth, G. S. (2007). Update in type 1 diabetes. *The Journal of Clinical Endocrinology and Metabolism, 92*(7), 2403–2407.

Fallas, J. L., Tobin, H. M., Lou, O., Guo, D., Sant'Angelo, D. B., & Denzin, L. K. (2004). Ectopic expression of HLA-DO in mouse dendritic cells diminishes MHC class II antigen presentation. *Journal of Immunology, 173*(3), 1549–1560.

French, M. B., Allison, J., Cram, D. S., Thomas, H. E., Dempsey-Collier, M., Silva, A., et al. (1997). Transgenic expression of mouse proinsulin II prevents diabetes in nonobese diabetic mice. *Diabetes, 46*(1), 34–39.

Gianani, R., Campbell-Thompson, M., Sarkar, S. A., Wasserfall, C., Pugliese, A., Solis, J. M., et al. (2010). Dimorphic histopathology of long-standing childhood-onset diabetes. *Diabetologia, 53*(4), 690–698.

Gillet, L. C., Navarro, P., Tate, S., Rost, H., Selevsek, N., Reiter, L., et al. (2012). Targeted data extraction of the MS/MS spectra generated by data-independent acquisition: A new concept for consistent and accurate proteome analysis. *Molecular & Cellular Proteomics: MCP, 11*(6), O111 016717.

Gyotoku, T., Fukui, Y., & Sasazuki, T. (1998). An endogenously processed self peptide and the corresponding exogenous peptide bound to the same MHC class II molecule could be distinct ligands for TCR with different kinetic stability. *European Journal of Immunology, 28*(12), 4050–4061.

Han, B., Serra, P., Amrani, A., Yamanouchi, J., Maree, A. F., Edelstein-Keshet, L., et al. (2005). Prevention of diabetes by manipulation of anti-IGRP autoimmunity: High efficiency of a low-affinity peptide. *Nature Medicine, 11*(6), 645–652.

Hassainya, Y., Garcia-Pons, F., Kratzer, R., Lindo, V., Greer, F., Lemonnier, F. A., et al. (2005). Identification of naturally processed HLA-A2–restricted proinsulin epitopes by reverse immunology. *Diabetes, 54*(7), 2053–2059.

He, X. L., Radu, C., Sidney, J., Sette, A., Ward, E. S., & Garcia, K. C. (2002). Structural snapshot of aberrant antigen presentation linked to autoimmunity: The immunodominant epitope of MBP complexed with I-Au. *Immunity, 17*(1), 83–94.

Hetherington, S., Hughes, A. R., Mosteller, M., Shortino, D., Baker, K. L., Spreen, W., et al. (2002). Genetic variations in HLA-B region and hypersensitivity reactions to abacavir. *Lancet, 359*(9312), 1121–1122.

Illing, P. T., Vivian, J. P., Dudek, N. L., Kostenko, L., Chen, Z., Bharadwaj, M., et al. (2012). Immune self-reactivity triggered by drug-modified HLA-peptide repertoire. *Nature, 486*(7404), 554–558.

Imagawa, A., Hanafusa, T., Itoh, N., Waguri, M., Yamamoto, K., Miyagawa, J., et al. (1999). Immunological abnormalities in islets at diagnosis paralleled further deterioration of glycaemic control in patients with recent-onset Type I (insulin-dependent) diabetes mellitus. *Diabetologia*, *42*(5), 574–578.

Itoh, N., Hanafusa, T., Miyazaki, A., Miyagawa, J., Yamagata, K., Yamamoto, K., et al. (1993). Mononuclear cell infiltration and its relation to the expression of major histocompatibility complex antigens and adhesion molecules in pancreas biopsy specimens from newly diagnosed insulin-dependent diabetes mellitus patients. *The Journal of Clinical Investigation*, *92*(5), 2313–2322.

Kash, S. F., Condie, B. G., & Baekkeskov, S. (1999). Glutamate decarboxylase and GABA in pancreatic islets: Lessons from knock-out mice. *Hormone and Metabolic Research = Hormon- und Stoffwechselforschung = Hormones et metabolisme*, *31*(5), 340–344.

Kay, T. W., Parker, J. L., Stephens, L. A., Thomas, H. E., & Allison, J. (1996). RIP-beta 2-microglobulin transgene expression restores insulitis, but not diabetes, in beta 2-microglobulin null nonobese diabetic mice. *Journal of Immunology*, *157*(8), 3688–3693.

King, C., & Sarvetnick, N. (2011). The incidence of type-1 diabetes in NOD mice is modulated by restricted flora not germ-free conditions. *PLoS One*, *6*(2), e17049.

Kjer-Nielsen, L., Patel, O., Corbett, A. J., Le Nours, J., Meehan, B., Liu, L., et al. (2012). MR1 presents microbial vitamin B metabolites to MAIT cells. *Nature*, *491*(7426), 717–723.

Kooy-Winkelaar, Y., van Lummel, M., Moustakas, A. K., Schweizer, J., Mearin, M. L., Mulder, C. J., et al. (2011). Gluten-specific T cells cross-react between HLA-DQ8 and the HLA-DQ2alpha/DQ8beta transdimer. *Journal of Immunology*, *187*(10), 5123–5129.

Kriegel, M. A., Sefik, E., Hill, J. A., Wu, H. J., Benoist, C., & Mathis, D. (2011). Naturally transmitted segmented filamentous bacteria segregate with diabetes protection in nonobese diabetic mice. *Proceedings of the National Academy of Sciences of the United States of America*, *108*(28), 11548–11553.

Krishnamurthy, B., Dudek, N. L., McKenzie, M. D., Purcell, A. W., Brooks, A. G., Gellert, S., et al. (2006). Responses against islet antigens in NOD mice are prevented by tolerance to proinsulin but not IGRP. *The Journal of Clinical Investigation*, *116*(12), 3258–3265.

Kronenberg, D., Knight, R. R., Estorninho, M., Ellis, R. J., Kester, M. G., de Ru, A., et al. (2012). Circulating preproinsulin signal peptide-specific CD8 T cells restricted by the susceptibility molecule HLA-A24 are expanded at onset of type 1 diabetes and kill beta-cells. *Diabetes*, *61*(7), 1752–1759.

Kubosaki, A., Gross, S., Miura, J., Saeki, K., Zhu, M., Nakamura, S., et al. (2004). Targeted disruption of the IA-2beta gene causes glucose intolerance and impairs insulin secretion but does not prevent the development of diabetes in NOD mice. *Diabetes*, *53*(7), 1684–1691.

Kubosaki, A., Miura, J., & Notkins, A. L. (2004). IA-2 is not required for the development of diabetes in NOD mice. *Diabetologia*, *47*(1), 149–150.

Kubosaki, A., Nakamura, S., & Notkins, A. L. (2005). Dense core vesicle proteins IA-2 and IA-2beta: Metabolic alterations in double knockout mice. *Diabetes*, *54*(Suppl. 2), S46–S51.

Lieberman, S. M., Evans, A. M., Han, B., Takaki, T., Vinnitskaya, Y., Caldwell, J. A., et al. (2003). Identification of the beta cell antigen targeted by a prevalent population of pathogenic $CD8^+$ T cells in autoimmune diabetes. *Proceedings of the National Academy of Sciences of the United States of America*, *100*(14), 8384–8388.

Liljedahl, M., Winqvist, O., Surh, C. D., Wong, P., Ngo, K., Teyton, L., et al. (1998). Altered antigen presentation in mice lacking H2-O. *Immunity*, *8*(2), 233–243.

Lovitch, S. B., & Unanue, E. R. (2005). Conformational isomers of a peptide-class II major histocompatibility complex. *Immunological Reviews*, *207*, 293–313.

Lovitch, S. B., Walters, J. J., Gross, M. L., & Unanue, E. R. (2003). APCs present A beta(k)-derived peptides that are autoantigenic to type B T cells. *Journal of Immunology*, *170*(8), 4155–4160.

Mallal, S., Nolan, D., Witt, C., Masel, G., Martin, A. M., Moore, C., et al. (2002). Association between presence of HLA-B*5701, HLA-DR7, and HLA-DQ3 and hypersensitivity to HIV-1 reverse-transcriptase inhibitor abacavir. *Lancet, 359*(9308), 727–732.

Mannering, S. I., Harrison, L. C., Williamson, N. A., Morris, J. S., Thearle, D. J., Jensen, K. P., et al. (2005). The insulin A-chain epitope recognized by human T cells is posttranslationally modified. *The Journal of Experimental Medicine, 202*(9), 1191–1197.

Markovic-Plese, S., Fukaura, H., Zhang, J., al-Sabbagh, A., Southwood, S., Sette, A., et al. (1995). T cell recognition of immunodominant and cryptic proteolipid protein epitopes in humans. *Journal of Immunology, 155*(2), 982–992.

Matsuo, H., Batocchi, A. P., Hawke, S., Nicolle, M., Jacobson, L., Vincent, A., et al. (1995). Peptide-selected T cell lines from myasthenia gravis patients and controls recognize epitopes that are not processed from whole acetylcholine receptor. *Journal of Immunology, 155*(7), 3683–3692.

McCluskey, J. T., Hamid, M., Guo-Parke, H., McClenaghan, N. H., Gomis, R., & Flatt, P. R. (2011). Development and functional characterization of insulin-releasing human pancreatic beta cell lines produced by electrofusion. *The Journal of Biological Chemistry, 286*(25), 21982–21992.

Michels, A. W., Ostrov, D. A., Zhang, L., Nakayama, M., Fuse, M., McDaniel, K., et al. (2011). Structure-based selection of small molecules to alter allele-specific MHC class II antigen presentation. *Journal of Immunology, 187*(11), 5921–5930.

Mohan, J. F., Levisetti, M. G., Calderon, B., Herzog, J. W., Petzold, S. J., & Unanue, E. R. (2010). Unique autoreactive T cells recognize insulin peptides generated within the islets of Langerhans in autoimmune diabetes. *Nature Immunology, 11*(4), 350–354.

Mohan, J. F., Petzold, S. J., & Unanue, E. R. (2011). Register shifting of an insulin peptide-MHC complex allows diabetogenic T cells to escape thymic deletion. *The Journal of Experimental Medicine, 208*(12), 2375–2383.

Morgan, M. A., Muller, P. S., Mould, A., Newland, S. A., Nichols, J., Robertson, E. J., et al. (2013). The nonconventional MHC class II molecule DM governs diabetes susceptibility in NOD mice. *PLoS One, 8*(2), e56738.

Murri, M., Leiva, I., Gomez-Zumaquero, J. M., Tinahones, F. J., Cardona, F., Soriguer, F., et al. (2013). Gut microbiota in children with type 1 diabetes differs from that in healthy children: A case-control study. *BMC Medicine, 11*, 46.

Nakayama, M., Abiru, N., Moriyama, H., Babaya, N., Liu, E., Miao, D., et al. (2005). Prime role for an insulin epitope in the development of type 1 diabetes in NOD mice. *Nature, 435*(7039), 220–223.

Neefjes, J., Jongsma, M. L., Paul, P., & Bakke, O. (2011). Towards a systems understanding of MHC class I and MHC class II antigen presentation. *Nature Reviews. Immunology, 11*(12), 823–836.

Nejentsev, S., Howson, J. M., Walker, N. M., Szeszko, J., Field, S. F., Stevens, H. E., et al. (2007). Localization of type 1 diabetes susceptibility to the MHC class I genes HLA-B and HLA-A. *Nature, 450*(7171), 887–892.

Noble, J. A., & Erlich, H. A. (2012). Genetics of type 1 diabetes. *Cold Spring Harbor Perspectives in Medicine, 2*(1), a007732.

Peakman, M., Stevens, E. J., Lohmann, T., Narendran, P., Dromey, J., Alexander, A., et al. (1999). Naturally processed and presented epitopes of the islet cell autoantigen IA-2 eluted from HLA-DR4. *The Journal of Clinical Investigation, 104*(10), 1449–1457.

Pinkse, G. G., Tysma, O. H., Bergen, C. A., Kester, M. G., Ossendorp, F., van Veelen, P. A., et al. (2005). Autoreactive CD8 T cells associated with beta cell destruction in type 1 diabetes. *Proceedings of the National Academy of Sciences of the United States of America, 102*(51), 18425–18430.

Pociot, F., Akolkar, B., Concannon, P., Erlich, H. A., Julier, C., Morahan, G., et al. (2010). Genetics of type 1 diabetes: What's next? *Diabetes, 59*(7), 1561–1571.

Pu, Z., Carrero, J. A., & Unanue, E. R. (2002). Distinct recognition by two subsets of T cells of an MHC class II-peptide complex. *Proceedings of the National Academy of Sciences of the United States of America*, *99*(13), 8844–8849.

Pugliese, A., Zeller, M., Fernandez, A., Jr., Zalcberg, L. J., Bartlett, R. J., Ricordi, C., et al. (1997). The insulin gene is transcribed in the human thymus and transcription levels correlated with allelic variation at the INS VNTR-IDDM2 susceptibility locus for type 1 diabetes. *Nature Genetics*, *15*(3), 293–297.

Rewers, M., & Gottlieb, P. (2009). Immunotherapy for the prevention and treatment of type 1 diabetes: Human trials and a look into the future. *Diabetes Care*, *32*(10), 1769–1782.

Roep, B. O., & Peakman, M. (2011). Diabetogenic T lymphocytes in human Type 1 diabetes. *Current Opinion in Immunology*, *23*(6), 746–753.

Roep, B. O., & Peakman, M. (2012). Antigen targets of type 1 diabetes autoimmunity. *Cold Spring Harbor Perspectives in Medicine*, *2*(4), a007781.

Saric, T., Chang, S. C., Hattori, A., York, I. A., Markant, S., Rock, K. L., et al. (2002). An IFN-gamma-induced aminopeptidase in the ER, ERAP1, trims precursors to MHC class I-presented peptides. *Nature Immunology*, *3*(12), 1169–1176.

Semana, G., Gausling, R., Jackson, R. A., & Hafler, D. A. (1999). T cell autoreactivity to proinsulin epitopes in diabetic patients and healthy subjects. *Journal of Autoimmunity*, *12*(4), 259–267.

Serwold, T., Gonzalez, F., Kim, J., Jacob, R., & Shastri, N. (2002). ERAAP customizes peptides for MHC class I molecules in the endoplasmic reticulum. *Nature*, *419*(6906), 480–483.

Skowera, A., Ellis, R. J., Varela-Calvino, R., Arif, S., Huang, G. C., Van-Krinks, C., et al. (2008). CTLs are targeted to kill beta cells in patients with type 1 diabetes through recognition of a glucose-regulated preproinsulin epitope. *The Journal of Clinical Investigation*, *118*(10), 3390–3402.

Stadinski, B. D., Delong, T., Reisdorph, N., Reisdorph, R., Powell, R. L., Armstrong, M., et al. (2010). Chromogranin A is an autoantigen in type 1 diabetes. *Nature Immunology*, *11*(3), 225–231.

Suri, A., Walters, J. J., Gross, M. L., & Unanue, E. R. (2005). Natural peptides selected by diabetogenic DQ8 and murine I-A(g7) molecules show common sequence specificity. *The Journal of Clinical Investigation*, *115*(8), 2268–2276.

Suri, A., Walters, J. J., Rohrs, H. W., Gross, M. L., & Unanue, E. R. (2008). First signature of islet beta-cell-derived naturally processed peptides selected by diabetogenic class II MHC molecules. *Journal of Immunology*, *180*(6), 3849–3856.

Tan, C. T., Croft, N. P., Dudek, N. L., Williamson, N. A., & Purcell, A. W. (2011). Direct quantitation of MHC-bound peptide epitopes by selected reaction monitoring. *Proteomics*, *11*(11), 2336–2340.

Toma, A., Haddouk, S., Briand, J. P., Camoin, L., Gahery, H., Connan, F., et al. (2005). Recognition of a subregion of human proinsulin by class I-restricted T cells in type 1 diabetic patients. *Proceedings of the National Academy of Sciences of the United States of America*, *102*(30), 10581–10586.

Trudeau, J. D., Kelly-Smith, C., Verchere, C. B., Elliott, J. F., Dutz, J. P., Finegood, D. T., et al. (2003). Prediction of spontaneous autoimmune diabetes in NOD mice by quantification of autoreactive T cells in peripheral blood. *The Journal of Clinical Investigation*, *111*(2), 217–223.

Tsai, S., Shameli, A., Yamanouchi, J., Clemente-Casares, X., Wang, J., Serra, P., et al. (2010). Reversal of autoimmunity by boosting memory-like autoregulatory T cells. *Immunity*, *32*(4), 568–580.

Unger, W. W., Pearson, T., Abreu, J. R., Laban, S., van der Slik, A. R., der Kracht, S. M., et al. (2012). Islet-specific CTL cloned from a type 1 diabetes patient cause beta-cell destruction after engraftment into HLA-A2 transgenic NOD/scid/IL2RG null mice. *PLoS One*, 7(11), e49213.

Vafiadis, P., Ounissi-Benkalha, H., Palumbo, M., Grabs, R., Rousseau, M., Goodyer, C. G., et al. (2001). Class III alleles of the variable number of tandem repeat insulin polymorphism associated with silencing of thymic insulin predispose to type 1 diabetes. *The Journal of Clinical Endocrinology and Metabolism, 86*(8), 3705–3710.

van den Hoorn, T., Paul, P., Jongsma, M. L., & Neefjes, J. (2011). Routes to manipulate MHC class II antigen presentation. *Current Opinion in Immunology, 23*(1), 88–95.

van Lummel, M., van Veelen, P. A., Zaldumbide, A., de Ru, A., Janssen, G. M., Moustakas, A. K., et al. (2012). Type 1 diabetes-associated HLA-DQ8 transdimer accommodates a unique peptide repertoire. *The Journal of Biological Chemistry, 287*(12), 9514–9524.

Vehik, K., Beam, C. A., Mahon, J. L., Schatz, D. A., Haller, M. J., Sosenko, J. M., et al. (2011). Development of autoantibodies in the TrialNet Natural History Study. *Diabetes Care, 34*(9), 1897–1901.

Verdaguer, J., Schmidt, D., Amrani, A., Anderson, B., Averill, N., & Santamaria, P. (1997). Spontaneous autoimmune diabetes in monoclonal T cell nonobese diabetic mice. *The Journal of Experimental Medicine, 186*(10), 1663–1676.

Viner, N. J., Nelson, C. A., Deck, B., & Unanue, E. R. (1996). Complexes generated by the binding of free peptides to class II MHC molecules are antigenically diverse compared with those generated by intracellular processing. *Journal of Immunology, 156*(7), 2365–2368.

Viner, N. J., Nelson, C. A., & Unanue, E. R. (1995). Identification of a major I-Ek-restricted determinant of hen egg lysozyme: Limitations of lymph node proliferation studies in defining immunodominance and crypticity. *Proceedings of the National Academy of Sciences of the United States of America, 92*(6), 2214–2218.

Wegmann, D. R., Norbury-Glaser, M., & Daniel, D. (1994). Insulin-specific T cells are a predominant component of islet infiltrates in pre-diabetic NOD mice. *European Journal of Immunology, 24*(8), 1853–1857.

Wenzlau, J. M., Liu, Y., Yu, L., Moua, O., Fowler, K. T., Rangasamy, S., et al. (2008). A common nonsynonymous single nucleotide polymorphism in the SLC30A8 gene determines ZnT8 autoantibody specificity in type 1 diabetes. *Diabetes, 57*(10), 2693–2697.

Winer, S., Astsaturov, I., Gaedigk, R., Hammond-McKibben, D., Pilon, M., Song, A., et al. (2002). ICA69(null) nonobese diabetic mice develop diabetes, but resist disease acceleration by cyclophosphamide. *Journal of Immunology, 168*(1), 475–482.

Wong, F. S., Siew, L. K., Scott, G., Thomas, I. J., Chapman, S., Viret, C., et al. (2009). Activation of insulin-reactive CD8 T-cells for development of autoimmune diabetes. *Diabetes, 58*(5), 1156–1164.

Wu, H. J., Ivanov, I. I., Darce, J., Hattori, K., Shima, T., Umesaki, Y., et al. (2010). Gut-residing segmented filamentous bacteria drive autoimmune arthritis via T helper 17 cells. *Immunity, 32*(6), 815–827.

Yamamoto, T., Yamato, E., Tashiro, F., Sato, T., Noso, S., Ikegami, H., et al. (2004). Development of autoimmune diabetes in glutamic acid decarboxylase 65 (GAD65) knockout NOD mice. *Diabetologia, 47*(2), 221–224.

Yamanouchi, J., Verdaguer, J., Han, B., Amrani, A., Serra, P., & Santamaria, P. (2003). Cross-priming of diabetogenic T cells dissociated from CTL-induced shedding of beta cell autoantigens. *Journal of Immunology, 171*(12), 6900–6909.

Yi, W., Seth, N. P., Martillotti, T., Wucherpfennig, K. W., Sant'Angelo, D. B., & Denzin, L. K. (2010). Targeted regulation of self-peptide presentation prevents type I diabetes in mice without disrupting general immunocompetence. *The Journal of Clinical Investigation, 120*(4), 1324–1336.

Ziegler, A. G., Hummel, M., Schenker, M., & Bonifacio, E. (1999). Autoantibody appearance and risk for development of childhood diabetes in offspring of parents with type 1 diabetes: The 2-year analysis of the German BABYDIAB Study. *Diabetes, 48*(3), 460–468.

CHAPTER SIX

Autophagy and Pancreatic β-Cells

Simona Mazza, Tania Maffucci[1]

Queen Mary University of London, Barts and The London School of Medicine and Dentistry, Blizard Institute, Centre for Diabetes, Inositide Signalling Group, London, United Kingdom

[1]Corresponding author: e-mail address: t.maffucci@qmul.ac.uk

Contents

Abstract

Autophagy plays a key role in maintaining pancreatic β-cell homeostasis. Deregulation of this process is associated with loss of β-cell mass and function, and it is likely to be involved in Type 2 diabetes development and progression. Evidence that modulation of autophagy may be beneficial to preserve β-cell mass and function is beginning to accumulate although the complexity of this process, the intricate link between autophagy and apoptosis, and the fine balance between the protective and the disruptive role of autophagy make it very difficult to develop interventional strategies. This chapter provides an overview of the role of constitutive and adaptive autophagy in pancreatic β-cell and in the context of Type 2 diabetes.

Vitamins and Hormones, Volume 95
ISSN 0083-6729
http://dx.doi.org/10.1016/B978-0-12-800174-5.00006-5

1. INTRODUCTION

Pancreatic β-cells are responsible for insulin secretion and control of plasma glucose levels. There is currently a huge interest to understand the precise cellular mechanisms regulating β-cell proliferation and/or survival and β-cell function. Interest has been fueled by accumulating evidence indicating that β-cell death and/or dysfunction plays a major role not only in Type 1 diabetes (caused by disruption of islets of Langerhans) but also in Type 2 diabetes. Type 2 diabetes is characterized by reduced insulin sensitivity and impaired pancreatic β-cell function resulting from genetic and acquired factors. Although insulin resistance plays a key role, the impairment of β-cell function appears to be the critical event inducing progressive deterioration of glycemic control (Bagust & Beale, 2003; Del Prato, Bianchi, & Marchetti, 2007; Weyer, Tataranni, Bogardus, & Pratley, 2001). Both reduced β-cell mass and impaired insulin secretion are responsible for progression from hyperglycemic conditions to diabetes; therefore, preservation of β-cell is an important therapeutic goal to prevent diabetes development and progression. So far, reduced pancreatic β-cell mass has been generally attributed to increased cell death, mostly through apoptosis, not compensated by adequate β-cell regeneration. Accumulating evidence has now revealed a critical role for other cellular processes, in particular autophagy, in regulation of pancreatic β-cell mass and function.

2. AUTOPHAGY

Autophagy is a finely regulated cellular process responsible for degradation and recycling of macromolecules, long-lived proteins, protein aggregates, and for the turnover of organelles (Codogno, Mehrpour, & Proikas-Cezanne, 2011; Mehrpour, Esclatine, Beau, & Codogno, 2010a). Three types of autophagy exist: chaperone-mediated autophagy, microautophagy, and macroautophagy. Chaperone-mediated autophagy targets specific proteins to lysosomes for degradation (Kaushik & Cuervo, 2012; Li, Yang, & Mao, 2011). Microautophagy occurs through direct engulfment of cytosolic components into lysosomal compartments and degradation (Li, Li, & Bao, 2012). Macroautophagy (usually referred to simply as "autophagy," as in this chapter) involves sequestration of cytoplasmic components in double-membrane-bound vacuoles (autophagosomes) that eventually fuse with lysosomes where the autophagosomes cargos are degraded

(Klionsky, 2007). The process was originally described and characterized in yeast. The identification of mammalian counterparts revealed that autophagy is conserved among eukaryotes. This chapter discusses only autophagy related to mammalian cells.

2.1. Autophagic flux

Autophagy is an extremely complex and tightly regulated cellular process (He & Klionsky, 2009; Mehrpour, Esclatine, Beau, & Codogno, 2010b) which can be schematically summarized in the following steps:

1. *Initiation step*: Autophagy starts with the generation of cup-shaped structures named phagophores or isolation membranes. These membranes elongate to form double-membrane-bound vacuoles named autophagosomes which engulf cytoplasmic material to be degraded.
2. *Maturation step*: Autophagosomes can then directly fuse with lysosomes, or they can further receive inputs from the endocytic pathway and form hybrid organelles named amphisomes. Autophagosomes or amphisomes are then trafficked along the microtubules to the microtubule-organizing center where lysosomes are clustered.
3. *Fusion step*: Autophagosomes/amphisomes fuse with lysosomes to generate autolysosomes. Degradation of autophagosomes content can then occur and molecules (amino acids, carbohydrates, lipids, etc.) can be recycled.

2.2. Mechanisms of regulation I: Protein complexes

The formation of the autophagosome is a multistep process (Xie & Klionsky, 2007). Autophagy-related (Atg) proteins appear to be hierarchically recruited to the phagophore assembly site to control the different steps of this process (Mehrpour et al., 2010a). These proteins can be functionally divided into four groups:

1. the Atg1 complex that is required during the initiation, nucleation, and expansion steps of autophagosome formation;
2. the Beclin 1 (mammalian ortholog of yeast Atg6)/hVps34 complex, which is involved in the nucleation phase;
3. two ubiquitin-like conjugation systems: microtubule-associated protein 1 light chain 3 (LC3, the mammalian ortholog of yeast Atg8) and Atg12. During the initiation step, Atg7 initiates the conjugation of Atg12 with Atg5 which in turn promotes the conjugation of LC3 with phosphatidylethanolamine (PE), required for the elongation step;

4. Atg1 and Atg9 which control the recycling of Atg proteins during autophagosomes formation.

Several other proteins are required for this process, including RabGTPase, involved in the maturation steps and SNAREs, required for the fusion steps and formation of the autolysosomes (Mehrpour et al., 2010b). Lysosomal-associated membrane protein 2 (Lamp2) is critical for the autophagosomes/lysosomes fusion, and indeed, its depletion results in inhibition of autophagic degradation (Eskelinen et al., 2002). Finally, lipids also play a key role in this process (Dall'Armi, Devereaux, & Di Paolo, 2013), in particular, phosphatidylinositol 3-phosphate (PtdIns3*P*) which is specifically synthesized by class III phosphoinositide 3-kinase (PI3K), hVps34.

1. The Atg1 complex is responsible for the initiation steps during autophagosome formation. At least five kinases closely related to yeast Atg1 in their N-terminal region have been found in vertebrates with the UNC51-like kinase 1 (Ulk1) and Ulk2 being the most related (Alers, Löffler, Wesselborg, & Stork, 2012). The current model suggests that Ulk1/2 form a complex with Atg13, FIP200, Atg101 (which does not have a counterpart in yeast) and a protein complex containing the enzyme mechanistic target of rapamycin (mTOR), described below.
2. The precise role of the Beclin 1/hVps34 complex in autophagy is still not totally understood although it is generally accepted that this complex is important to recruit other Atg proteins and for synthesis of PtdIns3*P* (Kang, Zeh, Lotze, & Tang, 2011). Beclin 1 binds both activators and inhibitors of autophagy which in turn can reduce or enhance its association to hVps34. For instance, under nutrient-rich conditions, the antiapoptotic protein Bcl2 associates strongly to Beclin 1 and this results in disruption of the Beclin 1/hVps34 interaction and autophagy inhibition. During starvation, Bcl2 dissociates from Beclin 1 allowing association of Beclin 1 with hVps34 and autophagy initiation. In addition, Beclin 1 can also associate with UVRAG, and this potentiates the Beclin 1/hVps34 interaction and promotes autophagy. Other regulators able to bind Beclin 1 include Ambra 1 (autophagy activator) and ICP34.5 (autophagy inhibitor; Pattingre, Espert, Biard-Piechaczyk, & Codogno, 2008).
3. A key protein in the autophagic process and one of the few markers currently available to monitor autophagy is LC3. During autophagosome formation, an LC3 precursor is cleaved by Atg4 and LC3-I is then conjugated to PE (LC3-II) by the complex Atg5/Atg12. LC3 seems to have a role during the formation and elongation of autophagosomes, and it is

also important to recruit proteins such as the ubiquitin-binding protein p62 (or sequestosome 1) to the autophagosomes. This protein possesses a LC3-binding domain and can mediate degradation of ubiquitinated proteins through autophagy.

2.3. Mechanisms of regulation II: Signaling pathways

One of the key enzymes responsible for regulation of autophagy is mTOR (Meijer & Codogno, 2004; Yang & Klionsky, 2009, 2010). mTOR is a master kinase involved in the regulation of a plethora of cellular functions mainly through activation of protein synthesis and in response to several stimuli including growth factors, nutrients, energy status, and oxygen levels (Laplante & Sabatini, 2012). mTOR exists in two complexes (mTORC1 and mTORC2) and data so far mostly implicated mTORC1 in autophagy regulation. Under nutrient-rich conditions, mTOR is mainly activated through a signaling cascade involving activation of class I PI3K/Akt, phosphorylation of tuberous sclerosis complex 2 (TSC2), and activation of the GTP-binding protein Rheb which in turn activates mTOR (Sengupta, Peterson, & Sabatini, 2010). During starvation, the PI3K/Akt pathway is switched off therefore mTOR is inactive. Starvation further results in activation of AMP-activated protein kinase (AMPK), a key enzyme in energy control (Carling, 2004). An AMPK-dependent phosphorylation results in the activation of TSC2 and therefore inhibition of Rheb and mTOR (Kwiatkowski & Manning, 2005). In addition to this indirect mechanism, AMPK can also further prevent mTOR activation by directly phosphorylating raptor, a key component of the mTORC1 complex (Alers et al., 2012). It must be noted that this is a very simplistic model of mTOR regulation and of the AMPK/mTOR cross talk which can be regulated by several distinct and complex signaling cascades. One of the mechanisms by which mTOR and AMPK can control autophagy is through the regulation of the Atg1 complex. Under nutrient-rich conditions, mTORC1 is associated with the complex Ulk1/2–FIP200–Atg13–Atg101: the mTOR-mediated phosphorylation of Atg13 and Ulk1/2 inhibits autophagy (Alers et al., 2012; Yang & Klionsky, 2010). Under starvation conditions, mTORC1 dissociates from the complex and this results in autophagy initiation. AMPK is critically involved in autophagy regulation not only due to its inhibitory effect on mTOR but also because of its ability to directly phosphorylate (and activate) Ulk1/2 (Alers et al., 2012). Recently, a role for mTOR in Ambra1 inhibition and Ulk1 ubiquitylation/stabilization has been reported (Nazio et al., 2013), indicating a complex mechanism of regulation of the autophagic complexes.

2.4. Cellular roles

Autophagy occurs at a basal rate in many cells (sometimes indicated as "constitutive" autophagy), and it has a critical physiological role in maintaining cytoplasmic homeostasis through removal of protein aggregates, ubiquitinated proteins, and macromolecules. In addition, autophagy is responsible for clearance of damaged and/or senescent organelles, including ribosomes (ribophagy; Kraft, Deplazes, Sohrmann, & Peter, 2008), endoplasmic reticulum (ER-phagy or reticulophagy; Cebollero, Reggiori, & Kraft, 2012), and mitochondria (mytophagy; Gottlieb & Carreira, 2010).

When the supply of nutrients is reduced or under conditions of environmental stress, autophagy can be induced to support energy needs (sometimes referred to as "adaptive" autophagy). Activation of autophagy during starvation can supply molecules to maintain protein and glucose synthesis and substrates for oxidation and ATP production in the mitochondria. For instance, induction of autophagy is critical in newborn mice to maintain energy levels in various tissues after interruption of the maternal supply through the placenta (Kuma et al., 2004), with a central role for mTOR in this process (Efeyan et al., 2013). Alternatively, autophagy can have a cytoprotective effect to inhibit apoptosis induced by mitochondria during starvation or mitochondrial damage. Based on all these data, autophagy is usually considered a prosurvival, protective cellular process, often opposing cellular apoptosis.

On the other hand, autophagy is also known as "Type 2 programmed cell death" since extended degradation of cytosolic components and organelles can represent a mechanism to induce cellular death (Gozuacik & Kimchi, 2004). This "death-promoting" role of autophagy can be activated as an alternative to apoptosis, or it can act in conjunction to apoptosis by activating apoptosis signals or by contributing to the removal of apoptotic cells. Based on several data (only few of them mentioned in this paragraph), it is evident that autophagy must be tightly and precisely regulated in order to guarantee the proper activation of its protective/prosurvival or its death-promoting role. There is currently a growing interest in understanding the mechanisms of autophagy regulation, and several lines of evidence now support the conclusion that deregulation of autophagy is involved in several diseases (Choi, Ryter, & Levine, 2013; Rubinsztein, Codogno, & Levine, 2012).

3. AUTOPHAGY AND PANCREATIC β-CELL HOMEOSTASIS

3.1. *In vivo* studies

3.1.1 Knockout mice

To study the role of autophagy in pancreatic β-cell, mouse models with deficient autophagy have been generated by ablation of the *Atg7* gene selectively in these cells (Ebato et al., 2008; Jung et al., 2008; Wu et al., 2009). In 2008, two studies were published simultaneously and they provided the definitive demonstration that constitutive autophagy is a key process in the maintenance of pancreatic β-cell homeostasis. Both studies showed that ablation of autophagy in β-cell results in increased glucose intolerance (Ebato et al., 2008; Jung et al., 2008) which was later confirmed in a third study that used a similar knockout model (Wu et al., 2009). Fasting serum insulin concentration was significantly lower in autophagy-impaired mice compared to control, and this was mainly due to reduced β-cell mass resulting from both reduced β-cell proliferation and increased β-cell apoptosis (Jung et al., 2008). Total insulin content was also reduced in the pancreas of knockout mice compared to control mice, and some β-cells showed reduced numbers of insulin granules (Jung et al., 2008). These data indicated that autophagy is critical for β-cell proliferation/survival and mass (Hur, Jung, & Lee, 2010; Jung & Lee, 2009). In addition, *ex vivo* experiments using healthy primary islets revealed impaired basal and glucose-stimulated insulin secretion in knockout mice, indicating that autophagy has also a role in the regulation of normal β-cell function independently of its effects on cell mass (Jung et al., 2008). Consistent with this conclusion, the second study reported no difference in insulin sensitivity in knockout mice despite increased glucose intolerance, suggesting impairment of β-cell function (Ebato et al., 2008). These authors further showed that glucose-induced (but not KCl-induced) stimulation of insulin secretion was reduced in isolated islets from knockout mice (Ebato et al., 2008; Fujitani, Ebato, Uchida, Kawamori, & Watada, 2009). Results from all these studies demonstrate that autophagy has a central role in control of pancreatic β-cell homeostasis and that deregulation of autophagy impairs β-cell function resulting in glucose intolerance (Fujitani, Ueno, & Watada, 2010).

3.1.2 *Aging*

A recent study has investigated the physiological changes in β-cell function associated with aging and its potential correlation with alteration of autophagy. The study compared several autophagic markers in islets from young (4 months), adult (12 months), and old (24 months) mice and detected reduced LC3-II, Atg7, Lamp-2 levels as well as increased p62 levels in old mice (Liu et al., 2013). Parallel reduction of β-cell function and glucose tolerance was also detected. These data may suggest that declined islets autophagy can represent one of the mechanisms responsible for the impairment of β-cell function detected with aging.

3.2. Role of autophagy in β-cells

Once the key role for autophagy in regulation of β-cell mass, proliferation, survival, and function is established, the question is: how does autophagy control pancreatic β-cell homeostasis?

3.2.1 *Role of mitophagy in β-cells*

Mitochondria play a pivotal role in pancreatic β-cell not only for normal energy control but also to regulate proper response to glucose stimulation and β-cell function (Las & Shirihai, 2010). Autophagy (better defined as mitophagy) is responsible for removing damaged, depolarized mitochondria, and this is critical to prevent mitochondrial damage-induced apoptosis and accumulation of reactive oxygen species (Twig, Elorza, et al., 2008; Twig, Hyde, & Shirihai, 2008). *In vivo* studies confirmed that this "organelle quality control" function of autophagy is extremely important to guarantee β-cell homeostasis and function. Pancreatic β-cell-specific Atg7-deficient mice showed swelling of mitochondria and cisternal distension of rough ER and Golgi complex (Hur et al., 2010; Jung et al., 2008). Moreover, isolated islets from these mice showed reduced glucose-stimulated ATP production, suggesting accumulation of dysfunctional mitochondria (Ebato et al., 2008; Fujitani, Ebato, et al., 2009). Dysfunction of ER and mitochondria was therefore indicated as one of the main reasons for the impairment of β-cell function and increased apoptosis/reduced survival detected in these mice (Jung et al., 2008). Accumulation of swollen, dysmorphic mitochondria in Atg7-deficient β-cells was also reported in the third study (Wu et al., 2009) which further demonstrated that basal mitochondrial respiration and oxidative capacity were strongly impaired in the absence of autophagy. Swelling of mitochondria, disintegration of mitochondrial cistae together with significant increase of oxidative damaged were also observed in aged mice with impaired autophagy (Liu et al., 2013), supporting the conclusion that autophagy plays a central role in preservation of mitochondrial function.

3.2.2 Role of ER-phagy in β-cells

As mentioned earlier, pancreatic β-cell-specific Atg7-deficient mice showed cisternal distension of rough ER and Golgi complex (Hur et al., 2010; Jung et al., 2008) which was considered partly responsible for the impaired β-cell function and survival (Jung et al., 2008). Because of their highly secretory function, protein synthesis (mainly proinsulin synthesis) is elevated in β-cells which are therefore more prone to accumulation of unfolded or misfolded proteins that can induce ER stress. ER stress activates adaptive cellular responses including unfolded protein response (UPR) which prevents accumulation of unfolded/misfolded proteins mainly by upregulating antioxidant production or chaperone expression or by recruiting ubiquitin-conjugating enzymes to increase protein degradation (Back, Kang, Han, & Chung, 2012). In addition, ER stress can activate ER-associated degradation (ERAD) which allows ubiquitination and degradation of misfolded proteins by retro-translocating them across the ER (Back et al., 2012). A good "ER quality control" and perfectly functioning ER are required to avoid an unbalance between production and degradation of misfolded proteins. Downregulation of UPR genes and other genes involved in protection against ER stress was detected in autophagy-deficient β-cells (Quan, Hur, et al., 2012; Quan, Lim, & Lee, 2012), indicating that autophagy is required to guarantee a proper ER stress response. Consistent with this, it was further shown that free fatty acids (FFAs)-induced UPR was impaired in autophagy-deficient β-cells, and this resulted in more pronounced ER stress-induced death (Quan, Hur, et al., 2012; Quan, Lim, et al., 2012). Taken together, these data demonstrate that autophagy is critical for quality control of the ER and activation of proper cellular responses to ER stress.

3.2.3 Prevention of ubiquitinated-protein aggregation

Unfolded/misfolded proteins that cannot be degraded through UPR or ERAD (sometime defined terminally misfolded proteins) form aggregates intracellularly. While soluble aggregates, as well as short-lived proteins, are usually removed by the ubiquitin–proteasome pathway, studies have revealed that insoluble aggregates and long-lived proteins are degraded through autophagy (Kirkin, Lamark, Johansen, & Dikic, 2009; Komatsu et al., 2005). Consistent with this, accumulation of ubiquitin aggregates, p62, and large cystic structures was reported in islets of β-cell-specific Atg7 knockout mice (Ebato et al., 2008; Fujitani, Ebato, et al., 2009; Hur et al., 2010; Jung et al., 2008). This role of autophagy in preventing accumulation of protein aggregates seems to be critical for protection of pancreatic β-cells, especially in stressful environments, as discussed in more details below.

3.2.4 Proinsulin turnover

Autophagy is important for proper regulation of proinsulin/insulin synthesis and degradation. Indeed, the first indication that autophagy is a crucial process for pancreatic β-cell homeostasis came from a study on a mouse model with deficient insulin secretion (Rab3A$^{-/-}$). Electron microscopy (EM) analysis revealed an increase in the number and size of degradative compartments (multigranular bodies) in β-cells from Rab3A$^{-/-}$ compared to wild-type mice (Marsh et al., 2007). Microautophagy and macroautophagy as well as downregulation of Lamp2 were detected in islets and β-cells of Rab3A$^{-/-}$ but not in wild-type mice. The authors proposed that in the presence of defective insulin secretion autophagy could be increased to accelerate insulin degradation rate and maintain normal insulin content (Marsh et al., 2007). More recently, it has been suggested that autophagy is directly involved in normal regulation of insulin content through control of proinsulin disposal (Zhang et al., 2011). In this study, inhibition of autophagy using chemical drugs reduced proinsulin disposal by 20–37%. This observation led the authors to propose that autophagy contributes to the normal processing of insulin, and it may represent an important mechanism for proinsulin disposal.

4. ADAPTIVE AUTOPHAGY IN PANCREATIC β-CELL

4.1. Adaptive/protective role of β-cell autophagy during insulin resistance

Evidence of autophagy upregulation under insulin-resistant conditions has been reported. Increased number of large autophagosomes was detected by EM analysis in cells from *db/db* mice or C57BL/6 mice fed a high-fat diet (HFD) for 12 weeks (Ebato et al., 2008), and increased autophagic activity was also observed in a mouse model of obesity (*ob/ob*) mice (Quan, Hur, et al., 2012; Quan, Lim, et al., 2012). The key role of β-cell autophagy during insulin resistance was confirmed when 8-week-old control and β-cell-specific Atg7 knockout mice were fed HFD for 12 weeks. Significantly, higher nonfasting glucose levels and severely impaired glucose tolerance were detected in knockout mice compared to wild-type mice together with reduced β-cell proliferation and increased apoptosis, increase of degenerative vacuoles and p62 immunoreactivity (Ebato et al., 2008; Fujitani, Ebato, et al., 2009). Importantly, obese mice with deficient β-cell autophagy developed severe diabetes (discussed in more details below). These studies revealed that deficient autophagy results in worsened β-cell survival and function under insulin-resistant conditions and may possibly accelerate progression from hyperglycemic conditions to diabetes development. This has led to the hypothesis that autophagy is upregulated under insulin-resistant condition as a protective mechanism. Consistent with this hypothesis, it has been reported that further enhancement of autophagy (through mTOR inhibition) ameliorates the FFAs-induced apoptosis (Choi et al., 2009). This led the author to conclude that autophagy may have a protective role toward FFAs-induced cell death.

4.2. Role of β-cell autophagy during insulin resistance

Why should autophagy be upregulated under insulin-resistant conditions? The onset of peripheral insulin resistance, as in the obese state, is usually accompanied by a compensatory response whereby β-cell mass is increased to sustain the elevated insulin demand. Due to its role in regulation of β-cell mass and function, autophagy may be crucial to activate a proper compensatory response. Consistent with this hypothesis, the severe impairment of glucose tolerance detected in HFD-fed, autophagy-deficient mice (β-cell Atg7 knockout) was indeed due, at least in part, to impaired ability to induce compensatory hyperplasia of β-cells (Ebato et al., 2008; Fujitani, Ebato, et al., 2009).

In addition, increased proinsulin synthesis under insulin-resistant conditions can induce accumulation of protein aggregates, as observed in acinar and β-cells of 19-week Zucker diabetic fatty rats but not in control, nondiabetic rats (Kaniuk et al., 2007). Under these conditions, autophagy may be critical to remove these aggregates and protect from ER stress-induced cell death. Consistent with this hypothesis, it has been reported that stimulation of autophagy in INS 832/13 using the mTOR inhibitor rapamycin protected from apoptosis whereas autophagy inhibition increased apoptosis induced by accumulation of human islets amyloid polypeptide (Rivera et al., 2011). Similarly, autophagy inhibition in INS1 832/12 cells appeared to induce aggregates accumulation in cells in normal and in high glucose concentrations (Kaniuk et al., 2007). Whether the protective role of autophagy under insulin-resistant conditions is indeed due to increased protein aggregates degradation remains to be established since it has also been proposed that autophagy upregulation in *ob/ob* mice is mainly required to eliminate lipids through lipophagy (Quan, Hur, et al., 2012).

4.3. Regulation of adaptive autophagy—Lipotoxicity

The mechanisms involved in stimulation of the adaptive/protective autophagy are not totally defined although it has been suggested that long-chain FFAs may be involved (Fujitani, Kawamori, & Watada, 2009). Treatment of INS1 cells with FFAs induces autophagosomes formation and/or accumulation as assessed by EM, Western blotting, and immunofluorescence analysis (Choi et al., 2009). Similarly, exposure of human islets from nondiabetic individuals to NEFA increased the number of dead β-cells showing vacuole engulfment, increased density volume of autophagic vacuoles, increased autophagosomes, and reduced levels of Lamp2 gene expression (Masini, Bugliani, et al., 2009). Few studies have further reported that FFAs are able to increase autophagy in β-cells (Komiya et al., 2010; Martino et al., 2012) and isolated islets (Martino et al., 2012) although a clarification is needed at this point. As briefly mentioned before, two of the most used readouts for autophagy stimulation are Western blotting analysis of LC3 (conjugation of LC3 with PE results in the appearance of a second band of lower molecular weight, LC3-II) and immunofluorescence analysis of LC3 localization (LC3-II localizes to the autophagosome, detected as bright puncta in the cytoplasm). The interpretation of LC3 results, however, has sometimes created some confusion in the literature. Defective final steps in the autophagy flux (for instance, defective autolysosomes formation or lysosomal degradation of the autophagosomal content) would result in accumulation of LC3-II which can be mistakenly interpreted as enhanced autophagosomes formation. For this reason, when studying autophagy, it is important to establish whether accumulation of LC3-II is due to increased formation of autophagosomes or rather to defective fusion with lysosomes and/or lysosomal degradation. Some evidence indeed suggests that the accumulation of autophagosomes observed in FFAs-treated cells may not be due to increased autophagosomes formation but rather to reduced autophagic turnover in β-cells (Las, Serada, Wikstrom, Twig, & Shirihai, 2011). This would support the hypothesis that FFAs are involved in deregulation of the normal autophagic process which would be probably more consistent with the observation that deregulation of autophagy occurs in Type 2 diabetic patients (see below).

4.4. Regulation of adaptive autophagy—Glucotoxicity

Contrasting evidence exists in the literature on the role of high glucose levels in autophagy regulation. Increased autophagy flux has been observed in INS1 and rat islets treated with high glucose concentrations, and blockade of autophagic degradation has been reported to increase high glucose-induced apoptosis (Han et al., 2010). Similarly, it has been proposed that oxidative stress induced by high glucose is mainly responsible for accumulation of ubiquitinated-protein aggregates which colocalizes with GFP-LC3 (Kaniuk et al., 2007). However, in another study, high glucose did not seem to have any effect on autophagy in INS1E, rat, and human islets (Martino et al., 2012).

5. AUTOPHAGY AND DIABETES

Data summarized so far have established that (1) autophagy is critical for normal pancreatic β-cell homeostasis, specifically β-cell proliferation/survival and function; (2) autophagy can be induced in stressful environments (such as under insulin-resistant conditions) to preserve pancreatic β-cell; (3) deregulation of autophagy (induced in animal models by genetic manipulation or as detected under physiological conditions as in aging) results in impairment of β-cell proliferation/survival and function under normal conditions; and (4) deregulation of autophagy exacerbates β-cell dysfunction and death under stressful conditions. It is therefore not surprising that several lines of evidence now support the conclusion that autophagy may play a critical role in Type 2 diabetes progression (Fujitani et al., 2010; Gonzalez et al., 2011). Only a couple of the most compelling evidence are discussed here.

As briefly mentioned before, crossing of β-cell Atg7 knockout with *ob/ob* mice revealed that obese mice with deficient β-cell autophagy developed severe diabetes with highly elevated nonfasting and fasting glucose levels and aggravated glucose intolerance (Quan, Hur, et al., 2012; Quan, Lim, et al., 2012). In contrast, mice with β-cell autophagy deficiency alone or obese mice alone only developed hyperglycaemia (Quan, Hur, et al., 2012; Quan, Lim, et al., 2012), supporting the conclusion that autophagy deregulation may accelerate the progression from hyperglycemic conditions to diabetes (Quan, Jung, & Lee, 2013), and therefore that deregulated autophagy may play a critical role in Type 2 diabetes progression.

Alteration of autophagy has, indeed, been detected in β-cells from Type 2 diabetic subjects (Marchetti & Masini, 2009; Masini, Bugliani, et al., 2009; Masini, Lupi, et al., 2009). A comparison of islets from Type 2 diabetic patients and a matched group of nondiabetic subjects showed increased number of dead β-cells in diabetic patients than in controls (Masini, Bugliani, et al., 2009). While almost 50% of the dead β-cells showed clear sign of apoptosis, the remaining 50% of cells showed accumulation of vacuoles in the cytoplasm with no sign of nuclear alterations, suggesting autophagy-associated cell death. Analysis of mRNA from these groups revealed that expression of Beclin-1 and Ulk1 was not affected in diabetic patients, whereas reduced transcription of Lamp2, cathepsin B, and cathepsin D was observed (Masini, Bugliani, et al., 2009), suggesting that defect in the late stage of autophagy occurs in β-cells of Type 2 diabetic patients.

6. MODULATION OF AUTOPHAGY AS THERAPEUTIC STRATEGY

Several studies are currently investigating the possibility of developing novel therapeutic strategies by targeting autophagy (Rubinsztein et al., 2012). Emerging evidence supports the hypothesis that modulation of autophagy may be beneficial to protect pancreatic β-cells and possibly counteract the progression toward diabetes.

In cellular systems, it has been shown that transferring of INS1 cells to normal glucose concentration after 48 h incubation in 30 mM glucose reduced the percentage of cells containing ubiquitinated-protein aggregates (Kaniuk et al., 2007), suggesting that accumulation of ubiquitinated-protein aggregates may be reversible. Consistent with this, data seem to suggest that stimulation of autophagy reduces apoptosis induced by FFAs and increases cell survival of β-cells (Choi et al., 2009; Las et al., 2011). Furthermore, treatment with the antioxidant *N*-acetylcysteine restored normal glucose tolerance in β-cell-specific Atg7-deficient mice (Wu et al., 2009), suggesting that oxidative stress induced by impaired mitochondrial function may also be reversible.

More importantly, a recent study has suggested that stimulation of autophagy may ameliorate diabetes induced by ER stress (Bachar-Wikstrom, Wikstrom, Ariav, et al., 2013). In this study, the authors used the *Akita* mice which possess the *C(A7)Y proinsulin* mutation. In this animal model, increased proinsulin misfolding (due to the mutation) leads to elevated ER stress and severe congenital diabetes. The authors first showed that basal autophagic flux was also increased in *Akita* β-cells (Bachar-Wikstrom, Wikstrom, Ariav, et al., 2013), suggesting that ER stress is able to stimulate autophagy. Treatment of *Akita* mice with rapamycin (which inhibits mTOR and therefore further stimulates autophagy) reduced β-cell apoptosis and it ameliorated ER stress. As a result, fed blood glucose levels in rapamycin-treated *Akita* mice were reduced to levels detected in control mice while both insulin content and insulin serum level were increased (Bachar-Wikstrom, Wikstrom, Ariav, et al., 2013). These data suggested that stimulation of autophagy can improve the ER stress-induced diabetes (Bachar-Wikstrom, Wikstrom, Ariav, et al., 2013; Bachar-Wikstrom, Wikstrom, Kaiser, Cerasi, & Leibowitz, 2013).

Due to the complexity of the process, it is still not clear whether stimulation of autophagy may always represent a clear interventional strategy (Chen et al., 2011). For instance, stimulation of autophagy by rapamycin has also been reported to reduce islets viability, mitochondrial integrity, and β-cell function (Tanemura et al., 2012). Similarly, beneficial effects were observed by inhibiting autophagy in the context of reduced expression of pancreas duodenal homeobox 1 (Fujimoto et al., 2008). It is very likely that rather than simply stimulating autophagy, a more appropriate interventional strategy should aim at preventing or overcoming autophagy deregulation. Based on evidence from human islets, it appears that deregulated autophagy might mainly derive from defects in the late steps of the process, that is, autolysosomes formation or lysosomal degradation (Masini, Bugliani, et al., 2009). In this respect, a strategy aimed at simply increasing autophagosomes formation probably would not be beneficial at all (in fact, possibly detrimental), whereas preventing or counteracting autophagy deregulation would be more appropriate. Some evidence supports the possibility that deregulation of autophagy can be reversible. Indeed, it has been shown that alteration detected in human islets from nondiabetic individuals exposed to NEFA was ameliorated by treatment of cells with metformin (Masini, Bugliani, et al., 2009).

It may also be worth mentioning that one study has also suggested that modulation of autophagy can be beneficial to preserve islets for transplantation. During isolation, blood vessels inside islets are destroyed. It has been speculated that autophagy can have an important role during this starvation time. A recent study reported that induction of autophagy (using trehalose, rapamycin, or amino acids deprivation) increased apoptosis of isolated human islets under hypoxic conditions. On the other hand, preincubation of islets with these autophagic inducers prior transferring of islets under hypoxic conditions was indeed able to protect them from apoptosis. These results led the authors to propose that autophagy manipulation during culturing of islets before transplantation may be beneficial (Wang, Crager, & Pugazhenthi, 2012).

7. CONCLUSIONS AND FUTURE DIRECTIONS

Several studies have now established the key role of autophagy in maintaining pancreatic β-cell homeostasis. Emerging evidence is also supporting the conclusion that deregulation of this process occurs in Type 2 diabetes, and it is likely to be associated with loss of β-cell mass and function. While modulation of autophagy may potentially represent an important novel therapeutic strategy our still limited and scarce understanding of this process and of the mechanisms of its regulation in β-cells is preventing a proper exploitation of autophagy. More studies are needed to better clarify if autophagy deregulation indeed occurs in diabetes, if this is partly responsible for β-cell dysfunction associated with this disease and, more importantly, whether modulation of autophagy may indeed be beneficial to develop potential therapeutic strategies.

ACKNOWLEDGMENTS

Simona Mazza and work in the laboratory are supported by Diabetes UK (Grant BDA:09/0003971 to Tania Maffucci).

REFERENCES

Alers, S., Löffler, A. S., Wesselborg, S., & Stork, B. (2012). Role of AMPK-mTOR-Ulk1/2 in the regulation of autophagy: Cross talk, shortcuts, and feedbacks. *Molecular and Cellular Biology*, *32*, 2–11.

Bachar-Wikstrom, E., Wikstrom, J. D., Ariav, Y., Tirosh, B., Kaiser, N., Cerasi, E., et al. (2013). Stimulation of autophagy improves endoplasmic reticulum stress-induced diabetes. *Diabetes*, *62*, 1227–1237.

Bachar-Wikstrom, E., Wikstrom, J. D., Kaiser, N., Cerasi, E., & Leibowitz, G. (2013). Improvement of ER stress-induced diabetes by stimulating autophagy. *Autophagy*, *9*, 626–628.

Back, S. H., Kang, S. W., Han, J., & Chung, H. T. (2012). Endoplasmic reticulum stress in the β-cell pathogenesis of type 2 diabetes. *Experimental Diabetes Research*, *2012*, 618396.

Bagust, A., & Beale, S. (2003). Deteriorating beta-cell function in type 2 diabetes: A long-term model. *QJM*, *96*, 281–288.

Carling, D. (2004). The AMP-activated protein kinase cascade—A unifying system for energy control. *Trends in Biochemical Sciences*, *29*, 18–24.

Cebollero, E., Reggiori, F., & Kraft, C. (2012). Reticulophagy and ribophagy: Regulated degradation of protein production factories. *International Journal of Cell Biology*, *2012*, 182834.

Chen, Z. F., Li, Y. B., Han, J. Y., Wang, J., Yin, J. J., Li, J. B., et al. (2011). The double-edged effect of autophagy in pancreatic beta cells and diabetes. *Autophagy*, *7*, 12–16.

Choi, S. E., Lee, S. M., Lee, Y. J., Li, L. J., Lee, S. J., Lee, J. H., et al. (2009). Protective role of autophagy in palmitate-induced INS-1 beta-cell death. *Endocrinology*, *150*, 126–134.

Choi, A. M., Ryter, S. W., & Levine, B. (2013). Autophagy in human health and disease. *The New England Journal of Medicine*, *368*, 651–662.

Codogno, P., Mehrpour, M., & Proikas-Cezanne, T. (2011). Canonical and non-canonical autophagy: Variations on a common theme of self-eating? *Nature Reviews. Molecular Cell Biology*, *13*, 7–12.

Dall'Armi, C., Devereaux, K. A., & Di Paolo, G. (2013). The role of lipids in the control of autophagy. *Current Biology*, *23*, R33–R45.

Del Prato, S., Bianchi, C., & Marchetti, P. (2007). beta-cell function and anti-diabetic pharmacotherapy. *Diabetes/Metabolism Research and Reviews*, *23*, 518–527.

Ebato, C., Uchida, T., Arakawa, M., Komatsu, M., Ueno, T., Komiya, K., et al. (2008). Autophagy is important in islet homeostasis and compensatory increase of beta cell mass in response to high-fat diet. *Cell Metabolism*, *8*, 325–332.

Efeyan, A., Zoncu, R., Chang, S., Gumper, I., Snitkin, H., Wolfson, R. L., et al. (2013). Regulation of mTORC1 by the Rag GTPases is necessary for neonatal autophagy and survival. *Nature*, *493*, 679–683.

Eskelinen, E. L., Illert, A. L., Tanaka, Y., Schwarzmann, G., Blanz, J., Von Figura, K., et al. (2002). Role of LAMP-2 in lysosome biogenesis and autophagy. *Molecular Biology of the Cell*, *13*, 3355–3368.

Fujimoto, K., Hanson, P. T., Tran, H., Ford, E. L., Han, Z., Johnson, J. D., et al. (2008). Autophagy regulates pancreatic beta cell death in response to Pdx1 deficiency and nutrient deprivation. *The Journal of Biological Chemistry*, *284*, 27664–27673.

Fujitani, Y., Ebato, C., Uchida, T., Kawamori, R., & Watada, H. (2009). β-cell autophagy: A novel mechanism regulating β-cell function and mass: Lessons from β-cell-specific Atg7-deficient mice. *Islets*, *1*, 151–153.

Fujitani, Y., Kawamori, R., & Watada, H. (2009). The role of autophagy in pancreatic beta-cell and diabetes. *Autophagy*, *5*, 280–282.

Fujitani, Y., Ueno, T., & Watada, H. (2010). Autophagy in health and disease. 4. The role of pancreatic beta-cell autophagy in health and diabetes. *American Journal of Physiology Cell Physiology*, *299*, C1–C6.

Gonzalez, C. D., Lee, M. S., Marchetti, P., Pietropaolo, M., Towns, R., Vaccaro, M. I., et al. (2011). The emerging role of autophagy in the pathophysiology of diabetes mellitus. *Autophagy*, *7*, 2–11.

Gottlieb, R. A., & Carreira, R. S. (2010). Autophagy in health and disease. 5. Mitophagy as a way of life. *American Journal of Physiology Cell Physiology*, *299*, C203–C210.

Gozuacik, D., & Kimchi, A. (2004). Autophagy as a cell death and tumor suppressor mechanism. *Oncogene*, *23*, 2891–2906.

Han, D., Yang, B., Olson, L. K., Greenstein, A., Baek, S. H., Claycombe, K. J., et al. (2010). Activation of autophagy through modulation of 5′-AMP-activated protein kinase protects pancreatic beta-cells from high glucose. *Biochemical Journal*, *425*, 541–551.

He, C., & Klionsky, D. J. (2009). Regulation mechanisms and signaling pathways of autophagy. *Annual Review of Genetics*, *43*, 67–93.

Hur, K. Y., Jung, H. S., & Lee, M. S. (2010). Role of autophagy in β-cell function and mass. *Diabetes, Obesity and Metabolism, 12*(Suppl. 2), 20–26.
Jung, H. S., Chung, K. W., Won Kim, J., Kim, J., Komatsu, M., Tanaka, K., et al. (2008). Loss of autophagy diminishes pancreatic beta cell mass and function with resultant hyperglycemia. *Cell Metabolism, 8*, 318–324.
Jung, H. S., & Lee, M. S. (2009). Macroautophagy in homeostasis of pancreatic beta-cell. *Autophagy, 5*, 241–243.
Kang, R., Zeh, H. J., Lotze, M. T., & Tang, D. (2011). The Beclin 1 network regulates autophagy and apoptosis. *Cell Death & Differentiation, 18*, 571–580.
Kaniuk, N. A., Kiraly, M., Bates, H., Vranic, M., Volchuk, A., & Brumell, J. H. (2007). Ubiquitinated-protein aggregates form in pancreatic beta-cells during diabetes-induced oxidative stress and are regulated by autophagy. *Diabetes, 56*, 930–939.
Kaushik, S., & Cuervo, A. M. (2012). Chaperone-mediated autophagy: A unique way to enter the lysosome world. *Trends in Cell Biology, 22*, 407–417.
Kirkin, V., Lamark, T., Johansen, T., & Dikic, I. (2009). NBR1 cooperates with p62 in selective autophagy of ubiquitinated targets. *Autophagy, 5*, 732–733.
Klionsky, D. J. (2007). Autophagy: From phenomenology to molecular understanding in less than a decade. *Nature Reviews Molecular Cell Biology, 8*, 931–937.
Komatsu, M., Waguri, S., Ueno, T., Iwata, J., Murata, S., Tanida, I., et al. (2005). Impairment of starvation-induced and constitutive autophagy in Atg7-deficient mice. *The Journal of Cell Biology, 169*, 425–434.
Komiya, K., Uchida, T., Ueno, T., Koike, M., Abe, H., Hirose, T., et al. (2010). Free fatty acids stimulate autophagy in pancreatic β-cells via JNK pathway. *Biochemical and Biophysical Research Communications, 401*, 561–567.
Kraft, C., Deplazes, A., Sohrmann, M., & Peter, M. (2008). Mature ribosomes are selectively degraded upon starvation by an autophagy pathway requiring the Ubp3p/Bre5p ubiquitin protease. *Nature Cell Biology, 10*, 602–610.
Kuma, A., Hatano, M., Matsui, M., Yamamoto, A., Nakaya, H., Yoshimori, T., et al. (2004). The role of autophagy during the early neonatal starvation period. *Nature, 432*, 1032–1036.
Kwiatkowski, D. J., & Manning, B. D. (2005). Tuberous sclerosis: A GAP at the crossroads of multiple signaling pathways. *Human Molecular Genetics, 14*, R251–R258.
Laplante, M., & Sabatini, D. M. (2012). mTOR signaling in growth control and disease. *Cell, 149*, 274–293.
Las, G., Serada, S. B., Wikstrom, J. D., Twig, G., & Shirihai, O. S. (2011). Fatty acids suppress autophagic turnover in β-cells. *The Journal of Biological Chemistry, 286*, 42534–42544.
Las, G., & Shirihai, O. S. (2010). The role of autophagy in β-cell lipotoxicity and type 2 diabetes. *Diabetes, Obesity and Metabolism, 12*(Suppl. 2), 15–19.
Li, W. W., Li, J., & Bao, J. K. (2012). Microautophagy: Lesser-known self-eating. *Cellular and Molecular Life Sciences, 69*, 1125–1136.
Li, W., Yang, Q., & Mao, Z. (2011). Chaperone-mediated autophagy: Machinery, regulation and biological consequences. *Cellular and Molecular Life Sciences, 68*, 749–763.
Liu, Y., Shi, S., Gu, Z., Du, Y., Liu, M., Yan, S., et al. (2013). Impaired autophagic function in rat islets with aging. *Age (Dordrecht, Netherlands), 35*, 1531–1544.
Marchetti, P., & Masini, M. (2009). Autophagy and the pancreatic beta-cell in human type 2 diabetes. *Autophagy, 5*, 1055–1056.
Marsh, B. J., Soden, C., Alarcón, C., Wicksteed, B. L., Yaekura, K., Costin, A. J., et al. (2007). Regulated autophagy controls hormone content in secretory-deficient pancreatic endocrine beta-cells. *Molecular Endocrinology, 21*, 2255–2269.
Martino, L., Masini, M., Novelli, M., Beffy, P., Bugliani, M., Marselli, L., et al. (2012). Palmitate activates autophagy in INS-1E β-cells and in isolated rat and human pancreatic islets. *PLoS One*, 7, e36188.

Masini, M., Bugliani, M., Lupi, R., del Guerra, S., Boggi, U., Filipponi, F., et al. (2009). Autophagy in human type 2 diabetes pancreatic beta cells. *Diabetologia*, *52*, 1083–1086.
Masini, M., Lupi, R., Bugliani, M., Boggi, U., Filipponi, F., Masiello, P., et al. (2009). A role for autophagy in β-cell life and death. *Islets*, *1*, 157–159.
Mehrpour, M., Esclatine, A., Beau, I., & Codogno, P. (2010a). Autophagy in health and disease. 1. Regulation and significance of autophagy: An overview. *American Journal of Physiology. Cell Physiology*, *298*, C776–C785.
Mehrpour, M., Esclatine, A., Beau, I., & Codogno, P. (2010b). Overview of macroautophagy regulation in mammalian cells. *Cell Research*, *20*, 748–762.
Meijer, A. J., & Codogno, P. (2004). Regulation and role of autophagy in mammalian cells. *The International Journal of Biochemistry & Cell Biology*, *36*, 2445–2462.
Nazio, F., Strappazzon, F., Antonioli, M., Bielli, P., Cianfanelli, V., Bordi, M., et al. (2013). mTOR inhibits autophagy by controlling ULK1 ubiquitylation, self-association and function through AMBRA1 and TRAF6. *Nature Cell Biology*, *15*, 406–416.
Pattingre, S., Espert, L., Biard-Piechaczyk, M., & Codogno, P. (2008). Regulation of macroautophagy by mTOR and Beclin 1 complexes. *Biochimie*, *90*, 313–323.
Quan, W., Hur, K. Y., Lim, Y., Oh, S. H., Lee, J. C., Kim, K. H., et al. (2012). Autophagy deficiency in beta cells leads to compromised unfolded protein response and progression from obesity to diabetes in mice. *Diabetologia*, *55*, 392–403.
Quan, W., Jung, H. S., & Lee, M. S. (2013). Role of autophagy in the progression from obesity to diabetes and in the control of energy balance. *Archives of Pharmacal Research*, *36*, 223–229.
Quan, W., Lim, Y. M., & Lee, M. S. (2012). Role of autophagy in diabetes and endoplasmic reticulum stress of pancreatic β-cells. *Experimental and Molecular Medicine*, *44*, 81–88.
Rivera, J. F., Gurlo, T., Daval, M., Huang, C. J., Matveyenko, A. V., Butler, P. C., et al. (2011). Human-IAPP disrupts the autophagy/lysosomal pathway in pancreatic β-cells: Protective role of p62-positive cytoplasmic inclusions. *Cell Death & Differentiation*, *18*, 415–426.
Rubinsztein, D. C., Codogno, P., & Levine, B. (2012). Autophagy modulation as a potential therapeutic target for diverse diseases. *Nature Reviews. Drug Discovery*, *11*, 709–730.
Sengupta, S., Peterson, T. R., & Sabatini, D. M. (2010). Regulation of the mTOR complex 1 pathway by nutrients, growth factors, and stress. *Molecular Cell*, *40*, 310–322.
Tanemura, M., Ohmura, Y., Deguchi, T., Machida, T., Tsukamoto, R., Wada, H., et al. (2012). Rapamycin causes upregulation of autophagy and impairs islets function both in vitro and in vivo. *American Journal of Transplantation*, *12*, 102–114.
Twig, G., Elorza, A., Molina, A. J., Mohamed, H., Wikstrom, J. D., Walzer, G., et al. (2008). Fission and selective fusion govern mitochondrial segregation and elimination by autophagy. *The EMBO Journal*, *27*, 433–446.
Twig, G., Hyde, B., & Shirihai, O. S. (2008). Mitochondrial fusion, fission and autophagy as a quality control axis: The bioenergetic view. *Biochimica et Biophysica Acta*, *1777*, 1092–1097.
Wang, M., Crager, M., & Pugazhenthi, S. (2012). Modulation of apoptosis pathways by oxidative stress and autophagy in β cells. *Experimental Diabetes Research*, *2012*, 647914.
Weyer, C., Tataranni, P. A., Bogardus, C., & Pratley, R. E. (2001). Insulin resistance and insulin secretory dysfunction are independent predictors of worsening of glucose tolerance during each stage of type 2 diabetes development. *Diabetes Care*, *24*, 89–94.
Wu, J. J., Quijano, C., Chen, E., Liu, H., Cao, L., Fergusson, M. M., et al. (2009). Mitochondrial dysfunction and oxidative stress mediate the physiological impairment induced by the disruption of autophagy. *Aging*, *1*, 425–437.
Xie, Z., & Klionsky, D. J. (2007). Autophagosome formation: Core machinery and adaptations. *Nature Cell Biology*, *9*, 1102–1109.

Yang, Z., & Klionsky, D. J. (2009). An overview of the molecular mechanism of autophagy. *Current Topics in Microbiology and Immunology, 335*, 1–32.
Yang, Z., & Klionsky, D. J. (2010). Mammalian autophagy: Core molecular machinery and signaling regulation. *Current Opinion in Cell Biology, 22*, 124–131.
Zhang, X., Yuan, Q., Tang, W., Gu, J., Osei, K., & Wang, J. (2011). Substrate-favored lysosomal and proteasomal pathways participate in the normal balance control of insulin precursor maturation and disposal in β-cells. *PLoS One, 6*, e27647.

CHAPTER SEVEN

The Somatostatin Receptor in Human Pancreatic β-Cells

Matthias Braun[1,✠]
Alberta Diabetes Institute, Department of Pharmacology, Faculty of Medicine and Dentistry, University of Alberta, Edmonton, Alberta, Canada
[1]Corresponding author: e-mail address: mbraun1@ualberta.ca

Contents

Abstract

The peptide hormone somatostatin (SST) is produced in the brain, the gut, and in δ-cells in pancreatic islets of Langerhans. SST secretion from δ-cells is stimulated by glucose, amino acids, and glucagon-like peptide-1. Exogenous SST strongly inhibits the secretion of the blood glucose-regulating hormones insulin and glucagon from pancreatic β-cells and α-cells, respectively. Endogenous SST secreted from δ-cells is a paracrine regulator of insulin and glucagon secretion, although the exact physiological significance of this

✠Deceased

Vitamins and Hormones, Volume 95
ISSN 0083-6729
http://dx.doi.org/10.1016/B978-0-12-800174-5.00007-7

regulation is unclear. Secreted SST binds to specific receptors (SSTRs), which are coupled to $G_{i/o}$ proteins. In both β- and α-cells, activation of SSTRs suppresses hormone secretion by reducing cAMP levels, inhibiting electrical activity, decreasing Ca^{2+} influx through voltage-gated Ca^{2+} channels and directly reducing exocytosis in a Ca^{2+} and cAMP-independent manner. In rodents, β-cells express predominantly SSTR5, whereas α-cells express SSTR2. In human islets, SSTR2 is the dominant receptor in both β- and α-cells, but other isoforms also contribute to the SST effects. Evidence from rodent models suggests that SST secretion from δ-cells is dysregulated in diabetes mellitus, which may contribute to the metabolic disturbances in this disease. SST analogues are currently used for the treatment of hyperinsulinism and other endocrine disorders, including acromegaly and Cushing's syndrome.

ABBREVIATIONS

K_{ATP} channel ATP-sensitive K^+ channel
GH growth hormone
GLP-1 glucagon-like peptide-1
GIRK G-protein gated inwardly rectifying K^+ channel
GPCR G-protein coupled receptor
SST somatostatin
SSTR somatostatin receptor
T1DM type 1 diabetes mellitus
T2DM type 2 diabetes mellitus

1. INTRODUCTION

Shortly after the discovery of somatostatin (SST) in 1973, the peptide hormone was found to be highly expressed in pancreatic islets and to have potent effects on the secretion of insulin and glucagon, two key hormones in the regulation of blood glucose homeostasis. Much effort has since been directed at elucidating the mechanisms of action and physiological roles of SST in islets and at finding ways to exploit these actions therapeutically. Most of this work has been performed in animal, in particular rodent, models. As a by-product of the more widespread use of islet transplantation in the treatment of type 1 diabetes in recent years (Shapiro et al., 2000), the availability of human islets for research purposes has also improved, and progress in the characterization of SST signaling in man has recently been made. This review summarizes the available literature on the function of SST in pancreatic islets. The focus therein will be on data obtained in man or using human tissue *in vitro*, and animal models will be discussed mainly when human data are not available or insufficient (for additional information on SST signaling in rodent islets see Strowski & Blake, 2008).

1.1. Discovery and physiological roles of SST

SST was first identified in 1973, when it was purified from hypothalamic extracts as an inhibitor of growth hormone (GH) secretion from cultured pituitary cells (Brazeau et al., 1973). SST is a peptide hormone that exists in two active forms consisting of 14 and 28 amino acids, respectively (SST-14 and SST-28). Both forms are processed from the same precursor (pro-SST).

SST-producing cells are most abundant in the brain, the gut, and the endocrine pancreas. In rats, the gut is responsible for 65% of the bodies SST production, with the brain contributing 25% and the pancreatic islets 5% (Patel & Reichlin, 1978). Hypothalamic neurons, D-cells in the gastric epithelium and δ-cells in pancreatic islets contain mostly SST-14, while SST-28 is mainly produced by D-cells in the intestinal epithelium (Patel, 1999). SST-14 has a short half-life in the plasma (<3 min) (Patel & Wheatley, 1983). Consequently, the circulating SST-like immunoreactivity, as detected by commonly used assays, mainly represents SST-28 and, to a lesser extent, SST-13, a biologically inactive cleavage product of SST-14 (D'Alessio & Ensinck, 1990; Ensinck et al., 1989). Based on these finding, it has been proposed that SST-28 may act as a hormone, whereas SST-14 functions as a paracrine transmitter (D'Alessio & Ensinck, 1990).

A well-known physiological role of SST is inhibition of GH secretion from the pituitary gland. Both GH itself and insulin-like growth factor 1, which is produced systemically in response to GH, stimulate SST release from hypothalamic neurons, thus constituting a negative feedback loop (Boron & Boulpaep, 2012). Hypothalamic SST also inhibits the secretion of thyroid-stimulating hormone from the pituitary (Patel, 1999). In the stomach, SST is likewise part of a negative feedback loop. It is secreted from D-cells in response to gastrin and luminal acidity and inhibits acid secretion both directly and indirectly by suppressing gastrin and histamin release (Boron & Boulpaep, 2012). Other gastrointestinal effects of SST include inhibition of gastrointestinal motility and bile flow and promotion of intestinal fluid absorption. SST can also act as a neurotransmitter in the CNS and is found in immune cells (Patel, 1999).

1.2. SST receptors

The first somatostatin receptors (SSTRs) were cloned in 1992 from human pancreatic islets, using degenerate primers against G-protein coupled receptor- (GPCR-) related sequences (Yamada et al., 1992). In total, five

SSTRs (SSTR1–5) encoded by different genes (*SSTR1–5*) have been found (Bruno, Xu, Song, & Berelowitz, 1992; O'Carroll, Lolait, Konig, & Mahan, 1992; Yamada et al., 1992, 1993; Yasuda et al., 1992). In addition, an alternatively spliced variant of SSTR2 with a 15 amino acid shorter C-terminus (SSTR2B) has been identified (Vanetti, Kouba, Wang, Vogt, & Hollt, 1992). SSTRs have the seven transmembrane domain structure that is typical of GPCRs. The receptors can exist as monomers, homodimers, or heterodimers. The dimerization status is influenced by ligand binding in an isoform-specific manner (Barbieri et al., 2013; Moller, Stidsen, Hartmann, & Holst, 2003). SSTRs can also interact with other GPCRs, including dopamine, opioid, and ghrelin receptors (Barbieri et al., 2013; Park, Jiang, Zhang, & Smith, 2012). SST binds to all SSTR isoforms with dissociation constants in the low nanomolar range (Table 7.1). While SSTR1–4 display slightly higher affinity for SST-14 than for SST-28, SSTR5 preferentially binds SST-28. Selective peptide and nonpeptide agonists have been developed for all receptor subtypes.

All five human SSTRs are coupled to $G_{i/o}$ proteins and inhibition of adenylate cyclase (Patel, Greenwood, Warszynska, Panetta, & Srikant, 1994). SSTRs also inhibit cellular secretion by activating K^+ channels (including voltage-gated, Ca^{2+} activated, and inwardly rectifying K^+ channels) and by inhibiting voltage-gated Ca^{2+} channels (Cervia & Bagnoli, 2007; Moller et al., 2003). In addition, SSTRs are coupled to the activation of protein–tyrosine phosphatases and to inhibition of mitogen-activated protein kinase. This underlies the inhibitory effects of SST on cell proliferation, via inhibition of cell cycle progression and induction of apoptosis

Table 7.1 Binding affinities of SST and SST analogues for human SSTR subtypes

Compound	Alternative names	SSTR1	SSTR2	SSTR3	SSTR4	SSTR5
SST-14[a]		0.1–2.26	0.2–1.3	0.3–1.6	0.3–1.8	0.2–0.9
SST-28[a]		0.1–2.2	0.2–4.1	0.3–6.1	0.3–7.9	0.05–0.4
Octreotide[b]	SMS201–995, Sandostatin	280	0.38	7.1	>1000	6.3
Lanreotide[b]	BIM23014, Somatuline	180	0.54	14	230	17
Pasireotide[b]	SOM230, Signifor	9.3	1	1.5	>100	0.16

Values represent IC_{50} in nmol/l.
[a]Data from Patel (1999).
[b]Data from Bruns, Lewis, Briner, Meno-Tetang, and Weckbecker (2002).

(Barbieri et al., 2013; Moller et al., 2003). SST also inhibits the Na^+/H^+ exchanger, and the resulting cytosolic acidification may contribute to its proapoptotic properties (Moller et al., 2003). These effects of SST are exploited in the treatment of neuroendocrine tumors.

SSTRs desensitize upon prolonged agonist exposure. This involves phosphorylation of C-terminal sites by G-protein coupled receptor kinases (GRKs) and binding of β-arrestins. Phosphorylation by protein kinase A or C may also play a role. The phosphorylated SSTRs are internalized by clathrin-dependent endocytosis, followed either by recycling through endosomal or trans-golgi pathways (typical for SSTR2) or by lysosomal degradation (SSTR3) (Csaba, Peineau, & Dournaud, 2012; Tulipano & Schulz, 2007).

2. SST IN PANCREATIC ISLETS

Shortly after the discovery of SST, it was demonstrated that the hormone is expressed in a population of endocrine cells in pancreatic islets, the δ-cells (Luft, Efendic, Hokfelt, Johansson, & Arimura, 1974). δ-Cells are the third most abundant endocrine cell type in islets, accounting for ~5% and ~10% of the endocrine cells in mouse and human islets, respectively (Brissova et al., 2005; Cabrera et al., 2006). The δ-cell fraction of human islets is similar in the different parts of the pancreas (Clark et al., 1988). Within δ-cells, SST is contained in secretory granules with a diameter of 100–200 nm (Gopel et al., 2004).

In rats and mice, δ-cells and glucagon-secreting α-cells are confined to the peripheral cell layer of pancreatic islets, while the islet core is composed of insulin-secreting β-cells. The blood flow in rodent islets is from central β-cells to peripheral non-β-cells (Samols, Stagner, Ewart, & Marks, 1988). This arrangement suggested that SST may act as a paracrine inhibitor of glucagon secretion without having a major effect on insulin secretion. However, recent studies have revealed significant differences between the architecture of rodent and human islets. With the exception of small islets, non-β-cells are not restricted to the islet periphery but distributed throughout human islets, allowing for frequent direct contact between β- and non-β-cells (Cabrera et al., 2006). Bosco et al. have proposed that the distribution of cell types in human islets is not random, but that islet cells are organized in trilaminar plates consisting of a central β-cell layer surrounded by non-β-cell layers. Blood vessels were found to run adjacent to the non-β-cell layers

(Bosco et al., 2010). These findings support the possibility of paracrine interactions between islet cells, including δ- to β-cell signaling.

3. REGULATION OF SST SECRETION FROM PANCREATIC δ-CELLS

Plasma SST concentrations are in the low picomolar range and roughly double after meals, mainly due to an increase in SST-28 (D'Alessio & Ensinck, 1990; Ensinck et al., 1989; Gutniak, Grill, Wiechel, & Efendic, 1987). Both basal and postprandial SST levels are similar in pancreatectomized patients as in controls, suggesting that islets contribute little to circulating SST, and that the changes largely reflect SST secretion from the gut (Gutniak et al., 1987). SST-14, which only accounts for a small fraction of circulating SST (see above), has been measured separately and likewise increases in the circulation after meals (D'Alessio & Ensinck, 1990). There is evidence that plasma SST-14 mainly originates from gastric D-cells rather than pancreatic δ-cells (Ensinck et al., 1989).

The available knowledge about the regulation of SST secretion from pancreatic δ-cells is therefore largely derived from *in vitro* studies. Data from human preparations are limited. In isolated human islets, raising the glucose concentration from 1 to 6 or 20 mM increased SST secretion 1.5- and 3.2-fold, respectively (Ramracheya et al., 2010). A stimulatory effect of glucose was also observed in perfused human islets (Hellman, Salehi, Gylfe, Dansk, & Grapengiesser, 2009). Similar to β-cells, human δ-cells express ATP-sensitive K^+ (K_{ATP}) channels, and SST secretion is stimulated by the K_{ATP} channel blocker tolbutamide and inhibited by the K_{ATP} channel opener diazoxide (Braun et al., 2009). All these findings are in good agreement with previous observations in animal models (Efendic, Enzmann, Nylen, Uvnas-Wallensten, & Luft, 1979; Ipp et al., 1977; Zhang et al., 2007). In mouse islets, a clear stimulation of SST secretion was detected at a glucose concentration (5 mM) that is below the threshold for stimulation of insulin secretion, whereas in human islets the difference seems to be less pronounced if at all present (Walker et al., 2011).

It is well documented in animal models that SST secretion is increased by amino acids (Ipp et al., 1977). The incretin glucagon-like peptide-1 (GLP-1) stimulates SST release in both rat (de Heer, Rasmussen, Coy, & Holst, 2008) and human islets (R. Ramracheya & P. Rorsman, personal communication). Noradrenaline inhibited SST secretion from the perfused dog pancreas (Ahren & Taborsky, 1988) and from mouse islets (Hauge-Evans,

King, Fairhall, Persaud, & Jones, 2010), which may be relevant for counter-regulatory responses during hypoglycemia.

In the perfused human pancreas, glucose-stimulated SST secretion was inhibited by immunoneutralization of insulin, suggesting a stimulatory effect of the β-cell hormone (Brunicardi et al., 2001). This is at variance with isolated mouse islets, where SST secretion was unaffected by exogenous insulin or anti-insulin IgG (Hauge-Evans, Anderson, Persaud, & Jones, 2012), and with the perfused rat pancreas, where insulin suppressed stimulated SST secretion without affecting basal release (Gerber, Trimble, Wollheim, & Renold, 1981). SST secretion from the perfused dog pancreas and from mouse islets is potentiated by glucagon (Hauge-Evans et al., 2012; Patton et al., 1977). It has recently been reported that SST secretion from human islets is increased by the neurotransmitters glutamate and GABA (Braun et al., 2010; Molina, Fachado, Menegaz, Berggren, & Caicedo, 2012), which are secreted from α-cells and β-cells, respectively (Braun et al., 2010; Cabrera et al., 2008). These findings suggest that a complex network of paracrine interactions regulates the secretion of the three main islet hormones (Caicedo, 2012).

Like mouse δ-cells (Gopel, Kanno, Barg, & Rorsman, 2000), human δ-cells are electrically excitable and express voltage-gated Na^+, Ca^{2+}, and K^+ channels (Braun, Ramracheya, Amisten, et al., 2009). Human δ-cells displayed oscillations of the cytosolic Ca^{2+} concentration that were enhanced by glucose and glucagon (Berts, Liu, Gylfe, & Hellman, 1997). Human δ-cells express K_{ATP} currents, and the membrane potential is sensitive to the K_{ATP} modulators tolbutamide and diazoxide, but effects of glucose on these channels have not been detected so far (Braun, Ramracheya, Amisten, et al., 2009). Studies in mice have shown that Ca^{2+}-induced Ca^{2+} release from intracellular stores plays an important role in the generation and glucose modulation of cytosolic Ca^{2+} signals in δ-cells (Zhang et al., 2007).

4. EFFECTS OF EXOGENOUS SST ON HORMONE SECRETION FROM PANCREATIC ISLETS

Exogenous SST strongly suppresses the basal as well as glucose- or arginine-stimulated secretion of insulin and glucagon in man (Alberti et al., 1973; Efendic, Claro, & Laft, 1976). This effect is routinely exploited in clinical studies (pancreatic clamp) to allow the manipulation of plasma insulin and glucagon levels independently of blood glucose concentrations. Interestingly, inhibition of pancreatic hormone secretion by SST infusion initially results in a lowering of blood glucose levels, which is followed by hyperglycemia when the infusion is maintained for more than 2 h (Sherwin, Hendler, DeFronzo, Wahren, & Felic, 1977).

The inhibitory effect of SST on pancreatic hormone secretion has been confirmed *in vitro*. In the isolated perfused human pancreas, SST inhibited insulin secretion induced by 3.9 or 12.9 mM glucose by 45–60% (Kleinman et al., 1994). SST also suppressed insulin secretion from isolated human islets in the presence of 20 mM glucose (by ~50%; Zambre et al., 1999), of 20 mM glucose and exendin-4 (by ~80%; Singh et al., 2007) or of 15 mM glucose and isobutylmethylxanthine (by ~75%; Misler, Dickey, & Barnett, 2005). In these studies, SST had no effect at 2.8 mM glucose, which is below the stimulation threshold of insulin secretion in human islets (3 mM; Henquin, Dufrane, & Nenquin, 2006). In agreement with the *in vivo* experiments, SST also strongly inhibited arginine-induced glucagon secretion from isolated human islets (Singh et al., 2007).

5. CELLULAR MECHANISMS UNDERLYING SST INHIBITION OF PANCREATIC HORMONE SECRETION

Glucose stimulates insulin secretion by inhibiting plasmalemmal K_{ATP} channels. This results in membrane depolarization, electrical activity, and Ca^{2+} influx through voltage-gated Ca^{2+} channels, which represents the direct stimulus for insulin granule exocytosis (Rorsman & Braun, 2013). Ca^{2+}-evoked exocytosis is modulated by other second messengers (e.g., ATP, cAMP, diacylglycerol, NAPDH). The classical pathway by which SST inhibits exocytosis is via inhibition of adenylate cyclase and reduction of cAMP levels. A recent study has described three additional mechanisms by which SST suppresses insulin secretion from human β-cells (Kailey et al., 2012) (Fig. 7.1). First, SST hyperpolarized the β-cell membrane potential and inhibited electrical activity by activating G-protein gated inwardly rectifying K^+ (GIRK) channels. Second, SST directly reduced Ca^{2+} influx through P/Q-type Ca^{2+} channels. Third, SST inhibited insulin granule exocytosis downstream of Ca^{2+} influx in a cAMP-independent manner.

The SST-induced *membrane hyperpolarization* is consistent with previous observations in rodent β-cells (Renstrom, Ding, Bokvist, & Rorsman, 1996; Smith, Sellers, & Humphrey, 2001). The hyperpolarization was independent of K_{ATP} channels but sensitive to the GIRK antagonist tertiapin Q, and expression of GIRK subunits in human islets was confirmed by RT-PCR (Kailey et al., 2012). The SST effect on the membrane potential

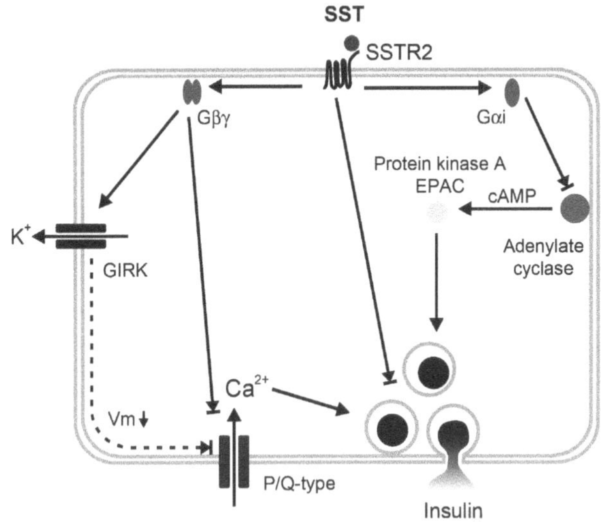

Figure 7.1 Cellular pathways involved in SST inhibition of insulin secretion in human β-cells. (For color version of this figure, the reader is referred to the online version of this chapter.)

tended to be transient, and action potential firing often resumed in the continued presence of the hormone. It has been suggested that this reflects the intrinsic properties of GIRK channels, rather than desensitization of SSTRs, as the GIRK currents show a similar spontaneous decay when activated in a receptor-independent manner (e.g., by cytosolic application of GTPγS) (Gromada et al., 2001). Receptor-dependent activation of GIRK is thought to be mediated by Gβγ subunits (Hibino et al., 2010), but this remains to be demonstrated in human β-cells.

SST stably suppresses insulin secretion *in vivo* even during prolonged application for several hours (Sherwin et al., 1977). It has been proposed that the direct effect of SST on *exocytosis* plays an important role in ensuring the continued inhibition of insulin release after electrical activity has resumed (Kailey et al., 2012). The effect on exocytosis was robust, strong (~80% reduction) and, at variance with the effect on membrane potential, showed no desensitization during the experiments (up to 10 min; Kailey et al., 2012).

cAMP is an important second messenger in β-cells and potentiates Ca^{2+}-induced insulin secretion by direct effects on the exocytotic machinery (Ämmälä, Ashcroft, & Rorsman, 1993; Tengholm & Gylfe, 2009). It has been clearly demonstrated that SST inhibits adenylate cyclase and lowers cAMP levels in rodent islets and purified β-cells (Claro, Grill, Efendic, & Luft, 1977;

Schuit & Pipeleers, 1985). In the study by Kailey et al. (2012), exocytosis was monitored by measuring the cell capacitance (which is proportional to the cell surface area) using the patch-clamp technique. During the experiments, the cells were infused with a buffer containing a high cAMP concentration (0.1 mM), which should effectively clamp the intracellular cAMP levels. This suggests that the inhibition of exocytosis under these conditions was independent of cAMP. This is in agreement with a previous study showing inhibition of insulin secretion by SST without lowering of cAMP levels under some experimental conditions in rat islets (Hahn, Gottschling, & Woltanski, 1978). Under voltage-clamp conditions (to prevent SST-evoked changes of the membrane potential), SST moderately reduced Ca^{2+} entry in isolated human β-cells (by 15%), but restoring Ca^{2+} influx to control levels by prolonging the stimulation rescued exocytosis only to a small extent (Kailey et al., 2012). A similar, Ca^{2+}- and cAMP-independent inhibition of insulin secretion has also been described for other hormones, including adrenaline and galanin (Renstrom et al., 1996; Zhao, Fang, Straub, Lindau, & Sharp, 2010). The signal transduction pathways underlying this inhibition are not well understood. Among the proposed mechanisms are activation of the protein phosphatase calcineurin (Renstrom et al., 1996), activation of protein acylation (Cheng, Straub, & Sharp, 2003), and direct interaction of Gα and Gβγ subunits with the exocytotic machinery (Chen et al., 2005; Zhao et al., 2010). In preliminary experiments, the SST inhibition of exocytosis in human β-cells was not prevented by the calcineurin-inhibitor cyclosporin A or the Gβγ inhibitor gallein (B. Kailey & M. Braun, unpublished data), but further studies are clearly required.

In human β-cells, SST inhibited *Ca^{2+} influx* specifically through voltage-gated P/Q-type Ca^{2+} channels (Kailey et al., 2012). This finding is at variance with rodent β-cells, where inhibition of N-type Ca^{2+} channels (Smith, 2009), L- and R-type Ca^{2+} channels (Mergler et al., 2008) or no effect on Ca^{2+} currents (Renstrom et al., 1996) have been reported. SST inhibition of P/Q-type channels has previously been observed neurons (Viana & Hille, 1996). GPCR inhibition of P/Q-type channels is thought to be mediated by Gβγ subunits (Catterall, 2011).

Evidence regarding direct effects of SST on *β-cell metabolism* is conflicting. In one study, SST was found to inhibit the glucose-induced oxygen consumption in mouse islets (Daunt, Dale, & Smith, 2006), whereas a more recent paper reported an increase of NADPH levels (an indicator of glucose metabolism) upon SST treatment (Schwetz, Ustione, & Piston, 2013).

The possible role of SST signaling in *pancreatic islet development* has been studied in transgenic mice. Islets from animals lacking SSTR5 (the predominant isoform in mouse β-cells, see below) have an increased insulin contents (Strowski et al., 2003; Zhou et al., 2012). By contrast, in mice with deletion of the SST gene, the number, size, architecture, and insulin and glucagon contents of the islets were all normal (Hauge-Evans et al., 2008). As the knockouts are whole-body knockouts, the islet phenotype may be influenced by extrapancreatic effects.

The data in Kailey et al. (2012) suggest that direct inhibition of exocytosis is the overall dominant effect of SST. However, the *hierarchy* of SST effects may differ under more physiological conditions *in vivo*. For example, there is evidence that different signal transduction pathways are activated at different SST concentrations (Smith, 2009). Moreover, the desensitization of the SST effect on electrical activity may be less significant *in vivo* if SST is secreted by δ-cells in a pulsatile manner, allowing for recovery of the pathways during the troughs (Hellman et al., 2009). The experiments in isolated β-cells may also underestimate the significance of the Ca^{2+} current inhibition because there is evidence that P/Q-type are specifically coupled to exocytosis in intact islets but not in dispersed β-cell (Braun, Ramracheya, Johnson, & Rorsman, 2009).

In *human α-cells*, SST has similar effects as in β-cells by inhibiting Ca^{2+} influx and exocytosis (Kailey et al., 2012) and hyperpolarizing the membrane potential (Ramracheya et al., 2010). The effects on exocytosis and electrical activity are in agreement with previous findings in rodent α-cells, where the latter effect is likewise due to activation of GIRK channels (Gromada, Hoy, Buschard, Salehi, & Rorsman, 2001; Gromada, Hoy, Olsen, et al., 2001; Yoshimoto et al., 1999).

6. SSTRs IN PANCREATIC ISLET CELLS

6.1. Rodent islets

Early studies in rat islets found that SST-28 is a more potent inhibitor of insulin secretion than SST-14, whereas the reverse was the case for glucagon secretion (Mandarino et al., 1981). This suggested that β-cells and α-cells express different SSTRs. This conclusion was later supported by immunohistochemical studies showing that the SST-28-sensitive SSTR5 is expressed in rat β-cells while the SST-14-sensitive SSTR2 is present mainly in α-cells (Hunyady, Hipkin, Schonbrunn, & Mezey, 1997; Mitra et al., 1999). Experiments using isoform-selective agonists subsequently confirmed that in mouse islets SSTR2 and SSTR5 principally mediate the suppression of glucagon and insulin release, respectively (Rohrer & Schaeffer, 2000; Yang et al., 1998). Further evidence comes from transgenic mouse models. Deletion of SSTR2 reduced (although not abolished) the effect of SST on glucagon release without affecting the insulin responses (Strowski, Parmar, Blake, & Schaeffer, 2000). Knockout of SSTR5 lowered the potency of SST-28 to inhibit glucose-induced insulin secretion (Strowski et al., 2003).

6.2. Human β-cells

In the first paper that systematically examined SSTR expression in human islets using *PCR*, transcripts for SSTR1, 2, and 4 but not 3 and 5 were detected (Kubota et al., 1994) (Table 7.2). A subsequent study, using the same method, found expression of both SSTR2 and 5 (Zambre et al., 1999). Recently, quantitative PCR revealed that SSTR2 is most strongly expressed, with SSTR3, 1, and 5 present at 30%, 25%, and 5% of the SSTR2 levels, while SSTR4 was not detected (Kailey et al., 2012).

Results from *immunohistochemical studies* using isoform-specific antibodies are summarized in Table 7.2. All studies found expression of SSTR2 in β-cells (when no co-staining with insulin was performed a diffuse staining pattern of islets was taken as evidence for β-cell expression; Lupp et al., 2011; Taniyama et al., 2005). SSTR5 was also consistently detected; while several studies reported stronger signals compared to SSTR2, (Taniyama et al., 2005) did not detect this isoform in half of the donors studied. Expression of the other isoforms was observed at varying levels, with a tendency for SSTR1 > SSTR3 > SSTR4. The only paper that specifically looked at the SSTR2 splice variants found SSTR2A in all and SSTR2B in half of the samples (Taniyama et al., 2005). The antibody used in Lupp et al. (2011) and Kailey et al. (2012) is specific for SSTR2A.

The functional significance of the SSTR isoforms has been investigated using selective agonists (Table 7.2). The first of these studies reported that two different SSTR5 agonists inhibited *insulin release* from isolated human islets whereas four different SSTR2 agonists were without effect (Zambre et al., 1999). It is noteworthy that the SSTR2-selective agonists failed to reduce insulin release even at concentrations 10-fold higher than their IC_{50} values for SSTR5. Different agonists for the same receptors were tested in the perfused human pancreas, and insulin secretion was most potently inhibited by the SSTR2 agonist, while an SSTR5 agonist was only effective

Table 7.2 SSTR subtypes in human β-cells

SSTR1	SSTR2	SSTR3	SSTR4	SSTR5	Comments
PCR					
+	+	–	+	–	Islets (Kubota et al., 1994)
	+			+	Islets (Zambre et al., 1999)
+	++	+	–	(+)	qPCR; islets (Kailey et al., 2012)
Immunohistochemistry					
++	+	+	(+)	++	β-Cells (Kumar et al., 1999)
++	+	++	++	++	β-Cells (Portela-Gomes, Grimelius, Westermark, & Stridsberg, 2010)
	++	++		++	β-Cells (Papotti et al., 2002)
	++				β-Cells (Kimura, Schindler, Kasai, & Kimura, 2001)
	+				β-Cells (Kailey et al., 2012)
+	++	(+)	(+)	+	Islets (Taniyama et al., 2005)
	+			+	Islets, diffuse pattern (Lupp et al., 2011)
		(+)			Islets, α-cell pattern (Lupp et al., 2012)
Insulin secretion					
	–			++	Batch-incubated islets (Zambre et al., 1999)
	+	–		(+)	Perfused pancreas (Brunicardi et al., 2003)
(+)	++	–		+	Batch-incubated islets (Singh et al., 2007)
Exocytosis					
–	++	+	–	–	Isolated β-cells (Kailey et al., 2012)
Electrical activity					
	++			(+)	Isolated β-cells (Kailey et al., 2012)

++, Strong signal/effect; +, clear signal/effect; (+), weak signal/effect; –, no signal/effect; blank, no data

at high concentrations (Brunicardi et al., 2003). A third set of agonists was studied in isolated human islets and inhibited secretion with an order of potency SSTR2 > SSTR5 > SSTR1 (Singh et al., 2007).

In experiments in single human β-cells, an SSTR2 agonist showed the highest potency at inhibiting *exocytosis and electrical activity* of all selective agonists tested, but was less potent than SST-14 (Kailey et al., 2012). An SSTR5 agonist marginally reduced electrical activity but did not influence exocytosis. Exocytosis was moderately decreased by an SSTR3 agonist but not by SSTR1 or SSTR4 agonists.

Finally, in *clinical studies* in patients with acromegaly (see also below), the SST-analogue octreotide, which preferentially binds to SSTR2 (Table 7.1), suppressed plasma insulin levels much more potently than SOM230, which has a ~40-fold higher affinity for SSTR5 (van der Hoek et al., 2005).

Taken together, these data suggest that human β-cells differ from rodent β-cells and that SST effects are predominantly (but not exclusively) mediated by SSTR2. SSTR5 and SSTR1 are also involved, while data regarding SSTR3 are conflicting. SSTR4 does not seem to play a major role. There is evidence that different receptor subtypes couple to different downstream signaling pathways (Barnett, 2003). However, in human β-cells the SSTR2 agonist had the strongest effect on membrane potential and exocytosis (Kailey et al., 2012) as well as Ca^{2+} influx (M. Braun, unpublished data) of the agonists tested.

6.3. Human α-cells

Available data on SSTR isoform expression in human α-cells are summarized in Table 7.3. Similar as in rodents, histological and functional data clearly support a dominant role for SSTR2 in this cell type. Both glucagon secretion and exocytosis measurements also provide evidence for an involvement of SSTR1 and, to a lesser extent, SSTR5. Thus, α- and β-cells in humans are more similar compared to those in rodents in this respect, suggesting that specific targeting of one cell type with SSTR agonists will be difficult. The data also suggest that studies using SSTR2 antagonists to block SST signaling in α-cells should be considered with caution, as these antagonists may not fully prevent the SST effects.

7. PHYSIOLOGICAL ROLE OF SST SIGNALING IN PANCREATIC ISLETS

Infusion of SST-28 at concentrations mimicking those observed after meals inhibited glucose-induced insulin secretion in man, suggesting a possible physiological role for circulating SST (D'Alessio, Sieber, Beglinger, & Ensinck, 1989). The physiological role of islet-derived SST as a paracrine regulator of pancreatic hormone secretion in man is not well understood. Clinical studies with SSTR antagonists have not been performed. In the isolated perfused human pancreas, immunoneutralization of SST with specific

Table 7.3 SSTR subtypes in human α-cells

SSTR1	SSTR2	SSTR3	SSTR4	SSTR5	Comments
Immunohistochemistry					
+	++	(+)	–	+	(Kumar et al., 1999)
++	++	++	++	+	(Portela-Gomes et al., 2010)
	++	++		++	(Papotti et al., 2002)
	+	+			(Taniyama et al., 2005)
	+				(Kimura et al., 2001)
		+			Islets; α-cell pattern (Lupp et al., 2012)
	++				(Kailey et al., 2012)
Glucagon secretion					
+	++	–		(+)	Batch-incubated islets (Singh et al., 2007)
Exocytosis					
+	+	(+)		–	Isolated α-cells (Kailey et al., 2012)
Electrical activity					
	+				Isolated α-cells (Ramracheya et al., 2010)

++, strong signal/effect; +, clear signal/effect; (+), weak signal/effect; –, no signal/effect; blank, no data.

antibodies increased insulin secretion at both 3.9 and 11.5 mM extracellular glucose (corresponding to low fasting and high postprandial levels, respectively) (Brunicardi et al., 2001). Glucagon secretion was augmented at the lower glucose concentration only. This implies that SST tonically inhibits both insulin and glucagon secretion at fasting plasma glucose concentrations. The left-shifted glucose dose–response curve for SST secretion (compared to that of insulin) suggests that SST still may regulate glucagon release at glucose levels where insulin is fully suppressed. A SSTR2 antagonist had no effect on glucagon release from human islets at 1 or 6 mM glucose (Ramracheya et al., 2010); however, it must be kept in mind that blocking SSTR2 may not be sufficient to fully antagonize the SST effects.

Given the paucity of human data, it is worth considering some findings from *rodent models*. Many of these studies have focussed on the role of SST in the regulation of *glucagon secretion*. Mice with disruption of the SST gene have normal fasting glucagon levels but increased glucagon responses after arginine injection (Hauge-Evans et al., 2008). Similar changes were observed in isolated islets (with basal levels measured at 2 mM glucose). Interestingly, glucagon secretion tended to be stimulated rather than inhibited by glucose in islets from SST −/− mice. By contrast, using perfused islets from the same mouse model, others have found elevated glucagon levels at 1 and 7 mM glucose but a preserved inhibitory effect of glucose on glucagon release (Cheng-Xue et al., 2013). Islets from SSTR2 knockout mice released normal amounts of glucagon at 5.5 mM glucose but showed exaggerated responses to arginine stimulation (Strowski et al., 2000). SSTR2 antagonism (but not SST-antiserum) increased glucagon release from the rat pancreas under hypoglycemic conditions (Cejvan, Coy, & Efendic, 2003; de Heer et al., 2008). By contrast, an SSTR2 blocker reduced the glucagon response to insulin-induced hypoglycemia in rats *in vivo* (Yue et al., 2012). In the perfused rat pancreas, SST-antiserum, as well as an SSTR2 antagonist, prevented the inhibition of glucagon secretion by the incretin GLP-1, but not by glucose (de Heer et al., 2008). By contrast, in mouse islets the effect of GLP-1 appears to be independent of SST (De Marinis et al., 2010). Taken together, these data demonstrate that SST is a paracrine regulator of glucagon secretion in rodent islets, but the exact conditions under which this regulation occurs are controversial (i.e., during hypoglycemia, normoglycemia, hyperglycemia, amino acid and/or GLP-1 stimulation). Species differences may contribute to the discrepancies.

Insulin secretion from islets from both SST −/− mice and SSTR5 −/− mice is normal at low extracellular glucose levels and exaggerated at high glucose concentrations (Hauge-Evans et al., 2008; Strowski et al., 2003). SSTR5 knockout mice have improved glucose tolerance when fed a high-fat diet, but the interpretation of the phenotype is complicated by the increased insulin sensitivity of the animals. Overall, paracrine SST signaling appears to modulate insulin secretion during stimulation with glucose and other secretagogues but not during hypoglycemia. As discussed above, the architecture of mouse islets suggested that δ-cell to β-cell signaling is less relevant, but this cannot be assumed for human islets. Insulin and SST are generally released in response to the same stimuli, and it seems counterintuitive that SST should be a physiological paracrine inhibitor of β-cell function. It may be speculated that this arrangement helps to prevent insulin-induced hypoglycemia after protein meals.

Insulin and glucagon secretion *in vivo* is pulsatile (Menge et al., 2011), and *in vitro* data suggest that the same is true for SST (Hellman et al., 2009). Insulin pulses are in phase with SST pulses and out of phase with glucagon pulses. This suggests that the secretion of the islet hormones is highly coordinated. The coordination of β-cells within islets is largely mediated by direct cell-to-cell coupling via gap junctions, but for different cell types diffusible factors are likely to be involved (Tengholm & Gylfe, 2009). It seems plausible that SST participates in this coordination, but this needs to be demonstrated experimentally.

8. SST AND δ-CELLS IN DIABETES MELLITUS

Elevated basal plasma SST concentrations have been detected in patients with type 1 diabetes mellitus (T1DM) (Segers, De Vroede, Michotte, & Somers, 1989; Skare, Dahl-Jorgensen, Hanssen, & Norman, 1985). The patients showed a normal increase of plasma SST in response to arginine injection (Skare et al., 1985), whereas the response to tolbutamide was reduced compared to healthy controls (Segers et al., 1989). These studies measured total SST-like immunoreactivity; as discussed above, the data therefore likely represent SST-28 released from the gut. In type 2 diabetes mellitus (T2DM), normal basal SST-like immunoreactivity (D'Alessio & Ensinck, 1990; Grill, Gutniak, Roovete, & Efendic, 1984; Segers et al., 1989), normal basal SST-14 (D'Alessio & Ensinck, 1990) and lowered basal SST-28 levels (D'Alessio & Ensinck, 1990) have been found. A glucose load or tolbutamide administration increased SST-like immunoreactivity in healthy controls but not in T2DM patients (Grill et al., 1984; Gutniak, Grill, Roovete, & Efendic, 1989; Segers et al., 1989), whereas total SST, SST-28 and SST-14 all showed normal increases in response to a fat meal (D'Alessio & Ensinck, 1990).

A limited number of studies have examined the δ-cell contents in pancreatic sections from diabetic donors, using immunohistochemistry. These studies have not found changes in the total pancreatic δ-cell mass in T1DM (Orci et al., 1976, $n=2$; Saito, Yaginuma, & Takahashi, 1979, $n=5$; Stefan et al., 1982, $n=2$; Rahier, Goebbels, & Henquin, 1983, $n=4$) or in T2DM (Saito et al., 1979, $n=26$; Stefan et al., 1982, $n=2$; Rahier et al., 1983, $n=4$; Clark et al., 1988, $n=15$). Some studies reported an increased δ-cell density in islets in T1DM (Orci et al., 1976; Rahier et al., 1983) and T2DM (Iki & Pour, 2007), but there is no clear evidence that this was due to proliferation of δ-cells, rather than a reduction in β-cell mass.

In the perfused pancreas of streptozotocin-treated, mildly diabetic rats, the SST secretory response to glucose was lost, while SST secretion was exaggerated upon arginine stimulation (Ostenson, Efendic, & Grill, 1990). A loss of the glucose-effect on SST secretion was also observed by others in streptozotocin-treated animal models of diabetes (Hermansen, Orskov, & Christensen, 1979; Trimble, Gerber, & Renold, 1981). Failure of glucose to increase SST levels, both systemically and in islets, may therefore contribute to the impaired suppression of glucagon secretion in diabetes (Cooperberg & Cryer, 2009; Dunning & Gerich, 2007). It is not known if SST secretion in human islets from diabetic donors is impaired in a similar manner.

9. CLINICAL USES OF SSTR AGONISTS AND PANCREATIC ISLETS

Three SST analogues are currently approved for clinical use. Octreotide (SMS201–995, Sandostatin) and lanreotide (BIM23014, Somatuline) activate SSTR2, 3, and 5, while pasireotide (SOM230, Signifor) also acts on SSTR1 and has a higher affinity for SSTR5 (Table 7.1). Due to its short half-life, SST needs to be administered by continuous infusion, whereas the analogues are applied by subcutaneous injection at twice daily to monthly frequencies.

9.1. Type 1 diabetes mellitus

Octreotide has been tested in combination with insulin in the treatment of T1DM. A reduction of insulin requirements and stabilization of blood glucose levels was observed in short-term trials (Bruttomesso et al., 2001; Gerich, 1978). In addition to reduced glucagon secretion, lowering of GH levels (which is likewise a blood glucose-raising hormone), slowing of gastric emptying and improved insulin sensitivity also contributed to these improvements (Bruttomesso et al., 2001). In a long-term trial, octreotide infusion led to a moderate improvement of glucose homeostasis and reduction of GH levels but no improvement of diabetic retinopathy (the main aim of the trial), and some patients withdrew from the study because of gastrointestinal side effects (Kirkegaard et al., 1990). SST analogues have not been further pursued as diabetes drugs in recent years (Unger & Cherrington, 2012).

It has recently been suggested to use SSTR2 antagonists in the treatment of T1DM to improve the glucagon counterregulation during hypoglycemia; this possibility is supported by results obtained in rodent models of diabetes (Gaisano, Macdonald, & Vranic, 2012; Yue et al., 2012).

9.2. Hyperinsulinism

Hyperinsulinism, leading to hypoglycemia, can be congenital or acquired. The most common cause of congenital hyperinsulinism are inactivating mutations in K_{ATP} channel subunits (Arnoux et al., 2011). Mutations in other genes involved in glucose metabolism and insulin secretion, such as glutamate dehydrogenase and glucokinase, have also been identified. Octreotide is the medical treatment of second choice when the K_{ATP} channel activator diazoxide is not effective. The effect of octreotide tends to decline during the first days of treatment (Arnoux et al., 2011). The treatment is then effective long term, but may result in reduced growth of the children (Yorifuji et al., 2013).

Acquired hyperinsulinism can develop as a consequence of gastric bypass surgery, which is used to treat severe obesity. The surgery leads to the exposure of L-cells in the small intestine to higher than normal nutrient concentrations, resulting in often dramatically elevated plasma GLP-1 levels (Thaler & Cummings, 2009). Rapid glucose absorption followed by excessive insulin responses ("late dumping syndrome") may also contribute (Myint et al., 2012). Successful long-term treatment of a patient with octreotide has been described (Myint et al., 2012). The SST analogue does not only suppress insulin secretion directly but also has a strong inhibitory effect on GLP-1 secretion (Myint et al., 2012; Velasquez-Mieyer et al., 2004); in mice, this is mediated by activation of SSTR5 on L-cells (Moss et al., 2012). Octreotide is also used in the treatment of insulin-producing tumors (insulinomas).

9.3. Other endocrine disorders

Acromegaly is characterized by elevated plasma GH levels. The most common cause is a pituitary adenoma. Octreotide or lanreotide are the preferred pharmacological treatment when surgery is not possible or fails (Longo et al., 2012). As described above, octreotide potently inhibits insulin secretion. The effects of both SST analogues on glucose homeostasis in acromegaly patients were examined in a meta-analysis of the available clinical trials (Mazziotti et al., 2009). Although the treatment decreased plasma insulin levels and increased glucose values during glucose tolerance tests, no change in fasting plasma glucose or, importantly, hemoglobin A(1c), a long-term indicator of glucose homeostasis, was found. A similar outcome was obtained in patients with preexisting glucose intolerance or diabetes. This suggests that the inhibition of insulin secretion is compensated by other factors, notably the normalization of the increased GH levels. It could be argued that normalizing GH levels alone should improve glucose homeostasis.

Pituitary adenomas are also the most common cause of elevated plasma cortisol levels in Cushing's syndrome (Longo et al., 2012). Although the production of adrenocorticotropic hormone (ACTH) in the pituitary is not physiologically regulated by SST (Patel, 1999), ACTH secreting tumors are often sensitive to SST treatment. The tumors express mostly SSTR5 (de Bruin et al., 2009), and the SSTR5-preferring analogue SOM230 has recently been approved for the treatment of Cushing's syndrome. Interestingly, despite having a much weaker effect on insulin secretion than octreotide, SOM230 has stronger hyperglycemic effects (McKeage, 2013; van der Hoek et al., 2005). The reasons for this discrepancy are unclear, but SOM230 seems to lack the insulin-sensitizing properties that have been described for octreotide (van der Hoek et al., 2005).

10. CONCLUSIONS AND FUTURE DIRECTIONS

SST is secreted from pancreatic δ-cells in response to glucose, amino acids, tolbutamide, and GLP-1 stimulation. Exogenous SST potently suppresses insulin and glucagon secretion from pancreatic islets. The inhibition of secretion is due to inhibition of adenylate cyclase, activation of GIRK K^+ channels, inhibition of Ca^{2+} channels (P/Q-type in human β-cells) and Ca^{2+}/cAMP-independent suppression of exocytosis. In rodents, the effects on β-cells and α-cells are mediated by principally SSTR5 and SSTR2, respectively, whereas in man SSTR2 is the dominant isoform in both cell types. Endogenous SST affects pancreatic islet function both as a hormone and a paracrine transmitter. Important question for future research include:

- Which signal transduction pathways underlie the Ca^{2+}/cAMP-independent inhibition of exocytosis by SST?
- What is the role of SST in the complex network of paracrine interactions between islet cells, particularly in human islets?
- Is the regulation of SST secretion from human pancreatic δ-cells altered in diabetes?
- Are SSTRs potential targets for new diabetes drugs that may help to restore glucagon counterregulation during hypoglycemia?

ACKNOWLEDGMENTS

This work was supported by the Canadian Institutes of Health Research (MOP-106435), the Canadian Foundation for Innovation, and the Alberta Diabetes Foundation.

REFERENCES

Ahren, B., & Taborsky, G. J., Jr. (1988). Effects of pancreatic noradrenaline infusion on basal and stimulated islet hormone secretion in the dog. *Acta Physiologica Scandinavica*, *132*(2), 143–150.

Alberti, K. G., Christensen, N. J., Christensen, S. E., Hansen, A. P., Iversen, J., Lundbaek, K., et al. (1973). Inhibition of insulin secretion by somatostatin. *Lancet*, *2*(7841), 1299–1301.

Ämmälä, C., Ashcroft, F. M., & Rorsman, P. (1993). Calcium-independent potentiation of insulin release by cyclic AMP in single beta-cells. *Nature*, *363*(6427), 356–358.

Arnoux, J. B., Verkarre, V., Saint-Martin, C., Montravers, F., Brassier, A., Valayannopoulos, V., et al. (2011). Congenital hyperinsulinism: Current trends in diagnosis and therapy. *Orphanet Journal of Rare Diseases*, *6*, 63.

Barbieri, F., Bajetto, A., Pattarozzi, A., Gatti, M., Wurth, R., Thellung, S., et al. (2013). Peptide receptor targeting in cancer: The somatostatin paradigm. *International Journal of Peptide*, *2013*, 926295.

Barnett, P. (2003). Somatostatin and somatostatin receptor physiology. *Endocrine*, *20*(3), 255–264.

Berts, A., Liu, Y. J., Gylfe, E., & Hellman, B. (1997). Oscillatory Ca2+ signaling in somatostatin-producing cells from the human pancreas. *Metabolism*, *46*(4), 366–369.

Boron, W. F., & Boulpaep, E. L. (2012). *Medical Physiology: A Cellular and Molecular Approach* (2nd ed.). Philadelphia, PA: Saunders.

Bosco, D., Armanet, M., Morel, P., Niclauss, N., Sgroi, A., Muller, Y. D., et al. (2010). Unique arrangement of alpha- and beta-cells in human islets of Langerhans. *Diabetes*, *59*(5), 1202–1210.

Braun, M., Ramracheya, R., Amisten, S., Bengtsson, M., Moritoh, Y., Zhang, Q., et al. (2009). Somatostatin release, electrical activity, membrane currents and exocytosis in human pancreatic delta cells. *Diabetologia*, *52*(8), 1566–1578.

Braun, M., Ramracheya, R., Bengtsson, M., Clark, A., Walker, J. N., Johnson, P. R., et al. (2010). Gamma-aminobutyric acid (GABA) is an autocrine excitatory transmitter in human pancreatic beta-cells. *Diabetes*, *59*(7), 1694–1701.

Braun, M., Ramracheya, R., Johnson, P. R., & Rorsman, P. (2009). Exocytotic properties of human pancreatic beta-cells. *Annals of the New York Academy of Sciences*, *1152*, 187–193.

Brazeau, P., Vale, W., Burgus, R., Ling, N., Butcher, M., Rivier, J., et al. (1973). Hypothalamic polypeptide that inhibits the secretion of immunoreactive pituitary growth hormone. *Science*, *179*(4068), 77–79.

Brissova, M., Fowler, M. J., Nicholson, W. E., Chu, A., Hirshberg, B., Harlan, D. M., et al. (2005). Assessment of human pancreatic islet architecture and composition by laser scanning confocal microscopy. *The Journal of Histochemistry and Cytochemistry*, *53*(9), 1087–1097.

Brunicardi, F. C., Atiya, A., Moldovan, S., Lee, T. C., Fagan, S. P., Kleinman, R. M., et al. (2003). Activation of somatostatin receptor subtype 2 inhibits insulin secretion in the isolated perfused human pancreas. *Pancreas*, *27*(4), e84–e89.

Brunicardi, F. C., Kleinman, R., Moldovan, S., Nguyen, T. H., Watt, P. C., Walsh, J., et al. (2001). Immunoneutralization of somatostatin, insulin, and glucagon causes alterations in islet cell secretion in the isolated perfused human pancreas. *Pancreas*, *23*(3), 302–308.

Bruno, J. F., Xu, Y., Song, J., & Berelowitz, M. (1992). Molecular cloning and functional expression of a brain-specific somatostatin receptor. *Proceedings of the National Academy of Sciences of the United States of America, 89*(23), 11151–11155.

Bruns, C., Lewis, I., Briner, U., Meno-Tetang, G., & Weckbecker, G. (2002). SOM230: A novel somatostatin peptidomimetic with broad somatotropin release inhibiting factor (SRIF) receptor binding and a unique antisecretory profile. *European Journal of Endocrinology, 146*(5), 707–716.

Bruttomesso, D., Fongher, C., Silvestri, B., Barberio, S., Marescotti, M. C., Iori, E., et al. (2001). Combination of continuous subcutaneous infusion of insulin and octreotide in Type 1 diabetic patients. *Diabetes Research and Clinical Practice, 51*(2), 97–105.

Cabrera, O., Berman, D. M., Kenyon, N. S., Ricordi, C., Berggren, P. O., & Caicedo, A. (2006). The unique cytoarchitecture of human pancreatic islets has implications for islet cell function. *Proceedings of the National Academy of Sciences of the United States of America, 103*(7), 2334–2339.

Cabrera, O., Jacques-Silva, M. C., Speier, S., Yang, S. N., Kohler, M., Fachado, A., et al. (2008). Glutamate is a positive autocrine signal for glucagon release. *Cell Metabolism*, 7(6), 545–554.

Caicedo, A. (2012). Paracrine and autocrine interactions in the human islet: More than meets the eye. *Seminars in Cell & Developmental Biology, 24*(1), 11–21.

Catterall, W. A. (2011). Voltage-gated calcium channels. *Cold Spring Harbor Perspectives in Biology, 3*(8), a003947.

Cejvan, K., Coy, D. H., & Efendic, S. (2003). Intra-islet somatostatin regulates glucagon release via type 2 somatostatin receptors in rats. *Diabetes, 52*(5), 1176–1181.

Cervia, D., & Bagnoli, P. (2007). An update on somatostatin receptor signaling in native systems and new insights on their pathophysiology. *Pharmacology & Therapeutics, 116*(2), 322–341.

Chen, X. K., Wang, L. C., Zhou, Y., Cai, Q., Prakriya, M., Duan, K. L., et al. (2005). Activation of GPCRs modulates quantal size in chromaffin cells through G(betagamma) and PKC. *Nature Neuroscience, 8*(9), 1160–1168.

Cheng, H., Straub, S. G., & Sharp, G. W. (2003). Protein acylation in the inhibition of insulin secretion by norepinephrine, somatostatin, galanin, and PGE2. *American Journal of Physiology Endocrinology and Metabolism, 285*(2), E287–E294.

Cheng-Xue, R., Gomez-Ruiz, A., Antoine, N., Noel, L. A., Chae, H. Y., Ravier, M. A., et al. (2013). Tolbutamide controls glucagon release from mouse islets differently than glucose: Involvement of KATP channels from both alpha-cells and delta-cells. *Diabetes, 62*, 1612–1622.

Clark, A., Wells, C. A., Buley, I. D., Cruickshank, J. K., Vanhegan, R. I., Matthews, D. R., et al. (1988). Islet amyloid, increased A-cells, reduced B-cells and exocrine fibrosis: Quantitative changes in the pancreas in type 2 diabetes. *Diabetes Research, 9*(4), 151–159.

Claro, A., Grill, V., Efendic, S., & Luft, R. (1977). Studies on the mechanisms of somatostatin action on insulin release. IV. Effect of somatostatin on cyclic AMP levels and phosphodiesterase activity in isolated rat pancreatic islets. *Acta Endocrinologica, 85*(2), 379–388.

Cooperberg, B. A., & Cryer, P. E. (2009). Beta-cell-mediated signaling predominates over direct alpha-cell signaling in the regulation of glucagon secretion in humans. *Diabetes Care, 32*(12), 2275–2280.

Csaba, Z., Peineau, S., & Dournaud, P. (2012). Molecular mechanisms of somatostatin receptor trafficking. *Journal of Molecular Endocrinology, 48*(1), R1–R12.

D'Alessio, D. A., & Ensinck, J. W. (1990). Fasting and postprandial concentrations of somatostatin-28 and somatostatin-14 in type II diabetes in men. *Diabetes, 39*(10), 1198–1202.

D'Alessio, D. A., Sieber, C., Beglinger, C., & Ensinck, J. W. (1989). A physiologic role for somatostatin 28 as a regulator of insulin secretion. *The Journal of Clinical Investigation, 84*(3), 857–862.
Daunt, M., Dale, O., & Smith, P. A. (2006). Somatostatin inhibits oxidative respiration in pancreatic beta-cells. *Endocrinology, 147*(3), 1527–1535.
de Bruin, C., Pereira, A. M., Feelders, R. A., Romijn, J. A., Roelfsema, F., Sprij-Mooij, D. M., et al. (2009). Coexpression of dopamine and somatostatin receptor subtypes in corticotroph adenomas. *The Journal of Clinical Endocrinology and Metabolism, 94*(4), 1118–1124.
de Heer, J., Rasmussen, C., Coy, D. H., & Holst, J. J. (2008). Glucagon-like peptide-1, but not glucose-dependent insulinotropic peptide, inhibits glucagon secretion via somatostatin (receptor subtype 2) in the perfused rat pancreas. *Diabetologia, 51*(12), 2263–2270.
De Marinis, Y. Z., Salehi, A., Ward, C. E., Zhang, Q., Abdulkader, F., Bengtsson, M., et al. (2010). GLP-1 inhibits and adrenaline stimulates glucagon release by differential modulation of N- and L-type Ca2+ channel-dependent exocytosis. *Cell Metabolism, 11*(6), 543–553.
Dunning, B. E., & Gerich, J. E. (2007). The role of alpha-cell dysregulation in fasting and postprandial hyperglycemia in type 2 diabetes and therapeutic implications. *Endocrine Reviews, 28*(3), 253–283.
Efendic, S., Claro, A., & Laft, R. (1976). Studies on the mechanism of somatostatin action on insulin release. III. Effect of somatostatin on arginine induced release of insulin and glucagon in man and perfused rat pancreas. *Acta Endocrinologica, 81*(4), 753–761.
Efendic, S., Enzmann, F., Nylen, A., Uvnas-Wallensten, K., & Luft, R. (1979). Effect of glucose/sulfonylurea interaction on release of insulin, glucagon, and somatostatin from isolated perfused rat pancreas. *Proceedings of the National Academy of Sciences of the United States of America, 76*(11), 5901–5904.
Ensinck, J. W., Laschansky, E. C., Vogel, R. E., Simonowitz, D. A., Roos, B. A., & Francis, B. H. (1989). Circulating prosomatostatin-derived peptides. Differential responses to food ingestion. *The Journal of Clinical Investigation, 83*(5), 1580–1589.
Gaisano, H. Y., Macdonald, P. E., & Vranic, M. (2012). Glucagon secretion and signaling in the development of diabetes. *Frontiers in Physiology, 3*, 349.
Gerber, P. P., Trimble, E. R., Wollheim, C. B., & Renold, A. E. (1981). Effect of insulin on glucose- and arginine-stimulated somatostatin secretion from the isolated perfused rat pancreas. *Endocrinology, 109*(1), 279–283.
Gerich, J. E. (1978). Somatostatin modulation of glucagon secretion and its importance in human glucose homeostasis. *Metabolism, 27*(9 Suppl. 1), 1283–1290.
Gopel, S. O., Kanno, T., Barg, S., & Rorsman, P. (2000). Patch-clamp characterisation of somatostatin-secreting -cells in intact mouse pancreatic islets. *The Journal of Physiology, 528*(Pt 3), 497–507.
Gopel, S., Zhang, Q., Eliasson, L., Ma, X. S., Galvanovskis, J., Kanno, T., et al. (2004). Capacitance measurements of exocytosis in mouse pancreatic {alpha}-, {beta}- and {delta}-cells studied in intact islets of Langerhans. *The Journal of Physiology, 556*, 711–726.
Grill, V., Gutniak, M., Roovete, A., & Efendic, S. (1984). A stimulating effect of glucose on somatostatin release is impaired in noninsulin-dependent diabetes mellitus. *The Journal of Clinical Endocrinology and Metabolism, 59*(2), 293–297.
Gromada, J., Hoy, M., Buschard, K., Salehi, A., & Rorsman, P. (2001). Somatostatin inhibits exocytosis in rat pancreatic alpha-cells by G(i2)-dependent activation of calcineurin and depriming of secretory granules. *The Journal of Physiology, 535*(Pt 2), 519–532.
Gromada, J., Hoy, M., Olsen, H. L., Gotfredsen, C. F., Buschard, K., Rorsman, P., et al. (2001). Gi2 proteins couple somatostatin receptors to low-conductance K+channels in rat pancreatic alpha-cells. *Pflügers Archiv, 442*(1), 19–26.

Gutniak, M., Grill, V., Roovete, A., & Efendic, S. (1989). Impaired somatostatin response to orally administered glucose in type II diabetes entails both somatostatin-28 and -14 and is associated with deranged metabolic control. *Acta Endocrinologica*, *121*(3), 322–326.

Gutniak, M., Grill, V., Wiechel, K. L., & Efendic, S. (1987). Basal and meal-induced somatostatin-like immunoreactivity in healthy subjects and in IDDM and totally pancreatectomized patients. Effects of acute blood glucose normalization. *Diabetes*, *36*(7), 802–807.

Hahn, H. J., Gottschling, H. D., & Woltanski, P. (1978). Effect of somatostatin on insulin secretion and cAMP content of isolated pancreatic rat islets. *Metabolism*, *27*(9 Suppl. 1), 1291–1294.

Hauge-Evans, A. C., Anderson, R. L., Persaud, S. J., & Jones, P. M. (2012). Delta cell secretory responses to insulin secretagogues are not mediated indirectly by insulin. *Diabetologia*, *55*(7), 1995–2004.

Hauge-Evans, A. C., King, A. J., Carmignac, D., Richardson, C. C., Robinson, I. C., Low, M. J., et al. (2008). Somatostatin secreted by islet {delta}-cells fulfils multiple roles as a paracrine regulator of islet function. *Diabetes*, *58*, 403–411.

Hauge-Evans, A. C., King, A. J., Fairhall, K., Persaud, S. J., & Jones, P. M. (2010). A role for islet somatostatin in mediating sympathetic regulation of glucagon secretion. *Islets*, *2*(6), 341–344.

Hellman, B., Salehi, A., Gylfe, E., Dansk, H., & Grapengiesser, E. (2009). Glucose generates coincident insulin and somatostatin pulses and antisynchronous glucagon pulses from human pancreatic islets. *Endocrinology*, *150*(12), 5334–5340.

Henquin, J. C., Dufrane, D., & Nenquin, M. (2006). Nutrient control of insulin secretion in isolated normal human islets. *Diabetes*, *55*(12), 3470–3477.

Hermansen, K., Orskov, H., & Christensen, S. E. (1979). Streptozotocin diabetes: A glucoreceptor dysfunction affecting D cells as well as B and A cells. *Diabetologia*, *17*(6), 385–389.

Hibino, H., Inanobe, A., Furutani, K., Murakami, S., Findlay, I., & Kurachi, Y. (2010). Inwardly rectifying potassium channels: Their structure, function, and physiological roles. *Physiological Reviews*, *90*(1), 291–366.

Hunyady, B., Hipkin, R. W., Schonbrunn, A., & Mezey, E. (1997). Immunohistochemical localization of somatostatin receptor SST2A in the rat pancreas. *Endocrinology*, *138*(7), 2632–2635.

Iki, K., & Pour, P. M. (2007). Distribution of pancreatic endocrine cells including IAPP-expressing cells in non-diabetic and type 2 diabetic cases. *The Journal of Histochemistry and Cytochemistry*, *55*(2), 111–118.

Ipp, E., Dobbs, R. E., Arimura, A., Vale, W., Harris, V., & Unger, R. H. (1977). Release of immunoreactive somatostatin from the pancreas in response to glucose, amino acids, pancreozymin-cholecystokinin, and tolbutamide. *The Journal of Clinical Investigation*, *60*(3), 760–765.

Kailey, B., van de Bunt, M., Cheley, S., Johnson, P. R., Macdonald, P. E., Gloyn, A. L., et al. (2012). SSTR2 is the functionally dominant somatostatin receptor in human pancreatic beta- and alpha-cells. *American Journal of Physiology Endocrinology and Metabolism*, *303*, E1107–E1116.

Kimura, N., Schindler, M., Kasai, N., & Kimura, I. (2001). Immunohistochemical localization of somatostatin receptor type 2A in rat and human tissues. *Endocrine Journal*, *48*(1), 95–102.

Kirkegaard, C., Norgaard, K., Snorgaard, O., Bek, T., Larsen, M., & Lund-Andersen, H. (1990). Effect of one year continuous subcutaneous infusion of a somatostatin analogue, octreotide, on early retinopathy, metabolic control and thyroid function in Type I (insulin-dependent) diabetes mellitus. *Acta Endocrinologica*, *122*(6), 766–772.

Kleinman, R., Ohning, G., Wong, H., Watt, P., Walsh, J., & Brunicardi, F. C. (1994). Regulatory role of intraislet somatostatin on insulin secretion in the isolated perfused human pancreas. *Pancreas*, *9*(2), 172–178.
Kubota, A., Yamada, Y., Kagimoto, S., Shimatsu, A., Imamura, M., Tsuda, K., et al. (1994). Identification of somatostatin receptor subtypes and an implication for the efficacy of somatostatin analogue SMS 201-995 in treatment of human endocrine tumors. *The Journal of Clinical Investigation*, *93*(3), 1321–1325.
Kumar, U., Sasi, R., Suresh, S., Patel, A., Thangaraju, M., Metrakos, P., et al. (1999). Subtype-selective expression of the five somatostatin receptors (hSSTR1-5) in human pancreatic islet cells: A quantitative double-label immunohistochemical analysis. *Diabetes*, *48*(1), 77–85.
Longo, D. L., Fauci, S., Kasper, D. L., Hauser, S. L., Jameson, J. L., & Loscalzo, J. (Eds.), (2012). *Harrison's Principles of Internal Medicine*. (18th ed.). New York, NY: McGraw-Hill.
Luft, R., Efendic, S., Hokfelt, T., Johansson, O., & Arimura, A. (1974). Immunohistochemical evidence for the localization of somatostatin—Like immunoreactivity in a cell population of the pancreatic islets. *Medical Biology*, *52*(6), 428–430.
Lupp, A., Hunder, A., Petrich, A., Nagel, F., Doll, C., & Schulz, S. (2011). Reassessment of sst(5) somatostatin receptor expression in normal and neoplastic human tissues using the novel rabbit monoclonal antibody UMB-4. *Neuroendocrinology*, *94*(3), 255–264.
Lupp, A., Nagel, F., Doll, C., Rocken, C., Evert, M., Mawrin, C., et al. (2012). Reassessment of sst3 somatostatin receptor expression in human normal and neoplastic tissues using the novel rabbit monoclonal antibody UMB-5. *Neuroendocrinology*, *96*(4), 301–310.
Mandarino, L., Stenner, D., Blanchard, W., Nissen, S., Gerich, J., Ling, N., et al. (1981). Selective effects of somatostatin-14, -25 and -28 on in vitro insulin and glucagon secretion. *Nature*, *291*(5810), 76–77.
Mazziotti, G., Floriani, I., Bonadonna, S., Torri, V., Chanson, P., & Giustina, A. (2009). Effects of somatostatin analogs on glucose homeostasis: A metaanalysis of acromegaly studies. *The Journal of Clinical Endocrinology and Metabolism*, *94*(5), 1500–1508.
McKeage, K. (2013). Pasireotide: A review of its use in Cushing's disease. *Drugs*, *73*, 563–574.
Menge, B. A., Gruber, L., Jorgensen, S. M., Deacon, C. F., Schmidt, W. E., Veldhuis, J. D., et al. (2011). Loss of inverse relationship between pulsatile insulin and glucagon secretion in patients with type 2 diabetes. *Diabetes*, *60*(8), 2160–2168.
Mergler, S., Singh, V., Grotzinger, C., Kaczmarek, P., Wiedenmann, B., & Strowski, M. Z. (2008). Characterization of voltage operated R-type Ca2+ channels in modulating somatostatin receptor subtype 2 and 3-dependent inhibition of insulin secretion from INS-1 cells. *Cellular Signalling*, *20*(12), 2286–2295.
Misler, S., Dickey, A., & Barnett, D. W. (2005). Maintenance of stimulus-secretion coupling and single beta-cell function in cryopreserved-thawed human islets of Langerhans. *Pflügers Archiv*, *450*(6), 395–404
Mitra, S. W., Mezey, E., Hunyady, B., Chamberlain, L., Hayes, E., Foor, F., et al. (1999). Colocalization of somatostatin receptor sst5 and insulin in rat pancreatic beta-cells. *Endocrinology*, *140*(8), 3790–3796.
Molina, J., Fachado, A., Menegaz, D., Berggren, P. O., & Caicedo, A. (2012). Paracrine regulation of human delta-cells is impaired in type 2 diabetes. *Diabetes*, *61*(Suppl. 1A), 145-LB.
Moller, L. N., Stidsen, C. E., Hartmann, B., & Holst, J. J. (2003). Somatostatin receptors. *Biochimica et Biophysica Acta*, *1616*(1), 1–84.
Moss, C. E., Marsh, W. J., Parker, H. E., Ogunnowo-Bada, E., Riches, C. H., Habib, A. M., et al. (2012). Somatostatin receptor 5 and cannabinoid receptor 1 activation inhibit

secretion of glucose-dependent insulinotropic polypeptide from intestinal K cells in rodents. *Diabetologia, 55*(11), 3094–3103.

Myint, K. S., Greenfield, J. R., Farooqi, I. S., Henning, E., Holst, J. J., & Finer, N. (2012). Prolonged successful therapy for hyperinsulinaemic hypoglycaemia after gastric bypass: The pathophysiological role of GLP1 and its response to a somatostatin analogue. *European Journal of Endocrinology, 166*(5), 951–955.

O'Carroll, A. M., Lolait, S. J., Konig, M., & Mahan, L. C. (1992). Molecular cloning and expression of a pituitary somatostatin receptor with preferential affinity for somatostatin-28. *Molecular Pharmacology, 42*(6), 939–946.

Orci, L., Baetens, D., Rufener, C., Amherdt, M., Ravazzola, M., Studer, P., et al. (1976). Hypertrophy and hyperplasia of somatostatin-containing D-cells in diabetes. *Proceedings of the National Academy of Sciences of the United States of America, 73*(4), 1338–1342.

Ostenson, C. G., Efendic, S., & Grill, V. (1990). Abnormal regulation by glucose of somatostatin secretion in the perfused pancreas of NIDDM rats. *Pancreas, 5*(3), 347–353.

Papotti, M., Bongiovanni, M., Volante, M., Allia, E., Landolfi, S., Helboe, L., et al. (2002). Expression of somatostatin receptor types 1-5 in 81 cases of gastrointestinal and pancreatic endocrine tumors. A correlative immunohistochemical and reverse-transcriptase polymerase chain reaction analysis. *Virchows Archiv, 440*(5), 461–475.

Park, S., Jiang, H., Zhang, H., & Smith, R. G. (2012). Modification of ghrelin receptor signaling by somatostatin receptor-5 regulates insulin release. *Proceedings of the National Academy of Sciences of the United States of America, 109*(46), 19003–19008.

Patel, Y. C. (1999). Somatostatin and its receptor family. *Frontiers in Neuroendocrinology, 20*(3), 157–198.

Patel, Y. C., Greenwood, M. T., Warszynska, A., Panetta, R., & Srikant, C. B. (1994). All five cloned human somatostatin receptors (hSSTR1-5) are functionally coupled to adenylyl cyclase. *Biochemical and Biophysical Research Communications, 198*(2), 605–612.

Patel, Y. C., & Reichlin, S. (1978). Somatostatin in hypothalamus, extrahypothalamic brain, and peripheral tissues of the rat. *Endocrinology, 102*(2), 523–530.

Patel, Y. C., & Wheatley, T. (1983). In vivo and in vitro plasma disappearance and metabolism of somatostatin-28 and somatostatin-14 in the rat. *Endocrinology, 112*(1), 220–225.

Patton, G. S., Ipp, E., Dobbs, R. E., Orci, L., Vale, W., & Unger, R. H. (1977). Pancreatic immunoreactive somatostatin release. *Proceedings of the National Academy of Sciences of the United States of America, 74*(5), 2140–2143.

Portela-Gomes, G. M., Grimelius, L., Westermark, P., & Stridsberg, M. (2010). Somatostatin receptor subtypes in human type 2 diabetic islets. *Pancreas, 39*(6), 836–842.

Rahier, J., Goebbels, R. M., & Henquin, J. C. (1983). Cellular composition of the human diabetic pancreas. *Diabetologia, 24*(5), 366–371.

Ramracheya, R., Ward, C., Shigeto, M., Walker, J. N., Amisten, S., Zhang, Q., et al. (2010). Membrane potential-dependent inactivation of voltage-gated ion channels in alpha-cells inhibits glucagon secretion from human islets. *Diabetes, 59*(9), 2198–2208.

Renstrom, E., Ding, W. G., Bokvist, K., & Rorsman, P. (1996). Neurotransmitter-induced inhibition of exocytosis in insulin-secreting beta cells by activation of calcineurin. *Neuron, 17*(3), 513–522.

Rohrer, S. P., & Schaeffer, J. M. (2000). Identification and characterization of subtype selective somatostatin receptor agonists. *Journal of Physiology, Paris, 94*(3–4), 211–215.

Rorsman, P., & Braun, M. (2013). Regulation of insulin secretion in human pancreatic islets. *Annual Review of Physiology, 75*, 155–179.

Saito, K., Yaginuma, N., & Takahashi, T. (1979). Differential volumetry of A, B and D cells in the pancreatic islets of diabetic and nondiabetic subjects. *The Tohoku Journal of Experimental Medicine, 129*(3), 273–283.

Samols, E., Stagner, J. I., Ewart, R. B., & Marks, V. (1988). The order of islet microvascular cellular perfusion is B——A——D in the perfused rat pancreas. *The Journal of Clinical Investigation*, *82*(1), 350–353.

Schuit, F. C., & Pipeleers, D. G. (1985). Regulation of adenosine 3',5'-monophosphate levels in the pancreatic B cell. *Endocrinology*, *117*(3), 834–840.

Schwetz, T. A., Ustione, A., & Piston, D. W. (2013). Neuropeptide Y and somatostatin inhibit insulin secretion through different mechanisms. *American Journal of Physiology. Endocrinology and Metabolism*, *304*(2), E211–E221.

Segers, O., De Vroede, M., Michotte, Y., & Somers, G. (1989). Basal and tolbutamide-induced plasma somatostatin in healthy subjects and in patients with diabetes and impaired glucose tolerance. *Diabetic Medicine*, *6*(3), 232–238.

Shapiro, A. M., Lakey, J. R., Ryan, E. A., Korbutt, G. S., Toth, E., Warnock, G. L., et al. (2000). Islet transplantation in seven patients with type 1 diabetes mellitus using a glucocorticoid-free immunosuppressive regimen. *The New England Journal of Medicine*, *343*(4), 230–238.

Sherwin, R. S., Hendler, R., DeFronzo, R., Wahren, J., & Felic, P. (1977). Glucose homeostasis during prolonged suppression of glucagon and insulin secretion by somatostatin. *Proceedings of the National Academy of Sciences of the United States of America*, *74*(1), 348–352.

Singh, V., Brendel, M. D., Zacharias, S., Mergler, S., Jahr, H., Wiedenmann, B., et al. (2007). Characterization of somatostatin receptor subtype-specific regulation of insulin and glucagon secretion: An in vitro study on isolated human pancreatic islets. *The Journal of Clinical Endocrinology and Metabolism*, *92*(2), 673–680.

Skare, S., Dahl-Jorgensen, K., Hanssen, K. F., & Norman, N. (1985). Increased peripheral venous somatostatin concentration and decreased glucagon response to arginine in patients with insulin dependent diabetes mellitus without residual B-cell function. Increased plasma SRIF in IDDM. *Acta Endocrinologica*, *109*(4), 517–521.

Smith, P. A. (2009). N-type Ca(2+) -channels in murine pancreatic beta-cells are inhibited by an exclusive coupling with somatostatin receptor subtype 1. *Endocrinology*, *150*(2), 741–748.

Smith, P. A., Sellers, L. A., & Humphrey, P. P. (2001). Somatostatin activates two types of inwardly rectifying K+channels in MIN-6 cells. *The Journal of Physiology*, *532*(Pt 1), 127–142.

Stefan, Y., Orci, L., Malaisse-Lagae, F., Perrelet, A., Patel, Y., & Unger, R. H. (1982). Quantitation of endocrine cell content in the pancreas of nondiabetic and diabetic humans. *Diabetes*, *31*(8 Pt 1), 694–700.

Strowski, M. Z., & Blake, A. D. (2008). Function and expression of somatostatin receptors of the endocrine pancreas. *Molecular and Cellular Endocrinology*, *286*(1–2), 169–179.

Strowski, M. Z., Kohler, M., Chen, H. Y., Trumbauer, M. E., Li, Z., Szalkowski, D., et al. (2003). Somatostatin receptor subtype 5 regulates insulin secretion and glucose homeostasis. *Molecular Endocrinology*, *17*(1), 93 106.

Strowski, M. Z., Parmar, R. M., Blake, A. D., & Schaeffer, J. M. (2000). Somatostatin inhibits insulin and glucagon secretion via two receptors subtypes: An in vitro study of pancreatic islets from somatostatin receptor 2 knockout mice. *Endocrinology*, *141*(1), 111–117.

Taniyama, Y., Suzuki, T., Mikami, Y., Moriya, T., Satomi, S., & Sasano, H. (2005). Systemic distribution of somatostatin receptor subtypes in human: An immunohistochemical study. *Endocrine Journal*, *52*(5), 605–611.

Tengholm, A., & Gylfe, E. (2009). Oscillatory control of insulin secretion. *Molecular and Cellular Endocrinology*, *297*(1–2), 58–72.

Thaler, J. P., & Cummings, D. E. (2009). Minireview: Hormonal and metabolic mechanisms of diabetes remission after gastrointestinal surgery. *Endocrinology*, *150*(6), 2518–2525.

Trimble, E. R., Gerber, P. P., & Renold, A. E. (1981). Abnormalities of pancreatic somatostatin secretion corrected by in vivo insulin treatment of streptozotocin-diabetic rats. *Diabetes*, *30*(10), 865–867.

Tulipano, G., & Schulz, S. (2007). Novel insights in somatostatin receptor physiology. *European Journal of Endocrinology*, *156*(Suppl. 1), S3–S11.

Unger, R. H., & Cherrington, A. D. (2012). Glucagonocentric restructuring of diabetes: A pathophysiologic and therapeutic makeover. *The Journal of Clinical Investigation*, *122*(1), 4–12.

van der Hoek, J., van der Lelij, A. J., Feelders, R. A., de Herder, W. W., Uitterlinden, P., Poon, K. W., et al. (2005). The somatostatin analogue SOM230, compared with octreotide, induces differential effects in several metabolic pathways in acromegalic patients. *Clinical Endocrinology*, *63*(2), 176–184.

Vanetti, M., Kouba, M., Wang, X., Vogt, G., & Hollt, V. (1992). Cloning and expression of a novel mouse somatostatin receptor (SSTR2B). *FEBS Letters*, *311*(3), 290–294.

Velasquez-Mieyer, P. A., Umpierrez, G. E., Lustig, R. H., Cashion, A. K., Cowan, P. A., Christensen, M., et al. (2004). Race affects insulin and GLP-1 secretion and response to a long-acting somatostatin analogue in obese adults. *International Journal of Obesity and Related Metabolic Disorders*, *28*(2), 330–333.

Viana, F., & Hille, B. (1996). Modulation of high voltage-activated calcium channels by somatostatin in acutely isolated rat amygdaloid neurons. *The Journal of Neuroscience*, *16*(19), 6000–6011.

Walker, J. N., Ramracheya, R., Zhang, Q., Johnson, P. R., Braun, M., & Rorsman, P. (2011). Regulation of glucagon secretion by glucose: Paracrine, intrinsic or both? *Diabetes, Obesity and Metabolism*, *13*(Suppl. 1), 95–105.

Yamada, Y., Kagimoto, S., Kubota, A., Yasuda, K., Masuda, K., Someya, Y., et al. (1993). Cloning, functional expression and pharmacological characterization of a fourth (hSSTR4) and a fifth (hSSTR5) human somatostatin receptor subtype. *Biochemical and Biophysical Research Communications*, *195*(2), 844–852.

Yamada, Y., Post, S. R., Wang, K., Tager, H. S., Bell, G. I., & Seino, S. (1992). Cloning and functional characterization of a family of human and mouse somatostatin receptors expressed in brain, gastrointestinal tract, and kidney. *Proceedings of the National Academy of Sciences of the United States of America*, *89*(1), 251–255.

Yamada, Y., Reisine, T., Law, S. F., Ihara, Y., Kubota, A., Kagimoto, S., et al. (1992). Somatostatin receptors, an expanding gene family: Cloning and functional characterization of human SSTR3, a protein coupled to adenylyl cyclase. *Molecular Endocrinology*, *6*(12), 2136–2142.

Yang, L., Berk, S. C., Rohrer, S. P., Mosley, R. T., Guo, L., Underwood, D. J., et al. (1998). Synthesis and biological activities of potent peptidomimetics selective for somatostatin receptor subtype 2. *Proceedings of the National Academy of Sciences of the United States of America*, *95*(18), 10836–10841.

Yasuda, K., Rens-Domiano, S., Breder, C. D., Law, S. F., Saper, C. B., Reisine, T., et al. (1992). Cloning of a novel somatostatin receptor, SSTR3, coupled to adenylylcyclase. *The Journal of Biological Chemistry*, *267*(28), 20422–20428.

Yorifuji, T., Kawakita, R., Hosokawa, Y., Fujimaru, R., Matsubara, K., Aizu, K., et al. (2013). Efficacy and safety of long-term, continuous subcutaneous octreotide infusion for patients with different subtypes of KATP -channel hyperinsulinism. *Clinical Endocrinology*, *78*(6), 891–897.

Yoshimoto, Y., Fukuyama, Y., Horio, Y., Inanobe, A., Gotoh, M., & Kurachi, Y. (1999). Somatostatin induces hyperpolarization in pancreatic islet alpha cells by activating a G protein-gated K+channel. *FEBS Letters*, *444*(2–3), 265–269.

Yue, J. T., Burdett, E., Coy, D. H., Giacca, A., Efendic, S., & Vranic, M. (2012). Somatostatin receptor type 2 antagonism improves glucagon and corticosterone

counterregulatory responses to hypoglycemia in streptozotocin-induced diabetic rats. *Diabetes*, *61*(1), 197–207.
Zambre, Y., Ling, Z., Chen, M. C., Hou, X., Woon, C. W., Culler, M., et al. (1999). Inhibition of human pancreatic islet insulin release by receptor-selective somatostatin analogs directed to somatostatin receptor subtype 5. *Biochemical Pharmacology*, *57*(10), 1159–1164.
Zhang, Q., Bengtsson, M., Partridge, C., Salehi, A., Braun, M., Cox, R., et al. (2007). R-type Ca(2+)-channel-evoked CICR regulates glucose-induced somatostatin secretion. *Nature Cell Biology*, *9*(4), 453–460.
Zhao, Y., Fang, Q., Straub, S. G., Lindau, M., & Sharp, G. W. (2010). Noradrenaline inhibits exocytosis via the G protein betagamma subunit and refilling of the readily releasable granule pool via the alpha(i1/2) subunit. *The Journal of Physiology*, *588*(Pt 18), 3485–3498.
Zhou, G., Liu, S. H., Shahi, K. M., Wang, H., Duan, X., Lin, X., et al. (2012). Negative regulation of pancreatic and duodenal homeobox-1 by somatostatin receptor subtype 5. *Molecular Endocrinology*, *26*(7), 1225–1234.

CHAPTER EIGHT

Modulation of the Pancreatic Islet-Stress Axis as a Novel Potential Therapeutic Target in Diabetes Mellitus

Barbara Ludwig[*,†,‡,1,2], **Andreas Barthel**[*,††,1], **Andreas Reichel**[*], **Norman L. Block**[§,||,#], **Stefan Ludwig**[**], **Andrew V. Schally**[§,¶,||,#], **Stefan R. Bornstein**[*,†,‡]

[*]Department of Medicine III, University Hospital Carl Gustav Carus, Dresden, Germany
[†]The Paul Langerhans Institute, Dresden, Germany
[‡]Center for Regenerative Therapies Dresden, Dresden University of Technology, Dresden, Germany
[§]Department of Pathology, University of Miami Miller School of Medicine, Miami, Florida, USA
[¶]Department of Medicine, Division of Endocrinology, University of Miami Miller School of Medicine, Miami, Florida, USA
[||]Department of Medicine, Division of Hematology-Oncology, University of Miami Miller School of Medicine, Miami, Florida, USA
[#]Veterans Administration Medical Center, Miami, Florida, USA
[**]Department of Visceral, Thorax and Vascular Surgery, University Hospital Carl Gustav Carus, Dresden, Germany
[††]Endokrinologikum Ruhr, Bochum, Germany
[1]These authors contributed equally to this work
[2]Corresponding author: e-mail address: barbara.ludwig@uniklinikum-dresden.de

Contents

Vitamins and Hormones, Volume 95
ISSN 0083-6729
http://dx.doi.org/10.1016/B978-0-12-800174-5.00008-9

Abstract

Loss of pancreatic islet function and insulin-producing beta cell mass is a central hallmark in the pathogenesis of both type 1 and type 2 diabetes. While in type 1 diabetes this phenomenon is due to an extensive destruction of beta cells caused by an autoimmune process, the mechanisms resulting in beta cell failure in type 2 diabetes are different and less clear. Also, beta cell destruction in type 1 diabetes occurs early and is the initial step in the pathogenetic process, while beta cell loss in type 2 diabetes after an initial phase of hyperinsulinemia due to the underlying insulin resistance occurs relatively late and it is less pronounced. Since diabetes mellitus is the most frequent endocrine disease, with an increasing high prevalence worldwide, huge efforts have been made over the past many decades to identify predisposing genetic, environmental, and nutritional factors in order to develop effective strategies to prevent the disease. In parallel, extensive studies in different cell systems and animal models have helped to elucidate our understanding of the physiologic function of islets and to gain insight into the immunological and non-immunological mechanisms of beta cell destruction and failure. Furthermore, currently emerging concepts of beta cell regeneration (e.g., the restoration of the beta cell pool by regenerative, proliferative and antiapoptotic processes, and recovery of physiologic islet function) apparently is yielding the first promising results.

Recent insights into the complex endocrine and paracrine mechanisms regulating the physiologic function of pancreatic islets, as well as beta cell life and death, constitute an essential part of this new and exciting area of diabetology. For example, understanding of the physiological role of glucagon-like peptide 1 has resulted in the successful clinical implementation of incretin-based therapies over the last years. Further, recent data suggesting paracrine effects of growth hormone-releasing hormone and corticotropin-releasing hormone on the regulation of pancreatic islet function, survival, and proliferation as well as on local glucocorticoid metabolism provide evidence for a potential role of the pancreatic islet-stress axis in the pathophysiology of diabetes mellitus.

In this chapter, we provide a comprehensive overview of current preventive and regenerative concepts as a basis for the development of novel therapeutic approaches to the treatment of diabetes mellitus. A particular focus is given on the potential of the pancreatic islet-stress axis in the development of novel regenerative strategies.

1. INTRODUCTION

Currently, we are observing globally a dramatically increasing prevalence of diabetes mellitus and its associated complications. For example, the cardiovascular morbidity and mortality related to the disease is a limiting prognostic factor for patients suffering from diabetes and a major burden for our health systems. Although substantial progress has been made over the past several decades with regard to our understanding of the pathophysiology of the disease, there is currently no curative approach for the treatment of diabetes mellitus. This implies that, apart from optimizing the currently available therapies, an effective prevention is of major importance to the limitation of the disease burden (Mayor, 2007; von Boehmer, 2004). Earlier therapeutic regimens for the treatment of diabetes were almost entirely glucocentric, meaning that the focus was put on glycemic control alone. However, since many diabetic patients develop cardiovascular morbidity despite sufficient glycemic control, current therapies must also consider other important aspects of the disease such as hormonal (e.g., the renin–angiotensin–aldosterone system) and inflammatory processes, each of which may play a major role in the development of the cardiovascular complications (Reichard, Nilsson, & Rosenqvist, 1993; UK Prospective Diabetes Study (UKPDS) Group, 1998). Further, during the last decade, some pharmacologic concepts have led to questions regarding drug safety and efficacy, resulting in the withdrawal of marketing authorization for several antidiabetic drugs by regulatory authorities (Massi-Benedetti, 2006). Therefore, in order to improve our therapeutic armamentarium for the treatment of diabetes, the development of sophisticated and safe therapeutic regimens is urgently required.

Based on this background and with increasing understanding of the disease, beta cell protection and regeneration became a major focus of research interest (Meier, 2008). It has been recognized that pancreatic islet inflammation and loss of insulin-producing beta cells is not only a central event in the pathogenesis of type 1 diabetes mellitus (T1DM) but also a characteristic in the pathophysiological development of type 2 diabetes (Donath et al., 2008). While in type 1 diabetes, beta cell loss is due to an autoimmune destruction of pancreatic beta cells, it was revealed that destruction of pancreatic islets is also commonly observed in the later stages of type 2 diabetes. Traditionally, type 2 diabetes was regarded as a disease almost exclusively affecting older individuals, whereas manifestation of type 1 diabetes was typically seen in adolescents or young adults. However, due to the dramatically increasing prevalence of type 2 diabetes in younger people and the approximation of the age of disease onset between each of the two disease entities, the clear contrast between type 1 and type 2 diabetes has apparently become "blurred" (Kempf, Rathmann, & Herder, 2008).

Since current data provide evidence for the regenerative potential of functional islets, even in later stages of life, both type 1 and type 2 diabetes may be attacked by novel anti-inflammatory and regenerative therapies aiming at the preservation and restoration of beta cell mass and function (Meier, 2008). Although future, novel preventive and regenerative approaches may offer attractive potential in the treatment of diabetes, and despite some similarities shared by type 1 and type 2 diabetes, a common therapeutic strategy addressing both, type 1 and type 2 diabetes, appears to be fictional today.

2. FACTORS AND CONDITIONS PREDISPOSING TO THE DEVELOPMENT OF DIABETES MELLITUS

2.1. Type 1 diabetes

The overall prevalence of T1DM is about 0.5%, with strong regional differences, and affects about 2 million individuals, or 10%, of all diabetic patients in North America and Western Europe. Pathophysiologically, the autoimmune response underlying the development of T1DM is characterized by the complex interplay between antigen-presenting cells, auto-reactive and adaptive regulatory T cells and is histologically reflected by macrophage- and T-cell infiltration of the islets which results finally in beta cell destruction and insulin deficiency of the organism (Achenbach, Bonifacio, Koczwara, & Ziegler, 2005; Foulis, McGill, & Farquharson, 1991). Both genetic and environmental factors have been extensively investigated to identify the mechanisms triggering the auto-destructive response (Baisch et al., 1990).

2.1.1 Genetic factors predisposing for type 1 diabetes

Although the vast majority of patients suffering from T1DM have a negative family history of diabetes, a number of genetic studies have identified an association of T1DM with some major susceptibility loci that are related either to the individual's immunologic responsiveness and identity or to the beta cell itself (Thivolet, 2001).

2.1.1.1 Association with human leukocyte antigens

Genetic linkage analysis of quantitative trait loci in families with T1DM has led to the identification of particular susceptibility loci on chromosome 6. These are related to specific HLA-genotypes which, in turn, are associated with more than half of the cases of familial T1DM (Todd, 1995). The strongest associations with T1DM has been described for the two haplotypes, DR4-DQ8 and DR3-DQ2, with the highest risk for the development of T1DM in subjects carrying both haplotypes (Caillat-Zucman et al., 1992).

2.1.1.2 Insulin

Another, less strong susceptibility locus associated with about 10% of the genetic background contributing to the development of T1DM is located on chromosome 11 in the region which encodes the promoter of the gene encoding for insulin (Bell, Horita, & Karam, 1984). Interestingly, the risk of developing T1DM is inversely associated with the length of specific repetitive tandem sequences in the insulin gene promoter region (Bennett et al., 1995).

2.1.1.3 Regulators of T-cell activation

Genetic screening has led to the identification of two T1DM-susceptibility loci which are related to T-cell function and activation, and which thus attract particular attention as potential targets for preventive approaches. These two genes encode for PTPN22, a variant of the gene encoding for lymphoid tyrosine phosphatase and for the gene encoding for the cytotoxic T lymphocyte antigen 4 (Bottini et al., 2004; Ueda et al., 2003). Both gene products are functionally involved in the regulation of antigen presentation to T cells and may therefore possibly play a direct role in the pathogenesis of T1DM.

2.1.2 Environmental factors predisposing for type 1 diabetes

The fact that we can observe regional differences, as well as rapidly increasing T1DM prevalence in some individual countries (Zalutskaya, Bornstein, Mokhort, & Garmaev, 2004), suggests that environmental factors may contribute to the manifestation of the disease in individuals with a genetic predisposition for T1DM (Gillespie et al., 2004). Obvious environmental factors with a local specificity include nutritional differences and exposure to certain infectious agents.

2.1.2.1 Nutrition

Immunomodulatory factors relating to nutritional components relevant in the pathogenesis of T1DM, apart from breastfeeding in early life, appear to be of particular importance as priming and maturation of the immune system appear to be vulnerable to nutritional factors during the first year of childhood. For example, the timing of dietary exposure to cereals and bovine milk appears to be of particular importance in the context of beta cell autoimmunity (Norris et al., 2003; Paronen, Bjorksten, Hattevig, Akerblom, & Vaarala, 2000; Winkler, Mollenhauer, Hummel, Bonifacio, & Ziegler, 2008). Some studies suggest a protective effect of nutritional supplementation, during the first year of life, with omega-3 fatty acids, fish oil, and vitamin D, on the later manifestation of T1DM (Fronczak et al., 2003; Hypponen, Laara, Reunanen, Jarvelin, & Virtanen, 2001;

Norris et al., 2007; Stene & Joner, 2003; Stene, Ulriksen, Magnus, & Joner, 2000).

2.1.2.2 Infectious factors

Challenge by infectious pathogens also contributes to priming and maturation of the immune system. Interestingly, over the last few decades, we have observed increased prevalence of allergic and autoimmune diseases in the Western world on one hand, and on the other hand, this is inversely related to a decreased exposure to common infectious pathogens during childhood as a result of general improvements in hygiene and social welfare (Gale, 2002). Although the precise nature of this general coincidence with regard to the pathogenesis of T1DM is not yet clear, some studies have provided evidence for a potential association between T1DM and specific viral (e.g., enteroviral) infections (Elfaitouri et al., 2007; Lonnrot et al., 2000; Salminen et al., 2003).

2.2. Type 2 diabetes

The epidemic prevalence of obesity, that is a predisposition to insulin resistance and impairments of glucose metabolism, is directly related to the probability of development of type 2 diabetes (T2DM). An increase in the total prevalence from 2.8% in the year 2000 to 4.4% in 2030 is anticipated (Bornstein, Wong, & Licinio, 2006; Sharma, 2006; Wild, Roglic, Green, Sicree, & King, 2004). The development of this disease in the individual is characterized by a pathophysiologic sequence of events ranging from impairments of glucose and lipid metabolism, initial inadequate insulin secretion, hyperinsulinism due to insulin resistance, and then subsequent lack of insulin due to failure and loss of the insulin-producing pancreatic beta cells (Goldstein, 2007). The latter with a loss of beta cell mass of more than 50% is regarded as the irreversible result of longstanding T2DM (Butler, Janson, Soeller, & Butler, 2003). However, since slim subjects may also develop T2DM and since not every obese subject develops T2DM, there is a wide individual variation of disease instigation suggesting a strong influence of individual genetic, as well as environmental factors, as being crucial for the development of this disease.

2.2.1 Genetic factors predisposing to type 2 diabetes

Genome-wide association studies and consecutive meta-analyses have revealed multiple genetic susceptibility loci associated with the developmental risk of T2DM (Cauchi et al., 2008; Horikawa et al., 1997, 2000;

Schwarz et al., 2006; Schwarz, Lindstrom, et al., 2008; Schwarz, Odenbach, et al., 2008; Zeggini et al., 2008, 2007). However, although epidemiologic and genetic data provide ample evidence for a significant genetic background of T2DM, and despite huge epidemiologic efforts, the current data are only sufficient to explain about 10% of the genetic background of T2DM (Dupuis et al., 2010). The strongest association with the development of T2DM that has been described so far is located within the *TCF7L2* gene, which encodes for the transcription factor, Tcf-4, that is also related with the degree of sulfonylurea efficacy (Pearson, 2009). The current demographic circumstance of increasing age of the general population, on one hand, and changes in diet, lack of physical activity, and consequent obesity, on the other hand, provides the current background for the gene–environment interaction and further refinement of the susceptibility profile for T2DM (Gerstein et al., 2006; Hanefeld, Koehler, Gallo, Benke, & Ott, 2007; Korenblum et al., 2005; Schwarz, Reimann, et al., 2007; Yach, Stuckler, & Brownell, 2006).

2.2.2 Endocrine and paracrine factors predisposing for type 2 diabetes

Glucose homeostasis is regulated not only by the classical hormones such as insulin, glucagon, and glucocorticoids (GCs) but also by a variety of factors released from fat tissue, thereby linking T2DM and its complications to obesity. These factors, released from excessive fat tissue, include, for example, free fatty acids that may directly interfere with the signal transduction pathways propagating the insulin response within the cells (Mlinar, Marc, Janez, & Pfeifer, 2007). A panel of adipocyte derived cytokines (the so-called adipokines; e.g., tumor necrosis factor-alpha, interleukin-6, adiponectin, visfatin, leptin-retinol-binding protein 4) are also, at least in part, known as mediators of inflammation. This provides an interesting pathophysiologic link between obesity, impaired glucose metabolism, and "low grade" inflammatory processes that are related to diabetic comorbidities such as cardiovascular complications (Bornstein et al., 2000; Ehrhart-Bornstein et al., 2003; Lamounier-Zepter et al., 2006; Ulgen, Scherbaum, Partke, Bornstein, & Schinner, 2008).

2.2.3 Stress and type 2 diabetes: Genetic–environmental interactions

An important factor prevalent in our current lifestyle is psychosocial stress (e.g., lack of quality time, pressure, noise, conflicting relationship). Interestingly, this phenomenon has been linked to aberrations in glucose metabolism and psychosocial stress has also been described as a risk factor of T2DM

(Kaufman et al., 2007; Kyrou & Tsigos, 2007; Reichel et al., 2005; Tselmin, Korenblum, Reimann, Bornstein, & Schwarz, 2007). An obvious hormonal link between stress and the pathophysiology of T2DM is provided by the effects of the stress hormones, namely catecholamines and GCs, on glucose metabolism. Both categories of stress hormones provide a physiologic link between central nervous system functions and the regulation of peripheral nutrient metabolism. The hypothalamic–pituitary–adrenal (HPA) axis has attracted particular research interest as a model system for gene–environment interactions due to the well characterized effects of the GCs on gene expression. In addition, there is new and increasing evidence that dysregulation and dysfunction of the HPA axis potentially contributes to the pathology of T2DM (Bates et al., 2008; Bornstein, 1997; Bornstein, Uhlmann, Haidan, Ehrhart-Bornstein, & Scherbaum, 1997; Bornstein et al., 2006; Golden, 2007). Interestingly, recent data provide evidence for the existence of a local, paracrine mechanism, based on the expression of hypothalamic-releasing hormones (e.g., corticotropin-releasing hormone, CRH) and their corresponding receptors (CRH-receptor type 1, CRHR1) in the pancreatic islets, and also for local mechanisms of GC metabolism (Ludwig et al., 2012, 2010; Schmid et al., 2010). Furthermore, these mechanisms may possibly be involved in the physiologic regulation of beta cell function, survival and also regeneration, thereby providing evidence for a potential role of the pancreatic islet-stress axis in the pathophysiology of diabetes mellitus. This amplifies our understanding of the disease and these findings may serve as a rational basis for the development of novel therapeutic approaches to prevent and treat T2DM.

3. CURRENT OPTIONS AND CONCEPTS FOR THE PREVENTION AND TREATMENT OF DIABETES MELLITUS

3.1. Type 1 diabetes

The most important prerequisite for successful primary prevention strategies is the identification of individuals at risk, and then early and subsequent avoidance of objective risk factors (e.g., early exposure to certain nutrients). Currently, there are ongoing clinical trials (e.g., TRIGR Study Group, 2007) aimed at defining the role of specific nutritional factors for prevention of T1DM in individuals with a high genetic risk.

The goal of secondary prevention strategies in T1DM is the modulation of the anti-islet autoimmune response. Interestingly, autoantibodies directed against beta cell antigens such as insulin (Nakayama et al., 2005; Palmer, 1987), glutamic acid decarboxylase 65 (GAD65) (Baekkeskov et al., 1989), islet-associated antigen 2/ICA512 (IA-2/ICA512) (Baekkeskov et al., 1989; Lan, Wasserfall, Maclaren, & Notkins, 1996), and the cation efflux transporter (ZnT8) (Wenzlau et al., 2007) are frequently detectable years before the clinical manifestation of T1DM (Ziegler, Hummel, Schenker, & Bonifacio, 1999). Detection of these specific antibodies in the serum defines a predictive risk of the affected individuals' development of T1DM (Verge et al., 1996). Conversely, screening for predisposing HLA-constellations (DR3-DQ2; DR4-DQ8) and for autoantibodies to insulin, GAD65, IA-2 and ZnT8 should allow identification of high-risk individuals who are prone to develop T1DM. Several clinical trials (e.g., the type 1 Diabetes Prediction and Prevention, DIPP Study and the Primary Oral/Intranasal Insulin Trial, Pre-POINT; Achenbach, Barker, & Bonifacio, 2008; Nejentsev et al., 1999) have been performed in order to predict and prevent the onset of T1DM based on this strategy. In addition to Pre-POINT, the efficacy of insulin exposure as an antigen-specific preventive approach in the prevention of T1DM was tested in the Diabetes Prevention Trial—Type 1 (DPT-1) (Diabetes Prevention Trial–Type 1 Diabetes Study Group, 2002). However, this trial did not show any preventive effect in subjects at risk for T1DM. Since the efficacy of insulin exposure may also depend on more sophisticated factors such as the application route, other antigen-specific studies using insulin as a primary target antigen are continuing (e.g., the Intranasal Insulin Trial, INIT; Harrison et al., 2004; Kupila et al., 2003). Other, nonantigen-specific strategies testing the role of systemic immunomodulators such as cyclosporine and nicotinamide have been unsuccsessful in the secondary prevention of T1DM (Bach et al., 1990; Gale, Bingley, Emmett, & Collier, 2004; Lampeter et al., 1998). More specific immunomodulatory concepts (e.g., affecting T-cell activation using anti-CD3 antibodies) have been more promising. Some intervention trials in patients with recent-onset type 1 diabetes reported an improvement and maintenance of beta cell function over a time period of 1–2 years (Herold et al., 2005, 2002; Keymeulen et al., 2005). Other specific immunomodulatory approaches currently being tested in recent-onset T1DM include anti-thymocyte globulin, the monoclonal anti-CD20 antibody (Rituximab), or vaccines based on heat-shock protein 277, GAD65, and a modified peptide ligand of the insulin B epitope (Alleva et al., 2006; Lazar et al., 2007; Ludvigsson, 2007). Further, several combinations of different immunomodulatory agents together or with agents improving beta cell function (e.g., anti-CD3 + insulin peptide; anti-CD3 + exenatide, mycophenolate mofetil + anti-CD25 (daclizumab); rapamycin (sirolimus) + interleukin-10 rapamycin (sirolimus) + interleukin-2) are currently under investigation in prevention and treatment trials for type 1 diabetes (Alleva et al., 2006; Battaglia, Stabilini, Draghici, Gregori, et al., 2006; Battaglia, Stabilini, Draghici, Migliavacca, et al., 2006; Battaglia, Stabilini, Migliavacca, Horejs-Hoeck, et al., 2006; Bresson et al., 2006; Ciancio et al., 2008; Lazar et al., 2007; Ludvigsson, 2007; Sherry et al., 2007).

Novel cell-based approaches using regulatory T cells (Tregs) for immunomodulation have shown promising results in animals (Tang et al., 2004). Recent data, using umbilical cord blood as an autologous cell source, suggest a delay in progression of beta cell loss in children suffering from T1DM (Haller et al., 2008). However, the idea of autologous cell transfer apparently needs further refinement as the usual requirement of an accompanying potent immunosuppression may limit the therapy due to the associated potential complications and side effects (Voltarelli et al., 2007). These side effects are also of major relevance to the transplantation of pancreatic islets. Islet transplantation has improved considerably over the last decade and frequently results in stable graft function or even insulin-independence long term. However, in order to maintain the function and integrity of the transplant, potent immunosuppressive regimens usually combining rapamycin (an inhibitor of mTOR) and tacrolimus (a calcineurin inhibitor) or tacrolimus and the purine synthesis inhibitor mycophenolate mofetil are required and reported to work efficiently. As induction therapy most protocols nowadays switched from the originally reported daclizumab (an anti-IL-2 receptor monoclonal antibody) to a T-cell-depleting agent such as thymoglobulin or alemtuzumab (Kaplan et al., 2008; Monti et al., 2008; Ryan et al., 2005; Shapiro et al., 2000). Notably, most of the mentioned immunosuppressants such as rapamycin and tacrolimus not only affect T-cell function but also may have adverse effects on beta cell survival and regeneration. Further optimization of the immunosuppressive treatment regimens used in islet cell transplantation is therefore required (Serr et al., 2007; Vantyghem, Marcelli-Tourvielle, Pattou, & Noel, 2007).

The availability of islet transplantation is restricted due to a number of limitations (e.g., availability of donor organs, immunosuppression and associated morbidity, long-term survival of the transplant). Alternative approaches for the treatment of T1DM have been proposed and are in different stages of clinical development and application. These include the regeneration or neogenesis of beta cells from different sources. For example, in initial studies insulin-producing beta-like cells could be generated from pancreatic progenitor cells *in vitro* (Bonner-Weir et al., 2008, 2000; Seaberg et al., 2004). Other data suggesting that beta cells in mice retain proliferative capacities (Dor, Brown, Martinez, & Melton, 2004) provide encouragement for these regenerative concepts. This concept is enhanced by the identification of a number of growth factor signaling pathways and transcription factors (e.g., Wnt, FoxO, TCF7L2, and others) that are specifically involved in the regulation of beta cell proliferation and beta cell apoptosis (Ackermann & Gannon, 2007; Cozar-Castellano et al., 2006; Granata et al., 2007; Mziaut et al., 2008, 2006; Rulifson et al., 2007; Schrader et al., 2007; Shu et al., 2008; Ta, Choi, Atouf, Park, & Lumelsky, 2006; Vasavada et al., 2007; Wente et al., 2006; Zhang et al., 2006). Interestingly, GLP1-based therapies that are already successfully established in clinical practice for the treatment of type 2 diabetes have been proven to have some beta cell regeneration augmenting properties based on an impairment of TCF7L2-mediated Wnt signaling (Liu & Habener, 2008). Strategies specifically targeting these mechanisms and pathways may therefore be promising for future regenerative therapies in T1DM.

3.2. Type 2 diabetes

Currently, about 300 million people worldwide are affected by diabetes and more than 90% of these patients suffer from type 2 diabetes (T2DM) which is closely associated with obesity and consequent insulin resistance of organs (Goldstein, 2007). However, T2DM not only affects peripheral insulin-regulated organs such as muscle and fat but also beta cells. This results in an initial (compensatory) hyperinsulinemia and later, a decrease of insulin production due to significant loss of beta cell mass (Butler et al., 2003). Early disruption of this morbid process in order to avoid beta cell destruction is the principal goal of prevention in people at high risk, because in the early stages of the disease beta cell regeneration appears to be adequate to allow reversal of the organ damage (Meier, 2008). Clinically, the earlier stages are characterized by an impaired fasting glucose level or an impaired glucose tolerance (IGT) before finally resulting in overt T2DM.

Thus, the goal of primary prevention is to identify subjects at risk for T2DM and provide modifiable risk factor reduction. Several "risk scores" have been proposed in this context (Bergmann et al., 2007; Lindstrom & Tuomilehto, 2003; Schulze et al., 2007; Schwarz, Li, et al., 2007). Numerous trials have been carried out in order to test for feasibility and efficacy of risk scoring. Easily collectable clinical data such as age, family history, obesity as well as certain basic lab tests such as fasting plasma glucose, random plasma glucose, and HbA1c have been found useful in risk stratification, although the general efficacy of these strategies may depend highly on further definition of characteristics of the community at risk (Diabetes Prevention Program Research Group, 2005; Harding, Griffin, & Wareham, 2006; Sandbaek et al., 2008; Satterfield et al., 2003; Schwarz, Reimann, et al., 2007). Several large prevention trials base on lifestyle modifications (e.g., the Da Qing IGT and Diabetes Study and the Finnish Diabetes Prevention Study) have proven the efficacy of dietary and exercise interventions aiming at weight control in reducing the incidence of T2DM in high-risk subjects (Pan et al., 1997; Rasmussen, Glumer, Sandbaek, Lauritzen, & Borch-Johnsen, 2008; Tuomilehto et al., 2001). Further, the efficacy of pharmacologic intervention has been studied intensely in T2DM prevention. Clinical trials performed with oral antidiabetic agents (e.g., the Diabetes Prevention program, the "DREAM" study (Diabetes Reduction Assessment with ramipril and rosiglitazone Medication), the Study To Prevent Non-Insulin-Dependent Diabetes Mellitus (STOP-NIDDM), and the TRIPOD study) provided evidence for the efficacy of metformin, the α-glucosidase inhibitor, acarbose, and the PPARγ agonists, troglitazone and rosiglitazone, in the primary prevention of T2DM (Buchanan et al., 2002; Chiasson et al., 2002; Gerstein et al., 2006; Knowler et al., 2002). Interestingly, treatment with glitazones appeared to be also associated with preservation of beta cell function (Buchanan et al., 2002). Unfortunately, several PPARγ agonists, including troglitazone and rosiglitazone, have been withdrawn from the market due to safety concerns. Other therapeutic developments potentially relevant to the prevention of T2DM include inhibitors of 11β-HSD-1 and of GC receptor antagonists, antagonists of the glucagon receptor, and renal glucose reabsorption inhibitors (SGLT2 inhibitors) (Combettes & Kargar, 2007; Fischer & Bornstein, 2008). In summary, lifestyle as well as specific pharmacologic interventions, have documented and comparable efficacy in preventing T2DM (Gillies et al., 2007). With regard to a variety of factors, including costs, sustainability, and safety aspects, lifestyle modification appears to be the preferable intervention strategy (Gillies et al., 2008; Knowler et al., 2005).

Over the last two decades, a number of clinical trials (e.g., the United Kingdom Prospective Diabetes Study (UKPDS), ADVANCE (Action in Diabetes and Vascular Disease: PreterAx and DiamicroN Controlled Evaluation), and ADOPT (A Diabetes Outcome Progression Trial)) have provided strong evidence for the efficacy of current pharmacotherapeutic regimens in the prevention of T2DM-associated secondary complications (Dluhy & McMahon, 2008;Patel et al., 2008; Scheen, 2007; UK Prospective Diabetes Study Group, 1998; UK Prospective Diabetes Study (UKPDS) Group, 1998). Traditionally, antidiabetic treatment based on insulin, sulfonylureas, glitinides, acarbose, metformin, or glitazones aimed at attainment of glycemic control. In the long run however, most of the oral antidiabetic treatment options fail due to the loss of beta cell function and mass, and consequently require putting the patient on insulin treatment. Interestingly, the recently introduced GLP1-based agents have attracted attention due to a number of promising beneficial effects. These include potential protective and regenerative effects of GLP1 on beta cells; non-clinical data suggest an inhibition of apoptosis as well as a stimulation of differentiation, proliferation, and regeneration of beta cells (Ferdaoussi et al., 2008; Mu et al., 2006; Toyoda et al., 2008). These data are exciting because they have the potential for a completely new therapeutic approach, the introduction of regenerative medicine into the treatment of T2DM. Current data from clinical trials provide further evidence for the efficacy of incretin-based therapies to improve beta cell function in patients suffering from T2DM (Aschner et al., 2006; Brazg et al., 2007; DeFronzo et al., 2005; Garber et al., 2008; Hermansen et al., 2007; Kendall et al., 2005; Klonoff et al., 2008; Scherbaum et al., 2008). In addition, this approach is also interesting for tertiary prevention of T2DM. The goal of tertiary prevention is to avoid long-term vascular complications in patients with T2DM. Since diabetic patients are at particular risk for the development of cardiovascular complications, the control of accompanying risk factors such as elevated blood pressure and hyperlipidemia is essential. There is evidence that vascular complications are related, in particular, to postprandial hyperglycemia and agents targeting postprandial glucose control include the GLP1-mimetic, exenatide, α-glucosidase inhibitors such as acarbose, short-acting insulin derivatives, and pramlintide, a derivative of the beta cell peptide, amylin (Jellinger, Lebovitz, & Davidson, 2007; Pistrosch et al., 2005). However, since diabetic complications also depend on factors other than glycemic control, multimodal therapeutic concepts have been introduced into the clinical armentarium. For example, control of cholesterol synthesis with inhibitors of HMG-CoA (statins) in hyperlipidemic patients with T2DM reductase is currently standard treatment since multiple clinical endpoint trials have demonstrated the efficacy of statins in the prevention of vascular complications (Haffner, 2003; Heart Protection Study

Collaborative Group, 2002; Sacks et al., 1996; The Long-Term Intervention with Pravastatin in Ischaemic Disease (LIPID) Study Group, 1998). Also, the use of ACE inhibitors in the treatment of hypertension in patients with T2DM or with diabetic nephropathy has been proven beneficial and is currently recommended as initial therapy (Konzem, Devore, & Bauer, 2002; Lewis et al., 2001; Pitt, 2000). Low-dose aspirin is currently recommended by the American Diabetes Association (ADA) for the prevention of cardiovascular events in T2DM (Haffner, 2003).

4. IMPLICATION OF THE PANCREATIC ISLET-STRESS AXIS IN DIABETES MELLITUS: A POTENTIAL TARGET FOR PREVENTION AND THERAPY

Hormonal factors, including CRH and GC regulate the activity of the HPA axis in response to stress. This axis is kept in balance by the negative feedback effects of GC on CRH synthesis and secretion in the hypothalamus. Recently, CRH has been shown to promote beta cell proliferation and potentiate insulin secretion in a glucose-dependent manner. On the other hand, GCs are referred to as diabetogenic hormones due to the induction of gluconeogenesis, implication on development of insulin resistance, effects on adipocytes, and the functionally insulin-antagonizing effects. Therefore, an imbalance of the CRH/GC system may lead to metabolic dysfunction and diabetes. GC access to intracellular receptors is regulated by 11β-hydroxysteroid dehydrogenase (11β-HSD) which catalyzes the interconversion of physiologically active GC (corticosterone in rodents, cortisol in humans) to their inactive metabolites (11-dehydrocorticosterone and cortisone, respectively).

Obesity and the associated development of insulin resistance and type 2 diabetes constitute major public health problems in developed and developing countries. The epidemic of obesity reflects altered regulation of energy homeostasis and is the major cause of the rising incidence of serious diseases such as cardiovascular and cancer. Whereas the underlying causes of the obesity epidemic remain unknown, several studies associate this condition with "stress" development due to various factors including changes in the natural environment (noise, air pollution, etc.).

In mammals, the stress response is mediated by activation of the HPA axis resulting in increased secretion/release of hormonal factors, including CRH and GC.

CRH, a 41-amino acid hypothalamic peptide, plays a central regulatory role as a key mediator of the HPA axis (Owens & Nemeroff, 1991; Vale, Spiess, Rivier, & Rivier, 1981). This peptide acts via binding to CRHR1 which is a member of the G-protein coupled membrane receptor group with signal transduction being mediated through several intracellular signaling pathways such as cAMP, protein kinase C, and mitogen-activated protein kinases (Chen, Lewis, Perrin, & Vale, 1993; Cibelli, Corsi, Diana, Vitiello, & Thiel, 2001; Kostich, Chen, Sperle, & Largent, 1998; Li, Robinson, Kawashima, Funder, & Liu, 1998; Lovenberg et al., 1995; Perrin et al., 1995). Components of the CRH and CRH-receptor system have been identified in many tissues related to immune, cardiovascular, energy homeostasis, and reproductive systems (Audhya, Jain, & Hollander, 1991; Clifton, Owens, Robinson, & Smith, 1995; Perrin et al., 1995; Singh & Fudenberg, 1988) and also in primary pancreatic islets (Huising et al., 2010). However, their actual contribution in these processes remains largely unknown. CRH peptide belongs to the glucagon secretion–vasoactive intestinal polypeptide family controlling insulin secretion and glucose metabolism. Activation of the cAMP-dependent protein kinase A signaling pathway enhances the exocytosis of insulin granules in the islet beta cells of mice (Ammala, Ashcroft, & Rorsman, 1993; Ding & Gromada, 1997) and humans (Gromada et al., 1998) and increases intracellular Ca^{2+} concentration in rat (Kanno, Suga, Wu, Kimura, & Wakui, 1998; Suga et al., 1997) and human beta cells (Gromada et al., 1998). By this effect, CRH has been shown to potentiate pancreatic insulin secretion (Ammala et al., 1993; Huising et al., 2010). Recent experimental studies strongly support the importance of the CRH/CRH-receptor system as a potential therapeutic goal in obesity, insulin resistance, and type 2 diabetes. The existence of CRH and CRH receptors in human pancreatic islets has not yet been fully established however. Application of CRH for an antidiabetic drug therapy requires demonstration of the presence of CRH receptors and CRH effects on human pancreatic islets.

GCs, the most widely studied stress-related hormones, have been traditionally associated with stimulation of food intake and increased adiposity. The effects of GC in its target tissues are determined by the abundance of its receptors, glucocorticoid receptors (GR), and by the available levels of the biologically active hormone. GCs are regulated at the pre-receptor level by 11β-HSD, which interconverts inactive cortisone to active cortisol. Two different isoenzymes of 11β-HSD have been characterized (Stewart & Krozowski, 1999). The type 1 isoenzyme (11β-HSD-1) acts as a reductase (cortisone to cortisol in human) and is expressed in several organs, such as pancreas and insulin target tissues including adipose tissue and brain (Ricketts et al., 1998); it is largely localized to cells expressing GR but not mineralocorticoid (MC) receptors. Gluconeogenesis in the liver is reduced in knockout mice without the 11β-HSD-1 gene and results in lower blood sugar levels (Kotelevtsev et al., 1997). Recently, it has been shown that selective inhibition of 11β-HSD-1 decreases blood glucose concentrations in hyperglycemic mice (Alberts et al., 2002). Moreover, diabetic islets showed increased expression and activity of the 11β-HSD-1 enzyme (Duplomb et al., 2004). The type 2 isoenzyme (11β-HSD-2) converts active GC to its inactive form (cortisol to cortisone in human), hence protecting the MC receptor against occupancy by GC. The type 2 enzyme is mostly expressed in MC tissues such as kidney, colon, salivary glands, and the sodium-transporting epithelia of the lung, a nonclassical MC target organ (Diederich et al., 2000). The inhibition of 11β-HSD activity by carbenoxolone and thereby reduction in cortisol concentration causes an increase in insulin sensitivity and a decrease in glucose production (Lindsay, Lindsay, Waddell, & Seckl, 1996). These results demonstrate that basal 11β-HSD activity plays an important role in maintaining adequate exposure of GR.

The endocrine stress system therefore may have critical implications on triggering and sustaining metabolic dysfunction and obesity. Selective 11β-HSD-1 inhibitors might have the potential for treatment of metabolic disorders such as insulin resistance and obesity (Barf et al., 2002; Davani et al., 2000; Kotelevtsev et al., 1997).

5. CONCLUSIONS AND FUTURE DIRECTIONS

Diabetes mellitus, types 1 and 2, together constitute a major world health and financial affliction. Current therapies are not totally adequate and are fraught with problems and side effects. As research in these areas progresses we hope to be able to augment our armamentarium by elucidating further and more practical and useful biochemical pathways, introducing novel approaches and agents, and applying them to patients, with resultant improved therapeutic results.

ACKNOWLEDGMENTS

The work described in this publication was supported by the University Hospital Carl Gustav Carus, Dresden, Department of Medicine III, the Centre for Regenerative Therapies

Dresden; the Paul Langerhans Institute Dresden; and the German Center for Diabetes Research. Further support was provided by the Medical Research Service of the Department of Veterans Affairs (to A. V. S.), by the University of Miami, Miller School of Medicine, Departments of Medicine (Divisions of Hematology/Oncology and Endocrinology) and Pathology (to A. V. S. and N. L. B.), and by the L. Austin Weeks Endowment for Urologic Research (to N. L. B.).

REFERENCES

Achenbach, P., Barker, J., & Bonifacio, E. (2008). Modulating the natural history of type 1 diabetes in children at high genetic risk by mucosal insulin immunization. *Current Diabetes Reports*, *8*(2), 87–93.

Achenbach, P., Bonifacio, E., Koczwara, K., & Ziegler, A. G. (2005). Natural history of type 1 diabetes. *Diabetes*, *54*(Suppl. 2), S25–S31.

Ackermann, A. M., & Gannon, M. (2007). Molecular regulation of pancreatic beta-cell mass development, maintenance, and expansion. *Journal of Molecular Endocrinology*, *38*(1–2), 193–206.

Alberts, P., Engblom, L., Edling, N., Forsgren, M., Klingstrom, G., Larsson, C., et al. (2002). Selective inhibition of 11beta-hydroxysteroid dehydrogenase type 1 decreases blood glucose concentrations in hyperglycaemic mice. *Diabetologia*, *45*(11), 1528–1532.

Alleva, D. G., Maki, R. A., Putnam, A. L., Robinson, J. M., Kipnes, M. S., Dandona, P., et al. (2006). Immunomodulation in type 1 diabetes by NBI-6024, an altered peptide ligand of the insulin B epitope. *Scandinavian Journal of Immunology*, *63*(1), 59–69.

Ammala, C., Ashcroft, F. M., & Rorsman, P. (1993). Calcium-independent potentiation of insulin release by cyclic AMP in single beta-cells. *Nature*, *363*(6427), 356–358.

Aschner, P., Kipnes, M. S., Lunceford, J. K., Sanchez, M., Mickel, C., & Williams-Herman, D. E. (2006). Effect of the dipeptidyl peptidase-4 inhibitor sitagliptin as monotherapy on glycemic control in patients with type 2 diabetes. *Diabetes Care*, *29*(12), 2632–2637.

Audhya, T., Jain, R., & Hollander, C. S. (1991). Receptor-mediated immunomodulation by corticotropin-releasing factor. *Cellular Immunology*, *134*(1), 77–84.

Bach, J. F., Feutren, G., Noel, L. H., Hannedouche, T., Landais, P., Timsit, J., et al. (1990). Factors predictive of cyclosporine-induced nephrotoxicity: The role of cyclosporine blood levels. *Transplantation Proceedings*, *22*(3), 1296–1298.

Baekkeskov, S., Warnock, G., Christie, M., Rajotte, R. V., Larsen, P. M., & Fey, S. (1989). Revelation of specificity of 64K autoantibodies in IDDM serums by high-resolution 2-D gel electrophoresis. Unambiguous identification of 64K target antigen. *Diabetes*, *38*(9), 1133–1141.

Baisch, J. M., Weeks, T., Giles, R., Hoover, M., Stastny, P., & Capra, J. D. (1990). Analysis of HLA-DQ genotypes and susceptibility in insulin-dependent diabetes mellitus. *The New England Journal of Medicine*, *322*(26), 1836–1841.

Barf, T., Vallgarda, J., Emond, R., Haggstrom, C., Kurz, G., Nygren, A., et al. (2002). Arylsulfonamidothiazoles as a new class of potential antidiabetic drugs. Discovery of potent and selective inhibitors of the 11beta-hydroxysteroid dehydrogenase type 1. *Journal of Medicinal Chemistry*, *45*(18), 3813–3815.

Bates, H. E., Sirek, A. S., Kiraly, M. A., Yue, J. T., Goche Montes, D., Matthews, S. G., et al. (2008). Adaptation to mild, intermittent stress delays development of hyperglycemia in the Zucker diabetic fatty rat independent of food intake: Role of habituation of the hypothalamic-pituitary-adrenal axis. *Endocrinology*, *149*(6), 2990–3001.

Battaglia, M., Stabilini, A., Draghici, E., Gregori, S., Mocchetti, C., Bonifacio, E., et al. (2006). Rapamycin and interleukin-10 treatment induces T regulatory type 1 cells that mediate antigen-specific transplantation tolerance. *Diabetes*, *55*(1), 40–49.

Battaglia, M., Stabilini, A., Draghici, E., Migliavacca, B., Gregori, S., Bonifacio, E., et al. (2006). Induction of tolerance in type 1 diabetes via both CD4+CD25+ T regulatory cells and T regulatory type 1 cells. *Diabetes*, *55*(6), 1571–1580.

Battaglia, M., Stabilini, A., Migliavacca, B., Horejs-Hoeck, J., Kaupper, T., & Roncarolo, M. G. (2006). Rapamycin promotes expansion of functional CD4+CD25+FOXP3+ regulatory T cells of both healthy subjects and type 1 diabetic patients. *The Journal of Immunology*, *177*(12), 8338–8347.

Bell, G. I., Horita, S., & Karam, J. H. (1984). A polymorphic locus near the human insulin gene is associated with insulin-dependent diabetes mellitus. *Diabetes*, *33*(2), 176–183.

Bennett, S. T., Lucassen, A. M., Gough, S. C., Powell, E. E., Undlien, D. E., Pritchard, L. E., et al. (1995). Susceptibility to human type 1 diabetes at IDDM2 is determined by tandem repeat variation at the insulin gene minisatellite locus. *Nature Genetics*, *9*(3), 284–292.

Bergmann, A., Li, J., Wang, L., Schulze, J., Bornstein, S. R., & Schwarz, P. E. (2007). A simplified Finnish diabetes risk score to predict type 2 diabetes risk and disease evolution in a German population. *Hormone and Metabolic Research*, *39*(9), 677–682.

Bonner-Weir, S., Inada, A., Yatoh, S., Li, W. C., Aye, T., Toschi, E., et al. (2008). Transdifferentiation of pancreatic ductal cells to endocrine beta-cells. *Biochemical Society Transactions*, *36*(Pt 3), 353–356.

Bonner-Weir, S., Taneja, M., Weir, G. C., Tatarkiewicz, K., Song, K. H., Sharma, A., et al. (2000). In vitro cultivation of human islets from expanded ductal tissue. *Proceedings of the National Academy of Sciences of the United States of America*, *97*(14), 7999–8004.

Bornstein, S. R. (1997). Is leptin a stress related peptide? *Nature Medicine*, *3*(9), 937.

Bornstein, S. R., Abu-Asab, M., Glasow, A., Path, G., Hauner, H., Tsokos, M., et al. (2000). Immunohistochemical and ultrastructural localization of leptin and leptin receptor in human white adipose tissue and differentiating human adipose cells in primary culture. *Diabetes*, *49*(4), 532–538.

Bornstein, S. R., Uhlmann, K., Haidan, A., Ehrhart-Bornstein, M., & Scherbaum, W. A. (1997). Evidence for a novel peripheral action of leptin as a metabolic signal to the adrenal gland: Leptin inhibits cortisol release directly. *Diabetes*, *46*(7), 1235–1238.

Bornstein, S. R., Wong, M. L., & Licinio, J. (2006). 150 years of Sigmund Freud: What would Freud have said about the obesity epidemic? *Molecular Psychiatry*, *11*(12), 1070–1072.

Bottini, N., Musumeci, L., Alonso, A., Rahmouni, S., Nika, K., Rostamkhani, M., et al. (2004). A functional variant of lymphoid tyrosine phosphatase is associated with type I diabetes. *Nature Genetics*, *36*(4), 337–338.

Brazg, R., Xu, L., Dalla Man, C., Cobelli, C., Thomas, K., & Stein, P. P. (2007). Effect of adding sitagliptin, a dipeptidyl peptidase-4 inhibitor, to metformin on 24-h glycaemic control and beta-cell function in patients with type 2 diabetes. *Diabetes, Obesity & Metabolism*, *9*(2), 186–193.

Bresson, D., Togher, L., Rodrigo, E., Chen, Y., Bluestone, J. A., Herold, K. C., et al. (2006). Anti-CD3 and nasal proinsulin combination therapy enhances remission from recent-onset autoimmune diabetes by inducing Tregs. *The Journal of Clinical Investigation*, *116*(5), 1371–1381.

Buchanan, T. A., Xiang, A. H., Peters, R. K., Kjos, S. L., Marroquin, A., Goico, J., et al. (2002). Preservation of pancreatic beta-cell function and prevention of type 2 diabetes by pharmacological treatment of insulin resistance in high-risk Hispanic women. *Diabetes*, *51*(9), 2796–2803.

Butler, A. E., Janson, J., Soeller, W. C., & Butler, P. C. (2003). Increased beta-cell apoptosis prevents adaptive increase in beta-cell mass in mouse model of type 2 diabetes: Evidence for role of islet amyloid formation rather than direct action of amyloid. *Diabetes*, *52*(9), 2304–2314.

Caillat-Zucman, S., Garchon, H. J., Timsit, J., Assan, R., Boitard, C., Djilali-Saiah, I., et al. (1992). Age-dependent HLA genetic heterogeneity of type 1 insulin-dependent diabetes mellitus. *The Journal of Clinical Investigation, 90*(6), 2242–2250.

Cauchi, S., Meyre, D., Durand, E., Proenca, C., Marre, M., Hadjadj, S., et al. (2008). Post genome-wide association studies of novel genes associated with type 2 diabetes show gene-gene interaction and high predictive value. *PLoS One, 3*(5), e2031.

Chen, R., Lewis, K. A., Perrin, M. H., & Vale, W. W. (1993). Expression cloning of a human corticotropin-releasing-factor receptor. *Proceedings of the National Academy of Sciences of the United States of America, 90*(19), 8967–8971.

Chiasson, J. L., Josse, R. G., Gomis, R., Hanefeld, M., Karasik, A., & Laakso, M. (2002). Acarbose for prevention of type 2 diabetes mellitus: The STOP-NIDDM randomised trial. *Lancet, 359*(9323), 2072–2077.

Ciancio, G., Burke, G. W., Gaynor, J. J., Roth, D., Sageshima, J., Kupin, W., et al. (2008). Randomized trial of mycophenolate mofetil versus enteric-coated mycophenolate sodium in primary renal transplant recipients given tacrolimus and daclizumab/thymoglobulin: One year follow-up. *Transplantation, 86*(1), 67–74.

Cibelli, G., Corsi, P., Diana, G., Vitiello, F., & Thiel, G. (2001). Corticotropin-releasing factor triggers neurite outgrowth of a catecholaminergic immortalized neuron via cAMP and MAP kinase signalling pathways. *The European Journal of Neuroscience, 13*(7), 1339–1348.

Clifton, V. L., Owens, P. C., Robinson, P. J., & Smith, R. (1995). Identification and characterization of a corticotrophin-releasing hormone receptor in human placenta. *European Journal of Endocrinology, 133*(5), 591–597.

Combettes, M., & Kargar, C. (2007). Newly approved and promising antidiabetic agents. *Thérapie, 62*(4), 293–310.

Cozar-Castellano, I., Weinstock, M., Haught, M., Velazquez-Garcia, S., Sipula, D., & Stewart, A. F. (2006). Evaluation of beta-cell replication in mice transgenic for hepatocyte growth factor and placental lactogen: Comprehensive characterization of the G1/S regulatory proteins reveals unique involvement of p21cip. *Diabetes, 55*(1), 70–77.

Davani, B., Khan, A., Hult, M., Martensson, E., Okret, S., Efendic, S., et al. (2000). Type 1 11beta-hydroxysteroid dehydrogenase mediates glucocorticoid activation and insulin release in pancreatic islets. *The Journal of Biological Chemistry, 275*(45), 34841–34844.

DeFronzo, R. A., Ratner, R. E., Han, J., Kim, D. D., Fineman, M. S., & Baron, A. D. (2005). Effects of exenatide (exendin-4) on glycemic control and weight over 30 weeks in metformin-treated patients with type 2 diabetes. *Diabetes Care, 28*(5), 1092–1100.

Diabetes Prevention Program Research Group, (2005). Strategies to identify adults at high risk for type 2 diabetes: The Diabetes Prevention Program. *Diabetes Care, 28*(1), 138–144.

Diabetes Prevention Trial–Type 1 Diabetes Study Group, (2002). Effects of insulin in relatives of patients with type 1 diabetes mellitus. *The New England Journal of Medicine, 346*(22), 1685–1691.

Diederich, S., Quinkler, M., Burkhardt, P., Grossmann, C., Bahr, V., & Oelkers, W. (2000). 11Beta-hydroxysteroid-dehydrogenase isoforms: Tissue distribution and implications for clinical medicine. *European Journal of Clinical Investigation, 30*(Suppl. 3), 21–27.

Ding, W. G., & Gromada, J. (1997). Protein kinase A-dependent stimulation of exocytosis in mouse pancreatic beta-cells by glucose-dependent insulinotropic polypeptide. *Diabetes, 46*(4), 615–621.

Dluhy, R. G., & McMahon, G. T. (2008). Intensive glycemic control in the ACCORD and ADVANCE trials. *The New England Journal of Medicine, 358*(24), 2630–2633.

Donath, M. Y., Schumann, D. M., Faulenbach, M., Ellingsgaard, H., Perren, A., & Ehses, J. A. (2008). Islet inflammation in type 2 diabetes: From metabolic stress to therapy. *Diabetes Care, 31*(Suppl. 2), S161–S164.

Dor, Y., Brown, J., Martinez, O. I., & Melton, D. A. (2004). Adult pancreatic beta-cells are formed by self-duplication rather than stem-cell differentiation. *Nature*, *429*(6987), 41–46.

Duplomb, L., Lee, Y., Wang, M. Y., Park, B. H., Takaishi, K., Agarwal, A. K., et al. (2004). Increased expression and activity of 11beta-HSD-1 in diabetic islets and prevention with troglitazone. *Biochemical and Biophysical Research Communications*, *313*(3), 594–599.

Dupuis, J., Langenberg, C., Prokopenko, I., Saxena, R., Soranzo, N., Jackson, A. U., et al. (2010). New genetic loci implicated in fasting glucose homeostasis and their impact on type 2 diabetes risk. *Nature Genetics*, *42*(2), 105–116.

Ehrhart-Bornstein, M., Lamounier-Zepter, V., Schraven, A., Langenbach, J., Willenberg, H. S., Barthel, A., et al. (2003). Human adipocytes secrete mineralocorticoid-releasing factors. *Proceedings of the National Academy of Sciences of the United States of America*, *100*(24), 14211–14216.

Elfaitouri, A., Berg, A. K., Frisk, G., Yin, H., Tuvemo, T., & Blomberg, J. (2007). Recent enterovirus infection in type 1 diabetes: Evidence with a novel IgM method. *Journal of Medical Virology*, *79*(12), 1861–1867.

Ferdaoussi, M., Abdelli, S., Yang, J. Y., Cornu, M., Niederhauser, G., Favre, D., et al. (2008). Exendin-4 protects beta-cells from interleukin-1 beta-induced apoptosis by interfering with the c-Jun NH2-terminal kinase pathway. *Diabetes*, *57*(5), 1205–1215.

Fischer, S., & Bornstein, S. R. (2008). New oral antidiabetic agents—Clinical perspectives. *Internist (Berlin)*, *49*(4), 495–501.

Foulis, A. K., McGill, M., & Farquharson, M. A. (1991). Insulitis in type 1 (insulin-dependent) diabetes mellitus in man—Macrophages, lymphocytes, and interferon-gamma containing cells. *The Journal of Pathology*, *165*(2), 97–103.

Fronczak, C. M., Baron, A. E., Chase, H. P., Ross, C., Brady, H. L., Hoffman, M., et al. (2003). In utero dietary exposures and risk of islet autoimmunity in children. *Diabetes Care*, *26*(12), 3237–3242.

Gale, E. A. (2002). A missing link in the hygiene hypothesis? *Diabetologia*, *45*(4), 588–594.

Gale, E. A., Bingley, P. J., Emmett, C. L., & Collier, T. (2004). European Nicotinamide Diabetes Intervention Trial (ENDIT): A randomised controlled trial of intervention before the onset of type 1 diabetes. *Lancet*, *363*(9413), 925–931.

Garber, A. J., Foley, J. E., Banerji, M. A., Ebeling, P., Gudbjornsdottir, S., Camisasca, R. P., et al. (2008). Effects of vildagliptin on glucose control in patients with type 2 diabetes inadequately controlled with a sulphonylurea. *Diabetes, Obesity & Metabolism*, *10*(11), 1047–1056.

Gerstein, H. C., Yusuf, S., Bosch, J., Pogue, J., Sheridan, P., Dinccag, N., et al. (2006). Effect of rosiglitazone on the frequency of diabetes in patients with impaired glucose tolerance or impaired fasting glucose: A randomised controlled trial. *Lancet*, *368*(9541), 1096–1105.

Gillespie, K. M., Bain, S. C., Barnett, A. H., Bingley, P. J., Christie, M. R., Gill, G. V., et al. (2004). The rising incidence of childhood type 1 diabetes and reduced contribution of high-risk HLA haplotypes. *Lancet*, *364*(9446), 1699–1700.

Gillies, C. L., Abrams, K. R., Lambert, P. C., Cooper, N. J., Sutton, A. J., Hsu, R. T., et al. (2007). Pharmacological and lifestyle interventions to prevent or delay type 2 diabetes in people with impaired glucose tolerance: Systematic review and meta-analysis. *BMJ*, *334*(7588), 299.

Gillies, C. L., Lambert, P. C., Abrams, K. R., Sutton, A. J., Cooper, N. J., Hsu, R. T., et al. (2008). Different strategies for screening and prevention of type 2 diabetes in adults: Cost effectiveness analysis. *BMJ*, *336*(7654), 1180–1185.

Golden, S. H. (2007). A review of the evidence for a neuroendocrine link between stress, depression and diabetes mellitus. *Current Diabetes Reviews*, *3*(4), 252–259.

Goldstein, B. J. (2007). Clinical translation of "a diabetes outcome progression trial": ADOPT appropriate combination oral therapies in type 2 diabetes. *The Journal of Clinical Endocrinology and Metabolism, 92*(4), 1226–1228.

Granata, R., Settanni, F., Biancone, L., Trovato, L., Nano, R., Bertuzzi, F., et al. (2007). Acylated and unacylated ghrelin promote proliferation and inhibit apoptosis of pancreatic beta-cells and human islets: Involvement of 3′,5′-cyclic adenosine monophosphate/protein kinase A, extracellular signal-regulated kinase 1/2, and phosphatidyl inositol 3-kinase/Akt signaling. *Endocrinology, 148*(2), 512–529.

Gromada, J., Bokvist, K., Ding, W. G., Holst, J. J., Nielsen, J. H., & Rorsman, P. (1998). Glucagon-like peptide 1 (7–36) amide stimulates exocytosis in human pancreatic beta-cells by both proximal and distal regulatory steps in stimulus-secretion coupling. *Diabetes, 47*(1), 57–65.

Haffner, S. M. (2003). Management of dyslipidemia in adults with diabetes. *Diabetes Care, 26*(Suppl. 1(1)), S83–S86.

Haller, M. J., Viener, H. L., Wasserfall, C., Brusko, T., Atkinson, M. A., & Schatz, D. A. (2008). Autologous umbilical cord blood infusion for type 1 diabetes. *Experimental Hematology, 36*(6), 710–715.

Hanefeld, M., Koehler, C., Gallo, S., Benke, I., & Ott, P. (2007). Impact of the individual components of the metabolic syndrome and their different combinations on the prevalence of atherosclerotic vascular disease in type 2 diabetes: The Diabetes in Germany (DIG) study. *Cardiovascular Diabetology, 6*(13), 13.

Harding, A. H., Griffin, S. J., & Wareham, N. J. (2006). Population impact of strategies for identifying groups at high risk of type 2 diabetes. *Preventive Medicine, 42*(5), 364–368.

Harrison, L. C., Honeyman, M. C., Steele, C. E., Stone, N. L., Sarugeri, E., Bonifacio, E., et al. (2004). Pancreatic beta-cell function and immune responses to insulin after administration of intranasal insulin to humans at risk for type 1 diabetes. *Diabetes Care, 27*(10), 2348–2355.

Heart Protection Study Collaborative Group (2002). MRC/BHF Heart Protection Study of cholesterol lowering with simvastatin in 20,536 high-risk individuals: A randomised placebo-controlled trial. *Lancet, 360*(9326), 7–22.

Hermansen, K., Kipnes, M., Luo, E., Fanurik, D., Khatami, H., & Stein, P. (2007). Efficacy and safety of the dipeptidyl peptidase-4 inhibitor, sitagliptin, in patients with type 2 diabetes mellitus inadequately controlled on glimepiride alone or on glimepiride and metformin. *Diabetes, Obesity & Metabolism, 9*(5), 733–745.

Herold, K. C., Gitelman, S. E., Masharani, U., Hagopian, W., Bisikirska, B., Donaldson, D., et al. (2005). A single course of anti-CD3 monoclonal antibody hOKT3gamma1(Ala-Ala) results in improvement in C-peptide responses and clinical parameters for at least 2 years after onset of type 1 diabetes. *Diabetes, 54*(6), 1763–1769.

Herold, K. C., Hagopian, W., Auger, J. A., Poumian-Ruiz, E., Taylor, L., Donaldson, D., et al. (2002). Anti-CD3 monoclonal antibody in new-onset type 1 diabetes mellitus. *The New England Journal of Medicine, 346*(22), 1692–1698.

Horikawa, Y., Iwasaki, N., Hara, M., Furuta, H., Hinokio, Y., Cockburn, B. N., et al. (1997). Mutation in hepatocyte nuclear factor-1 beta gene (TCF2) associated with MODY. *Nature Genetics, 17*(4), 384–385.

Horikawa, Y., Oda, N., Cox, N. J., Li, X., Orho-Melander, M., Hara, M., et al. (2000). Genetic variation in the gene encoding calpain-10 is associated with type 2 diabetes mellitus. *Nature Genetics, 26*(2), 163–175.

Huising, M. O., van der Meulen, T., Vaughan, J. M., Matsumoto, M., Donaldson, C. J., Park, H., et al. (2010). CRHR1 is expressed on pancreatic beta cells, promotes beta cell proliferation, and potentiates insulin secretion in a glucose-dependent manner. *Proceedings of the National Academy of Sciences of the United States of America, 107*(2), 912–917.

Hypponen, E., Laara, E., Reunanen, A., Jarvelin, M. R., & Virtanen, S. M. (2001). Intake of vitamin D and risk of type 1 diabetes: A birth-cohort study. *Lancet*, *358*(9292), 1500–1503.

Jellinger, P. S., Lebovitz, H. E., & Davidson, J. A. (2007). Management of hyperglycemia in type 2 diabetes: A consensus algorithm for the initiation and adjustment of therapy: A consensus statement from the American Diabetes Association and the European Association for the Study of Diabetes: Response to Nathan et al. *Diabetes Care*, *30*(4), e16–e17, author reply e18–20, e21–12.

Kanno, T., Suga, S., Wu, J., Kimura, M., & Wakui, M. (1998). Intracellular cAMP potentiates voltage-dependent activation of L-type Ca^{2+} channels in rat islet beta-cells. *Pflügers Archiv*, *435*(4), 578–580.

Kaplan, B., West, P., Neeley, H., Martellotto, J., Iqbal, R., Gangemi, A., et al. (2008). Use of low dose tacrolimus, mycophenolate mofetil and maintenance IL-2 receptor blockade in an islet transplant recipient. *Clinical Transplantation*, *22*(2), 250–253.

Kaufman, D., Banerji, M. A., Shorman, I., Smith, E. L., Coplan, J. D., Rosenblum, L. A., et al. (2007). Early-life stress and the development of obesity and insulin resistance in juvenile bonnet macaques. *Diabetes*, *56*(5), 1382–1386.

Kempf, K., Rathmann, W., & Herder, C. (2008). Impaired glucose regulation and type 2 diabetes in children and adolescents. *Diabetes/Metabolism Research and Reviews*, *24*(6), 427–437.

Kendall, D. M., Riddle, M. C., Rosenstock, J., Zhuang, D., Kim, D. D., Fineman, M. S., et al. (2005). Effects of exenatide (exendin-4) on glycemic control over 30 weeks in patients with type 2 diabetes treated with metformin and a sulfonylurea. *Diabetes Care*, *28*(5), 1083–1091.

Keymeulen, B., Vandemeulebroucke, E., Ziegler, A. G., Mathieu, C., Kaufman, L., Hale, G., et al. (2005). Insulin needs after CD3-antibody therapy in new-onset type 1 diabetes. *The New England Journal of Medicine*, *352*(25), 2598–2608.

Klonoff, D. C., Buse, J. B., Nielsen, L. L., Guan, X., Bowlus, C. L., Holcombe, J. H., et al. (2008). Exenatide effects on diabetes, obesity, cardiovascular risk factors and hepatic biomarkers in patients with type 2 diabetes treated for at least 3 years. *Current Medical Research and Opinion*, *24*(1), 275–286.

Knowler, W. C., Barrett-Connor, E., Fowler, S. E., Hamman, R. F., Lachin, J. M., Walker, E. A., et al. (2002). Reduction in the incidence of type 2 diabetes with lifestyle intervention or metformin. *The New England Journal of Medicine*, *346*(6), 393–403.

Knowler, W. C., Hamman, R. F., Edelstein, S. L., Barrett-Connor, E., Ehrmann, D. A., Walker, E. A., et al. (2005). Prevention of type 2 diabetes with troglitazone in the Diabetes Prevention Program. *Diabetes*, *54*(4), 1150–1156.

Konzem, S. L., Devore, V. S., & Bauer, D. W. (2002). Controlling hypertension in patients with diabetes. *American Family Physician*, *66*(7), 1209–1214.

Korenblum, W., Barthel, A., Licinio, J., Wong, M. L., Wolf, O. T., Kirschbaum, C., et al. (2005). Elevated cortisol levels and increased rates of diabetes and mood symptoms in Soviet Union-born Jewish immigrants to Germany. *Molecular Psychiatry*, *10*(11), 974–975.

Kostich, W. A., Chen, A., Sperle, K., & Largent, B. L. (1998). Molecular identification and analysis of a novel human corticotropin-releasing factor (CRF) receptor: The CRF2gamma receptor. *Molecular Endocrinology*, *12*(8), 1077–1085.

Kotelevtsev, Y., Holmes, M. C., Burchell, A., Houston, P. M., Schmoll, D., Jamieson, P., et al. (1997). 11beta-Hydroxysteroid dehydrogenase type 1 knockout mice show attenuated glucocorticoid-inducible responses and resist hyperglycemia on obesity or stress. *Proceedings of the National Academy of Sciences of the United States of America*, *94*(26), 14924–14929.

Kupila, A., Sipila, J., Keskinen, P., Simell, T., Knip, M., Pulkki, K., et al. (2003). Intranasally administered insulin intended for prevention of type 1 diabetes—A safety study in healthy adults. *Diabetes/Metabolism Research and Reviews*, *19*(5), 415–420.

Kyrou, I., & Tsigos, C. (2007). Stress mechanisms and metabolic complications. *Hormone and Metabolic Research*, *39*(6), 430–438.

Lamounier-Zepter, V., Ehrhart-Bornstein, M., Karczewski, P., Haase, H., Bornstein, S. R., & Morano, I. (2006). Human adipocytes attenuate cardiomyocyte contraction: Characterization of an adipocyte-derived negative inotropic activity. *FASEB Journal*, *20*(10), 1653–1659.

Lampeter, E. F., Klinghammer, A., Scherbaum, W. A., Heinze, E., Haastert, B., Giani, G., et al. (1998). The Deutsche Nicotinamide Intervention Study: An attempt to prevent type 1 diabetes. DENIS Group. *Diabetes*, *47*(6), 980–984.

Lan, M. S., Wasserfall, C., Maclaren, N. K., & Notkins, A. L. (1996). IA-2, a transmembrane protein of the protein tyrosine phosphatase family, is a major autoantigen in insulin-dependent diabetes mellitus. *Proceedings of the National Academy of Sciences of the United States of America*, *93*(13), 6367–6370.

Lazar, L., Ofan, R., Weintrob, N., Avron, A., Tamir, M., Elias, D., et al. (2007). Heat-shock protein peptide DiaPep277 treatment in children with newly diagnosed type 1 diabetes: A randomised, double-blind phase II study. *Diabetes/Metabolism Research and Reviews*, *23*(4), 286–291.

Lewis, E. J., Hunsicker, L. G., Clarke, W. R., Berl, T., Pohl, M. A., Lewis, J. B., et al. (2001). Renoprotective effect of the angiotensin-receptor antagonist irbesartan in patients with nephropathy due to type 2 diabetes. *The New England Journal of Medicine*, *345*(12), 851–860.

Li, H., Robinson, P. J., Kawashima, S., Funder, J. W., & Liu, J. P. (1998). Differential regulation of MAP kinase activity by corticotropin-releasing hormone in normal and neoplastic corticotropes. *International Journal of Biochemistry and Cell Biology*, *30*(12), 1389–1401.

Lindsay, R. S., Lindsay, R. M., Waddell, B. J., & Seckl, J. R. (1996). Prenatal glucocorticoid exposure leads to offspring hyperglycaemia in the rat: Studies with the 11 beta-hydroxysteroid dehydrogenase inhibitor carbenoxolone. *Diabetologia*, *39*(11), 1299–1305.

Lindstrom, J., & Tuomilehto, J. (2003). The diabetes risk score: A practical tool to predict type 2 diabetes risk. *Diabetes Care*, *26*(3), 725–731.

Liu, Z., & Habener, J. F. (2008). Glucagon-like peptide-1 activation of TCF7L2-dependent Wnt signaling enhances pancreatic beta cell proliferation. *The Journal of Biological Chemistry*, *283*(13), 8723–8735.

Lonnrot, M., Korpela, K., Knip, M., Ilonen, J., Simell, O., Korhonen, S., et al. (2000). Enterovirus infection as a risk factor for beta-cell autoimmunity in a prospectively observed birth cohort. The Finnish Diabetes Prediction and Prevention Study. *Diabetes*, *49*(8), 1314–1318.

Lovenberg, T. W., Liaw, C. W., Grigoriadis, D. E., Clevenger, W., Chalmers, D. T., De Souza, E. B., et al. (1995). Cloning and characterization of a functionally distinct corticotropin-releasing factor receptor subtype from rat brain. *Proceedings of the National Academy of Sciences of the United States of America*, *92*(3), 836–840.

Ludvigsson, J. (2007). Immune intervention at diagnosis—Should we treat children to preserve beta-cell function? *Pediatric Diabetes*, *8*(Suppl. 6), 34–39.

Ludwig, B., Rotem, A., Schmid, J., Weir, G. C., Colton, C. K., Brendel, M. D., et al. (2012). Improvement of islet function in a bioartificial pancreas by enhanced oxygen supply and growth hormone releasing hormone agonist. *Proceedings of the National Academy of Sciences of the United States of America*, *109*(13), 5022–5027.

Ludwig, B., Ziegler, C. G., Schally, A. V., Richter, C., Steffen, A., Jabs, N., et al. (2010). Agonist of growth hormone-releasing hormone as a potential effector for survival and proliferation of pancreatic islets. *Proceedings of the National Academy of Sciences of the United States of America, 107*(28), 12623–12628.

Massi-Benedetti, M. (2006). Changing targets in the treatment of type 2 diabetes. *Current Medical Research and Opinion, 22*(Suppl. 2), S5–S13.

Mayor, S. (2007). International Diabetes Federation consensus on prevention of type 2 diabetes. *International Journal of Clinical Practice, 61*(10), 1773–1775.

Meier, J. J. (2008). Beta cell mass in diabetes: A realistic therapeutic target? *Diabetologia, 51*(5), 703–713.

Mlinar, B., Marc, J., Janez, A., & Pfeifer, M. (2007). Molecular mechanisms of insulin resistance and associated diseases. *Clinica Chimica Acta, 375*(1–2), 20–35.

Monti, P., Scirpoli, M., Maffi, P., Piemonti, L., Secchi, A., Bonifacio, E., et al. (2008). Rapamycin monotherapy in patients with type 1 diabetes modifies CD4+CD25+FOXP3+ regulatory T-cells. *Diabetes, 57*(9), 2341–2347.

Mu, J., Woods, J., Zhou, Y. P., Roy, R. S., Li, Z., Zycband, E., et al. (2006). Chronic inhibition of dipeptidyl peptidase-4 with a sitagliptin analog preserves pancreatic beta-cell mass and function in a rodent model of type 2 diabetes. *Diabetes, 55*(6), 1695–1704.

Mziaut, H., Kersting, S., Knoch, K. P., Fan, W. H., Trajkovski, M., Erdmann, K., et al. (2008). ICA512 signaling enhances pancreatic beta-cell proliferation by regulating cyclins D through STATs. *Proceedings of the National Academy of Sciences of the United States of America, 105*(2), 674–679.

Mziaut, H., Trajkovski, M., Kersting, S., Ehninger, A., Altkruger, A., Lemaitre, R. P., et al. (2006). Synergy of glucose and growth hormone signalling in islet cells through ICA512 and STAT5. *Nature Cell Biology, 8*(5), 435–445.

Nakayama, M., Abiru, N., Moriyama, H., Babaya, N., Liu, E., Miao, D., et al. (2005). Prime role for an insulin epitope in the development of type 1 diabetes in NOD mice. *Nature, 435*(7039), 220–223.

Nejentsev, S., Sjoroos, M., Soukka, T., Knip, M., Simell, O., Lovgren, T., et al. (1999). Population-based genetic screening for the estimation of Type 1 diabetes mellitus risk in Finland: Selective genotyping of markers in the HLA-DQB1, HLA-DQA1 and HLA-DRB1 loci. *Diabetic Medicine, 16*(12), 985–992.

Norris, J. M., Barriga, K., Klingensmith, G., Hoffman, M., Eisenbarth, G. S., Erlich, H. A., et al. (2003). Timing of initial cereal exposure in infancy and risk of islet autoimmunity. *JAMA, 290*(13), 1713–1720.

Norris, J. M., Yin, X., Lamb, M. M., Barriga, K., Seifert, J., Hoffman, M., et al. (2007). Omega-3 polyunsaturated fatty acid intake and islet autoimmunity in children at increased risk for type 1 diabetes. *JAMA, 298*(12), 1420–1428.

Owens, M. J., & Nemeroff, C. B. (1991). Physiology and pharmacology of corticotropin-releasing factor. *Pharmacological Reviews, 43*(4), 425–473.

Palmer, J. P. (1987). Insulin autoantibodies: Their role in the pathogenesis of IDDM. *Diabetes/Metabolism Reviews, 3*(4), 1005–1015.

Pan, X. R., Li, G. W., Hu, Y. H., Wang, J. X., Yang, W. Y., An, Z. X., et al. (1997). Effects of diet and exercise in preventing NIDDM in people with impaired glucose tolerance. The Da Qing IGT and Diabetes Study. *Diabetes Care, 20*(4), 537–544.

Paronen, J., Bjorksten, B., Hattevig, G., Akerblom, H. K., & Vaarala, O. (2000). Effect of maternal diet during lactation on development of bovine insulin-binding antibodies in children at risk for allergy. *The Journal of Allergy and Clinical Immunology, 106*(2), 302–306.

Patel, A., MacMahon, S., Chalmers, J., Neal, B., Billot, L., Woodward, M., et al. (2008). Intensive blood glucose control and vascular outcomes in patients with type 2 diabetes. *The New England Journal of Medicine, 358*(24), 2560–2572.

Pearson, E. R. (2009). Pharmacogenetics in diabetes. *Current Diabetes Reports, 9*(2), 172–181.

Perrin, M., Donaldson, C., Chen, R., Blount, A., Berggren, T., Bilezikjian, L., et al. (1995). Identification of a second corticotropin-releasing factor receptor gene and characterization of a cDNA expressed in heart. *Proceedings of the National Academy of Sciences of the United States of America*, *92*(7), 2969–2973.

Pistrosch, F., Herbrig, K., Kindel, B., Passauer, J., Fischer, S., & Gross, P. (2005). Rosiglitazone improves glomerular hyperfiltration, renal endothelial dysfunction, and microalbuminuria of incipient diabetic nephropathy in patients. *Diabetes*, *54*(7), 2206–2211.

Pitt, B. (2000). The anti-ischemic potential of angiotensin-converting enzyme inhibition: Insights from the heart outcomes prevention evaluation trial. *Clinical Cardiology*, *23*(7 Suppl. 4), IV9–IV14.

Rasmussen, S. S., Glumer, C., Sandbaek, A., Lauritzen, T., & Borch-Johnsen, K. (2008). Determinants of progression from impaired fasting glucose and impaired glucose tolerance to diabetes in a high-risk screened population: 3 year follow-up in the ADDITION study, Denmark. *Diabetologia*, *51*(2), 249–257.

Reichard, P., Nilsson, B. Y., & Rosenqvist, U. (1993). The effect of long-term intensified insulin treatment on the development of microvascular complications of diabetes mellitus. *The New England Journal of Medicine*, *329*(5), 304–309.

Reichel, A., Schwarz, J., Schulze, J., Licinio, J., Wong, M. L., & Bornstein, S. R. (2005). Depression and anxiety symptoms in diabetic patients on continuous subcutaneous insulin infusion (CSII). *Molecular Psychiatry*, *10*(11), 975–976.

Ricketts, M. L., Verhaeg, J. M., Bujalska, I., Howie, A. J., Rainey, W. E., & Stewart, P. M. (1998). Immunohistochemical localization of type 1 11beta-hydroxysteroid dehydrogenase in human tissues. *The Journal of Clinical Endocrinology and Metabolism*, *83*(4), 1325–1335.

Rulifson, I. C., Karnik, S. K., Heiser, P. W., ten Berge, D., Chen, H., Gu, X., et al. (2007). Wnt signaling regulates pancreatic beta cell proliferation. *Proceedings of the National Academy of Sciences of the United States of America*, *104*(15), 6247–6252.

Ryan, E. A., Paty, B. W., Senior, P. A., Bigam, D., Alfadhli, E., Kneteman, N. M., et al. (2005). Five-year follow-up after clinical islet transplantation. *Diabetes*, *54*(7), 2060–2069.

Sacks, F. M., Pfeffer, M. A., Moye, L. A., Rouleau, J. L., Rutherford, J. D., Cole, T. G., et al. (1996). The effect of pravastatin on coronary events after myocardial infarction in patients with average cholesterol levels. Cholesterol and Recurrent Events Trial Investigators. *The New England Journal of Medicine*, *335*(14), 1001–1009.

Salminen, K., Sadeharju, K., Lonnrot, M., Vahasalo, P., Kupila, A., Korhonen, S., et al. (2003). Enterovirus infections are associated with the induction of beta-cell autoimmunity in a prospective birth cohort study. *Journal of Medical Virology*, *69*(1), 91–98.

Sandbaek, A., Griffin, S. J., Rutten, G., Davies, M., Stolk, R., Khunti, K., et al. (2008). Stepwise screening for diabetes identifies people with high but modifiable coronary heart disease risk. The ADDITION study. *Diabetologia*, *51*(7), 1127–1134.

Satterfield, D. W., Volansky, M., Caspersen, C. J., Engelgau, M. M., Bowman, B. A., Gregg, E. W., et al. (2003). Community-based lifestyle interventions to prevent type 2 diabetes. *Diabetes Care*, *26*(9), 2643–2652.

Scheen, A. J. (2007). ADOPT study: Which first-line glucose-lowering oral medication in type 2 diabetes? *Revue Médicale de Liège*, *62*(1), 48–52.

Scherbaum, W. A., Schweizer, A., Mari, A., Nilsson, P. M., Lalanne, G., Wang, Y., et al. (2008). Evidence that vildagliptin attenuates deterioration of glycaemic control during 2-year treatment of patients with type 2 diabetes and mild hyperglycaemia. *Diabetes, Obesity & Metabolism*, *10*(11), 1114–1124.

Schmid, J., Ludwig, B., Schally, A. V., Steffen, A., Ziegler, C. G., Block, N. L., et al. (2010). Modulation of pancreatic islets-stress axis by hypothalamic releasing hormones and

11beta-hydroxysteroid dehydrogenase. *Proceedings of the National Academy of Sciences of the United States of America, 108*(33), 13722–13727.

Schrader, J., Rennekamp, W., Niebergall, U., Schoppet, M., Jahr, H., Brendel, M. D., et al. (2007). Cytokine-induced osteoprotegerin expression protects pancreatic beta cells through p38 mitogen-activated protein kinase signalling against cell death. *Diabetologia, 50*(6), 1243–1247.

Schulze, M. B., Hoffmann, K., Boeing, H., Linseisen, J., Rohrmann, S., Mohlig, M., et al. (2007). An accurate risk score based on anthropometric, dietary, and lifestyle factors to predict the development of type 2 diabetes. *Diabetes Care, 30*(3), 510–515.

Schwarz, P. E., Govindarajalu, S., Towers, W., Schwanebeck, U., Fischer, S., Vasseur, F., et al. (2006). Haplotypes in the promoter region of the ADIPOQ gene are associated with increased diabetes risk in a German Caucasian population. *Hormone and Metabolic Research, 38*(7), 447–451.

Schwarz, P. E., Li, J., Wegner, H., Bornstein, S. R., Lindstrom, J., & Tuomilehto, J. (2007). An accurate risk score based on anthropometric, dietary, and lifestyle factors to predict the development of type 2 diabetes: Response to Schulze et al. *Diabetes Care, 30*(8), e87, author reply e88.

Schwarz, P. E., Lindstrom, J., Kissimova-Scarbeck, K., Szybinski, Z., Barengo, N. C., Peltonen, M., et al. (2008). The European perspective of type 2 diabetes prevention: Diabetes in Europe-Prevention using lifestyle, physical activity and nutritional intervention (DE-PLAN) project. *Experimental and Clinical Endocrinology and Diabetes, 116*(3), 167–172.

Schwarz, P. E., Odenbach, C., Rothe, U., Bergmann, A., Bornstein, S. R., Kunath, H., et al. (2008). Prevention in occupational health care—A societal challenge. *Medizinische Klinik (Munich, Germany), 103*(4), 210–216.

Schwarz, P. E., Reimann, M., Li, J., Bergmann, A., Licinio, J., Wong, M. L., et al. (2007). The Metabolic Syndrome—A global challenge for prevention. *Hormone and Metabolic Research, 39*(11), 777–780.

Seaberg, R. M., Smukler, S. R., Kieffer, T. J., Enikolopov, G., Asghar, Z., Wheeler, M. B., et al. (2004). Clonal identification of multipotent precursors from adult mouse pancreas that generate neural and pancreatic lineages. *Nature Biotechnology, 22*(9), 1115–1124.

Serr, F., Lauer, H., Armann, B., Ludwig, S., Thiery, J., Fiedler, M., et al. (2007). Sirolimus improves early microcirculation, but impairs regeneration after pancreatic ischemia-reperfusion injury. *American Journal of Transplantation, 7*(1), 48–56.

Shapiro, A. M., Lakey, J. R., Ryan, E. A., Korbutt, G. S., Toth, E., Warnock, G. L., et al. (2000). Islet transplantation in seven patients with type 1 diabetes mellitus using a glucocorticoid-free immunosuppressive regimen. *The New England Journal of Medicine, 343*(4), 230–238.

Sharma, A. M. (2006). The obese patient with diabetes mellitus: From research targets to treatment options. *The American Journal of Medicine, 119*(5 Suppl. 1), S17–S23.

Sherry, N. A., Chen, W., Kushner, J. A., Glandt, M., Tang, Q., Tsai, S., et al. (2007). Exendin-4 improves reversal of diabetes in NOD mice treated with anti-CD3 monoclonal antibody by enhancing recovery of beta-cells. *Endocrinology, 148*(11), 5136–5144.

Shu, L., Sauter, N. S., Schulthess, F. T., Matveyenko, A. V., Oberholzer, J., & Maedler, K. (2008). Transcription factor 7-like 2 regulates beta-cell survival and function in human pancreatic islets. *Diabetes, 57*(3), 645–653.

Singh, V. K., & Fudenberg, H. H. (1988). Binding of [125I]corticotropin releasing factor to blood immunocytes and its reduction in Alzheimer's disease. *Immunology Letters, 18*(1), 5–8.

Stene, L. C., & Joner, G. (2003). Use of cod liver oil during the first year of life is associated with lower risk of childhood-onset type 1 diabetes: A large, population-based, case–control study. *The American Journal of Clinical Nutrition, 78*(6), 1128–1134.

Stene, L. C., Ulriksen, J., Magnus, P., & Joner, G. (2000). Use of cod liver oil during pregnancy associated with lower risk of Type I diabetes in the offspring. *Diabetologia, 43*(9), 1093–1098.

Stewart, P. M., & Krozowski, Z. S. (1999). 11 beta-Hydroxysteroid dehydrogenase. *Vitamins and Hormones, 57*, 249–324.

Suga, S., Kanno, T., Nakano, K., Takeo, T., Dobashi, Y., & Wakui, M. (1997). GLP-I(7–36) amide augments Ba^{2+} current through L-type Ca^{2+} channel of rat pancreatic beta-cell in a cAMP-dependent manner. *Diabetes, 46*(11), 1755–1760.

Ta, M., Choi, Y., Atouf, F., Park, C. H., & Lumelsky, N. (2006). The defined combination of growth factors controls generation of long-term-replicating islet progenitor-like cells from cultures of adult mouse pancreas. *Stem Cells, 24*(7), 1738–1749.

Tang, Q., Henriksen, K. J., Bi, M., Finger, E. B., Szot, G., Ye, J., et al. (2004). In vitro-expanded antigen-specific regulatory T cells suppress autoimmune diabetes. *The Journal of Experimental Medicine, 199*(11), 1455–1465.

The Long-Term Intervention with Pravastatin in Ischaemic Disease (LIPID) Study Group (1998). Prevention of cardiovascular events and death with pravastatin in patients with coronary heart disease and a broad range of initial cholesterol levels. *The New England Journal of Medicine, 339*(19), 1349–1357.

Thivolet, C. (2001). New therapeutic approaches to type 1 diabetes: From prevention to cellular or gene therapies. *Clinical Endocrinology, 55*(5), 565–574.

Todd, J. A. (1995). Genetic analysis of type 1 diabetes using whole genome approaches. *Proceedings of the National Academy of Sciences of the United States of America, 92*(19), 8560–8565.

Toyoda, K., Okitsu, T., Yamane, S., Uonaga, T., Liu, X., Harada, N., et al. (2008). GLP-1 receptor signaling protects pancreatic beta cells in intraportal islet transplant by inhibiting apoptosis. *Biochemical and Biophysical Research Communications, 367*(4), 793–798.

TRIGR Study Group, (2007). Study design of the Trial to Reduce IDDM in the Genetically at Risk (TRIGR). *Pediatric Diabetes, 8*(3), 117–137.

Tselmin, S., Korenblum, W., Reimann, M., Bornstein, S. R., & Schwarz, P. E. (2007). The health status of Russian-speaking immigrants in Germany. *Hormone and Metabolic Research, 39*(12), 858–861.

Tuomilehto, J., Lindstrom, J., Eriksson, J. G., Valle, T. T., Hamalainen, H., Ilanne-Parikka, P., et al. (2001). Prevention of type 2 diabetes mellitus by changes in lifestyle among subjects with impaired glucose tolerance. *The New England Journal of Medicine, 344*(18), 1343–1350.

Ueda, H., Howson, J. M., Esposito, L., Heward, J., Snook, H., Chamberlain, G., et al. (2003). Association of the T-cell regulatory gene CTLA4 with susceptibility to autoimmune disease. *Nature, 423*(6939), 506–511.

UK Prospective Diabetes Study Group, (1998). Tight blood pressure control and risk of macrovascular and microvascular complications in type 2 diabetes: UKPDS 38. *BMJ, 317*(7160), 703–713.

UK Prospective Diabetes Study (UKPDS) Group, (1998). Effect of intensive blood-glucose control with metformin on complications in overweight patients with type 2 diabetes (UKPDS 34). *Lancet, 352*(9131), 854–865.

Ulgen, F., Scherbaum, W. A., Partke, H. J., Bornstein, S. R., & Schinner, S. (2008). Intra-pancreatic adipocyte deposition in a mouse model of the metabolic syndrome. *Hormone and Metabolic Research, 40*(7), 507–509.

Vale, W., Spiess, J., Rivier, C., & Rivier, J. (1981). Characterization of a 41-residue ovine hypothalamic peptide that stimulates secretion of corticotropin and beta-endorphin. *Science, 213*(4514), 1394–1397.

Vantyghem, M. C., Marcelli-Tourvielle, S., Pattou, F., & Noel, C. (2007). Effects of non-steroid immunosuppressive drugs on insulin secretion in transplantation. *Annales d'endocrinologie, 68*(1), 21–27.

Vasavada, R. C., Wang, L., Fujinaka, Y., Takane, K. K., Rosa, T. C., Mellado-Gil, J. M., et al. (2007). Protein kinase C-zeta activation markedly enhances beta-cell proliferation: An essential role in growth factor mediated beta-cell mitogenesis. *Diabetes*, *56*(11), 2732–2743.

Verge, C. F., Gianani, R., Kawasaki, E., Yu, L., Pietropaolo, M., Jackson, R. A., et al. (1996). Prediction of type I diabetes in first-degree relatives using a combination of insulin, GAD, and ICA512bdc/IA-2 autoantibodies. *Diabetes*, *45*(7), 926–933.

Voltarelli, J. C., Couri, C. E., Stracieri, A. B., Oliveira, M. C., Moraes, D. A., Pieroni, F., et al. (2007). Autologous nonmyeloablative hematopoietic stem cell transplantation in newly diagnosed type 1 diabetes mellitus. *JAMA*, *297*(14), 1568–1576.

von Boehmer, H. (2004). Type 1 diabetes: Focus on prevention. *Nature Medicine*, *10*(8), 783–784.

Wente, W., Efanov, A. M., Brenner, M., Kharitonenkov, A., Koster, A., Sandusky, G. E., et al. (2006). Fibroblast growth factor-21 improves pancreatic beta-cell function and survival by activation of extracellular signal-regulated kinase 1/2 and Akt signaling pathways. *Diabetes*, *55*(9), 2470–2478.

Wenzlau, J. M., Juhl, K., Yu, L., Moua, O., Sarkar, S. A., Gottlieb, P., et al. (2007). The cation efflux transporter ZnT8 (Slc30A8) is a major autoantigen in human type 1 diabetes. *Proceedings of the National Academy of Sciences of the United States of America*, *104*(43), 17040–17045.

Wild, S., Roglic, G., Green, A., Sicree, R., & King, H. (2004). Global prevalence of diabetes: Estimates for the year 2000 and projections for 2030. *Diabetes Care*, *27*(5), 1047–1053.

Winkler, C., Mollenhauer, U., Hummel, S., Bonifacio, E., & Ziegler, A. G. (2008). Exposure to environmental factors in drinking water: Risk of islet autoimmunity and type 1 diabetes—The BABYDIAB study. *Hormone and Metabolic Research*, *40*(8), 566–571.

Yach, D., Stuckler, D., & Brownell, K. D. (2006). Epidemiologic and economic consequences of the global epidemics of obesity and diabetes. *Nature Medicine*, *12*(1), 62–66.

Zalutskaya, A., Bornstein, S. R., Mokhort, T., & Garmaev, D. (2004). Did the Chernobyl incident cause an increase in Type 1 diabetes mellitus incidence in children and adolescents? *Diabetologia*, *47*(1), 147–148.

Zeggini, E., Scott, L. J., Saxena, R., Voight, B. F., Marchini, J. L., Hu, T., et al. (2008). Meta-analysis of genome-wide association data and large-scale replication identifies additional susceptibility loci for type 2 diabetes. *Nature Genetics*, *40*(5), 638–645.

Zeggini, E., Weedon, M. N., Lindgren, C. M., Frayling, T. M., Elliott, K. S., Lango, H., et al. (2007). Replication of genome-wide association signals in UK samples reveals risk loci for type 2 diabetes. *Science*, *316*(5829), 1336–1341.

Zhang, W., Patil, S., Chauhan, B., Guo, S., Powell, D. R., Le, J., et al. (2006). FoxO1 regulates multiple metabolic pathways in the liver: Effects on gluconeogenic, glycolytic, and lipogenic gene expression. *The Journal of Biological Chemistry*, *281*(15), 10105–10117.

Ziegler, A. G., Hummel, M., Schenker, M., & Bonifacio, E. (1999). Autoantibody appearance and risk for development of childhood diabetes in offspring of parents with type 1 diabetes: The 2-year analysis of the German BABYDIAB Study. *Diabetes*, *48*(3), 460–468.

CHAPTER NINE

Regenerative Medicine for Diabetes: Differentiation of Human Pluripotent Stem Cells into Functional β-Cells *In Vitro* and Their Proposed Journey to Clinical Translation

Bipasha Bose[*,1,2], **Kishore Reddy Katikireddy**[†,2], **Sudheer Shenoy P**[*,2]

[*]Nanyang Technological University, School of Biological Sciences, NTU Lab Location @ Level 2 Singapore Institute for Clinical Sciences, Brenner Centre for Molecular Medicine, Singapore, Singapore
[†]Schepens Eye Research Institute, Harvard Medical School, Boston, Massachusetts, USA
[1]Corresponding author: e-mail address: Bipasha.bose@gmail.com
[2]Equally contributing authors.

Contents

Vitamins and Hormones, Volume 95
ISSN 0083-6729
http://dx.doi.org/10.1016/B978-0-12-800174-5.00009-0

Abstract

Diabetes is a group of metabolic diseases, rising globally at an alarming rate. Type 1 (juvenile diabetes) is the autoimmune version of diabetes where the pancreas is unable to produce insulin, whereas Type 2 (adult onset diabetes) is caused due to insulin resistance of the cells. In either of the cases, elevated blood glucose levels are observed which leads to progressive comorbidity like renal failure, cardiovascular disease, retinopathy, etc. Metformin, sulphonyl urea group of drugs, as well as insulin injections are the available therapies. In advanced cases of diabetes, the drug alone or drug in combination with insulin injections are not able to maintain a steady level of blood glucose. Moreover, frequent insulin injections are rather cumbersome for the patient. So, regenerative medicine could be a permanent solution for fighting diabetes. Islet transplantation has been tried with a limited amount of success on a large population of diabetics because of the shortage of cadaveric pancreas. Therefore, the best proposed alternative is regenerative medicine involving human pluripotent stem cell (hPSC)-derived beta islet transplantation which can be obtained in large quantities. Efficient protocols for *in vitro* differentiation of hPSC into a large number of sustained insulin-producing beta cells for transplantation will be considered to be a giant leap to address global rise in diabetic cases. Although most of the protocols mimic *in vivo* pancreatic development in humans, considerable amount of lacuna persists for near-perfect differentiation strategies. Moreover, beta islets differentiated from hPSC have not yet been successfully translated under clinical scenario.

1. INTRODUCTION

As per classical methods of available therapies a specific disease is treated with a compound, often known as a drug. Such a drug has properties to modify biological processes, thereby leading to a total elimination or reduction in severity of a disease. More often than not, it is a reduction in the severity of a disease rather than total elimination of diseased conditions. In order to overcome such a limitation of classical therapeutic methods, concept and practice of regenerative medicine was introduced in the field of medical science. Regenerative medicine involves replacing damaged or degenerated tissues and organs with healthier tissues and organs which are capable to restore the normal function or stimulate the weaker tissues of the body to restore normal function.

The term "Regenerative Medicine" was first coined by William Haseltine (founder of Human Genome Sciences) (Viola, Lal, & Grad, 2003). This term was first referred in 1992 in an article on hospital administration by Leland Kaiser. Kaiser's paper closes with a series of short paragraphs on future technologies that will impact hospitals. One such paragraph had "Regenerative Medicine" as a bold print title and went on to state, "A new branch of medicine will develop that attempts to change the course of chronic disease and in many instances will regenerate tired and failing organ systems" (Kaiser, 1992; Lysaght & Crager, 2009). More often than not, regenerative medicine refers to a group of biomedical approaches to clinical therapies that may involve the use of stem cells (Riazi, Kwon, & Stanford, 2009).

The history of first successful incidence of tissue engineering and regenerative medicine is relatively new which spans over just less than two decades. In 1998, the US Food and Drug Administration (FDA) granted its first approval for an allogeneic tissue-engineered product in the form of Apligraf®, which was described originally as a living-skin equivalent by Organogenesis, a company started by Eugene Bell's laboratory. The launch of Apligraf® followed the autologous burns treatment, Epicel®, which originated from Green's laboratory and was at first unregulated by the FDA and treated as a tissue graft. Following this, a lot of other cell-based products, which were approved by FDA, were into clinical trials, as well as, therapy in the market for the treatment of various diseases, or disorders, namely, autologous bone marrow cells for treatment of long bone fracture and diabetic limb ischemia, allogeneic fibroblasts for the treatment of diabetic ulcers, cultured keratinocytes for the treatment of burns, microencapsulated allogeneic islet cells for the treatment of Type I diabetes, cultured autologous skeletal muscle myoblasts for the treatment of myocardial infarction and congestive heart failure, etc.

As far as pluripotent stem cell (PSC)-based therapies are concerned, there have been safety issues relating to the teratoma-formation potential of the cells as well as an ethical issue regarding destruction of human embryos to obtain human embryonic stem cells (hESCs). However, overcoming all such issues, a California-based company, Geron Corporation on January 23, 2009, got the US FDA clearance for the initiation of the first clinical trial of an embryonic stem cell-based therapy on humans. The trial aimed to evaluate the drug GRNOPC1, embryonic stem cell-derived oligodendrocyte progenitor cells, on patients with acute spinal cord injury. The trial was later discontinued on account of being too expensive and company's decision to channelize the funding for some other projects (Lebkowski, 2011).

2. DIABETES AND ITS HISTORY

2.1. Discovery of diabetes

Diabetes was identified and narrated in a book named *Diabetes: Its Various Forms and Different Treatments*, as early as, in the year 1866 by English Physician George Harley (1829–1896) (Harley, 1866). At that time, Harley attributed the disease due to excess formation of sugar by the liver because the role of β-islets in pancreas in insulin biogenesis was not known then. Later on, in 1889, Oskar Minkowski, working in Strasbourg discovered serendipitously that pancreatectomy in dogs caused a severe wasting type of diabetes (Mering & Minkowski, 1889) (first publication on experimental pancreatic diabetes) which was translated later by Rachmiel Levine during centenary celebration of the work and published in *Diabetes* journal (Minkowski, 1989). One possible explanation to this was that pancreas destroyed a toxin which interfered with glucose metabolism but Minkowski and others believed that something is produced as an internal secretion. This something was later found to be insulin. Moreover, in 1894, Gustave Laguesse (1861–1927) suggested that this was produced by small irregularly polygonal cells, with brilliant cytoplasm, diffusely scattered in the pancreatic parenchyma. These cells were earlier discovered in 1861 by a medical student named Paul Langerhans (1847–1888) and hence were named islets of Langerhans. Eventually, two types of diabetes were identified as those which affect a person at an early age and cannot be managed with lifestyle changes, and the ones which affects a person at a later age and can be managed with lifestyle-related changes.

2.2. Discovery of insulin

One of the earliest and most dramatic in the history of modern medicine achievements was the isolation and use of insulin to treat diabetes in 1923. For this, the Nobel Prize in Physiology and Medicine was awarded to Fredrick Grant Banting (1891–1941) and John James Rickard Macleod (1876–1935). Use of insulin as a therapy for diabetes was first unsuccessfully tried in the form of feeding the cell extracts of pancreas to the diabetic patients. Thereafter, in January 1922, a diabetic teenager, a boy named

Leonard Thompson, in a Toronto hospital became the first person to receive an injection of insulin. At that time, insulin was not purified, rather it was directly the cell extract made from pancreas and the slurry was directly injected into the patient. Initially, the patient was given a single shot of insulin injection, which did show an initial decrease in his blood sugar levels, and blood sugar levels of the same patient again got elevated. However, after a couple of days, the same patient was given two insulin injections over a span of 12 h in response to which the patient showed a drastic improvement. Thereafter, he was cured of diabetes and lived a healthy life and died later due to pneumonia. The University of Toronto immediately gave pharmaceutical companies license to produce insulin free of royalties. In early 1923, about 1 year after the first test injection, insulin became widely available and saved countless lives.

In the intermediate phase of insulin era, insulin was purified from animals like porcine and bovine origin and was administered to the diabetic patients. Insulin was one of the first proteins to be crystallized in pure form, in 1926. The crystalline form of insulin allowed researchers to study its structure with a technique called X-ray crystallography and approximate its three-dimensional (3D) shape. These studies facilitated to look into the mechanisms of action of insulin, as well. In 1955, insulin became the first protein to be fully sequenced. That work resulted in a 1959 Nobel Prize for Frederick Sanger. In fact, insulin was the first protein to be chemically synthesized in a laboratory, in 1963, but researchers were unable to produce much of it. For 60 years after Banting's group isolated insulin, diabetics relied on hormone purified from animals, primarily cattle and pigs, which had adverse reactions on human like skin rashes, etc., for being from animal origin.

In 1978, insulin became the first human protein to be manufactured through biotechnology by scientific collaborators from the City of Hope National Medical Center and the biotech company Genentech, in USA, who first time made recombinant human insulin using bacteria and launched it successfully into the market. The presently available insulin is also recombinant human insulin used to treat diabetics globally.

2.3. History of cell or tissue transplantation as a treatment for diabetes

Simultaneously, with the treatment of diabetes with insulin, a permanent cure of diabetes was intriguing to scientists in the field. Accordingly, cell or tissue transplantation to replace damaged or degenerated islets with the healthy and active pancreas/islets was thought about as the most relevant alternative. The aim of such transplantation was to cure the diabetics, especially, Type 1 diabetics from the secondary complications like diabetic retinopathy, kidney failure, etc., by maintaining the homeostatic levels of glucose in the body.

The goal of islet transplantation (IT) is to infuse enough islets to control the blood glucose level removing the need for insulin injections. For an average-size person (70 kg), a typical transplant requires about one million islets, isolated from two donor pancreases. Because good control of blood glucose can slow or prevent the progression of complications associated with diabetes, such as nerve or eye damage, a successful transplant may reduce the risk of these complications. A transplant recipient will need to take immunosuppressive drugs that stop the immune system from rejecting the transplanted islets.

The two possible options to cell and tissue transplantation for diabetics are (1) pancreas graft or pancreas transplantation (PT) and (2) IT. Three types of PTs are there: in the first one, in a single dose of immunosuppression, pancreas and kidney transplantations are carried out simultaneously; in the second, PT is done after kidney transplantation; and in the third one, PT alone is done. All types of PTs require donor organs. The history of PT dates back to December 17, 1966 in University of Minnesota. It was a simultaneous pancreas and kidney transplantation in a female aged 28 years who was suffering from Type 1 diabetic nephropathy. Initially, the patient did require insulin just after transplantation but eventually developed graft pancreatitis. Because of graft pancreatitis, the grafted pancreas had to be removed from the patient on February 14, 1967. The patient died 13 days after the graft removal, suffering from pulmonary embolism.

2.4. Islet transplantation and possibility of use of pluripotent stem cell-derived islets

The concept of IT is not new. English surgeon Charles Pybus (1882–1975) was the first to attempt to graft pancreatic tissue to cure diabetes. In 1967, Paul Lacy's group described a novel collagenase-based method (later modified by Dr. Camillo Ricordi, Tzakis et al., 1990, then working with Dr. Lacy) to isolate islets, paving the way for future *in vitro* and *in vivo* islet experiments (Lacy & Kostianovsky, 1967). However, further studies confirmed that transplanted islets could reverse diabetes in both rodents and nonhuman primates (Kemp, Knight, Scharp, Lacy, & Ballinger, 1973; Scharp, Murphy, Newton, Ballinger, & Lacy, 1975).

In a summary, of the 1977 Workshop on Pancreatic Islet Cell Transplantation in Diabetes, Lacy commented on the feasibility of "islet cell transplantation as a therapeutic approach for the possible prevention of the complications of diabetes in man" (Lacy, 1978). Improvements in isolation techniques and immunosuppressive regimens ushered in the first human IT clinical trials in the mid-1980s. The first successful trial of human islet allotransplantation resulting in long-term reversal of diabetes was performed at the University of Pittsburgh in 1990 (Tzakis et al., 1990). Yet, despite continued procedural improvements, only about 10% of islet recipients in the late 1990s achieved euglycemia (normal blood glucose). In 2000, Dr. James Shapiro and colleagues published a report describing seven consecutive patients who achieved euglycemia following IT using a steroid-free protocol and large numbers of donor islets since referred to as the Edmonton protocol (Shapiro et al., 2000). This protocol has been adapted by islet transplant centers around the world and has tremendously increased islet transplant success.

Accordingly, as far as IT is concerned, it is a safer and less invasive procedure, which has resulted in more success as compared to pancreatic transplantation, but the availability of more than one donor pancreas is the only concern, apart from the immunosuppressive regime. So, *in vitro*-generated islets from human pluripotent stem cells (hPSCs) would be the best option for the regenerative medicine for diabetes.

3. DIFFERENTIATION PROTOCOLS FOR HUMAN PLURIPOTENT STEM CELLS TO β-CELLS

In the direction of generation of a large number of transplantable beta islets from hPSCs, scientists have been working globally since a decade or so using various strategies. The strategies for large-scale *in vitro* differentiation and purification of beta islets (Fig. 9.1) were designed to mimic *in vivo* pancreatic development and are summarized under the following subheads.

3.1. Evolution of differentiation protocols based on developmental biology of pancreas: Olden days to recent advances

The development of adult pancreas is quite complex. The complexity of development of adult pancreas is primarily attributed to the composition of adult pancreas, which includes the exocrine and endocrine parts (pancreatic islets). The exocrine cells produce digestive enzymes, and the endocrine

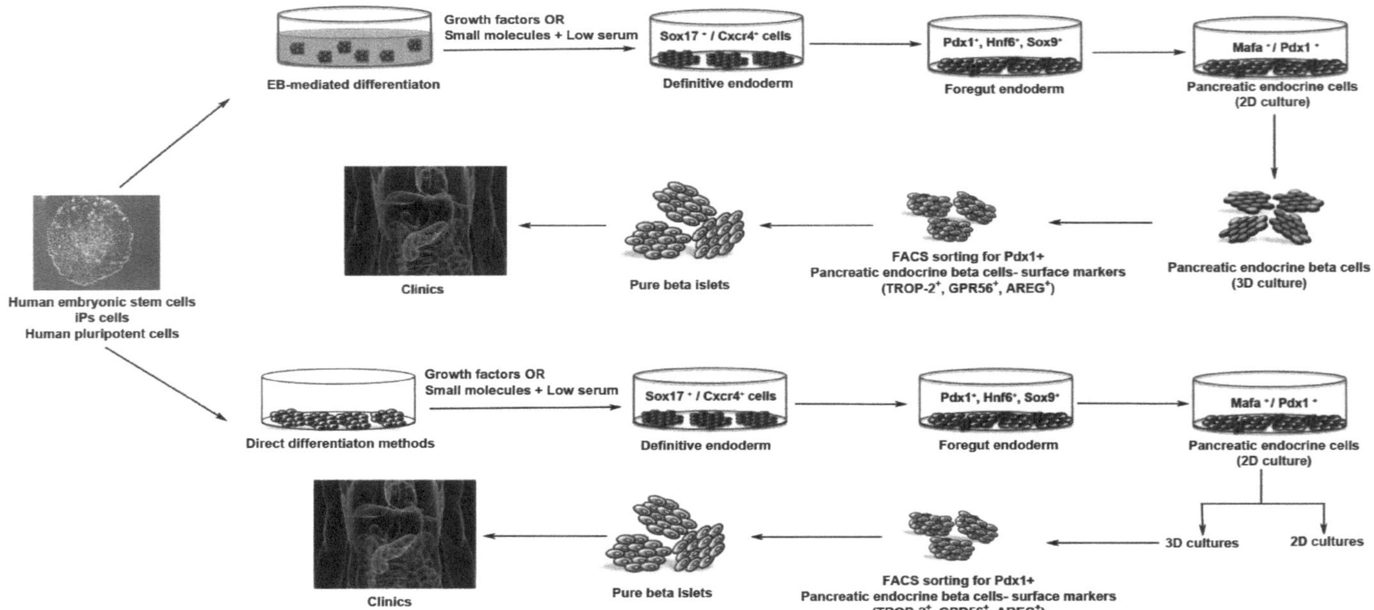

Figure 9.1 Strategies for *in vitro* pancreatic beta cell differentiation. (See the color plate.)

cells produce insulin (β-cells), glucagon (α-cells), somatostatin (δ-cells), and pancreatic polypeptide cells (Slack, 1995). hESCs, which are immortal and capable of self-renewal and differentiation into any cell types of the body, can be a potential source for indefinite supply of insulin-producing β-cells for transplantation into diabetic patients (Soria, Skoudy, & Martín, 2001). Initial efforts to generate functional beta islets *in vitro* were taken using mouse embryonic stem cells (Lumelsky et al., 2001). Till date, all the *in vitro* differentiation protocols have been rather aimed to mimic pancreatic organogenesis *in vivo*.

Pancreatic islets contain many cell types of multiple developmental origins. Exocrine, as well as, endocrine cells, such as β-cells, arise from a region of foregut endoderm that expresses the transcription factor, *Pdx1* (Stoffers, Heller, Miller, & Habener, 1999). Islets are also innervated by neurons (Kirchgessner & Gershon, 1990) and surrounded by Schwann cells (Sunami et al., 2001). Moreover, neurons and Schwann cells, which are interspersed, within the islets, are originated from neural crest. During organogenesis of pancreas, the neural crest-derived cells in pancreas like neurons and Schwann cells have been shown to influence proliferation and maturation of β-islets (Plank et al., 2011). Islets are also vascularized with β-cells in direct contact with endothelial cells of mesodermal origin, as well (Ranjan, Joglekar, & Hardikar, 2009).

More than a decade back, researchers found that the pancreatic endoderm and neural ectoderm cells coexpress a large number of markers, suggesting that they share a common pathway of differentiation. Accordingly, differentiation protocols involved "Nestin selection pathway" which is common for both neural and pancreatic differentiation (Lumelsky et al., 2001). As a consequence of this strategy, the insulin-producing cells generated by Lumelsky and colleagues did not result in the formation of bonafide β-cells, but likely cells with the combination of neuronal lineage. Although such cells stained positive for insulin, it was subsequently shown to be a result of uptake of insulin from the culture medium rather than activation of robust insulin transcription (Rajagopal, Anderson, Kume, Martinez, & Melton, 2003). As a result, such a protocol failed and was no longer acceptable to the scientific community by and large. Eventually, workers identified a rare population of cells in the adult pancreas that are capable of proliferation *in vitro* and differentiation to multiple pancreatic and neural cell types—a pancreas-derived multipotent precursor (PMP). These precursors express multiple pancreatic and neural markers and are capable of differentiating into endocrine and neural cells *in vitro* and *in vivo* (Seaberg et al., 2004;

Smukler et al., 2011). Subsequent lineage-tracing experiments suggested that the majority of PMPs were derived from pancreatic lineage. More recently, it was, however, reported that adult mammalian pancreas contains separate precursors of pancreatic and neural crest developmental origins (Arntfield & Van der Kooy, 2013). After the failure of nestin selection protocol, researches working on *in vitro* pancreatic differentiation started to focus more on the chronological development of embryonic pancreas and followed typical embryonic development pattern like definitive endoderm formation preceding pancreatic endoderm, the transcriptional hierarchy of factors regulating β-cell identity during embryogenesis, various cytokines secreted which facilitated *in vivo* pancreatic development.

3.2. Protocols mimicking *in vivo* embryonic pancreas development and transcriptional hierarchy of factors regulating β-cell identity

Despite the fact that pancreas has multiple cell types and complex developmental origin, overlapping gene expression emerges when we consider the origin of these cells within the embryo. Most of the studies in the past decade were done based on the transcriptional hierarchy of factors regulating β-cell identity during embryogenesis. Results of such studies on the transcriptional hierarchy of factors regulating β-cell identity during embryogenesis prompted a number of groups to test whether forced expression of such factors, including *Pdx1, Pax4,* and *Nkx2.2,* was sufficient to drive ESCs toward the β-cell (Blyszczuk et al., 2003; Miyazaki, Yamato, & Miyazaki, 2004; Shiroi et al., 2005).

D'Amour et al. (2005) and colleagues, in 2005, published that the hESC differentiation into β-cells is possible when the culture conditions used replicate embryonic development as closely as possible. Taking a stepwise approach, this group set out to first differentiate hESCs toward definitive endoderm, a prerequisite for all pancreatic cell types. This stepwise approach for endodermal differentiation was followed by the differentiation into pancreatic β-islet cells through the use of various growth factors (Shi et al., 2005). D'Amour et al. (2006) described a five-step and a four-step two-dimensional (or monolayer) hESC differentiation protocol that leads to efficient *Pdx1* activation by day 12 and 15, respectively, and the impressive formation of up to 12% insulin-containing cells. Other protocols, which also mimicked *in vivo* pancreatic development resulted in the formation of *in vivo* transplantable functional β-islet cells by day 18 (Madsen & Serup, 2006) and day 25 (Jiang, Au, et al., 2007; Jiang, Shi, et al., 2007).

The use of different model systems to understand early embryonic development had shown that nodal, a soluble molecule of the TGFβ/activin-signaling family, was required for mesoderm and definitive endoderm formation during gastrulation, with higher levels of nodal-promoting endoderm specification (Conlon et al., 1994; Lowe, Yamada, & Kuehn, 2001; Osada & Wright, 1999; Vincent, Dunn, Hayashi, Norris, & Robertson, 2003). Based on these observations, D'Amour and colleagues implemented a protocol in which hESCs were exposed to distinct soluble signaling factors. Activin A, another member of the TGFβ signaling family, was used together with Wnt3a to generate cells expressing markers of definitive endoderm (D'Amour et al., 2005, 2006). The approach of using embryonic signals to instruct hESCs to definitive endoderm and subsequently to β-cells was validated by several other groups using modifications of this procedure (Eshpeter et al., 2008; Jiang, Au, et al., 2007; Jiang, Shi, et al., 2007; Mao, Chen, Bai, Song, & Wang, 2009). These cells were generated by Shi et al. (2005). D'Amour et al. (2006) responded to a variety of insulin secretagogues, but only showed limited glucose responsiveness. Modified pancreatic differentiation by Kroon et al. (2008) reported the production of insulin-producing cells from hESC which were also *in vivo* responsive to glucose. Recently, Nostro et al. (2011) reported improved efficiency (25%) of insulin-producing cells by stage-specific *in vitro* regulation of TGFβ family members.

During organogenesis within the mouse embryonic foregut, pancreatic fate is first specified by the expression of the homoeobox gene *Pdx1* (pancreatic and duodenal homoeobox-1) (Guz et al., 1995; Jonsson, Carlsson, Edlund, & Edlund, 1994). Thus, activation of *Pdx1* is considered a prerequisite for pancreatic differentiation *in vitro* and should precede the progressive expression of more mature markers of the endocrine lineage including *Ngn3, Nkx2.2, Nkx6.1, MafA*, and *MafB* (Jensen, 2004). Moreover, *MafA* has been identified as the master regulator of glucose-stimulated insulin secretion in functional β-islet cells (Hang & Stein, 2011; Matsuoka et al., 2004; Wang, Brun, Kataoka, Sharma, & Wollheim, 2007; Zhang et al., 2005). This transcription factor, which is expressed, last among all β-islet transcription factors has been involved in regulating β-cell function by activating the insulin gene promoter via Pdx1 and positive regulation of essential β-cell genes such as *Glut2, Pdx1, Nkx6.1*, and *Glp1* (glucagon-like peptide 1). Also, MafA and MafB have been implicated in functional maturation of pancreatic β-islet cells from hESC (Guz et al., 1995;Jonsson et al., 1994; Wang et al., 2007). Thus, in vitro pancreatic differentiation strategies from

ES cells, which are recently developed, involve *Pdx1* activation, in order to, mimic β cell organogenesis.

3.3. 3D culture protocols as more efficient than 2D *in vitro* pancreatic differentiation protocols

Most of the protocols described above relied on two-dimensional culture techniques in which cells are grown as monolayers throughout the differentiation process. However, a few groups have used 3D methods in which ESCs are first aggregated to form embryoid bodies (EB) that have the potential to give rise to cells of all three germ layers, including the endoderm that forms the pancreas (Ku et al., 2004; Kubo et al., 2004). Modifications of the EB culture protocol include separation of cells followed by fluorescence-activated cell sorting (FACS) and reaggregation (Gadue, Huber, Paddison, & Keller, 2006; Gouon-Evans et al., 2006). The advantage of 3D culture over monolayer cultures is the better ability of cells to differentiate in a 3D space in EB cultures. 3D culture conditions are likely to strengthen interactions between β-cells and could enhance insulin-secretory dynamics that may be directly affected by electrical coupling between insulin-producing cells (Speier et al., 2007). Thus, signals provided through cell–cell interactions or via interactions with extracellular matrices are likely more prominent under these conditions. Extracellular interactions have been shown to optimize β-cell functions and proliferation (Hammar et al., 2005; Parnaud et al., 2009; Weber, Hayda, & Anseth, 2008). Experiments will need to be performed to determine whether 2D versus EB/3D conditions have intrinsic benefits in generating fully matured β-cells from human stem cell populations. Contemporarily, 3D, β-islets were also generated from mouse ES cells (mESCc), iPS cells and mouse fetal pancreatic cells, which gave rise to 60% insulin-producing cells (Saito, Takeuchi, Chida, & Miyajima, 2011; Wang & Ye, 2009). However, very recently Bose, Shenoy, Konda, and Wangikar (2012) reported generation of pancreatic β-islet cells which produced 65% insulin-producing cells in 3D *in vitro* culture systems from human ES cells.

The 2D islets, as well as, 3D islets expressed high amounts of mature β-islet marker gene *MafA*. Furthermore, the 2D islets continued to coexpress non-β-cell endocrine pancreatic markers, for example, glucagon and somatostatin. However, 3D islet cultures upon analysis for the presence of other exocrine or endocrine hormone-producing cells of pancreas other than β-islet cells had a much lower expression of glucagon and somatostatin. 3D islet-like clusters (ILC) did not express amylase, a marker of exocrine pancreas. This observation regarding negligible expression of non-β-cell endocrine pancreatic markers by 3D ILC proved a purer population of β ILC (Bose et al., 2012).

3.4. Mimicking specific signaling cues from embryonic development for *in vitro* pancreatic differentiation protocols

During embryonic development, numerous signaling cues aid in the specification of the definitive endoderm that is progressively segregated into cells carrying distinct differentiation potential along the anterior–posterior axis followed by the development of foregut endoderm and finally pancreatic endoderm and insulin-producing cells. Based on the results of such basic studies on pancreatic endodermal developmental biology, various *in vitro* pancreatic differentiation protocols from hPSCs were designed. For example, application of fibroblast growth factor 4 (FGF4) protein in the chick induces posterior endodermal markers in anterior (foregut) endoderm (Wells & Melton, 2000). Activin and FGF2, which function to suppress endodermal sonic hedgehog signaling, are permissive for pancreas formation, similar to the role of the embryonic notochord (Hebrok, Kim, & Melton, 1998). For this important role, Activin A has been used, in the very first step of most of the *in vitro* differentiation protocols, to obtain definitive endoderm cells (Bose et al., 2012; Jiang, Au, et al., 2007; Kroon et al., 2008). Kumar and colleagues (Kumar, Jordan, Melton, & Grapin-Botton, 2003) used chick explant cultures to show that pancreatic markers are induced in the anterior endoderm by lateral plate mesoderm from the prepancreatic region. They also showed that activin, bone morphogenetic proteins, or retinoic acid (RA) can all induce pancreatic markers in the anterior endoderm cocultured with anterior mesoderm.

FGF signaling promotes the formation of endodermal cells slated to give rise to organs along the foregut, including the pancreas that forms at the fore-midgut border. Adding FGF10 or FGF7 to cultures of differentiating hESCs promotes the formation of foregut endodermal cells. Treatment with RA and inhibition of hedgehog signaling further defines the foregut endoderm cells to assume a pancreatic fate as a result of which the cytokines RA has been included in the third step of most of the pancreatic differentiation protocols (D'Amour et al., 2006; Kroon et al., 2008). RA synthesized in the anterior paraxial mesoderm adjacent to the foregut is necessary for the development of insulin-expressing cells *in vivo* in all vertebrates, and RA receptor function is exclusively required in the foregut endoderm for insulin expression but not in mesoderm and ectoderm (Stafford et al., 2006).

Importantly, the stepwise differentiation states of hESCs can be monitored via expression of transcription factors that are expressed at distinct stages during normal embryonic pancreas and β-cell differentiation. For example, cells within the foregut anlage destined to give rise to the pancreas, termed the pancreas progenitors, express Pdx1, Foxa2, and Hnf6, and eventually fully differentiated hormone-producing cells. The validity of this approach was shown when pancreas progenitor cells were transplanted into recipient immune-compromised mice. Interestingly, considering that hESC-derived pancreas progenitors are transplanted into different, non-pancreatic host tissues, including the fat pad and under the kidney capsule, these *in vivo* matured cells are capable of restoring normoglycemia in streptozotocin-treated diabetic mice and secreted insulin at concentrations similar to what was observed in control mice transplanted with human islets (Kroon et al., 2008).

Streptozotocin preferentially depletes murine β-cells as it is mainly taken up into cells via the Glut2 glucose transporter expressed in mouse insulin-producing cells. In contrast, human β-cells express Glut1 as the main glucose transporter and consequently are less susceptible to streptozotocin (Eizirik et al., 1994; Hosokawa, Dolci, & Thorens, 2001; Yang & Wright, 2002). This experimental "trick" is quite effective as it generates a scenario in which hESC-derived β-cells can be evaluated in animals for their ability to regulate glucose levels under physiological conditions as well as under stress, for example, during a glucose challenge. Importantly, removal of the human cell transplant in streptozotocin-treated mice resulted in rapid appearance of hyperglycemia and diabetes, strongly supporting the argument that normoglycemia in these animals was regulated by the hESC-derived β-cells (Kroon et al., 2008). Thus, all these *in vivo* validations of *in vitro*-differentiated hPSCs prove the accuracy of *in vitro* differentiation protocols in mimicking *in vivo* pancreas development.

3.5. Chemicals employed for *in vitro* pancreatic differentiation from human pluripotent stem cells

Many of the currently employed differentiation protocols rely on the sequential activation or inhibition of embryonic signaling pathways through treatment with the receptor ligands of the respective cell types in the form of cytokines. Since these cytokines are protein-based material, they are difficult to obtain and not cost effective for large-scale differentiation. Alternative cost-effective approaches have been undertaken to identify biologically active small chemical compounds that can functionally mimic cellular signaling molecules. Identification of such small molecules/biologically active compounds and their successful application in pancreatic differentiation protocols thereby replacing expensive cytokines not only open door for large-scale differentiation for clinical applications but also shed light on various molecular mechanisms essential for stem cell differentiation.

Based on screening chemical libraries ranging from 4000 to 20,000 compounds, only four small molecules, IDE1, IDE2, (−)-Indolactam V (ILV), and Stauprimide (Spd), were found highly effective in priming or promoting ESC differentiation to pancreatic lineage (Borowiak et al., 2009; Chen et al., 2009). Moreover, such small molecules are less than 1000 Dalton in molecular weight, can be easily synthesized in large quantities, and can serve as agonists or antagonists for specific signaling pathways for hPSC differentiation.

mESCs expressing a reporter driven by the *Sox17* promoter were used to assess the activity of such screened compounds to differentiate toward the definitive endoderm lineage in the absence of Activin A (Borowiak et al., 2009). The mechanisms for promoting ESC differentiation to endoderm/pancreatic lineage were found to be different among these molecules. Both IDE1 and IDE2 acted as agonist to upregulate the activin/nodal signaling pathway, the pathway which is known to be essential for inducing endoderm fate. ES cells treated with IDE1 or IDE2 had twice as many $Sox17^+$ endoderm cells than with Activin A treatment. Molecularly, both compounds phosphorylated Smad2, a critical mediator of activin signaling, and their activity was blocked by the activin receptor-like kinase inhibitor SB43125. ILV induced ESC differentiation from endoderm to Pdx1-expressing pancreatic progenitors by activating the protein kinase C signaling pathway. In addition, the effect of ILV was found to be substantially improved in the presence of FGF10. ILV promoted differentiation to $Pdx1^+$ pancreatic progenitor from ES cells that had been instructed to become definitive endoderm by natural molecules (Activin A or nodal) or by small chemicals (IDE1 or IDE2). Unlike IDE1, IDE2, and ILV, which promoted differentiation toward a specific fate, Spd acted to disrupt the pluripotent state of ES cells, which, in turn, primed the ES cells for differentiation. A transcription factor that regulates *c-Myc* expression called NME2 (nonmetastatic cells 2, protein [NM23B] expressed in; Gene ID 4831) was also shown to be a direct target of Spd. Affinity-based experiment revealed that Spd interacted with NME2 and inhibited its nuclear localization resulting in downregulation of *c-Myc*, a key factor in the maintenance of ESC self-renewal (Zhu et al., 2009). Thus, Spd is dependent on the subsequent treatment with Activin A for the differentiation of Spd-primed ESC to definitive endoderm. Importantly, all of these small molecules exerted similar effect on both mouse and hESCs. Altogether, these findings represent a significant step toward controlling stem cell differentiation into pancreatic lineage.

3.6. Identification of various cell-surface markers for isolating stepwise *in vitro*-differentiated progenitors (definitive endoderm, foregut, pancreatic, and endocrine precursors, etc.)

As a strategy for cell-based therapy in diabetes, it would be necessary to transplant a large population of stepwise differentiated progenitors into the individual. This might aid in efficient engraftment of the large population of progenitors in the form of Pdx1$^+$ cells rather than terminally differentiated cells (Sui, Geens, Sermon, Bouwens, & Mfopou, 2013). By slightly altering differentiation conditions, Cai et al. (2010) reported the generation of 95% Pdx1$^+$ cells from hESC. In order to facilitate such a process, sorting/isolation of progenitors at various stages of differentiation would be essential. However, Pdx1 is a transcription factor which is expressed in the nucleus. Accordingly, it is difficult to FACS sort the cells based on only Pdx1 staining of the cells. Until recently, no specific cell-surface marker was known for Pdx1$^+$ or else other pancreatic progenitor cells. More recently, Fishman et al. (2012) generated hESC clones harboring BAC GFP reporter constructs of *Sox17*, a definitive endoderm marker, and *Pdx1*, a pancreatic marker, and identified subpopulations of GFP-expressing cells. Using this approach, they isolated a highly enriched population of pancreatic progenitor cells from hESCs and examined their gene expression with an emphasis on the expression of stage-specific cell-surface markers. They were able to identify novel molecules that are involved in the pancreatic differentiation process, as well as, stage-specific cell markers that may serve to define (alone or in combination with other markers) a specific pancreatic progenitor cell. These findings might be helpful in optimizing conditions for ultimately generating and isolating beta cells (by FACS sorting) for transplantation therapy. The interesting outcome of this study was an association of different cell-surface proteins with different progenitor cell populations, for example, (1) Sox17$^+$ cells, (2) Pdx1$^+$ cells, (3) Sox17$^+$/Pdx1$^+$ cells, and (4) Pdx1$^+$ pancreas-specific cells. It was furthermore reported that, the cell-surface proteins that were highly enriched only in the $Sox17^+$ cells were follicle-stimulating hormone receptor, frizzled homolog 5, and Cholecystokinin B receptor. Cell-surface proteins that were highly enriched only in the $Pdx1^+$ cells were identified as Frizzled-3, G protein-coupled receptor 50, and matrix metalloproteinase 16. Delta-like 1 homolog, low-density lipoprotein receptor-related protein 2, and bone marrow stromal cell antigen 2 were enriched in both $Pdx1^+$ and $Sox17^+$ cells, while tumor-associated calcium signal transducer 2, G protein-coupled receptor 56, and amphiregulin were enriched in both $Pdx1^+$ cells and pancreatic cells (Fishman et al., 2012).

4. hESC/hPSC-DERIVED BETA ISLETS-BASED CELL THERAPY FOR DIABETES

4.1. Will this cell therapy hit the clinics? Various roadblocks

Cellular therapies in recent years have grown dramatically in sophistication, power, and scope. The promise of stem cell-derived therapies holds particularly high hopes for diabetes. The first successful transplantation of islet cells into the liver in 1989 established the proof-of-principle for islet cell transplantation (IT) in diabetic patients (Melkman-Zehavi et al., 2011). Despite considerable clinical success of the IT in 1989, beta cell transplantation is still considered being experimental rather than a routine treatment in most countries. The foremost challenges in IT are finding an adequate supply, large-scale purification and storage, insulin responsiveness of transplantable islets to increased glycemia, and finally preventing transplanted or regenerated cells from being killed by immune destruction from autoimmunity and/or transplant rejection. The various approaches that might lead to an adequate supply of beta cells for replacement therapy could be (a) embryonic or induced PSCs, (b) adult stem/progenitor cells (islet neogenesis from duct cells or other precursor cells in the pancreas, or from nonpancreatic precursor cells), (c) beta cell replication, (d) genetic engineering (conditional expression of specific genes in beta cells or generation of cells that resist immune destruction), (e) reprogramming (e.g., acinar, liver, intestine, others), and (f) xeno-transplants (porcine fetal, neonatal, or adult; or other species). Understanding fundamental development of islets and ductal cells has given us open thoughts for regeneration of the endocrine pancreas *in vivo*, and this approach can be achieved by stimulation of neogenesis, replication, or reprogramming. All the approaches listed above have certain limitations based on severity/condition of diabetes. Discussing limitations

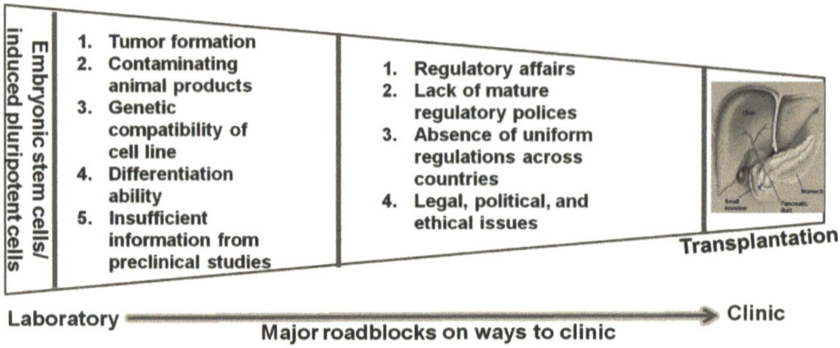

Figure 9.2 Schematic representation of major roadblocks for clinical application of embryonic and induced pluripotent cells. (See the color plate.)

of each approach is beyond the scope of this chapter. Accordingly, we have highlighted various challenges and roadblocks to hit this technology to clinic (Fig. 9.2).

hESCs/human induced pluripotent stem cells (hiPSC), also termed in common, hPSCs have advantages over other potential sources because hPSCs are now readily available and highly expandable under *in vitro* conditions. Accordingly, the path to successful hPSC therapies seems to be straightforward in making the desired cell type from hPSCs, such as neurons to treat neurodegenerative disease (Keirstead et al., 2005) or pancreatic β-cells to treat type I diabetes, and then transfer these cells to the desired site *in vivo*. A large body of literature already exists on differentiation of hES cell to pancreatic β-cells (Bose et al., 2012; Jiang, Au, et al., 2007; Kroon et al., 2008). The advances of embryonic stem cell biology are truly remarkable and have brought us a crucial step closer to developing novel sources of human beta cells for transplantation therapy and drug discovery.

4.2. Challenges in setting up new islets program?

Important challenges remain as the pathways regulating the development of the progenitors of the second transition and their maturation to functional cells *in vitro* are not well understood. Based on developmental scheme, the initial steps of pancreatic development from hPSCs should involve a loss of pluripotency, the formation of definitive endoderm, the development of the equivalent of the primitive gut tube, and the specification of pancreatic endothelium. Under certain optimal conditions, these developmental steps should proceed at the expense of the other germ layers (mesoderm and ectoderm) and of the other endoderm lineages. Differentiation to pancreatic pathway will involve specification of the first and second transition populations and ultimately the development and maturation of the beta cell lineage, by manipulating appropriate signaling pathways in control stepwise fashion. As discussed in this chapter by using a variety of modifications, different groups have reported on the generation of pancreatic lineage cells from a range of different hESC and hiPSC lines. The findings from above studies collectively give insights into pancreatic development from hPSCs by (1) definitive endoderm formation, (2) endoderm patterning, (3) pancreatic epithelium specification, and finally (4) endocrine commitment. Most prominent and difficult challenges remain such as the pathways regulating the development of the progenitors of the second transition and their maturation to functional cells *in vitro* are not well understood. In particular, epigenetic and expression profiling of the different PSCs could provide novel information on their "pancreatic propensity" and on signaling pathways that regulate the generation and maturation of beta cell progenitors *in vitro*. Current differentiation protocols try to mimic pancreatic organogenesis by sequential treatment of ES cells with defined growth and differentiation factors in chemically defined medium. However, differentiation protocols follow insights gained from mouse models of pancreatic development and may not be fully suitable for human *in vitro* systems. Despite all efforts, none of the protocols established so far generate fully functional insulin-producing cells comparable with mature beta cells *in vivo*. Beta cells resembling human fetal pancreas were generated instead, using most of the protocols. The challenge of most pancreatic differentiation protocols remains as the heterogeneity of the ES progeny.

Other major challenge is the presence of contaminating animal products (Fig. 9.2). Any cell-based therapeutic agent used in humans must be free of animal contaminants that may contain pathogens or elicit an immune reaction after transfer to a host. All hES cell lines on the NIH registry were derived in the presence of animal products. Studies have developed novel approaches for removing animal products from existing lines (Amit, Shariki, Margulets, & Itskovitz-Eldor, 2004; Xu et al., 2001). In addition, ES cell lines, mouse and human, are generally grown on mouse-derived feeders, a layer of fibroblasts treated so that they no longer proliferate, that provide additional factors that promote both ES cell proliferation and inhibit their differentiation. All of the hES cell lines on the NIH registry approved for use by government-sponsored laboratories were isolated under conditions that included animal serum and mouse feeders.

Studies conducted much after the derivation of the NIH-registered hES lines demonstrate the ability of FGF-2 to replace the need for feeder coculture of hES lines (Xu, Peck, et al., 2005; Xu, Rosler, et al., 2005). Followed by the establishment of use of FGF-2 under feeder-free conditions, another study documented the derivation of hES cell lines under animal product-free conditions (Ludwig et al., 2006). This progress suggests that the problem of animal product contamination is being solved. However, the journey to eliminating this roadblock may have been more direct and faster if federal funding had been available for generating uncontaminated cell lines.

The *in vitro*-generated pancreatic cells have to be capable of engrafting and surviving *in vivo* for extended periods of time under successful control of immune responses without forming tumors. All ES and iPS cell-based approaches will have to ensure complete absence of pluripotent cells after transplantation to circumvent teratoma formation. Finally, clinical application of stem cell-based cell therapies requires that all procedures necessary to generate insulin-secreting cells follow the guidelines of good manufacturing practice. Apart from above mentioned challenges in the field of stem cells, the current roadblocks for stem cell-based therapy include legal, political, and ethical issues, lack of mature regulatory policy, absence of uniform regulations and activity across countries, and uniform global patent interpretations on PSCs (Fig. 9.2). Most noteworthy aspect is the presence of limited expertise in scaled-up cell manufacturing. Apart from above mentioned challenges for stem cell-based therapy for diabetes, current roadblocks include legal, political, and ethical issues, lack of mature regulatory policy, absence of uniform regulations and activity across countries, and uniform global patent interpretations on pluripotent.

4.3. Limitations in bench to bed side for hESC/hiPSC-derived beta islets cells, highlighting with major regulatory bodies (FDA in USA, European regulations, etc.)

In the United Kingdom, and in all other countries, in Europe, and worldwide, production of cell-based products must be carried out under good medical practice in a specifically licensed laboratory. In order to obtain a license, the entire production process (including raw materials, manufacturing, supply, and storage) must be assessed and approved, and there must be stringent ongoing quality control and inspections. These new regulations impact on this field of research because in order to obtain a license, a huge input of validation, time, and funding is required. The cost of treating each patient will also rise due to this. FDA has considerable experience in the evaluation of investigational cell therapy products and has published several relevant guidance documents to facilitate safe progress in this field. However, the use of cellular products derived from hESCs present unique challenges worthy of further consideration.

The most distinguished feature for preclinical application of hESC according to Title 21 of the Code of Federal Regulations (CFR) Part 312.23 (a) (8), the sponsor of a clinical trial should provide "*...adequate information about the pharmacological and toxicological studies... on the basis of which the sponsor has concluded that it is reasonably safe to conduct the proposed clinical investigations. The kind, duration, and scope of animal and other tests required vary with the duration and nature of the proposed clinical investigations.*" The designs and conduct of the preclinical studies are thus critical to the regulatory decisions made in allowing the administration of a cellular therapy into humans. To evaluate the safety of a hESC-derived cellular product *in vivo* adequately, comprehensive preclinical studies to identify and understand potential toxicities need to be conducted before entering clinical trials. Based on the biological properties of these cells, both the potential for tumorigenicity and the potential for inappropriate differentiation at a nontarget location are significant safety concerns. It is, therefore, indispensable to consider the biological relevance of the animal species and animal models used to assess the *in vivo* safety of the hESC-derived cellular product, very carefully.

4.4. Different approaches to overcome roadblocks

Advanced tissue engineering, cell culture, differentiation techniques developed by the scientific community has led path to eliminate certain difficulties. One of leading challenge in stem cell research is the development of pure differentiated cells without undifferentiated and other cell types (other than target-specific differentiated cell). This can be achieved by (1) destroying the remaining undifferentiated hESC/hiPSC in the differentiated tissue population with specific agents or antibodies, (2) separating or removing the undifferentiated hESC/hiPSC from the differentiated cell population, by flow cytometry, with most specific markers, (3) eliminating pluripotent cells during the differentiation process, by using effective high-percentage driving protocols, and (4) inducing further differentiation of left-over rogue undifferentiated pluripotent cells.

5. CONCLUSION

As diabetes, more often, the Type 1 diabetes becomes life threatening due to its severity, the transplantation of beta islets would be particularly giving hope to Type 1 diabetics. Currently, most of the diabetics are managing the disease at a drug level which comprises mainly on insulin, and metformin and sulfonylurea group of drugs. IT into the portal vein of the patients is relatively a less invasive, less complicated, and well-standardized procedure as compared to whole PT. However, IT has not gained so much of popularity due to the resource constraint in the form of availability of beta islets. As such, the advent of PSCs has revolutionized the field of medicine for their cell therapy potential. Definitely, diabetics also have ample hopes to depend on PSC-based transplantation therapy. Scientists are in the right direction of having devised various *in vitro* differentiation protocols for generating β-cells from hPSCs which are *in vivo* responsive in mice models, although the efficiency of differentiation beta cells from hPSC is not as high as efficiency of hPSC differentiation into other cell types like neurons. Furthermore, finer tuning still needs to be done regarding the starting material, that is, clinical-grade generation of hPSCs and *in vitro* beta cell differentiation also under GMP settings and, scaling up of beta cells and testing on primate models of diabetes. In conclusion, once the aforementioned are achieved, the hPSC-based beta islets should be ready for clinical trials.

REFERENCES

Amit, M., Shariki, C., Margulets, V., & Itskovitz-Eldor, J. (2004). Feeder layer- and serum-free culture of human embryonic stem cells. *Biology of Reproduction*, *70*, 837–845.

Arntfield, M. E., & Van der Kooy, D. (2013). The adult mammalian pancreas contains separate precursors of pancreatic and neural crest developmental origins. *Stem Cells and Development*, *22*, 2145–2157.

Blyszczuk, P., Czyz, J., Kania, G., Wagner, M., Roll, U., St-Onge, L., et al. (2003). Expression of Pax4 in embryonic stem cells promotes differentiation of nestin-positive progenitor and insulin-producing cells. *Proceedings of the National Academy of Sciences*, *100*, 998–1003.

Borowiak, M., Maehr, R., Chen, S., Chen, A. E., Tang, W., Fox, J. L., et al. (2009). Small molecules efficiently direct endodermal differentiation of mouse and human embryonic stem cells. *Cell Stem Cell*, *4*, 348–358.

Bose, B., Shenoy, P. S., Konda, S., & Wangikar, P. (2012). Human embryonic stem cell differentiation into insulin secreting β-cells for diabetes. *Cell Biology International*, *36*, 1013–1020.

Cai, J., Yu, C., Liu, Y., Chen, S., Guo, Y., Yong, J., et al. (2010). Generation of homogeneous Pdx1(+) pancreatic progenitors from human ES cell derived endoderm cells. *Journal of Molecular Cell Biology*, *2*, 50–60.

Chen, S., Borowiak, M., Fox, J. L., Maehr, R., Osafune, K., Davidow, L., et al. (2009). A small molecule that directs differentiation of human ESCs into the pancreatic lineage. *Nature Chemical Biology*, *4*, 258–265.

Conlon, F. L., Lyons, K. M., Takaesu, N., Barth, K. S., Kispert, A., Herrmann, B., et al. (1994). A primary requirement for nodal in the formation and maintenance of the primitive streak in the mouse. *Development*, *120*, 1919–1928.

D'Amour, K. A., Agulnick, A. D., Eliazer, S., Kelly, O. G., Kroon, E., & Baetge, E. E. (2005). Efficient differentiation of human embryonic stem cells to definitive endoderm. *Nature Biotechnology*, *23*, 1534–1541.

D'Amour, K. A., Bang, A. G., Eliazer, S., Kelly, O. G., Agulnick, A. D., Smart, N. G., et al. (2006). Production of pancreatic hormone-expressing endocrine cells from human embryonic stem cells. *Nature Biotechnology*, *24*, 1392–1401.

Eizirik, D. L., Pipeleers, D. G., Ling, Z., Welsh, N., Hellerstrom, C., & Andersson, A. (1994). Major species differences between humans and rodents in the susceptibility to pancreatic b-cell injury. *Proceedings of the National Academy of Sciences*, *91*, 9253–9256.

Eshpeter, A., Jiang, J., Au, M., Rajotte, R. V., Lu, K., Lebkowski, J. S., et al. (2008). In vivo characterization of transplanted human embryonic stem cell-derived pancreatic endocrine islet cells. *Cell Proliferation*, *41*, 843–858.

Fishman, B., Segev, H., Kopper, O., Nissenbaum, J., Schulman, M., Benvenisty, N., et al. (2012). Targeting pancreatic progenitor cells in human embryonic stem cell differentiation for the identification of novel cell surface markers. *Stem Cell Reviews and Reports*, *8*, 792–802.

Gadue, P., Huber, T. L., Paddison, P. J., & Keller, G. M. (2006). Wnt and TGF-b signaling are required for the induction of an in vitro model of primitive streak formation using embryonic stem cells. *Proceedings of the National Academy of Sciences*, *103*, 16806–16811.

Gouon-Evans, V., Boussemart, L., Gadue, P., Nierhoff, D., Koehler, C. I., Kubo, A., et al. (2006). BMP-4 is required for hepatic specification of mouse embryonic stem cell-derived definitive endoderm. *Nature Biotechnology*, *24*, 1402–1411.

Guz, Y., Montminy, M. R., Stein, R., Leonard, J., Gamer, L. W., Wright, C. V., et al. (1995). Expression of murine STF-1, a putative insulin gene transcription factor, in beta cells of pancreas, duodenal epithelium and pancreatic exocrine and endocrine progenitors during ontogeny. *Development*, *121*, 11–18.

Hammar, E. B., Irminger, J. C., Rickenbach, K., Parnaud, G., Ribaux, P., Bosco, D., et al. (2005). Activation of NF-kB by extracellular matrix is involved in spreading and glucose-stimulated insulin secretion of pancreatic b cells. *The Journal of Biological Chemistry*, *280*, 30630–30637.

Hang, Y., & Stein, R. (2011). MafA and MafB activity in pancreatic b cells. *Trends in Endocrinology and Metabolism*, *22*, 364–373.

Harley, G. (1866). *Diabetes: Its various forms and different treatments*. London: Walton and Maberly.

Hebrok, M., Kim, S. K., & Melton, D. A. (1998). Notochord repression of endodermal Sonic hedgehog permits pancreas development. *Genes & Development*, *12*, 1705–1713.

Hosokawa, M., Dolci, W., & Thorens, B. (2001). Differential sensitivity of GLUT1- and GLUT2-expressing b cells to streptozotocin. *Biochemical and Biophysical Research Communications*, *289*, 1114–1117.

Jensen, J. (2004). Gene regulatory factors in pancreatic development. *Developmental Dynamics*, *229*, 176–200.

Jiang, J., Au, M., Lu, K., Eshpeter, A., Korbutt, G., Fisk, G., et al. (2007). Generation of insulin-producing islet-like clusters from human embryonic stem cells. *Stem Cells*, *25*, 1940–1953.

Jiang, W., Shi, Y., Zhao, D., Chen, S., Yong, J., Zhang, J., et al. (2007). In vitro derivation of functional insulin-producing cells from human embryonic stem cells. *Cell Research*, *17*, 333–344.

Jonsson, J., Carlsson, L., Edlund, T., & Edlund, H. (1994). Insulin-promoter-factor 1 is required for pancreas development in mice. *Nature*, *371*, 606–609.

Kaiser, L. R. (1992). The future of multihospital systems. *Topics in Health Care Financing*, *18*, 32–45.

Keirstead, H. S., Nistor, G., Bernal, G., Totoiu, M., Cloutier, F., Sharp, K., et al. (2005). Human embryonic stem cell-derived oligodendrocyte progenitor cell transplants remyelinate and restore locomotion after spinal cord injury. *The Journal of Neuroscience*, *25*, 4694–4705.

Kemp, C., Knight, M., Scharp, D., Lacy, P., & Ballinger, W. (1973). Transplantation of isolated pancreatic islets into the portal vein of diabetic rats. *Nature*, *244*, 447.

Kirchgessner, A. L., & Gershon, M. D. (1990). Innervations of the pancreas by neurons in the gut. *The Journal of Neuroscience*, *10*, 1626–1642.

Kroon, E., Martinson, L. A., Kadoya, K., Bang, A. G., Kelly, O. G., Eliazer, S., et al. (2008). Pancreatic endoderm derived from human embryonic stem cells generates glucose-responsive insulin-secreting cells in vivo. *Nature Biotechnology*, *26*, 443–452.

Ku, H. T., Zhang, N., Kubo, A., O'Connor, R., Mao, M., Keller, G., et al. (2004). Committing embryonic stem cells to early endocrine pancreas in vitro. *Stem Cells*, *22*, 1205–1217.

Kubo, A., Shinozaki, K., Shannon, J. M., Kouskoff, V., Kennedy, M., Woo, S., et al. (2004). Development of definitive endoderm from embryonic stem cells in culture. *Development*, *131*, 1651–1662.

Kumar, M., Jordan, N., Melton, D., & Grapin-Botton, A. (2003). Signals from lateral plate mesoderm instruct endoderm toward a pancreatic fate. *Developmental Biology*, *259*, 109–122.

Lacy, P. (1978). Workshop on Pancreatic Islet Cell Transplantation in Diabetes sponsored by the National Institute of Arthritis, Metabolism, and Digestive Diseases and held at the National Institutes of Health in Bethesda, Maryland, on November 29 and 30, 1977. *Diabetes*, *27*, 427–429.

Lacy, P., & Kostianovsky, M. (1967). Method for the isolation of intact islets of Langerhans from the rat pancreas. *Diabetes*, *16*, 35–39.

Lebkowski, J. (2011). GRNOPC1: The world's first embryonic stem cell-derived therapy. Interview with Jane Lebkowski. *Regenerative Medicine*, 6, 11–13.

Lowe, L. A., Yamada, S., & Kuehn, M. R. (2001). Genetic dissection of nodal function in patterning the mouse embryo. *Development*, *128*, 1831–1843.

Ludwig, T. E., Levenstein, M. E., Jones, J. M., Berggren, W. T., Mitchen, E. R., Frane, J. L., et al. (2006). Derivation of human embryonic stem cells in defined conditions. *Nature Biotechnology*, *24*, 185–187.

Lumelsky, N., Blondel, O., Laeng, P., Velasco, I., Ravin, R., & McKay, R. (2001). Differentiation of embryonic stem cells to insulin-secreting structures similar to pancreatic islets. *Science*, *292*, 1389–1394.

Lysaght, M. J., & Crager, J. (2009). Origins. *Tissue Engineering Part A*, *15*, 1449–1450.

Madsen, O. D., & Serup, P. (2006). Towards cell therapy for diabetes. *Nature Biotechnology*, *24*, 1481–1483.

Mao, G. H., Chen, G. A., Bai, H. Y., Song, T. R., & Wang, Y. X. (2009). The reversal of hyperglycemia in diabetic mice using PLGA scaffolds seeded with islet-like cells derived from human embryonic stem cells. *Biomaterials*, *30*, 1706–1714.

Matsuoka, T. A., Artner, I., Henderson, E., Means, A., Sander, M., & Stein, R. (2004). The MafA transcription factor appears to be responsible for tissue specific expression of insulin. *Proceedings of the National Academy of Sciences of the United States of America, 101*, 2930–2933.

Melkman-Zehavi, T., Oren, R., Kredo-Russo, S., Shapira, T., Mandelbaum, A. D., Rivkin, N., et al. (2011). miRNAs control insulin content in pancreatic beta-cells via downregulation of transcriptional repressors. *The EMBO Journal, 30*, 835–845.

Mering, J. V., & Minkowski, O. (1889). Diabetes Mellitus nach Pankreas Extirpation Z. *Zentrabl Klinik Medizinische, 10*, 393–403.

Minkowski, O. (1989). Historical development of theory of pancreatic diabetes. *Diabetes, 38*, 1–6.

Miyazaki, S., Yamato, E., & Miyazaki, J. (2004). Regulated expression of pdx-1 promotes in vitro differentiation of insulin producing cells from embryonic stem cells. *Diabetes, 53*, 1030–1037.

Nostro, M. C., Sarangi, F., Ogawa, S., Holtzinger, A., Corneo, B., Li, X., et al. (2011). Stage-specific signaling through TGFb family members and WNT regulates patterning and pancreatic specification of human pluripotent stem cells. *Development, 138*, 861–871.

Osada, S. I., & Wright, C. V. (1999). Xenopus nodal-related signaling is essential for mesendodermal patterning during early embryogenesis. *Development, 126*, 3229–3240.

Parnaud, G., Hammar, E., Ribaux, P., Donath, M. Y., Berney, T., & Halban, P. A. (2009). Signaling pathways implicated in the stimulation of b-cell proliferation by extracellular matrix. *Molecular Endocrinology, 23*, 1264–1271.

Plank, J. L., Mundell, N. A., Frist, A. Y., LeGrone, A. W., Kim, T., Musser, M. A., et al. (2011). Influence and timing of arrival of murine neural crest on pancreatic beta cell development and maturation. *Developmental Biology, 349*, 321–330.

Rajagopal, J., Anderson, W. J., Kume, S., Martinez, O. I., & Melton, D. A. (2003). Insulin staining of ES cell progeny from insulin uptake. *Science, 299*, 363.

Ranjan, A. K., Joglekar, M. V., & Hardikar, A. A. (2009). Endothelial cells in pancreatic islet development and function. *Islets, 1*, 2–9.

Riazi, A. M., Kwon, S. Y., & Stanford, W. L. (2009). Stem cell sources for regenerative medicine. *Methods in Molecular Biology, 482*, 55–90.

Saito, H., Takeuchi, M., Chida, K., & Miyajima, A. (2011). Generation of glucose responsive functional islets with a three-dimensional structure from mouse fetal pancreatic cells and iPS cells in vitro. *PLoS One, 6*, e28209.

Scharp, D., Murphy, J., Newton, W., Ballinger, W., & Lacy, P. (1975). Transplantation of islets of Langerhans in diabetic rhesus monkeys. *Surgery, 77*, 100–105.

Seaberg, R. M., Smukler, S. R., Kieffer, T. J., Enikolopov, G., Asghar, Z., Wheeler, M. B., et al. (2004). Clonal identification of multipotent precursors from adult mouse pancreas that generate neural and pancreatic lineages. *Nature Biotechnology, 22*, 1115–1124.

Shapiro, A., Lakey, J., Ryan, E., Korbutt, G., Toth, E., Warnock, G., et al. (2000). Islet transplantation in seven patients with type 1 diabetes mellitus using a glucocorticoid-free immunosuppressive regimen. *The New England Journal of Medicine, 343*, 230–238.

Shi, Y., Hou, L., Tang, F., Jiang, W., Wang, P., Ding, M., et al. (2005). Inducing Embryonic stem cells to differentiate into pancreatic beta cells by a novel three step approach using activin A and all-trans retinoic acid. *Stem Cells, 23*, 93–110.

Shiroi, A., Ueda, S., Ouji, Y., Saito, K., Moriya, K., Sugie, Y., et al. (2005). Differentiation of embryonic stem cells into insulin-producing cells promoted by Nkx2.2 gene transfer. *World Journal of Gastroenterology, 11*, 4161–4166.

Slack, J. M. (1995). Developmental biology of the pancreas. *Development, 121*, 1569–1580.

Smukler, S. R., Arntfield, M. E., Razavi, R., Bikopoulos, G., Karpowicz, P., Seaberg, R., et al. (2011). The adult mouse and human pancreas contain rare multipotent stem cells that express insulin. *Cell Stem Cell, 8*, 281–293.

Soria, B., Skoudy, A., & Martín, F. (2001). From stem cells to beta cells: New strategies in cell therapy of diabetes mellitus. *Diabetologia, 44*, 407–415.

Speier, S., Gjinovci, A., Charollais, A., Meda, P., & Rupnik, M. (2007). Cx36-mediated coupling reduces beta-cell heterogeneity, confines the stimulating glucose concentration range, and affects insulin release kinetics. *Diabetes, 56*, 1078–1086.

Stafford, D., White, R. J., Kinkel, M. D., Linville, A., Schilling, T. F., & Prince, V. E. (2006). Retinoids signal directly to zebrafish endoderm to specify *insulin*-expressing cells. *Development, 133*, 949–956.

Stoffers, D. A., Heller, R. S., Miller, C. P., & Habener, J. F. (1999). Developmental expression of the homeodomain protein IDX-1 in mice transgenic for an IDX-1 promoter/lacZ transcriptional reporter. *Endocrinology, 140*, 5374–5381.

Sui, L., Geens, M., Sermon, K., Bouwens, L., & Mfopou, J. K. (2013). Role of BMP signaling in pancreatic progenitor differentiation from human embryonic stem cells. *Stem Cells Reviews and Reports, 9*, 569–577.

Sunami, E., Kanazawa, H., Hashizume, H., Takeda, M., Hatakeyama, K., & Ushiki, T. (2001). Morphological characteristics of Schwann cells in the islets of Langerhans of the murine pancreas. *Archives of Histology and Cytology, 64*, 191–201.

Tzakis, A., Ricordi, C., Alejandro, R., Zeng, Y., Fung, J., Todo, S., et al. (1990). Pancreatic islet transplantation after upper abdominal exenteration and liver replacement. *Lancet, 336*, 402–405.

Vincent, S. D., Dunn, N. R., Hayashi, S., Norris, D. P., & Robertson, E. J. (2003). Cell fate decisions within the mouse organizer are governed by graded Nodal signals. *Genes & Development, 17*, 1646–1662.

Viola, J., Lal, B., & Grad, O. (2003). *The emergence of tissue engineering as a research field.* Arlington, VA: National Science Foundation.

Wang, H., Brun, T., Kataoka, K., Sharma, A. J., & Wollheim, C. B. (2007). MAFA controls genes implicated in insulin biosynthesis and secretion. *Diabetologia, 50*, 348–358.

Wang, X., & Ye, K. (2009). Three dimensional differentiations of embryonic stem cells into islet-like insulin producing clusters. *Tissue Engineering Part A, 15*, 1941–1952.

Weber, L. M., Hayda, K. N., & Anseth, K. S. (2008). Cell-matrix interactions improve b-cell survival and insulin secretion in three-dimensional culture. *Tissue Engineering Part A, 14*, 1959–1968.

Wells, J. M., & Melton, D. A. (2000). Early mouse endoderm is patterned by soluble factors from adjacent germ layers. *Development, 127*, 1563–1572.

Xu, C., Inokuma, M. S., Denham, J., Golds, K., Kundu, P., Gold, J. D., et al. (2001). Feeder-free growth of undifferentiated human embryonic stem cells. *Nature Biotechnology, 19*, 971–974.

Xu, R. H., Peck, R. M., Li, D. S., Feng, X., Ludwig, T., & Thomson, J. A. (2005). Basic FGF and suppression of BMP signaling sustain undifferentiated proliferation of human ES cells. *Nature Methods, 2*, 185–190.

Xu, C., Rosler, E., Jiang, J., Lebkowski, J. S., Gold, J. D., O'Sullivan, C., et al. (2005). Basic fibroblast growth factor supports undifferentiated human embryonic stem cell growth without conditioned medium. *Stem Cells, 23*, 315–323.

Yang, H., & Wright, J. R., Jr. (2002). Human b cells are exceedingly resistant to streptozotocin in vivo. *Endocrinology, 143*, 2491–2495.

Zhang, C., Moriguchi, T., Kajihara, M., Esaki, R., Harada, A., Shimohata, H., et al. (2005). MafA is a key regulator of glucose stimulated insulin secretion. *Molecular and Cellular Biology, 25*, 4969–4976.

Zhu, S., Wurdak, H., Wang, J., Lyssiotis, C. A., Peters, E. C., Cho, C. Y., et al. (2009). A small molecule primes embryonic stem cells for differentiation. *Cell Stem Cell, 4*, 416–426.

CHAPTER TEN

The Calcium-Sensing Receptor and β-Cell Function

Paul E. Squires[*,1], **Peter M. Jones**[†], **Mustafa Y.G. Younis**[*], **Claire E. Hills**[*]

[*]School of Life Sciences, University of Warwick, Coventry, United Kingdom

[†]Diabetes & Nutritional Sciences Division, School of Medicine, King's College London, London, United Kingdom

[1]Corresponding author: e-mail address: P.E.Squires@warwick.ac.uk

Contents

Abstract

In addition to its central role controlling systemic calcium homeostasis, the extracellular calcium-sensing receptor (CaSR) can be found on multiple cell types not associated with controlling plasma calcium. The endocrine pancreas is one such tissue, and it is apparent that the receptor plays an important role in regulating β-cell function. During exocytosis, divalent cations are coreleased with insulin and their concentration within the restricted intercellular compartments of the pancreatic islet increases sufficiently to activate the CaSR on neighboring cells. Acute and chronic activation of the receptor has multiple effects on the β-cell, from increasing cadherin-based cell–cell adhesion to directly altering the expression and function of various potassium and voltage-dependent calcium channels. The promiscuous activation of multiple binding partners improves cell adhesion, cell coupling, and cell-to-cell communication within the islet and is the basis for the effect of the CaSR on β-cell function and improved glucose responsiveness.

Vitamins and Hormones, Volume 95
ISSN 0083-6729
http://dx.doi.org/10.1016/B978-0-12-800174-5.00010-7

1. INTRODUCTION

Transplantation of pancreas or islets/β-cells isolated from human pancreata offers a potential cure for type 1 diabetes, but the limited availability of donor tissue means that this approach is unlikely to make a significant impact as a major clinical treatment. For this reason, much attention is now being directed toward the generation *in vitro* of suitable material for transplantation therapy. The problem is more complex than merely generating large numbers of insulin-secreting β-cells. Pancreatic islets are the functional unit of secretion where activity between β-cells is coordinated to permit the synchronous release of insulin. The secretory response of an intact islet is greater than the sum of the responses of the individual β-cells in isolation, and dispersed β-cells exhibit reduced glucose responsiveness (Hauge-Evans, Squires, Persaud, & Jones, 1999). Within the islet, the intrinsic control of insulin secretion is mediated by a complex interplay between cell–cell contact, cell coupling, and cell-to-cell communication.

Individual β-cells show very different responses to nutrient activation. The heterogeneity of responsiveness, at least in terms of changes in intracellular calcium ($[Ca^{2+}]_i$), can be greatly reduced by forming β-cells into highly coupled three-dimensional, islet-like structures. In these "pseudoislets," glucose-induced elevations in $[Ca^{2+}]_i$ are synchronized across the bulk mass of the islet (Squires, Hauge-Evans, Persaud, & Jones, 2000). In contrast, only a relatively small proportion of isolated cells exhibit glucose-evoked changes in $[Ca^{2+}]_i$ (Hauge-Evans et al., 1999), and even within small cell clusters, some cells respond to depolarizing stimuli much earlier than their immediate neighbors (Squires et al., 2002). These studies suggest that only a subpopulation of cells are required to sense appropriate stimuli and that communication between responsive and nonresponsive cells allows the entire population to evoke a simultaneous response. Neighboring β-cells are coupled by gap junctions, which allow the direct transfer of solutes, metabolic precursors, and electrical currents. These junctions are composed of connexins (Cxs), and gap-junction intercellular communication (GJIC) between β-cells is an important mechanism for coordinating effective responses to physiological stimuli (recently reviewed by Cigliola, Chellakudam, Arabieter, & Meda, 2012). However, this direct cell–cell communication is not the only mechanism by which β-cells recruit their immediate neighbors. Grapengiesser, Gylfe, and Hellman (1999) suggested the idea that a "diffusible synchronizer" might mediate the coordination of activity between cells within the islet. Certainly, insulin secretion is associated with the corelease of a number of intragranular factors with the potential to act as paracrine mediators. Adenosine and/or adenosine triphosphate (ATP) has commonly been linked to this role (Hazama, Hayashi, & Okada, 1998; Obermuller et al., 2005). It has been proposed that intermittent release of ATP, combined with gap-junction coupling, could propagate messages between adjacent cells (Hellman et al., 2004). ATP is present in insulin-containing granules of mouse β-cells (Detimary, Jonas, & Henquin, 1996) and human β-cells readily respond to purinergic signals (Squires, James, London, & Dunne, 1994). However, despite this seductive hypothesis, there are conflicting data concerning the precise role of adenosine and ATP in regulating β-cell function. Enzyme-coated electrode biosensors have recently been used to show that glucose actually reduces extracellular adenosine in mouse pancreatic islets (Yang et al., 2012), and in MIN6 pseudoislets, enhanced secretory efficiency of the islet was not inhibited by purinergic receptor antagonists, suggesting that the response could not be attributed to the action of adenine nucleotides (Hauge-Evans et al., 2002). Therefore, the precise role for the local release of adenosine and/or ATP in orchestrating cell–cell communication to enhance β-cell function needs further investigation.

In addition to adenosine and ATP, insulin secretory granules also contain high concentrations of divalent cations (Ca^{2+}, Mg^{2+}, and Zn^{2+}), which are coreleased with insulin during exocytosis (Hutton, 1989). Local fluctuations in extracellular calcium have been recorded using calcium-selective microelectrodes inserted into the restricted spaces that immediately surround pancreatic β-cells (Gerino et al., 2012; Perez-Armendariz & Atwater, 1986). These elegant studies suggest that glucose produces a dramatic increase in the concentration of extracellular calcium and that the concentration of the ion at these local intercellular "hot-spots" can increase within the millimolar range. It has been known for some time that the extracellular calcium-sensing receptor (CaSR) is expressed on rodent (Rasschaert & Malaisse, 1999) and human pancreatic β-cells (Gray et al., 2006; Squires, Harris, et al., 2000; Squires, Hauge-Evans, et al., 2000). The receptor is able to detect small local changes in free calcium, which occur immediately following nutrient and/or non-nutrient stimulation. The data support the intriguing possibility that the CaSR provides an alternative mechanism for autocrine/paracrine cell-to-cell communication between β-cells and may help regulate islet function.

2. THE CALCIUM-SENSING RECEPTOR (CASR)

The CaSR is a seven transmembrane spanning G-protein-coupled receptor found on many tissues involved in the regulation of systemic mineral ion homeostasis (reviewed in Brown & MacLeod, 2001). Activation of the CaSR is coupled to multiple, tissue-specific, downstream signaling protein partners that regulate a variety of biological processes, including secretion and proliferation (reviewed by Chakravarti, Chattopadhyay, & Brown, 2012; Magno, Ward, & Ratajczak, 2011). First cloned in bovine parathyroid hormone (PTH)-secreting cells (Brown et al., 1993), activation of the receptor reduces PTH secretion but increases secretion from calcitonin-secreting C-cells of the thyroid. Together with its actions on osteoclasts, osteoblasts, osteocytes, as well as the kidney and intestine, the receptor helps maintain systemic normocalcaemia.

In addition to the accepted role of the CaSR in regulating systemic calcium homeostasis, the receptor is also found on a large number of tissue types not associated with the control of plasma [Ca^{2+}] including oesophageal (Justinich et al., 2008) and colonic epithelia (Cheng, Giebel, & Herbert, 2004), the cardiovascular system (reviewed in Smajilovic & Tfelt-Hansen, 2007), hypothalamic neurons (Vizard et al., 2008), and pancreatic ducts (Racz et al., 2002). The significance of the receptor in these tissues is still not fully understood. In exocrine pancreas, it has been suggested that the CaSR might monitor extracellular Ca^{2+} in pancreatic juice to limit the risk of Ca^{2+} carbonate stone formation (Bruce et al., 1999), while it may act to detect changes in levels of dietary Ca^{2+} in gastrin-secreting cells of the human antrum (Buchan, Squires, Ring, & Meloche, 2001; Ray, Squires, Curtis, Meloche, & Buchan, 1997; Squires, Meloche, & Buchan, 1999). However, a more expansive explanation for the role of the CaSR could be in its ability to detect local fluctuations in Ca^{2+}-release from one cell to propagate a response into a neighboring cell. The phenomenon of local paracrine signaling for calcium was beautifully demonstrated in a model kidney epithelium system in which Ca^{2+}-extrusion from fibroblasts was found to activate the CaSR expressed on cocultured HEK cells. HEK cells were then able to elicit their own response to fibroblast-derived changes in extracellular calcium (Hofer, Curci, Doble, Brown, & Soybel, 2000; Hofer, Gerbino, Caroppo, & Curci, 2004). The ability of cells to detect local Ca^{2+} fluctuations and use this information to propagate a response between neighboring cells suggests that the CaSR may have an important role in cell–cell coupling, communication, and function. The proposed mechanism of CaSR-mediated propagation of signals across the islet is illustrated in Fig. 10.1. Glucose-evoked changes in insulin secretion in one cell are associated with the corelease of divalent cations, which activate the CaSR expressed on neighboring cells to help propagate the response. The net effect enhances the functional coupling between β-cells and improves the secretory function of the intact islet.

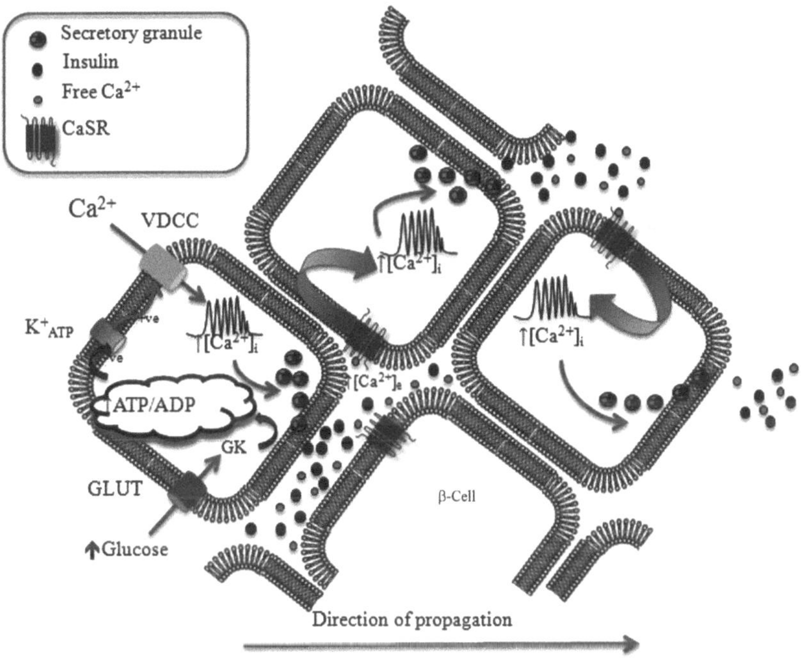

Figure 10.1 CaSR-mediated cell-to-cell communication between pancreatic β-cells: Following uptake by the glucose transporter (GLUT) glucose metabolism is controlled by the low-affinity glucokinase (GK). The resultant rise in ATP/ADP ratio closes the ATP-sensitive potassium channels (K^+_{ATP}), depolarizing the cell membrane, and opening voltage-dependent Ca^{2+}-channels (VDCC). Calcium enters the cell down a steep concentration gradient and stimulates insulin secretion. Divalent cations, including free Ca^{2+}, are coreleased with insulin, increasing the local concentration of extracellular calcium ($[Ca^{2+}]_e$) in the intraislet space. These local changes create "hot-spots" of high $[Ca^{2+}]_e$ in the restricted space immediately surrounding the β-cells and activate the CaSRs on adjacent cells in a paracrine manner. CaSR-mediated increases in intracellular calcium ($[Ca^{2+}]_i$) propagate the signal across the islet, thus coordinating whole islet activity and enhancing glucose-induced insulin secretion. (For color version of this figure, the reader is referred to the online version of this chapter.)

3. EFFECTS OF CaSR ON β-CELL ADHESION, COUPLING, AND COMMUNICATION

Epithelial (E)-cadherin is a transmembrane protein whose extracellular domain forms calcium-dependent homodimers with cadherins expressed on neighboring cells facilitating cell-to-cell adhesion in a variety of systems, including the pancreatic β-cell. Cadherins are important in forming the multiprotein adherens junction that links cell–cell contact to the actin cytoskeleton and various signaling molecules. As can be seen from Fig. 10.2, the extracellular domain mediates ligation with epithelial (E)-cadherin on adjacent cells, while the cytoplasmic domain binds to β-catenin linking cadherin to the actin cytoskeleton via α-catenin. Interaction of cadherin with F-actin, via the catenins, not only serves to increase adhesive strength of the junction but also acts as a signaling "node" for proteins that influence adhesiveness and/or initiate intracellular signaling.

In developing mouse pancreas, E-cadherin plays an essential role in allowing β-cells to cluster into islet structures (Dahl, Sjodin, & Semb, 1996).

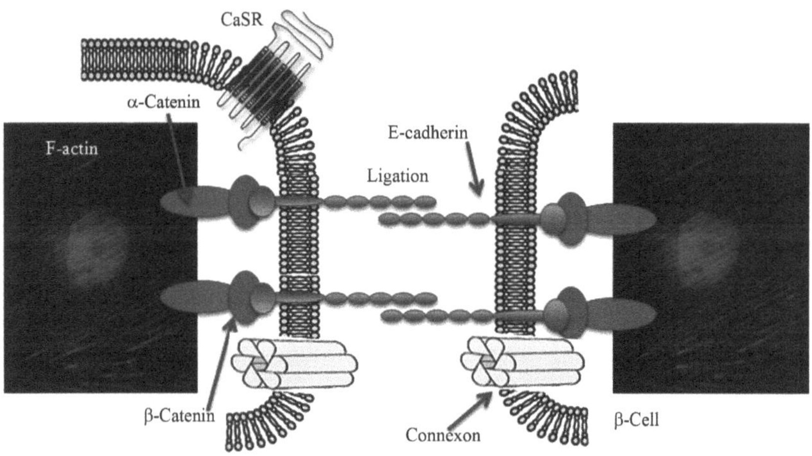

Figure 10.2 E-cadherin and the adherens junction: E-cadherin is a transmembrane protein with multiple adhesion and signaling roles in the pancreatic β-cell. The extracellular domains of E-cadherin homodimers enter homotypic Ca^{2+}-dependent-binding interactions with those of dimers on adjacent cells. The intracellular domain of E-cadherin interacts with F-actin via α-catenin and β-catenin. Cadherin–catenin complexes constitute the adherens junction and this represents not only a point of cell–cell contact, but also a signaling node for various binding partners that can include connexins and various ion channels. (For color version of this figure, the reader is referred to the online version of this chapter.)

Overexpression of dominant-negative hepatocyte nuclear factor-1 in mouse β-cells (the gene responsible for type 3 MODY) results in downregulation of E-cadherin, abnormal islet architecture, and reduced insulin secretion (Shih et al., 2002; Yamagata et al., 2002). Similarly, in the MIN6 cell line subclone (C3), downregulated E-cadherin expression is associated with reduced glucose-evoked insulin secretion (Lilla et al., 2003), while in rat pancreatic islets, increased expression of the adherens proteins α-catenin and β-catenin is correlated with increased glucose-evoked insulin secretion (Collares-Buzato, Carvalho, Furtado, & Boschero, 2004). Therefore, it is clear that E-cadherin plays an important role not only in islet development but also in the continued function of the islet in terms of glucose responsiveness and insulin secretion.

The clonal mouse insulin-secreting cell line (MIN6) expresses the CaSR (Jones, Kitsou-Mylona, Gray, Squires, & Persaud, 2007), and 48-h activation of the receptor using a phenylalkylamine agonist (calcimimetic), which activates the receptor by allosterically increasing its affinity for Ca^{2+}, without using nonphysiological increases in extracellular calcium, significantly increases the expression of E-cadherin (Hills, Younis, et al., 2012). The CaSR-evoked increase in cadherin-based adhesion has been confirmed using atomic force microscopy, single-cell force spectroscopy, which demonstrated that the energy required to uncouple CaSR-treated cells was significantly elevated, while the maximum force required to physically detach the cells from one another also increased (Hills, Younis, et al., 2012). These novel data provide compelling evidence that the activation of the receptor increases expression of the epithelial (E) adhesion protein E-cadherin and functional increases tethering between β-cells.

The use of MIN6 cells as a homogenous insulin-secreting population avoids confounding cross talk between β-cells and other endocrine cell types of the islet. This is particularly important considering that α-cells from human islets also express the CaSR (Squires, Harris, et al., 2000). Activation of the CaSR in α-cells stimulates glucagon secretion from human islets (Gray et al., 2006). Despite the counter-regulatory effect of glucagon on energy homeostasis, within the islet, glucagon actually increases insulin secretion and may play a supportive role in augmenting insulin secretion in terms of the whole islet response to local changes in intercellular calcium. Somatostatin-secreting δ-cells act to inhibit insulin secretion and do not express the CaSR (Squires, Harris, et al., 2000).

Various partner proteins are colocalized with E-cadherin and β-catenin at the sites of cell–cell contact. Of particular interest are the Cxs (Fujimoto et al., 1997). Cxs oligomerize into hexameric hemichannels (connexons) connecting the cytoplasm of adjoining cells and forming gap junctions. Inhibiting cadherin-based cell adhesion inhibits gap-junction assembly (Kanno, Sasaki, Shiba, Yoshida-Noro, & Takeichi, 1984), while expression of recombinant cadherins into cells lacking strong coupling increases Cx phosphorylation at the adherens junction (Musil, Cunningham, Edelman, & Goodenough, 1990) and increases cell-to-cell communication (Mege et al., 1988). Since intercellular adhesion precedes gap-junction-formation and inhibiting cadherin-based cell adhesion inhibits gap-junction assembly, it seems reasonable to assume that enhanced cell adhesion would improve cell-to-cell communication and the functional responsiveness of β-cells (Rogers, Hodgkin, & Squires, 2007). In renal proximal tubule epithelial cells, high glucose and the activated downstream proinflammatory cytokine transforming growth factor beta (TGFβ) have been shown to impair E-cadherin-mediated cell–cell adhesion, reduce Cx expression, and inhibit gap-junction-mediated intercellular communication in diabetic nephropathy (Hills, Siamantouras, et al., 2012). Even activation of the cadherin-switch, which attempts to upregulate N-cadherin as a compensatory mechanism to maintain cell–cell adhesion, failed to restore cell communication (Hills, Siamantouras, et al., 2012). The effects were mimicked by immunoneutralizing E-cadherin ligation. Therefore, it would appear as though activation of the CaSR in β-cells is able to increase cell–cell adhesion and improve direct coupling of cellular activity to facilitate cell–cell communication. Given the increased probability for restricted intercellular spaces and the increased number of local "hot-spots" of high-extracellular calcium in three-dimensional islets, the data could help explain why the secretory efficiency of an intact islet is greater than the sum of its composite β-cells when studied in isolation (Hauge-Evans et al., 1999).

4. EFFECTS OF THE CaSR ON INSULIN SECRETION

The primary regulator of insulin release is a change in the plasma glucose concentration. Metabolism of glucose within the β-cell alters the ATP/ADP ratio and closes ATP-dependent K^+ channels (K^+_{ATP}), which depolarizes the cell membrane and opens L-type voltage-dependent Ca^{2+} channels (VDCCs), elevating intracellular calcium ($[Ca^{2+}]_i$), and evoking pulses of insulin release (Hellman et al., 1994). Each voltage-dependent spike in membrane potential permits Ca^{2+} entry across the plasma membrane and links glucose metabolism with changes in $[Ca^{2+}]_i$ (Santos et al.,

1991). Extracellular Ca^{2+} has been generally assumed to play a passive role in the regulation of insulin secretion, merely acting as a sink from which Ca^{2+} enters the cell down a steep concentration gradient. However, after glucose-induced secretion from pancreatic β-cells, intraislet Ca^{2+} concentration can increase in the millimolar range (Gerino et al., 2012). Following the identification of the CaSR, Ca^{2+} could have important role in autocrine and/or intercellular communication within the islet, where close cell-to-cell contact improves the functional responsiveness of cells and augments insulin secretion. Activation of the CaSR enhances insulin secretion from human islets (Gray et al., 2006) and provides an obvious link by which glucose-evoked release of calcium-rich secretory granules feeds forward to synchronize secretion and perpetuate the whole islet response.

Activation of the CaSR initiates rapid, transient stimulation of insulin secretion from human islets of Langerhans (Gray et al., 2006). In the absence of extracellular calcium, calcimimetics have little effect on insulin secretion and the magnitude of the secretory response in the presence of calcium depends upon the concentration of the cation rather than that of the calcimimetic *per se*, consistent with Ca^{2+} being the agonist for the receptor. In MIN6 pseudoislets, activation of the CaSR using supraphysiological concentrations of extracellular calcium (10 mM) produces an initial rapid increase in insulin secretion, followed by a prolonged inhibition, as reported for human (Squires, Harris, et al., 2000) and rodent (Malaisse et al., 1999) islets. However, in both MIN6 cells and primary human islets, specific activation of the CaSR using calcimimetics produces rapid, transient stimulation of insulin secretion, without the secondary inhibitory phase, perhaps suggesting that the inhibition is a response to nonphysiological concentrations of extracellular calcium, rather than any effect mediated through the CaSR (Gray et al., 2006).

It should be noted that it is extremely unusual for receptor-operated stimuli to initiate an insulin-secretory response in the absence of a stimulatory concentration of glucose. However, activation of the CaSR initiates insulin secretion from human and rodent β-cells without a concomitant need for nutrient stimulation (Gray et al., 2006). This fact alone suggests that the receptor is important in regulating insulin secretion. The observation that calcimimetics further enhance the maximal secretory response to glucose in human islets agrees with a previous report in rat islets (Straub, Kornreich, Oswald, Nemeth, & Sharp, 2000) and implies that CaSR activation enhances exocytosis through separate transduction pathways to those used by glucose and other nutrient secretagogues. There are numerous reports from different tissues that link the CaSR to a variety of intracellular transduction cascades (reviewed by Chakravarti et al., 2012; Magno et al., 2011), suggesting that the intracellular effector systems may be tissue-type dependent. Grey and colleagues suggested that CaSR-dependent insulin secretion was only partially inhibited by blocking phospholipase C, a finding that suggests the involvement of another signal transduction systems beyond PLC activation of inositol trisphosphate (IP_3) and Ca^{2+}-release in β-cells (Gray et al., 2006). The nonselective inhibition of protein kinase activity inhibited CaSR-induced insulin secretion, while more selective kinase inhibition implicated CAMK II (Gray et al., 2006). Together, these observations are consistent with elevation in $[Ca^{2+}]_i$ through IP_3-induced increases in $[Ca^{2+}]_i$, or an influx of $[Ca^{2+}]_e$ activating CAMK to initiate an exocytotic response. The diacylglycerol (DAG) generated by PLC activation may also play an important role in the stimulation of insulin secretion by receptor-operated stimuli, such as acetylcholine, by activating one or more of the DAG-sensitive isoforms of PKC that are expressed in β-cells (Jones & Persaud, 1998). Some of these downstream signaling cascades are illustrated in Fig. 10.3. As with other cell types, activation of the CaSR in pancreatic β-cells is also associated with a rapid increase in p42/44 MAPK

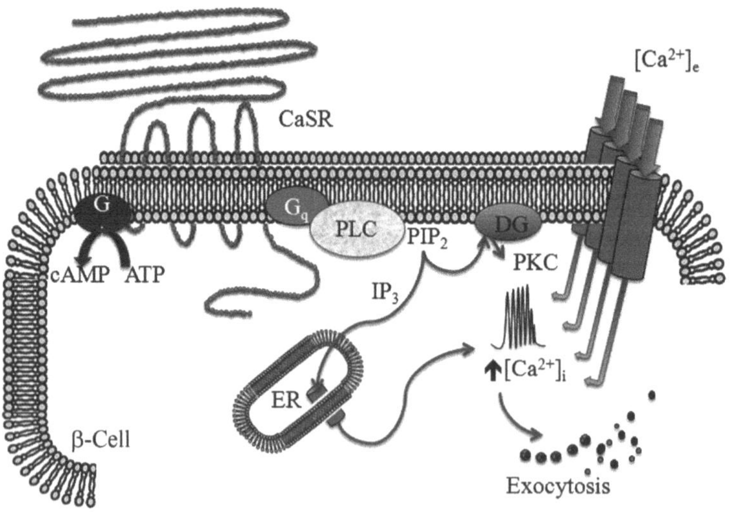

Figure 10.3 CaSR signaling in pancreatic β-cells: Activation of the CaSR initiates a number of intercellular effector systems, including phospholipase C (PLC)-activation of IP_3 and Ca^{2+}-release, and an elevation in cAMP. The DAG generated by PLC activation may also play an important role in the stimulation of insulin secretion by activating one or more of the DAG-sensitive isoforms of PKC that are expressed in β-cells. Expression of L-type VDCCs is also linked to CaSR activation and provides an intriguing explanation to explain how the CaSR could augments glucose-evoked insulin secretion. (For color version of this figure, the reader is referred to the online version of this chapter.)

phosphorylation, consistent with MAPK activation being involved in insulin secretion. Inhibition of p42/44 MAPK abolishes CaSR-mediated secretion from human islets (Gray et al., 2006). These observations suggest that the β-cell CaSR initiates insulin secretion by a process that is dependent on the activation of both p42/44 MAPK and other intracellular pathways, including CAMK II activation. The involvement of p42/44 MAPK in initiating an insulin-secretory response to a receptor-operated, G-protein-coupled stimulus comprises a novel β-cell signaling pathway.

As discussed in Section 3, chronic 48-h activation of the CaSR increases E-cadherin expression and improves functional tethering between β-cells (Hills, Younis, et al., 2012). In the same study, CaSR activation also increased expression of L-type VDCCs. As shown in Fig. 10.1, L-type VDCCs are a major route of Ca^{2+}-entry in pancreatic β-cells and are integral to the glucose-evoked exocytotic process. Any increase in VDCC expression might be expected to enhance glucose-evoked Ca^{2+}-entry and augment glucose-evoked secretion (see Fig. 10.3), an effect supported by studies in which glucose-evoked insulin secretion from MIN6 pseudoislets was reduced when CaSR expression was knocked down (Kitsou-Mylona, Burns, Squires, Persaud, & Jones, 2008). Various molecular complexes, such as protein kinases and G-protein-coupled receptors, regulate VDCC activity and distribution within the cell (Yang & Berggren, 2005) and channel expression changes in various physiological and pathophysiological conditions. The C-terminus of the CaSR has been shown to interact with ion channels in other cell systems, including inwardly rectifying potassium channels on the distal nephron (Huang et al., 2007), and it appears as though the CaSR also interacts with VDCCs in pancreatic β-cells (Parkash, 2008), providing the intriguing possibility that the receptor can control Ca^{2+}-channel activity via direct protein–protein interaction. However, the only study examining spatial interaction of the CaSR with VDCC in β-cells suggests that as the association increases, Ca^{2+}-channel activity actually decreases, thus attenuating glucose-induced changes in $[Ca^{2+}]_i$ and decreasing first phase insulin secretion (Parkash & Asotra, 2011). Clearly, the possibility that this G-protein receptor is able to regulate the expression and function of this major route for glucose-evoked Ca^{2+}-influx is an exciting area of study that may identify future targets for therapeutic intervention.

5. EFFECTS OF THE CaSR ON β-CELL PROLIFERATION

Numerous studies have investigated the proliferative effect of the CaSR in cells as diverse as fibroblasts (McNeil, Hobson, Nipper, &

Rodland, 1998), astrocytoma (Chattopadhyay et al., 1999), and osteoblasts (Huang, Cheng, & Slatopolsky, 2001). Activation of the CaSR in the colon upregulates the expression of proteins in the adherens junction, while a loss of receptor expression is associated with abnormal differentiation and progression of carcinomas (Bhagavathula et al., 2007). In parathyroid tissue, CaSR expression has been linked to proliferation of both carcinomas and adenomas (Yano et al., 2003), while loss of receptor expression was associated with downregulation of the adherens junction and apoptosis in keratinocytes (Tu, Chang, Xie, & Bikle, 2008). It therefore appears that a reduction in CaSR expression downregulates adherens junction proteins and reduces proliferative capacity in skin and colon.

The low mitotic index of primary β-cells leads to considerable technical difficulties in measuring β-cell proliferation in cells from primary islets. Previous studies demonstrate that although MIN6 cells are a transformed cell line, their proliferative capacity is regulated by extracellular signals, validating these clonal β-cells as a representative experimental model of β-cell proliferation. Elevated $[Ca^{2+}]_e$ can activate p38 and p42/44 MAPkinases (Burns, Squires, & Persaud, 2000; Sakwe, Larsson, & Rask, 2004) and increase cell proliferation (Liao, Schneider, Datta, & McCauley, 2006), and we recently demonstrated that calcimimetic activation of the CaSR enhances MAPK-mediated β-cell proliferation at physiologically appropriate concentrations of extracellular calcium (Hills, Younis, et al., 2012). These data suggest the intriguing possibility that the CaSR may act to maintain and even increase β-cell mass.

As catenins are known regulators of gene transcription and drive cell proliferation, the effect of the receptor on localization of catenin within the cell is of particular interest (Jin, 2008; Lui & Habener, 2008). It has been suggested that compared to their monolayer counterparts, β-TC6 pseudoislets exhibit increased E-cadherin expression, but a reduction in the nuclear expression of nuclear β-catenin and cyclin D2 (Wakae-Takada, Xuan, Watanabe, Meda, & Leibel, 2013). This change in cellular localization decreased proliferation and suggests that E-cadherin negatively regulates β-cell proliferation by reducing the amount of β-catenin at the nucleus, resulting in reduced levels of D-cyclin. If correct, these data should link CaSR-evoked increases in E-cadherin to reduce the proliferative capacity in β-cells. However, activation of the CaSR in MIN6 monolayers increases expression of E-cadherin (Hills, Younis, et al., 2012) and increases cell proliferation (Kitsou-Mylona et al., 2008). Similarly, cell turnover in CaSR-depleted pseudoislets was reduced. The balance between β-catenin at the adherens junction and the cytosolic destruction complex (part of the Wnt signaling pathway) ultimately regulates how the catenins govern proliferative/apoptotic responses versus differentiated functions such as adhesion/secretion (Jin, 2008), and clearly, more information is needed to uncover how the CaSR acts to alter β-cell proliferation. As an additional observation to the mix, it should also be noted that β-catenin also colocalizes to insulin-secretory granules at the cell periphery and the association could provide an additional and novel role for the adherens junction protein in β-cell function (Hodgkin, Rogers, & Squires, 2007).

6. THE CaSR AND DIABETES MELLITUS

As indicated in the preceding discussion, the CaSR has multiple effects on normal β-cell function. It therefore seems reasonable to expect that changes in receptor expression and/or function may be linked to evidence of dysregulated function in diabetes mellitus (see Ward, Mangno, Walsh, & Ratajczak, 2012). In the streptozotocin (STZ) model of type 1 diabetes, expression of the CaSR in the kidney was halved, while serum levels of 1,25-dihydroxy vitamin D_3 fell by almost 80% (Ward et al., 2001). Changes in these parameters could be rectified by subcutaneous insulin implantation and the effect used to partly explain hypercalciuria seen in experimental diabetes (Anwand & Garland, 1990). Decreased expression of the CaSR is also seen in progression of diabetic cardiomyopathy in STZ-treated animals, where loss of the receptor coincides with abnormal cardiac structure and systolic and diastolic dysfunction (Bai et al., 2012). These progressive changes could be slowed, and even prevented, by application of the CaSR agonist spermine. A similar loss of CaSR expression and function in mesenteric arteries in the Zucker diabetic fatty rat suggests that long-term development of high vascular tone could contribute to vascular complications associated with type 2 diabetes (Weston et al., 2008).

In the pancreatic islet, the potassium inwardly rectifying channel, subfamily J, member 15 (*KCNJ15*) is a type 2 diabetes-associated risk gene (Okamoto, Iwasaki, Nishimura, Doi, Noiri, et al., 2010), which suppresses insulin secretion when overexpressed in rat insulinoma cells (INS-1). In individuals with type 2 diabetes, islet mRNA expression of *KCNJ15* has been found to be higher (Okamoto et al., 2012). KCNJ15 inhibits CaSR in Xenopus oocytes (Huang et al., 2007), and it has been shown to functionally associate with the receptor in the INS-1 cells. Knockdown and loss of CaSR expression has been shown to decrease glucose-evoked insulin secretion (Okamoto et al., 2012), and increases in insulin secretion evoked by inactivation of KCNJ15 disappeared when CaSR was coinactivated, suggesting a direct interaction between the potassium channel and the receptor as previously reported in the kidney (Huang, Handlogten, & Miller, 2002). Linking model data to the clinical scenario is often complex; however, case studies have suggested an association between missense mutations in the CaSR in familial hypocalciuric hypercalcemia (FHH) and type 2 diabetes (Ohkubo et al., 2000). The study suggested that coexistence of nuclear gene and mitochondrial DNA mutations may have caused or modified the development of abnormal glucose tolerance in the family. In a separate case study using the arterial stimulation and venous sampling technique to localize an insulinoma in a patient with concurrent FHH (Ono et al., 2008), there was no significant change in plasma levels of insulin or C-peptide during the test, even though CaSR expression was confirmed. This discrepancy may reflect the fact that normal islets and insulinoma cells respond differently to changes in the concentration of extracellular calcium (Komoto et al., 2003). Although the available data are persuasive, we still lack definitive evidence that changes in CaSR expression/function are directly linked to diabetes mellitus, and this topic remains a hotbed of continued investigation.

7. CONCLUSION

This review of the current literature supports the notion that calcium receptor-mediated cell-to-cell communication permits local changes in coreleased calcium to synchronize responses to nutrient and nonnutrient secretagogues in the intact islet. It seems likely that local changes in extracellular calcium provide a paracrine mechanism to support GJIC, to ensure efficient and appropriate glucose responsiveness. Calcimimetics are used to activate the CaSR and block PTH secretion and have been developed to treat hyperparathyroidism, while calcilytic compounds provide an anabolic therapy for osteoporosis (reviewed in Nemeth, 2004). However, the functional expression of the CaSR within pancreatic α- and β-cells suggests that these therapies may have wider implications for tissue regulation outside the normal targets for controlling systemic calcium. The evidence supports an important role for the receptor in orchestrating a synchronized response from the whole islet. It suggests several key mechanisms by which the CaSR might affect β-cell function, including an increase in cell–cell adhesion, cell coupling, and cell-to-cell communication. Activation of the CaSR in the β-cell can modify proliferation and glucose-evoked insulin secretion. These effects can be linked to the direct association of the receptor to various partner proteins, which include E-cadherin, L-type VDCCs, and potassium channels. The data suggest that the CaSR plays a promiscuous but vital role in modifying β-cell function and that dysregulation of the system is likely to have implications in disease. Greater understanding of these complex processes may well identify targets for future therapeutic intervention.

ACKNOWLEDGMENT

This work was supported by the generous support of Diabetes UK (BDA:09/0003913 and 12/0004546).

REFERENCES

Anwand, A. B., & Garland, H. O. (1990). Renal calcium and magnesium handling in experimental diabetes mellitus in the rat. *Acta Endocrinologica, 122*, 479–486.

Bai, S.-Z., Sun, J., Wu, H., Zhang, N., Li, H.-X., Li, G. W., et al. (2012). Decrease in calcium-sensing receptor in the progress of diabetic cardiomyopathy. *Diabetes Research and Clinical Practice, 95*, 378–385.

Bhagavathula, N., Hanosh, A. W., Nerusu, K. C., Appelman, H., Chakrabarty, S., & Varani, J. (2007). Regulation of E-cadherin and beta-catenin by Ca^{2+} in colon carcinoma is dependent on calcium-sensing receptor expression and function. *International Journal of Cancer, 121*, 1455–1462.

Brown, E. M., Gamba, G., Riccardi, D., Lombardi, M., Butters, R., Kifor, O., et al. (1993). Cloning and characterization of an extracellular Ca2+-sensing receptor from bovine parathyroid. *Nature, 366*, 575–580.

Brown, E. M., & MacLeod, R. J. (2001). Extracellular calcium sensing and extracellular calcium signaling. *Physiological Reviews, 81*, 239–297.

Bruce, J. I. E., Yang, X., Ferguson, C. J., Elliot, A. C., Steward, M. C., Maynard-Case, R., et al. (1999). Molecular and functional identification of a Ca^{2+} (polyvalent cation)-sensing receptor in rat pancreas. *Journal of Biological Chemistry, 274*, 20561–20568.

Buchan, A. M. J., Squires, P. E., Ring, M., & Meloche, R. M. (2001). Mechanism of action of the calcium-sensing receptor in human antral gastrin cells. *Gastroenterology, 120*, 1128–1139.

Burns, C. J., Squires, P. E., & Persaud, S. J. (2000). Signaling through the p38 and p42/44 mitogen-activated kinases in pancreatic β-cell proliferation. *Biochemical and Biophysical Research Communications, 268*, 541–546.

Chakravarti, B., Chattopadhyay, N., & Brown, E. M. (2012). Signaling through the extracellular calcium-sensing receptor (CaSR). *Advances in Experimental Medicine and Biology, 740*, 103–142.

Chattopadhyay, N., Ye, C. P., Yamaguchi, T., Kerner, R., Vassilev, P. M., & Brown, E. M. (1999). Extracellular calcium-sensing receptor induces cellular proliferation and activation of a nonselective cation channel in U373 human astrocytoma cells. *Brain Research, 851*, 116–124.

Cheng, S. X., Giebel, J. P., & Herbert, S. C. (2004). Extracellular polyamines regulate fluid secretion in rat colonic crypts via the extracellular calcium-sensing receptor. *Gastroenterology, 126*, 148–158.

Cigliola, V., Chellakudam, V., Arabieter, W., & Meda, P. (2012). Connexins and β-cell function. *Diabetes Research and Clinical Practice, 99*, 250–259.

Collares-Buzato, C. B., Carvalho, C. P. F., Furtado, A. G., & Boschero, A. C. (2004). Up-regulation of the expression of tight and adherens junction-associated proteins during maturation of neonatal pancreatic islets in vitro. *Journal of Molecular Histology, 35*, 811–822.
Dahl, U., Sjodin, A., & Semb, H. (1996). Cadherins regulate aggregation of pancreatic β-cells in vivo. *Development, 122*, 2895–2902.
Detimary, P., Jonas, J. C., & Henquin, J. C. (1996). Stable and diffusible pools of nucleotides in pancteatic islet cells. *Endocrinology, 137*, 4671–4676.
Fujimoto, K., Nagafuchi, A., Tsukita, S., Kuraoka, A., Ohokuma, A., & Shibata, Y. (1997). Dynamics of connexins, E-cadherin and alpha-catenin on cell membranes during gap junction formation. *Journal of Cell Science, 110*, 311–322.
Gerino, A., Maiellaro, I., Carmone, C., Caroppo, R., Debellis, L., Barile, M., et al. (2012). Glucose increases extracellular [Ca2+] in rat insulinoma (INS-1E) pseudoislets as measured with Ca2+-sensitive microelectrodes. *Cell Calcium, 51*, 393–401.
Grapengiesser, E., Gylfe, E., & Hellman, B. (1999). Synchronisation of glucose-induced Ca^{2+} transients in pancreatic β-cells by a diffusible factor. *Biochemical and Biophysical Research Communications, 254*, 436–439.
Gray, E., Squires, P. E., Muller, D., Asare-Anane, H., Cai Huang, G., Amiel, S., et al. (2006). Activation of the extracellular calcium sensing receptor initiates insulin secretion from human islets of Langerhans: Involvement of protein kinases. *Journal of Endocrinology, 190*, 711–718.
Hauge-Evans, A. C., Squires, P. E., Belin, V. D., Roderigo-Milne, H., Ramracheya, R. D., Persaud, S. J., et al. (2002). Role of adenosine nucleotides in insulin secretion from MIN6 pseudoislets. *Molecular and Cellular Endocrinology, 191*, 167–176.
Hauge-Evans, A. C., Squires, P. E., Persaud, S. J., & Jones, P. M. (1999). Pancreatic β-cell-β-cell interactions are required for integrated responses to nutrient stimuli: Enhanced Ca^{2+} and insulin secretory responses of MIN6 pseudoislets. *Diabetes, 48*, 1402–1408.
Hazama, A., Hayashi, S., & Okada, Y. (1998). Cell surface measurement of ATP release from single pancreatic β-cells using a novel biosensor technique. *Pflugers Archiv: European Journal of Physiology, 437*, 31–35.
Hellman, B., Dansk, H., & Grapengiesser, E. (2004). Pancreatic β-cells communicate via intermittent release of ATP. *American Journal of Physiology, 286*, E759–E765.
Hellman, B., Gylfe, E., Bergsten, P., Grapengiesser, E., Lund, P. E., Berts, A., et al. (1994). Glucose induces oscillatory Ca2+ signalling and insulin release in human pancreatic beta cells. *Diabetologia, 37*, S11–S20.
Hills, C. E., Siamantouras, E., Smith, S. W., Cockwell, P., Liu, K.-K., & Squires, P. E. (2012). TGFβ modulates cell-cell communication in early epithelial-to-mesenchymal transition. *Diabetologia, 55*, 812–824.
Hills, C. E., Younis, M. Y. G., Bennett, J., Siamantouras, E., Liu, K.-K., & Squires, P. E. (2012). Calcium-sensing receptor activation increases cell-cell adhesion and β-cell function. *Cellular Physiology and Biochemistry, 30*, 575–586.
Hodgkin, M. H., Rogers, G. J., & Squires, P. E. (2007). Co-localisation between β-catenin and insulin suggests a novel role for the adherens junction in β-cell function. *Pancreas, 34*, 170–171.
Hofer, A. M., Curci, S., Doble, M. A., Brown, E. M., & Soybel, D. I. (2000). Intercellular communication mediated by the extracellular calcium-sensing receptor. *Nature Cell Biology, 2*, 392–398.
Hofer, A. M., Gerbino, A., Caroppo, R., & Curci, S. (2004). The extracellular calcium-sensing receptor and cell-cell signaling in epithelia. *Cell Calcium, 35*, 297–306.
Huang, Z., Cheng, S. L., & Slatopolsky, E. (2001). Sustained activation of the extracellular signal-regulated kinase pathway is required for extracellular calcium stimulation of human osteoblast proliferation. *Journal of Biological Chemistry, 276*, 21351–21358.

Huang, C., Handlogten, M. E., & Miller, R. T. (2002). Parallel activation of phosphatidylinositol 4-kinase and phospholipase C by the extracellular calcium-sensing receptor. *Journal of Biological Chemistry, 277*, 20293–20300.

Huang, C., Sindic, A., Hill, C. E., Hujer, K. M., Chan, K. W., Sassen, M., et al. (2007). Interaction of the Ca2+-sensing receptor with the inwardly rectifying potassium channels Kir4.1 and Kir4.2 results in inhibition of channel function. *American Journal of Physiology. Renal Physiology, 292*, F1073–F1081.

Hutton, J. C. (1989). The insulin secretory granule. *Diabetologia, 32*, 271–281.

Jin, T. (2008). The WNT signaling pathway and diabetes mellitus. *Diabetologia, 51*, 1771–1780.

Jones, P. M., Kitsou-Mylona, I., Gray, E., Squires, P. E., & Persaud, S. J. (2007). Expression and function of the extracellular calcium-sensing receptor in pancreatic β-cells. *Archives of Physiology and Biochemistry, 113*, 98–103.

Jones, P. M., & Persaud, S. J. (1998). Protein kinases, protein phosphorylation, and the regulation of insulin secretion from pancreatic β-cells. *Endocrine Reviews, 19*, 429–461.

Justinich, C. J., Mak, N., Pacheco, I., Mulder, D., Wells, R. W., Blennerhassett, M. G., et al. (2008). The extracellular calcium-sensing receptor (CaSR) on human esophagus and evidence of expression of the CaSR on the esophageal epithelial cell line (HET-1A). *American Journal of Physiology, 294*, G120–G129.

Kanno, Y., Sasaki, Y., Shiba, Y., Yoshida-Noro, C., & Takeichi, M. (1984). Monoclonal antibody ECCD-1 inhibits intercellular communication in teratocarcinoma PCC3 cells. *Experimental Cell Research, 152*, 270–274.

Kitsou-Mylona, I., Burns, C. J., Squires, P. E., Persaud, S. J., & Jones, P. M. (2008). A role for the extracellular calcium-sensing receptor in cell-cell communication in pancreatic islets of Langerhans. *Cellular Physiology and Biochemistry, 22*, 557–566.

Komoto, I., Kato, M., Itami, A., Shimada, Y., Doi, R., Hosotani, R., et al. (2003). Expression and function of the calcium-sensing receptor in pancreatic islets and insulinoma cells. *Pancreas, 26*, 178–184.

Liao, J., Schneider, A., Datta, N. S., & McCauley, L. K. (2006). Extracellular calcium as a candidate mediator of prostate cancer skeletal metastasis. *Cancer Research, 66*, 9065–9073.

Lilla, V., Webb, G., Rickenbach, K., Maturana, A., Steiner, D. F., Halban, P. A., et al. (2003). Differential gene expression in well-regulated and dysregulated pancreatic beta-cell (MIN6) sub-lines. *Endocrinology, 144*, 1368–1379.

Lui, Z., & Habener, J. F. (2008). Glucagon like peptide-1 activation of TCFL2-dependent Wnt signaling enhances pancreatic beta cell proliferation. *Journal of Biological Chemistry, 283*, 8723–8735.

Magno, A. L., Ward, B. K., & Ratajczak, T. (2011). The calcium sensing receptor: A molecular perspective. *Endocrine Reviews, 32*, 3–30.

Malaisse, W. J., Louchami, K., Lagmich, A., Ladriere, L., Morales, M., Villaneuva-Penacarrillo, M. L., et al. (1999). Possible participation of an islet β-cell calcium-sensing receptor in insulin release. *Endocrinology, 111*, 293–300.

McNeil, S. E., Hobson, S. A., Nipper, V., & Rodland, K. D. (1998). Functional calcium-sensing receptors in rat fibroblasts are required for activation of SRC kinase and mitogen-activated protein kinase in response to extracellular calcium. *Journal of Biological Chemistry, 273*, 1114–1120.

Mege, R. M., Matsuzaki, F., Gallin, W. J., Goldberg, J. I., Cunningham, B. A., & Edelman, G. M. (1988). Construction of epithelioid sheets by transfection of mouse sarcoma cells with cDNAs for chicken cell adhesion molecules. *Proceedings of the National Academy of Sciences of the United States of America, 85*, 7274–7278.

Musil, L. S., Cunningham, B. A., Edelman, G. M., & Goodenough, D. A. (1990). Differential phosphorylation of the gap junction protein connexin43 in junctional communication-competent and -deficient cell lines. *Journal of Cell Biology, 111*, 2077–2081.

Nemeth, E. F. (2004). Calcimimetic and calcilytic drugs: Just for parathyroid cells? *Cell Calcium*, *35*, 283–289.

Obermuller, S., Lindqvist, A., Karanauskaite, J., Galvanovskis, J., Rorsman, P., & Barg, S. (2005). Selective nucleotide-release from dense core granules in insulin-secreting cells. *Journal of Cell Science*, *118*, 4271–4282.

Ohkubo, E., Aida, K., Chen, J., Hayashi, J.-I., Isobe, K., Tawata, M., et al. (2000). A patient with type 2 diabetes mellitus associated with mutations in calcium sensing receptor gene and mitochondrial DNA. *Biochemical and Biophysical Research Communications*, *278*, 808–813.

Okamoto, K., Iwasaki, N., Doi, K., Noiri, E., Iwamoto, Y., Uchigata, Y., et al. (2012). Inihibition of glucose-stimulated insulin secretion by KCJN15, a newly identified susceptibility gene for type2 diabetes. *Diabetes*, *61*, 1734–1741.

Okamoto, K., Iwasaki, N., Nishimure, C., Doi, K., Noiri, E., Nakamura, S., et al. (2010). Identification of KCNJ15 as a susceptibility gene in Asian patients with type 2 diabetes mellitus. *American Journal of Human Genetics*, *86*, 54–64.

Ono, Y., Oda, N., Ishihara, S., Shimomura, A., Hayakawa, N., Suzuki, A., et al. (2008). Insulinoma cell calcium-sensing receptor influences insulin secretion in a case with concurrent familial hypocalciuric hypercalccmia and malignant metastatic insulinoma. *European Journal of Endocrinology*, *159*, 81–86.

Parkash, J. (2008). Inflammatory cytokine signaling in insulin producing β-cells enhances the colocalization correlation coefficient between L-type voltage-dependent calcium channel and calcium-sensing receptor. *International Journal of Molecular Medicine*, *22*, 155–163.

Parkash, J., & Asotra, K. (2011). L-histidine sensing by calcium sensing receptor inhibits voltage-dependent calcium channel activity and insulin secretion in β-cells. *Life Sciences*, *88*, 440–446.

Perez-Armendariz, E., & Atwater, I. (1986). Glucose-evoked changes in $[K^+]$ and $[Ca^{2+}]$ in intercellular spaces of the mouse islet of Langerhans. *Advances in Experimental Medicine and Biology*, *211*, 31–51.

Racz, G. Z., Kittel, A., Riccardi, D., Case, R. M., Elliot, A. C., & Varga, G. (2002). Extracellular calcium sensing receptor in human pancreatic cells. *Gut*, *51*, 705–711.

Rasschaert, J., & Malaisse, W. J. (1999). Expression of the calcium-sensing receptor in pancreatic β-cells. *Biochemical and Biophysical Research Communications*, *264*, 615–618.

Ray, J. M., Squires, P. E., Curtis, S. B., Meloche, R. M., & Buchan, A. M. J. (1997). Expression of the calcium-sensing receptor on human antral gastrin cells in culture. *Journal of Clinical Investigation*, *99*, 2328–2333.

Rogers, G. J., Hodgkin, M. N., & Squires, P. E. (2007). E-cadherin and cell adhesion: A role in architecture and function in the pancreatic islet. *Cellular Physiology and Biochemistry*, *20*, 987–994.

Sakwe, A. M., Larsson, M., & Rask, L. (2004). Involvement of protein kinase C-alpha and -epsilon in extracellular $Ca(^{2+})$ signalling mediated by the calcium sensing receptor. *Experimental Cell Research*, *297*, 560–573.

Santos, R. M., Rosario, L. M., Nadal, A., Garcia-Sancho, J., Soria, B., & Valdeolmillos, M. (1991). Widespread synchronous $[Ca^{2+}]_i$ oscillations due to bursting electrical activity in single pancreatic islets. *Pflugers Archiv: European Journal of Physiology*, *418*, 417–422.

Shih, D. Q., Heimesaat, M., Kuwajima, S., Stein, R., Wright, C. V. E., & Stoffel, M. (2002). Profound defects in pancreatic beta-cell function in mice with combined heterozygous mutations in Pdx-1, Hnf-1alpha, and Hnf-3beta. *Proceedings of the National Academy of Sciences of the United States of America*, *99*, 3818–3823.

Smajilovic, S., & Tfelt-Hansen, J. (2007). Calcium acts as a first messenger through the calcium-sensing receptor in the cardiovascular system. *Cardiovascular Research*, *75*, 457–467.

Squires, P. E., Harris, T. E., Persaud, S. J., Curtis, S. B., Buchan, A. M. J., & Jones, P. M. (2000). The extracellular calcium-sensing receptor on human β-cells negatively modulates insulin secretion. *Diabetes*, *49*, 409–417.

Squires, P. E., Hauge-Evans, A. C., Persaud, S. J., & Jones, P. M. (2000). The synchronization of Ca^{2+}-signals within insulin-secreting pseudoislets: Effects of gap-junctional uncouplers. *Cell Calcium*, *27*, 287–296.

Squires, P. E., James, R. F. L., London, N. J. M., & Dunne, M. J. (1994). ATP-induced intracellular Ca2+-signals in isolated human insulin-secreting cells. *Pflugers Archiv: European Journal of Physiology*, *427*, 181–183.

Squires, P. E., Meloche, R. M., & Buchan, A. M. J. (1999). Bombesin-evoked gastrin release and calcium signalling in human antral G-cells in culture. *American Journal of Physiology*, *276*, G227–G237.

Squires, P. E., Persaud, S. J., Hauge-Evans, A. C., Gray, E., Ratcliff, H., & Jones, P. M. (2002). Co-ordinated Ca^{2+}-signaling within pancreatic islets: Does β-cell entrainment require a secreted messenger. *Cell Calcium*, *31*, 209–219.

Straub, S. G., Kornreich, B., Oswald, R. E., Nemeth, E. F., & Sharp, G. W. G. (2000). The calcimimetic R-467 potentiates insulin secretion in pancreatic β cells by activation of a non-specific cation channel. *Journal of Biological Chemistry*, *275*, 18777–18784.

Tu, C.-L., Chang, W., Xie, Z., & Bikle, D. D. (2008). Inactivation of the calcium sensing receptor inhibits E-cadherin-mediated cell-cell adhesion and calcium-induced differentiation in human epidermal keratinocytes. *Journal of Biological Chemistry*, *283*, 3519–3528.

Vizard, T. N., O'Keeffe, G. W., Gutierrez, H., Kos, C. H., Riccardi, D., & Davies, A. M. (2008). Regulation of axonal and dendritic growth by the extracellular calcium-sensing receptor. *Nature Neuroscience*, *11*, 285–291.

Wakae-Takada, N., Xuan, S., Watanabe, K., Meda, P., & Leibel, R. L. (2013). Molecular basis for the regulation of islet beta cell mass in mice: The role of E-cadherin. *Diabetologia*, *56*, 856–866.

Ward, B. K., Mangno, A. L., Walsh, J. P., & Ratajczak, T. (2012). The role of the calcium-sensing receptor in human disease. *Clinical Biochemistry*, *45*, 943–953.

Ward, D. T., Yau, S. K., Mee, A. P., Mawer, E. B., Miller, C. A., Garland, H. O., et al. (2001). Functional, molecular, and biochemical characterization of streptozotocin-induced diabetes. *Journal of the American Society of Nephrology*, *12*, 779–790.

Weston, A. H., Absi, M., Harno, E., Geraghty, A. R., Ward, D. T., Ruat, M., et al. (2008). The expression and function of Ca2+-sensing receptors in rat mesenteric artery; comparative studies using a model of type II diabetes. *British Journal of Pharmacology*, *154*, 652–662.

Yamagata, K., Nammo, T., Moriwaki, M., Ihara, A., Iizuka, K., Yang, Q., et al. (2002). Overexpression of dominant-negative mutant hepatocyte nuclear factor-1 alpha in pancreatic beta-cells causes abnormal islet architecture with decreased expression of E cadherin, reduced beta-cell proliferation, and diabetes. *Diabetes*, *51*, 114–123.

Yang, S. N., & Berggren, P. O. (2005). B-cell CaV channel regulation in physiology and pathophysiology. *American Journal of Physiology*, *288*, E16–E28.

Yang, G. K., Squires, P. E., Tian, F., Kieffer, T. J., Kwok, Y. N., & Dale, N. (2012). Glucose decreases extracellular adenosine levels in isolated mouse and rat pancreatic islets. *Islets*, *4*, 64–70.

Yano, S., Sugimoto, T., Tsukamoto, T., Chihara, K., Kobayashi, A., Kitazawa, S., et al. (2003). Decrease in vitamin D receptor and calcium-sensing receptor in highly proliferative parathyroid adenomas. *European Journal of Endocrinology*, *148*, 403–411.

CHAPTER ELEVEN

Cellular Inhibitor of Apoptosis Protein-1 and Survival of Beta Cells Undergoing Endoplasmic Reticulum Stress

Pu Xia[*,†,1], **Yanfei Qi**[*]

[*]Signal Transduction Program, Centenary Institute, Sydney, Australia
[†]Department of Endocrinology and Metabolism, Zhongshan Hospital, Fudan University, Shanghai, PR China
[1]Corresponding author: e-mail address: xiapu_fudan@163.com

Contents

Abstract

Pancreatic beta cells rely heavily on the endoplasmic reticulum (ER) to process folding and posttranslational modification of a large amount of insulin and many other proteins and are therefore vulnerable to ER stress. The role of the ER is thus crucial in the regulation of beta cell function and survival through the unfolded protein response (UPR) pathways. However, the UPR can either allow cells to survive by adapting to stress or kill cells through apoptosis in a context-dependent manner. How cell fate is determined following UPR activation remains enigmatic. In this review, we discuss the molecular mechanisms linking ER stress to beta cell survival or apoptosis. Specifically, we focus on the role of the cellular inhibitor of apoptosis protein-1 and propose a new model for understanding survival of beta cells undergoing ER stress.

1. INTRODUCTION

Pancreatic beta cell dysfunction and destruction caused by apoptosis are regarded as fundamental pathogenic events in the development of both type 1 and type 2 diabetes. Beta cell apoptosis resulting from autoimmune

Vitamins and Hormones, Volume 95
ISSN 0083-6729
http://dx.doi.org/10.1016/B978-0-12-800174-5.00011-9

reactions has been well characterized as a central mechanism causing type 1 diabetes. Two principal pathways are proposed in this pathogenic process, that is, (i) cytotoxic T-cells activated by beta cell autoantigens kill beta cells through direct cell–cell contacts, and (ii) beta cell death is provoked by cytokines and other soluble death mediators produced by activated T-cells, macrophages, or the beta cell itself. In type 2 diabetes, although beta cell death was observed in diabetic individuals, there is a long-standing controversy as to whether beta cell death is a causative factor or merely a coincidence of diabetes. Evidence is accumulating that the loss of functional beta cell mass is crucial in determining whether an individual who has insulin resistance develops diabetes. Although the mechanism remains unclear, the recent consensus is that beta cell apoptosis is a key contributor to the loss of functional beta cell mass (Ashcroft & Rorsman, 2012; Cerasi, 2011; Donath et al., 2005; Eizirik, Cardozo, & Cnop, 2008; Prentki & Nolan, 2006). Thus, attempting to promote beta cell survival and rescue insulin secretory function is emerging as a strategy for the management of type 2 diabetes.

Survival is obviously essential for any type of cell to maintain normal function. Apart from this simple relationship, there are multiple direct connections between the molecular pathways controlling cell survival and those that regulate insulin secretion in beta cells. One such connection is the mitochondrion. It is here that glucose is metabolized and where the signals coupling glucose metabolism to insulin secretion are generated, but it is also a key center of the apoptotic machinery (Maechler & Wollheim, 2001). So, it is not surprising that many apoptotic or antiapoptotic agonists eventually affect insulin secretion. For instance, cytokines TNFα, IL1, or INFγ have been shown to cause beta cell apoptosis and also to inhibit insulin secretion (Dunger et al., 1996; Igoillo-Esteve et al., 2010). In light of this, interventions that inhibit beta cell apoptosis may have considerable potential to preserve insulin secretion and other cellular functions. Surprisingly, although overexpression of the antiapoptotic protein Bcl-x_L in pancreatic beta cells protected the cells from apoptosis, it paradoxically resulted in a severe defect in insulin secretion and hyperglycemia in the Bcl-x_L transgenic mice (Zhou et al., 2000). These unexpected phenotypic and functional changes associated with the overexpression of Bcl-x_L in beta cells present a challenge against the development of strategies in related to Bcl-x_L or other antiapoptotic proteins for therapeutic purposes.

Apart from mitochondria, the endoplasmic reticulum (ER) is another principal organelle linking beta cell survival and insulin production. As a prototypical, professional secretory cell type, pancreatic beta cells have a highly developed ER to facilitate the folding of large amounts of insulin and various glycoproteins for secretion and are thus vulnerable to ER stress. Notably, the cellular response to ER stress, often referred to as the unfolded protein response (UPR), is critically involved in regulating both insulin production and beta cell survival, either under physiological or disease conditions (Eizirik et al., 2008; Hotamisligil, 2010; Ron & Walter, 2007). Especially, under obese and insulin-resistant conditions, beta cells are confronted with a dramatically enhanced demand for insulin production, accompanied by multiple pathological factors such as elevated levels of free fatty acids (FFA). Such insults place a strain on the cell and cause prolonged or chronic activation of the UPR pathways, ultimately leading to beta cell dysfunction and cell death. This has been suggested to be a key pathogenic event contributing to the development of type 2 diabetes. Several excellent reviews have recently summarized the evidence for the role of ER stress in the pathogenesis of beta cell dysfunction and diabetes (Ashcroft & Rorsman, 2012; Eizirik et al., 2008; Hetz, 2012; Hotamisligil, 2010; Tabas & Ron, 2011). In this review, we discuss the molecular mechanisms that promote the survival of beta cells undergoing ER stress. Specifically, we focus on the role of cellular inhibitor of apoptosis protein-1 (cIAP1) in the control of beta cell survival.

2. ER STRESS IN THE BALANCE BETWEEN CELL DEATH AND SURVIVAL

The ER system is a membranous network of branching tubules and flattened sacs, in which mRNA and their encoded proteins are properly folded and posttranslational modifications take place, such as asparagine-linked glycosylation, disulfide bond formation, lipidation, hydroxylation, and oligomerization (Kaufman, 1999; Schroder & Kaufman, 2005). Normal ER function is critical for the maturation, assembly, and delivery of secretory and membrane proteins (Lai, Teodoro, & Volchuk, 2007). The ER is also a metabolic organelle that regulates intracellular Ca^{2+} homeostasis, vesicle trafficking, gluconeogenesis, glycogen synthesis and breakdown, fat storage, and biogenesis of membrane lipids (Fagone & Jackowski, 2009; Mandl, Meszaros, Banhegyi, Hunyady, & Csala, 2009). Any insults that perturb ER homeostasis will impair the protein folding machinery, resulting in accumulation of unfolded and misfolded proteins in the ER lumen, leading to ER stress.

Beta cells, like many other cell types, can efficiently sense and respond to ER stress through the UPR pathway (Fig. 11.1), in order to maintain normal cellular function. The UPR is triggered by three sensor proteins, including protein kinase-like ER kinase (PERK), activating transcription factor 6 (ATF6), and inositol-requiring enzyme 1 (IRE1; Kawaguchi & Ng, 2011).

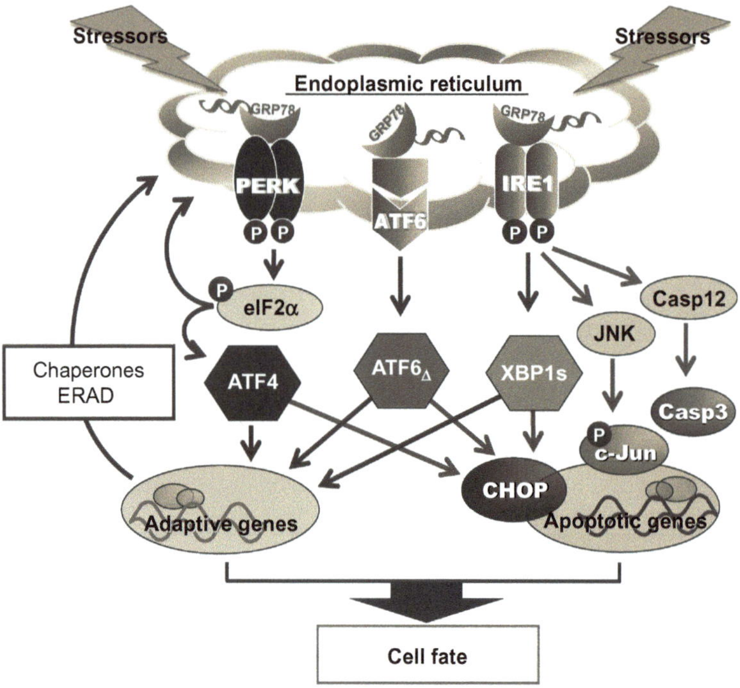

Figure 11.1 ER stress response—the UPR. Upon the challenges from various stressors on ER causing accumulation of unfolded and/or misfolded proteins in the ER lumen, the chaperone GRP78 dissociates from the luminal domain of the three ER transmembrane stress sensors: PERK, ATF6, and IRE1, leading to their activation. Both IRE1 and PERK are oligomerized and autophosphorylated. PERK induces phosphorylation of eIF2a, which blocks new protein synthesis and enables translation of ATF4 transcription factor, promoting the transcription of genes required to restore ER homeostasis. Activated ATF6 is cleaved as a cytosolic fragment that migrates to the nucleus, which regulates the expression of ER chaperones and X-box-binding protein 1 (XBP1). XBP1 mRNA spliced by IRE1 codes for the active transcription factor XBP1s that controls the transcription of chaperones and ERAD components. This concerted action of the UPR pathways restores the folding capacity of the ER by blocking further buildup of client proteins, enhancing its folding capacity and eliminating terminally misfolded proteins. Sustained or unresolved ER stress activates apoptotic mechanisms, including activation of JNK, caspase-12, and induction of CHOP, leading to cell death. (See the color plate.)

In unstressed cells, the sensor proteins are maintained in an inactive state by association with the ER chaperone protein BiP/GRP78 via their luminal domains (Kohno, Normington, Sambrook, Gething, & Mori, 1993). In a stressed state, accumulation of unfolded proteins provokes dissociation of BiP/GRP78 from the sensors (Rutkowski & Kaufman, 2007), as BiP/GRP78 has higher affinity binding to unfolded proteins than stress sensors (Schroder & Kaufman, 2005). Dissociation leads to the autophosphorylation of PERK and IRE1 and the transactivation of ATF6 (Xu, Bailly-Maitre, & Reed, 2005), which in turn initiate the activation of the UPR (Szegezdi, Logue, Gorman, & Samali, 2006). Activation of these pathways culminates in transcriptional regulation of a range of genes that improve ER homeostasis through the following mechanisms: (i) translational attenuation to reduce further loading of newly synthesized proteins to the ER lumen; (ii) transcriptional induction of ER chaperone genes; and (iii) ER-associated degradation (ERAD) of unfolded and misfolded proteins (Hotamisligil, 2010; Ron & Walter, 2007). Intriguingly, gene expression profiling has demonstrated that numerous cellular processes beyond ER homeostasis are also regulated by UPR activation (Harding, Zhang, Bertolotti, Zeng, & Ron, 2000; Novoa et al., 2003; Rutkowski et al., 2006). Indeed, it is now acknowledged that cellular UPR is programmed for both adaptation to stress and commitment to cell death by apoptosis (Hetz, 2012; Hotamisligil, 2010; Rutkowski & Kaufman, 2007; Tabas & Ron, 2011; Xu et al., 2005) (Fig. 11.1). Thus far, a major question that remains is how cells decide to either adapt or undergo apoptosis following UPR activation.

2.1. Adaptive UPR leading to cell survival

The UPR-mediated translational attenuation is mainly attributable to PERK activation, which serves as an emergency response (Wu & Kaufman, 2006). PERK is a type I ER-resident transmembrane protein, possessing kinase activity. Following dissociation from BiP/GRP78, PERK undergoes dimerization and transautophosphorylation, which induce the activation of its Ser/Thr protein kinase domain (Shi et al., 1998). Activated PERK can further phosphorylate a series of substrates, including eukaryotic initiation factors-2α (eIF2α) (Shi et al., 1999). Phosphorylation of Ser51 in the α-unit of eIF2α greatly reduces its efficiency in initiating protein translation, because phosphorylated eIF2α no longer exchanges GDP for GTP, or brings methionyl-transfer RNA to the 40S ribosome, and thus the 80S initiation complex for protein translation cannot be formed (Harding, Calfon, Urano, Novoa, & Ron, 2002).

Although phospho-eIF2α attenuates global protein translation, it selectively upregulates the expression of transcription factor ATF4 that relieves ER stress by inducing the expression of ER chaperones, amino acid transporters, and redox controllers (Lai et al., 2007). In addition to ATF4, the IRE1 and ATF6 branches of UPR pathways are also responsible for the transcriptional regulation of ER chaperones. IRE1 is an atypical type I ER residential transmembrane protein, possessing kinase and endoribonuclease activity (Nikawa & Yamashita, 1992). Once released from BiP/GRP78, IRE1 undergoes oligomerization and autophosphorylation, leading to the activation of its RNase activity (Gardner & Walter, 2011; Schroder & Kaufman, 2005; Zhou et al., 2006). Activated IRE1 allows activation of X-box DNA-binding protein-1 (XBP1) by removing a 26-nucleotide intron from XBP1 mRNA (Yoshida, Matsui, Yamamoto, Okada, & Mori, 2001). The sliced XBP1 mRNA binds to and upregulates ER stress response element (ERSE) promoter in the genes encoding UPR chaperones, such as BiP/GRP78, which assist protein folding (Rao & Bredesen, 2004). ATF6 is a type II ER residential transmembrane protein (Wu & Kaufman, 2006). Dissociation from BiP/GRP78 induces translocation of ATF6 from ER to the Golgi apparatus. Subsequently, site-1 and site-2 proteases in the Golgi apparatus cleave ATF6 into an N-terminal cytosolic portion that contains a basic zipper transcription factor (Ye et al., 2000). The truncated ATF6 will further translocate to the nucleus and bind to the ERSE promoter, inducing the expression of XBP1 and BiP/GRP78 (Li et al., 2000; Nadanaka, Yoshida, Sato, & Mori, 2006).

If attenuation of protein translation or induction of ER chaperones is not sufficient to relieve ER stress, ERAD is then activated to remove unfolded or misfolded proteins in the ER lumen (Lai et al., 2007; Meusser, Hirsch, Jarosch, & Sommer, 2005; Smith, Ploegh, & Weissman, 2011). This process involves the following subsequent steps. (i) The substrate proteins are specifically selected by ER chaperones, for example, BiP/GRP78 (Nishikawa, Brodsky, & Nakatsukasa, 2005). (ii) After selection, unfolded proteins translocate into the cytoplasm through the ER membrane channels constituted with Sec61p, which are also involved in protein import to the ER (Friedlander, Jarosch, Urban, Volkwein, & Sommer, 2000; Vembar & Brodsky, 2008). (iii) Following export, substrate proteins will be ubiquitylated and degraded by the proteasomes (Richly et al., 2005).

Collectively, the three branches of the UPR promote immense adaptive responses that work together in a highly coordinative way to restore ER function and maintain cell survival. Although activation of the three UPR pathways often leads to adaptation, the UPR does not always result in successful alleviation of ER stress but triggers apoptotic program leading to cell death (see below).

2.2. Switch from the adaptive UPR to apoptosis

Under physiological conditions, beta cells that demand a high rate of insulin production and secretion must sustain activation of the adaptive UPR without damaging the cells. However, under certain circumstances, such as prolonged or unresolved ER stress, the UPR will switch from the adaptive prosurvival mode to proapoptotic mode, resulting in apoptosis. ER stress-induced apoptosis often correlates with the expression of CCAAT/enhancer-binding protein homologous protein (CHOP) (Szegezdi et al., 2006). CHOP, also known as growth arrest and DNA damage gene 153 (GADD153), is the major prodeath transcription factor implicated in ER stress-mediated apoptosis. CHOP transcription is highly induced under prolonged ER stress via the transcription factors ATF4, ATF6, and XBP1; thus, all three arms of the UPR pathway converge at the upregulation of CHOP. Of the three, the PERK–eIF2α–ATF4 pathway is essential (Oyadomari & Mori, 2004). Cells deficient in PERK or ATF4, and those expressing mutant eIF2α (S51A), fail to induce CHOP in response to ER stressors, although other UPR pathways remain activated (Xu et al., 2005). The *Chop* promoter contains two elements, ERSE and C/EBP-ATF composite site, which are directly regulated by transactivation of ATF4 (Bruhat et al., 2000; Ma, Brewer, Diehl, & Hendershot, 2002). In addition to transcriptional regulation, the protein expression and activity of CHOP are subject to posttranslational regulation. The p38 mitogen-activated protein kinase (MAPK) phosphorylates CHOP on Ser78 and Ser81, which increases the transcriptional activity of CHOP (Wang & Ron, 1996). Furthermore, the protein levels of CHOP are also determined by ubiquitination and proteasomal degradation. Treatment with the proteasome inhibitor MG-132 results in accumulation of endogenous CHOP in cells. Mutation of a lysine residue at position aa50 on CHOP (K50R) induces CHOP augmentation similar to that caused by MG-132, indicating a possible polyubiquitin binding site in CHOP (Ohoka, Hattori, Kitagawa, Onozaki, & Hayashi, 2007).

The role of CHOP in promoting cell death has been demonstrated in a diverse range of cell types, including beta cells, both *in vitro* and *in vivo* (Tabas & Ron, 2011). Notably, several recent studies from *chop*-deficient mice indicate that CHOP is critically required for ER stress-induced apoptosis in pancreatic beta cells (Song, Scheuner, Ron, Pennathur, & Kaufman, 2008), hepatocytes (Oyadomari, Harding, Zhang, Oyadomari, & Ron, 2008), and cardiomyocytes (Fu et al., 2010) under certain stress conditions. Overexpression of CHOP leads to translocation of Bax to the mitochondrial membrane and potentiates cell death in response to the chemical ER stressors thapsigargin and tunicamycin (McCullough, Martindale, Klotz, Aw, & Holbrook, 2001). Microinjection of CHOP was reported to induce apoptosis by downregulation of Bcl-2 (Matsumoto, Minami, Takeda, Sakao, & Akira, 1996; McCullough et al., 2001). The proapoptotic effects of CHOP are often associated with its transcriptional regulation (Tabas & Ron, 2011). The heterodimer of CHOP with C/EBPα is reported to bind directly to an element in the first intron of the gene encoding the BH3-only protein Bim, promoting its expression and leading to apoptosis (Puthalakath et al., 2007). Another transcription substrate for CHOP is GADD34. It interacts with protein phosphatase 1 to dephosphorylate eIF2α during ER stress. As phosphorylation of eIF2α is an emergency response in shutting-off protein translation, induction of GADD34 releases the translational block, leading to greatly increased synthesis of proapoptotic regulators (Brush, Weiser, & Shenolikar, 2003). Furthermore, CHOP impairs redox cycling, induces cytotoxic reactive oxygen species (ROS), and activates oxidative stress and apoptosis by its transcriptional target ER oxidase 1α (Marciniak et al., 2004).

In addition to the role of CHOP in promoting apoptosis, two important kinases including apoptosis signal-regulating kinase 1 (ASK1) and c-Jun NH2-terminal kinase (JNK) play important roles in ER stress-associated apoptosis. In response to ER stress, ASK1 is activated by recruitment into a complex consisting of the oligomerized IRE1 and TRAF2 on the ER membrane, which subsequently activates JNK and p38 MAPK (Nishitoh et al., 2002). JNK activation leads to phosphorylation of Bcl-2, which in turn relieves its inhibition of the proapoptotic Bcl-2 family members and efflux of Ca^{2+} from the ER lumen (Bassik, Scorrano, Oakes, Pozzan, & Korsmeyer, 2004). Meanwhile, activated JNK expedites Bim activation due to dissociation from dynein motor complex (Lei & Davis, 2003). In addition, JNK activation facilitates the formation of a CHOP and c-Jun heterodimer, leading to upregulation of PUMA and activation of Bax (Cazanave et al., 2010). Of importance, JNK activation positively regulates

CHOP expression. Inhibition of JNK phosphorylation by the inhibitor SP600125 attenuates CHOP levels during ER stress (Ramirez-Alcantara, LoGuidice, & Boelsterli, 2009). As the induction of CHOP occurs later than the phosphorylation of JNK, it is believed that CHOP activation is an "advanced stage" of ER stress-associated apoptosis (Ramirez-Alcantara et al., 2009).

Caspase-12 is a well-known prodeath protease involved in ER stress-associated apoptosis. It is located on the outer surface of the ER membrane, and it can be specifically activated by ER stressors such as tunicamycin and thapsigargin (Momoi, 2004). It is proposed that ER stressors may induce the depletion of ER luminal Ca^{2+}, leading to the activation of calpain that subsequently activates caspase-12 (Tan et al., 2006). *Capn1* (mouse gene encoding calpain)-knockout MEFs lack casapse-12 activation and thus are resistant to ER stress-induced apoptosis (Tan et al., 2006). Translocation of caspase-7 from the cytosol to the ER membrane during ER stress is also attributed to caspase-12 cleavage (Yoneda et al., 2001). Cleaved caspase-12 activates caspase-9 and caspase-3 in a cytochrome *c*-independent manner during ER stress (Morishima, Nakanishi, Takenouchi, Shibata, & Yasuhiko, 2002). However, the involvement of caspase-12 in ER stress-mediated apoptosis has been controversial, as *Casp12* deficiency does not induce any resistance to ER stress-induced apoptosis in mice (Saleh et al., 2006). Furthermore, inhibition of calpain, but not caspase-12, prevents tunicamycin-induced cell death (Sanges & Marigo, 2006).

3. ER STRESS AND LIPOTOXICITY IN BETA CELL FAILURE

As professional secretory cells, the ER system in pancreatic beta cells needs to process the folding and posttranslational modification of a large amount of insulin and many other proteins (Scheuner & Kaufman, 2008). The role of the ER is crucial to beta cells, which relies heavily on this organelle not only to process proinsulin into mature insulin for secretion but also to regulate cell survival through the UPR pathways.

Indeed, it has emerged that beta cell ER stress and the UPR pathways play an important role in the development of diabetes (Eizirik et al., 2008; Hotamisligil, 2010). For instance, the formation of intramolecular disulfide bonds in insulin is required for insulin folding and subsequent trafficking from the ER to the Golgi apparatus for secretion. Mutation of Ins2 (C96Y) in Akita mice disables the Cys80–Cys96 bond causing ER stress, resulting in beta cell failure and the progression of diabetes (Izumi et al.,

2003; Oyadomari et al., 2001, 2002). *Perk*$^{-/-}$ neonates develop diabetes within 1 week of life due to defects in beta cell proliferation and differentiation (Zhang et al., 2006). Homozygous mutation of eIF2α (S51A), downstream of the PERK branch of the UPR pathway, causes severe beta cell deficiency in mice, such that they die within 18 h of birth due to hypoglycemia derived from defective gluconeogenesis (Scheuner et al., 2001). The heterozygous eIF2α (S51A) mice perform normally on a regular chow diet, whereas on a high-fat diet they develop obesity and insulin resistance due to ER dysfunction (Scheuner et al., 2005). The defect in the PERK–eIF2a pathway is also implicated in beta cell dysfunction in humans. A loss-of-function mutation in PERK causes a heritable form of juvenile diabetes called Wallcot–Rallison syndrome, characterized by severe defects in pancreatic beta cells (Zhang et al., 2002). Additionally, mutations in the *WFS1* gene in humans, which encodes the ER transmembrane protein wolframin, have been linked to increased incidence of diabetes in Wolfram syndrome patients (Fonseca et al., 2005). In the IRE1 branch of UPR, preventing IRE1 phosphorylation in beta cells suppresses insulin biosynthesis (Lipson et al., 2006). Complete *Xbp1* deficiency causes embryonic lethality, while *Xbp1*$^{+/-}$ mice experience higher levels of ER stress and exhibit increased body weight and evident insulin resistance (Ozcan et al., 2004). In addition, the role of CHOP in mediating ER stress-associated beta cell death has been well documented in several animal models and diabetic patients. Elevated expression levels of CHOP in beta cells are shown in obese *db/db* mice (Song et al., 2008) and patients with type 2 diabetes (Huang et al., 2007). Treatment of *db/db* mice with the GLP-1 agonist exendin-4 improves hyperglycemia, which is correlated with a marked reduction in nuclear expression of CHOP (Yusta et al., 2006). Knockout of *Chop* delays the onset of diabetes by about 8 weeks in the Akita mouse model due to protection of beta cells from apoptosis (Oyadomari et al., 2002). When *Chop*-deficient animals are crossed with obese *db/db* mice, beta cell death and diabetes are prevented (Song et al., 2008).

Under obese and insulin-resistant conditions, beta cells are subjected to dramatically enhanced and sustained ER stress due to the increased demand for insulin. Additionally, many factors associated with obesity and type 2 diabetes, such as elevated levels of FFA, can further exacerbate ER stress, leading to beta cell dysfunction and death (Eizirik & Cnop, 2010). It is generally accepted that prolonged exposure to FFA and the accumulation of lipids have direct or indirect effects on both insulin secretory defects and a relative loss of beta cell mass due to apoptosis, namely, lipotoxicity (Giacca, Xiao,

Oprescu, Carpentier, & Lewis, 2011; Kusminski, Shetty, Orci, Unger, & Scherer, 2009; Newsholme, Keane, Welters, & Morgan, 2007; Prentki & Nolan, 2006). While both saturated and unsaturated FFA contributes to the secretory defects, specifically saturated species, such as palmitate, mediate lipotoxic apoptosis (Cnop, Hannaert, Hoorens, Eizirik, & Pipeleers, 2001; Laybutt et al., 2007; Maedler et al., 2001), and in fact unsaturated species are protective (Busch et al., 2005; Cnop et al., 2001; Maedler et al., 2001; Qi & Xia, 2012). However, it remains unclear how FFAs actually initiate ER stress and why different FFAs result in different outcomes through the same UPR pathways, beyond the knowledge that FFA metabolism is required and that esterification pathways are particularly associated with creation of toxic metabolites (Newsholme et al., 2007). Several mechanisms have been proposed to explain the ER stress-mediated lipotoxic effects of FFA. Carboxypeptidase E (CPE) is a key enzyme in the regulation of insulin biosynthesis. Exposure of human and rodent islets to palmitate causes downregulation of CPE and accumulation of unfolded insulin, leading to ER stress (Jeffrey et al., 2008). Palmitate also induces ER stress by depleting ER luminal Ca^{2+}, which disturbs insulin processing, resulting in insulin mal-secretion (Guest, Bailyes, & Hutton, 1997). Palmitate can also slow protein trafficking from the ER to the Golgi apparatus causing accumulation of secretory proteins in the ER lumen, leading to ER stress in beta cells (Preston, Gurisik, Bartley, Laybutt, & Biden, 2009). The transcription factor Pdx1 is a key regulator of beta cell differentiation, early islet development, as well as insulin production. Treatment of beta cells with palmitate decreases Pdx1 expression and nuclear location of the protein, which is suggested to contribute to CHOP induction and ER stress-mediated cell death (Hagman, Hays, Parazzoli, & Poitout, 2005; Martinez et al., 2008). In addition, FFA-induced increases in saturated phospholipids, particularly phosphatidylcholine, are proposed to contribute to lipotoxic ER stress (Ariyama, Kono, Matsuda, Inoue, & Arai, 2010; Borradaile et al., 2006; Newsholme et al., 2007). However, this has never been addressed in beta cells. Ceramide, a bioactive sphingolipid that has an established role as a proapoptotic lipid (Hannun & Obeid, 2008), is also suggested to account for palmitate-induced lipotoxicity (Paumen, Ishida, Muramatsu, Yamamoto, & Honjo, 1997; Shimabukuro et al., 1998). Inhibition of ceramide biosynthesis partially ablated the induction of cell death in lipotoxic beta cells (Lupi et al., 2002; Shimabukuro et al., 1998). However, the use of proximal inhibitors of *de novo* ceramide synthesis is unable to distinguish between the effects of ceramide itself or of its downstream metabolites.

Indeed, evidence for involvement of ceramide in beta cell lipotoxicity is less strong, nor is a putative mechanism for the proapoptotic function of ceramide readily apparent (Beeharry, Chambers, & Green, 2004; Lupi et al., 2002; Maedler et al., 2001). A recent study based on lipidomic analysis of palmitate-treated MIN6 β-cells shows no significant alteration in the amounts of either ceramide mass or sphingomyelin, although an enhancement of glucosylceramide mass was observed (Boslem et al., 2011). Sphingosine kinase 1 (SphK1), which catalyzes sphingosine to sphingosine 1-phosphate (S1P), is an important signaling enzyme that controls cell survival in a wide variety of cell types (Maceyka, Harikumar, Milstien, & Spiegel, 2012; Xia & Wadham, 2011). Recent studies suggest that SphK1 is also a key regulator of beta cell survival under lipotoxic ER stress (Qi et al., 2013; Veret et al., 2013). This has been supported by our recent studies both *in vitro* and *in vivo* (Qi et al., 2013). Enforced overexpression of SphK1 or addition of S1P prevents beta cells from lipotoxicity, while inhibition of SphK1 or transfection with a dominant negative mutant SphK1 potentiates FFA-induced cell death. Notably, SphK1 deficiency causes a significant loss of beta cell mass due to increased apoptosis in the mice fed a high-fat diet, leading to the onset of diabetes. As no accumulation of ceramide mass or sphingosine was found in the diabetic *Sphk1*$^{-/-}$ mice, the loss of functional beta cell mass is unlikely to be attributable to ceramide or sphingosine accumulation. Interestingly, administration of S1P prevents palmitate-induced beta cell apoptosis in the islets isolated from *Sphk1*$^{-/-}$ mice, highlighting a key role of S1P in promoting survival of beta cell undergoing lipotoxic ER stress.

While it is clear that ER stress is a critical mechanism for beta cell lipotoxicity, many other mechanisms and pathways contribute to FFA-induced cell death, including inflammation, oxidative stress, glucotoxicity, islet amyloid deposition, and epigenomic alterations, among others. For instance, exposure of beta cells to FFA induces the production of ROS in both a dose- and time-dependent manner (Poitout et al., 2010). FFA induces the expression of proinflammatory cytokines by activating the NF-κB pathway (Yuan et al., 2010). FFA can also induce JNK activation directly or indirectly. It has been noted that the deleterious effects of FFA occurs only in the presence of elevated glucose concentrations under certain circumstances, so-called glucolipotoxicity (Briaud, Harmon, Kelpe, Segu, & Poitout, 2001; El-Assaad et al., 2003; Giacca et al., 2011; Poitout et al., 2010). The "permissive" effect of glucose on FFA toxicity in the beta cell has been suggested to be secondary to a partitioning effect on lipid metabolism

(Giacca et al., 2011; Poitout et al., 2010), such that elevated glucose and FFA levels result in the accumulation of long-chain acyl CoA esters in the cytosol, which are detrimental to beta cell function (Prentki et al., 1992). The nature of the FFA themselves also appears to be relevant to glucolipotoxicity (Giacca et al., 2011), whereby saturated fatty acids (e.g., palmitic acid) confer the greatest toxicities and monounsaturated fatty acids (e.g., palmitoleic acid) might actually have a neutral or protective effect because they are more readily esterified into triglycerides (El-Assaad et al., 2003; Maedler et al., 2001; Mandl et al., 2009).

Irrespective of the early instigating mechanisms, cell death under ER stress depends on the core mitochondrial apoptotic machinery-integrated Bcl-2 protein family (Tait & Green, 2010). Bcl-2 family proteins contain one to four Bcl-2 homology (BH) domains (BH1–4), functioning as either proapoptotic or antiapoptotic signals in the face of cytotoxic insults (Adams & Cory, 1998). Of these, Bcl-2-associated X protein (Bax) and Bcl-2-antagonist/killer (Bak) form transmembrane transition pores via oligomerization in mitochondria. The conformational activation of the Bax/Bak complex is essential to trigger caspase activation. In the extrinsic apoptotic pathway, caspase-8 cleaves BH3-only protein, BH3-interacting domain death agonist (Bid), into a truncated form, t-Bid that induces the translocation and oligomerization of Bax and Bak, leading to cytochrome *c* release (Li, Zhu, Xu, & Yuan, 1998). In contrast, Bcl-2, Bcl-2-like protein 1 (Bcl-x_L), and myeloid cell leukemia sequence-1 (Mcl-1) exhibit antiapoptotic effects by inhibiting the transactivation of Bax and Bak. For example, Mcl-1 interacts with and suppresses Bak in healthy cells. During apoptosis, Mcl-1 undergoes rapid degradation through ubiquitination and the proteasomal pathway, which leads to the liberation of Bak and induction of the mitochondrial outer membrane permeabilization (Youle & Strasser, 2008). In response to death stimuli, BH3-only protein Bcl-2-associated agonist of cell death (Bad) is dephosphorylated and breaks away from its homeostatic binding protein 14-3-3. Then dephosphorylated Bad binds to and inhibits Bcl-2 or Bcl-x_L, leading to cytochrome *c* release (Zha, Harada, Yang, Jockel, & Korsmeyer, 1996). Enforced expression of BH3-only proteins, p53-upregulated modulator of apoptosis (Puma) and Noxa, also inhibits prosurvival Bcl-2 proteins, increases expression of Bax and Bak, and promotes pore-formation on mitochondria (Liu, Newland, & Jia, 2003; Oda et al., 2000). Chronic ER stress leads to BAX- and/or BAK-dependent apoptosis through the transcriptional upregulation of the BH3-only proteins BIM and PUMA, as well as the cell death sensitizer NOXA (Woehlbier & Hetz, 2011). CHOP promotes both the transcription of BIM and the downregulation of Bcl-2 expression, contributing to the induction of apoptosis (Hetz, 2012; Tabas & Ron, 2011). In addition to CHOP, ATF4 and p53 are also involved in the direct transcriptional upregulation of BH3-only proteins under ER stress (Hetz, 2012; Woehlbier & Hetz, 2011). Under certain conditions, activation of the IRE1α UPR pathway is also linked to apoptosis, through its ability to activate JNK and p38, as well as the degradation of mRNAs encoding for key-folding mediators via the IRE1-dependent decay of mRNA mechanism (Hetz, 2012).

4. ROLE OF cIAP1 IN BETA CELL SURVIVAL UNDER ER STRESS

Because the UPR can result in distinct and contrasting outputs, it is believed that additional mechanisms and pathways are required for cell fate decisions under ER stress. Emerging evidence from many different experimental systems reveals that the UPR cannot be considered as three linear and parallel pathways. Instead, the three major signaling branches of the UPR are interconnected with each other and interact with additional signal transduction networks, allowing cells to efficiently handle stress (Hetz, 2012). For example, our recent work demonstrates that cIAP1, a member of the inhibitor of apoptosis protein (IAP) family, plays an important role in the control of beta cell survival under lipotoxic stress through its interaction with the UPR pathways (Qi & Xia, 2012).

The IAP family is a group of endogenous negative regulators of apoptosis. The first IAP genes were identified in baculovirus as a substitute signal of p35, a pan-caspase inhibitor (Crook, Clem, & Miller, 1993). Soon after, the homologous proteins were found ubiquitously in nematodes, yeasts, and vertebrates (Uren, Coulson, & Vaux, 1998), and eight human IAPs identified, including NAIP/baculovirus IAP repeating (BIR)-containing protein 1 (BIRC1), cIAP1/BIRC2, cIAP2/BIRC3, X-linked IAP (XIAP)/BIRC4, survivin/BIRC5, BRUCE/BIRC6, livin/BIRC7, and IAP-like protein-2 (ILP-2)/BIRC8. In addition to inhibiting apoptosis, IAPs have recently emerged as important signaling molecules involved in a multitude of cellular processes, such as inflammation, immunity, cell migration, and cell proliferation (Gyrd-Hansen & Meier, 2010).

IAPs are featured as a typical structure consisting of four functional domains, including BIR domain, really interesting new gene (RING)

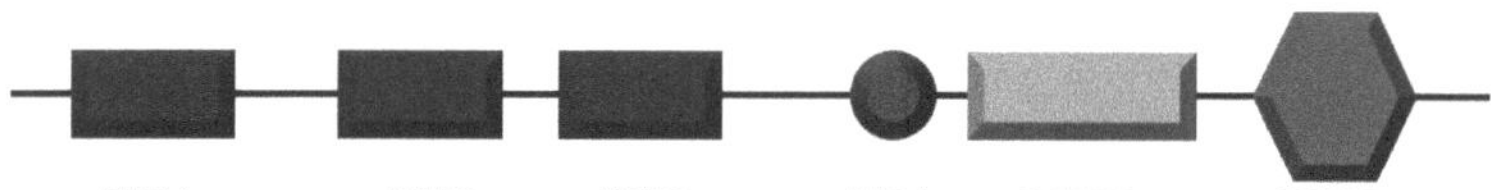

Figure 11.2 Domain structure of cIAP1. Three baculovirus IAP repeat (BIR) domains are located at the N-terminal of cIAP1 (indicated by red boxes). Along with the BIR domains, cIAP1 contains really interesting new gene (RING) domain at its C-terminus (indicated by green hexagon). cIAP1 also possesses a caspase activation and recruitment domain (CARD; indicated by yellow box) and a ubiquitin-associated (UBA) domain (indicated by blue circle) in the linker region between BIRs and CARD. (See the color plate.)

domain, ubiquitin-associated (UBA) domain, and caspase activation and recruitment domain (CARD) (Hunter, LaCasse, & Korneluk, 2007). cIAP1 contains three copies of the BIR domain (Fig. 11.2). The BIR domain is compacted as a surface groove by several α-helix, β-sheets, and chelated zinc (Hinds, Norton, Vaux, & Day, 1999). With these secondary structures, the BIR domain can mediate protein–protein interactions by directly interacting with IAP-binding motif in their partner proteins including caspase-9, caspase-3, caspase-7, Smac, and Omi (Dubrez-Daloz, Dupoux, & Cartier, 2008). Crystallographic studies reveal that BIR1 in cIAP1 is also required for the activation of NF-κB by interacting with TRAF2 (Samuel et al., 2006). Truncation of BIR2–BIR3 in cIAP1 inhibits the interaction of cIAP1 with the p12 subunit of caspase-9 and further suppresses apoptosome-mediated cleavage of caspase-3 (Abhari & Davoodi, 2008; Burke, Smith, & Smith, 2010; Gyrd-Hansen & Meier, 2010). In addition, BIR3 of cIAP1 can be recognized by Smac mimetics, leading to cIAP1 autoubiquitination (Cossu et al., 2010). The RING domain located at the C-terminus is critically required for the dimerization of cIAP1, which endows cIAP1 E3 ubiquitin ligase activity (Dueber et al., 2011; Silke et al., 2005). The UBA domain is located between the N-terminal BIR domains and the C-terminal RING domain, which binds to ubiquitin chains via a hydrophobic motif (Blankenship et al., 2009). The CARD domain structure has not been completely elucidated. However, based on the conserved properties, CARD is predicted to mediate the heterooligomerization of cIAP1 with other CARD-containing proteins, including Apaf-1, Bcl-10, and FADD (Hunter et al., 2007; Martin, 2001). Recently, CARD was shown to regulate E3 ligase activity of cIAP1 by preventing homodimerization and attachment of E2 ubiquitin-conjugating enzymes (Lopez et al., 2011).

The antiapoptotic property of IAPs is well documented, especially in cancer research fields. Overexpression of IAPs has been implicated in tumor cell survival (Hunter et al., 2007), and genetic amplification of cIAP1 can both promote tumorigenesis and sustain tumor growth in a mouse model of liver cancer (Zender et al., 2006). XIAP is able to directly bind to and inhibit caspase-9, caspase-3, and caspase-7, which accounts chiefly for its activity in antiapoptosis (Gyrd-Hansen & Meier, 2010). Unlike XIAP, although cIAP1 binds to caspase-7 and caspase-9, it cannot directly inhibit their proteolytic activity (Tenev, Zachariou, Wilson, Ditzel, & Meier, 2005). It is believed that the antiapoptotic activity of cIAP1 is attributable to its ability to modulate signaling pathways elicited by the tumor necrosis factor receptor (TNFR) superfamily (Li, Yang, & Ashwell, 2002; Samuel et al., 2006) and regulate NF-κB transcriptional activity (Bertrand et al., 2011; Samuel et al., 2006). Several mammalian IAPs may also utilize ubiquitination to regulate their own stability and, through cross-association, stability of other IAPs (Varfolomeev & Vucic, 2008). For example, treatment with glucocorticoids and etoposide results in both XIAP and cIAP1 autoubiquitination, and their subsequent degradation in the thymocytes (Yang, Fang, Jensen, Weissman, & Ashwell, 2000). cIAP1 also ubiquitinates cIAP2, leading to proteasomal degradation of cIAP2, and accordingly, cIAP1-null cells exhibit elevated levels of cIAP2 (Conze et al., 2005). In a similar fashion, cIAP1 can downregulate another interacting molecule, XIAP, by ubiquitination and subsequent proteasomal degradation (Silke et al., 2005).

As cIAP1 was initially found to associate with the TRAF1/2 heterodimer in TNFR2 complexes (Rothe, Pan, Henzel, Ayres, & Goeddel, 1995; Rothe, Wong, Henzel, & Goeddel, 1994), it is not surprising that cIAP1 possesses antiapoptotic activity by modulating TNFR signaling. Recruitment to the TNFR2 complex leads to cIAP1-mediated TRAF2 ubiquitination and degradation (Li et al., 2002). Reduction of TRAF2 protein levels blocks TNF-induced NFκB activation, resulting in enhanced caspase-8 activation and cell death (Li et al., 2002). In addition, cIAP1 activates NF-κB in response to TNFα stimulation by directly interacting with and ubiquitylating NEMO/IKKγ (Tang, Wang, Xiong, & Guan, 2003) or by regulating RIP1–4 ubiquitination (Bertrand et al., 2011). Apart from inhibiting death receptor-initiated apoptosis, cIAP1 has also been implicated in protection against the mitochondria-dependent apoptosis by its interaction with the apoptosomes and inhibition of caspases (Burke et al., 2010). Furthermore, cIAP1 can mediate polyubiquitination and proteasomal degradation of ASK1, which binds to TRAF2, leading to the inhibition of p38- and JNK-induced apoptosis as observed in cells undergoing oxidative stress and ER stress (Zhao, Conze, Hanover, & Ashwell, 2007).

Given the potent antiapoptotic activity of IAPs, it is surprising that there are only a few studies on the potential role of IAPs in regulating cell survival under ER stress conditions. An earlier study reports that treatment of MCF7 breast cancer cells with the chemical ER stressors tunicamycin and thapsigargin results in an increase in cIAP2 and XIAP expression through the PI3K–Akt signaling (Hu, Han, Couvillon, & Exton, 2004). Ablation of these IAPs by RNA interference sensitizes stressed cells to death, suggesting a role of IAPs in regulation of ER stress-mediated cell death (Hu et al., 2004). The expression of cIAP1 is also induced by the chemical ER stressors in HeLa cells and attenuates ER stress-induced cell death (Warnakulasuriyarachchi, Cerquozzi, Cheung, & Holcik, 2004). The induction of cIAP1 is executed at the level of protein synthesis and is mediated by an inducible internal ribosome entry site element, suggesting a mechanism by which cells upregulate cIAP during ER stress (Warnakulasuriyarachchi et al., 2004). By using PERK$^{-/-}$ fibroblasts, a recent study demonstrates that the chemical ER stressor induced upregulation of cIAP1 expression at both the transcriptional and translational levels and that both are dependent on activation of the PERK UPR pathway (Hamanaka, Bobrovnikova-Marjon, Ji, Liebhaber, & Diehl, 2009). Enforced overexpression of cIAP1 delays the early onset of apoptosis exhibited by PERK-deficient cells, highlighting the importance of cIAP1 induction for the survival following ER stress (Hamanaka et al., 2009). Interestingly, our recent studies show that cIAP1 is reduced in pancreatic beta cells undergoing apoptosis in response to ER stress induced by either FFA or the chemical ER stressor tunicamycin in both time-and dose-dependent manners (Qi & Xia, 2012). This is at variance with previous reports showing that ER stressors increased upregulation of IAPs in the transformed or cancer cell lines (Hamanaka et al., 2009; Hu et al., 2004; Warnakulasuriyarachchi et al., 2004). Such a conflicting finding could be attributable to the difference between experimental models applied in the studies. It is noted that although the mRNA levels of these IAPs are increased in the stressed beta cells, their protein levels are significantly reduced when cells are exposed to chronic ER stress and undergo apoptosis, suggesting that the reduced levels of cIAP1 might be a consequence of apoptosis. However, the reduction of cIAP1 occurs as early as 4 h after palmitate treatment in beta cells where no evident apoptosis is observed (Qi & Xia, 2012). Furthermore, cIAP1 reduction is insensitive to the pan-caspase inhibitor Z-VAD-fmk, placing it upstream of the caspase activation cascades and suggesting an active role of cIAP1 in ER stress-mediated apoptosis. Indeed, reintroduction of cIAP1 significantly prevents palmitate-induced beta cell death, whereas lipotoxicity is augmented in the cIAP1-knockdown beta cells or *cIap1*-deficient MEFs (Qi & Xia, 2012). Together, these data demonstrate that cIAP1 is a key endogenous protector against ER stress-mediated apoptosis in beta cells.

It is of interest to note that although both the saturated FFA palmitate and the unsaturated palmitoleate cause ER stress and CHOP induction in beta cells, only palmitate is capable of inducing cell death. Such a different fate of these stressed cells suggests that additional signals are required for the CHOP–UPR pathway to commit to apoptosis. The findings that cIAP1 is downregulated in ER stress-induced apoptotic cells suggest a key role of cIAP1 in determining beta cell fate during ER stress, which is supported by the following evidence (Qi & Xia, 2012): (i) the lipotoxic reagent palmitate or the chemical ER stressor tunicamycin, but not the nontoxic analog palmitoleate, induces cIAP1 reduction; (ii) cIAP1 expression levels are negatively correlated with CHOP expression; (iii) either the siRNA-mediated knockdown of cIAP1 in beta cells or knockout of *cIap1* in MEFs not only increases palmitate-induced apoptosis but also commits cells to death in response to the nontoxic palmitoleate treatment. Collectively, these findings highlight an essential role of cIAP1 for beta cell survival under ER stress.

As previously mentioned, cIAP1 has emerged as an E3 ubiquitin ligase that catalyzes both trans- and autoubiquitination, playing important roles in mitotic chromosome segregation, cellular morphogenesis, and cell signaling (Hunter et al., 2007; Mace, Shirley, & Day, 2010; Srinivasula & Ashwell, 2008). The E3 ubiquitin ligase activity is also implicated in the antiapoptotic activity of cIAP1 (Bertrand et al., 2011, 2008; Zhao et al., 2007). Interestingly, cIAP1 can mediate either nondegradative K63 or degradative K48 polyubiquitination of protein targets. For example, K63 polyubiquitination of RIP1 mediates TNFα-evoked NF-κB activation (Bertrand et al., 2008), whereas K48 auto- or transubiquitination mediates proteasomal degradation of cIAP1 itself or cIAP1-binding proteins such as caspase, Smac, TRAF2, ASK1, Mad1, cIAP2, and XIAP (Choi et al., 2009; Conze et al., 2005; Dueber et al., 2011; Hu & Yang, 2003; Silke et al., 2005; Wu et al., 2005; Xu et al., 2007; Zhao et al., 2007). Does the E3 activity of cIAP1 also account for its antiapoptotic effect in ER stress-associated apoptosis?

CHOP has been previously reported as a substrate for K48 polyubiquitination and proteasomal degradation (Hattori, Ohoka, Inoue, Hayashi, & Onozaki, 2003). Given the fact that cIAP1 is negatively correlated with CHOP expression in the stressed beta cells and that overexpression of cIAP1 prevents ER stressor-induced CHOP reduction, cIAP1 is thought to be responsible for CHOP degradation. Indeed, ubiquitination assays conducted in both cells and the cell-free systems clearly demonstrate that cIAP1 is an E3 ubiquitin ligase that catalyzes CHOP ubiquitination and degradation (Qi & Xia, 2012). Therefore, in addition to the well-documented antiapoptotic property, cIAP1 protects against cell death by promoting degradation of the proapoptotic protein CHOP, illustrating a new mechanism for cell fate decision under ER stress status (Fig. 11.3).

E3 ubiquitin ligases are classified as either RING or HECT type of ligases. cIAP1 belongs to RING domain-containing E3 ligases, which interact with both E2 enzymes and substrate proteins, and thus offers a platform for the transfer of ubiquitin from E2 enzymes directly to the lysine residue of the substrate (Deshaies & Joazeiro, 2009; Rotin & Kumar, 2009).

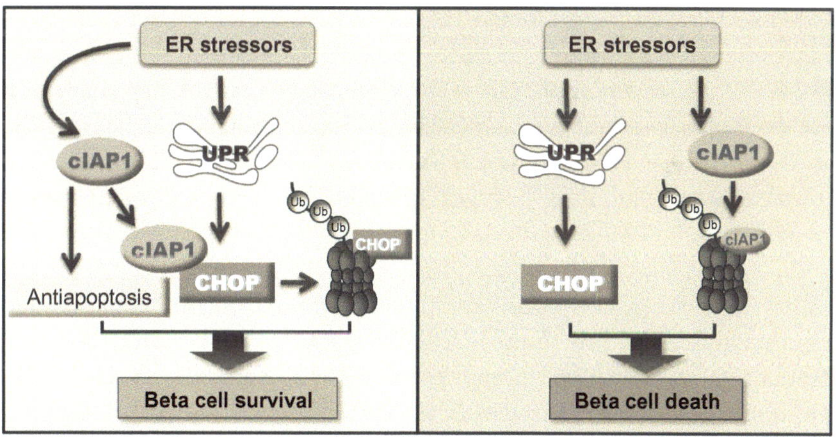

Figure 11.3 Model depicting the role of cIAP1 in determining beta cell fate under ER stress. For adaptation to ER stress, the UPR (e.g., induced by palmitoleate) activates survival pathways and increases the expression of cIAP1. cIAP1 functions through its antiapoptotic properties and the E3 ligase activity causing CHOP ubiquitination and degradation, ultimately leading to cell survival. Under certain ER stress conditions (e.g., exposure to palmitate), cIAP1 is quickly degraded through the apoptotic pathways, which relieves CHOP degradation and preserves its proapoptotic activity, resulting in cell death. (See the color plate.)

Accordingly, in contrast to full-length cIAP1, the recombinant cIAP1 lacking a RING domain fails to induce CHOP ubiquitination (Qi & Xia, 2012). The RING domain also determines the specificity of cIAP1 in selection of E2 enzymes, while different E2s mediate different forms of polyubiquitin chain linkage. For instance, Ubc13 mediates cIAP1-induced K63 polyubiquitination of RIP1 as a constitutive posttranslational modification, leading to NF-κB activation, but not degradation of RIP1 (Bertrand et al., 2008). On the other hand, some E2 enzymes evoke K48 polyubiquitination and proteasomal degradation of substrate proteins. For example, both Ubc5 and Ubc6 are implicated in cIAP1-mediated K48 ubiquitination and protein degradation. In the presence of Ubc5a, cIAP1 mediates proteasomal degradation of RIP1 (Park, Yoon, & Lee, 2004) and Smac (Hu & Yang, 2003). Incubation with Ubc5b leads to the autoubiquitination of cIAP1 (Feltham et al., 2011), and cIAP1-mediated transubiquitination of ASK1 (Zhao et al., 2007) and Mad1 (Xu et al., 2007). In addition, cIAP1 mediates K48 ubiquitination of caspase-3 and caspase-7 in cooperation with the Ubc5 family and Ubc6 (Choi et al., 2009). Furthermore, cIAP1 mediates K48 ubiquitination of TRAF2 at ER membranes in the presence of Ubc6e (Wu et al., 2005). We found that cIAP1 directly binds to and induces CHOP ubiquitination in the presence of UbcH5a, UbcH5b, and UbcH6 E2 enzymes, whereas other E2 enzymes that we tested are unable to mediate the cIAP1-dependent ubiquitination of CHOP (Qi & Xia, 2012). It is therefore likely that the key reaction is Lys 48 ubiquitination, by which cIAP1 promotes proteasomal degradation of CHOP. However, we cannot exclude the possibility that cIAP1 may also produce other ubiquitin linkages on CHOP, which requires further investigation.

In the model of FFA-induced ER stress in pancreatic beta cells, many studies have revealed a consistent phenomenon that both saturated and monounsaturated FFAs cause UPR activation and CHOP induction (Borradaile et al., 2006; Cnop et al., 2007; Karaskov et al., 2006; Kusminski et al., 2009; Maedler et al., 2001; Qi & Xia, 2012). However, only saturated FFAs are capable of inducing evident cell death, indicating that induction of CHOP during ER stress is necessary, but not sufficient, for triggering apoptosis. Indeed, overexpression of CHOP alone fails to reduce cell viability, but only sensitizes ER stressor-induced death in various cell types (McCullough et al., 2001; Qi & Xia, 2012; Zinszner et al., 1998). On the other hand, overexpression of CHOP undoubtedly promotes Bax translocation, downregulates Bcl-2, induces Bim, and potentiates cell death as reported previously (Oyadomari & Mori, 2004; Puthalakath et al., 2007). As discussed earlier, several mechanisms have been proposed to explain the cell fate decision following the UPR activation. We propose that CHOP probably functions as a sensitizer that decides the susceptibility of cells to the death stimuli, whereas cIAP1 acts as a scavenger of CHOP, which desensitizes cells from the stress-stimulated death. In this regard, the strength and duration of ER stressors are critical in regulating the balance between CHOP and cIAP1, which in turn determines cell fate, either adaptation to stress or commitment to death. This model provides a mechanistic insight into the cellular pathways utilized by cIAP1 to prevent cell death induced by ER stress. It is tempting to speculate that cIAP1 or its regulators may represent novel targets for therapeutic intervention to promote beta cell survival under lipotoxic and ER stress conditions, thereby providing an additional way to prevent and treat type 2 diabetes.

ACKNOWLEDGMENTS

We thank Dr. Carol Wadham for critical reading of the manuscript. This work was supported by grants from Australian National Health and Medical Research Council (NHMRC, Project #349348 and Program #571408). P. X. is a recipient of Cancer Institute NSW Research Fellowship, Australia, and Fudan Distinguished Professorship, China. Y. Q. is supported by NHMRC Scholarship, Australia.

REFERENCES

Abhari, B. A., & Davoodi, J. (2008). A mechanistic insight into SMAC peptide interference with XIAP-Bir2 inhibition of executioner caspases. *Journal of Molecular Biology*, *381*(3), 645–654.

Adams, J. M., & Cory, S. (1998). The Bcl-2 protein family: Arbiters of cell survival. *Science*, *281*(5381), 1322–1326.

Ariyama, H., Kono, N., Matsuda, S., Inoue, T., & Arai, H. (2010). Decrease in membrane phospholipid unsaturation induces unfolded protein response. *The Journal of Biological Chemistry*, *285*(29), 22027–22035.

Ashcroft, F. M., & Rorsman, P. (2012). Diabetes mellitus and the beta cell: The last ten years. *Cell*, *148*(6), 1160–1171.

Bassik, M. C., Scorrano, L., Oakes, S. A., Pozzan, T., & Korsmeyer, S. J. (2004). Phosphorylation of BCL-2 regulates ER Ca2+ homeostasis and apoptosis. *The EMBO Journal*, *23*(5), 1207–1216.

Beeharry, N., Chambers, J. A., & Green, I. C. (2004). Fatty acid protection from palmitic acid-induced apoptosis is lost following PI3-kinase inhibition. *Apoptosis*, *9*(5), 599–607.

Bertrand, M. J., Lippens, S., Staes, A., Gilbert, B., Roelandt, R., De Medts, J., et al. (2011). cIAP1/2 are direct E3 ligases conjugating diverse types of ubiquitin chains to receptor interacting proteins kinases 1 to 4 (RIP1-4). *PLoS One*, *6*(9), e22356.

Bertrand, M. J., Milutinovic, S., Dickson, K. M., Ho, W. C., Boudreault, A., Durkin, J., et al. (2008). cIAP1 and cIAP2 facilitate cancer cell survival by functioning as E3 ligases that promote RIP1 ubiquitination. *Molecular Cell*, *30*(6), 689–700.

Blankenship, J. W., Varfolomeev, E., Goncharov, T., Fedorova, A. V., Kirkpatrick, D. S., Izrael-Tomasevic, A., et al. (2009). Ubiquitin binding modulates IAP antagonist-stimulated proteasomal degradation of c-IAP1 and c-IAP2(1). *The Biochemical Journal*, *417*(1), 149–160.

Borradaile, N. M., Han, X., Harp, J. D., Gale, S. E., Ory, D. S., & Schaffer, J. E. (2006). Disruption of endoplasmic reticulum structure and integrity in lipotoxic cell death. *Journal of Lipid Research*, *47*(12), 2726–2737.

Boslem, E., MacIntosh, G., Preston, A. M., Bartley, C., Busch, A. K., Fuller, M., et al. (2011). A lipidomic screen of palmitate-treated MIN6 beta-cells links sphingolipid metabolites with endoplasmic reticulum (ER) stress and impaired protein trafficking. *The Biochemical Journal*, *435*(1), 267–276.

Briaud, I., Harmon, J. S., Kelpe, C. L., Segu, V. B., & Poitout, V. (2001). Lipotoxicity of the pancreatic beta-cell is associated with glucose-dependent esterification of fatty acids into neutral lipids. *Diabetes*, *50*(2), 315–321.

Bruhat, A., Jousse, C., Carraro, V., Reimold, A. M., Ferrara, M., & Fafournoux, P. (2000). Amino acids control mammalian gene transcription: Activating transcription factor 2 is essential for the amino acid responsiveness of the CHOP promoter. *Molecular and Cellular Biology*, *20*(19), 7192–7204.

Brush, M. H., Weiser, D. C., & Shenolikar, S. (2003). Growth arrest and DNA damage-inducible protein GADD34 targets protein phosphatase 1 alpha to the endoplasmic reticulum and promotes dephosphorylation of the alpha subunit of eukaryotic translation initiation factor 2. *Molecular and Cellular Biology*, *23*(4), 1292–1303.

Burke, S. P., Smith, L., & Smith, J. B. (2010). cIAP1 cooperatively inhibits procaspase-3 activation by the caspase-9 apoptosome. *The Journal of Biological Chemistry*, *285*(39), 30061–30068.

Busch, A. K., Gurisik, E., Cordery, D. V., Sudlow, M., Denyer, G. S., Laybutt, D. R., et al. (2005). Increased fatty acid desaturation and enhanced expression of stearoyl coenzyme A desaturase protects pancreatic beta-cells from lipoapoptosis. *Diabetes*, *54*(10), 2917–2924.

Cazanave, S. C., Elmi, N. A., Akazawa, Y., Bronk, S. F., Mott, J. L., & Gores, G. J. (2010). CHOP and AP-1 cooperatively mediate PUMA expression during lipoapoptosis. *American Journal of Physiology Gastrointestinal and Liver Physiology*, *299*(1), G236–G243.

Cerasi, E. (2011). β-Cell dysfunction vs insulin resistance in type 2 diabetes: The eternal "chicken and egg" question. *Medicographia*, *33*, 7.

Choi, Y. E., Butterworth, M., Malladi, S., Duckett, C. S., Cohen, G. M., & Bratton, S. B. (2009). The E3 ubiquitin ligase cIAP1 binds and ubiquitinates caspase-3 and -7 via unique mechanisms at distinct steps in their processing. *The Journal of Biological Chemistry*, *284*(19), 12772–12782.

Cnop, M., Hannaert, J. C., Hoorens, A., Eizirik, D. L., & Pipeleers, D. G. (2001). Inverse relationship between cytotoxicity of free fatty acids in pancreatic islet cells and cellular triglyceride accumulation. *Diabetes*, *50*(8), 1771–1777.

Cnop, M., Ladriere, L., Hekerman, P., Ortis, F., Cardozo, A. K., Dogusan, Z., et al. (2007). Selective inhibition of eukaryotic translation initiation factor 2 alpha dephosphorylation potentiates fatty acid-induced endoplasmic reticulum stress and causes pancreatic beta-cell dysfunction and apoptosis. *The Journal of Biological Chemistry*, *282*(6), 3989–3997.

Conze, D. B., Albert, L., Ferrick, D. A., Goeddel, D. V., Yeh, W. C., Mak, T., et al. (2005). Posttranscriptional downregulation of c-IAP2 by the ubiquitin protein ligase c-IAP1 in vivo. *Molecular and Cellular Biology*, *25*(8), 3348–3356.

Cossu, F., Malvezzi, F., Canevari, G., Mastrangelo, E., Lecis, D., Delia, D., et al. (2010). Recognition of Smac-mimetic compounds by the BIR domain of cIAP1. *Protein Science*, *19*(12), 2418–2429.

Crook, N. E., Clem, R. J., & Miller, L. K. (1993). An apoptosis-inhibiting baculovirus gene with a zinc finger-like motif. *Journal of Virology*, *67*(4), 2168–2174.
Deshaies, R. J., & Joazeiro, C. A. (2009). RING domain E3 ubiquitin ligases. *Annual Review of Biochemistry*, *78*, 399–434.
Donath, M. Y., Ehses, J. A., Maedler, K., Schumann, D. M., Ellingsgaard, H., Eppler, E., et al. (2005). Mechanisms of beta-cell death in type 2 diabetes. *Diabetes*, *54*(Suppl. 2), S108–S113.
Dubrez-Daloz, L., Dupoux, A., & Cartier, J. (2008). IAPs: More than just inhibitors of apoptosis proteins. *Cell Cycle*, 7(8), 1036–1046.
Dueber, E. C., Schoeffler, A. J., Lingel, A., Elliott, J. M., Fedorova, A. V., Giannetti, A. M., et al. (2011). Antagonists induce a conformational change in cIAP1 that promotes autoubiquitination. *Science*, *334*(6054), 376–380.
Dunger, A., Cunningham, J. M., Delaney, C. A., Lowe, J. E., Green, M. H., Bone, A. J., et al. (1996). Tumor necrosis factor-alpha and interferon-gamma inhibit insulin secretion and cause DNA damage in unweaned-rat islets. Extent of nitric oxide involvement. *Diabetes*, *45*(2), 183–189.
Eizirik, D. L., Cardozo, A. K., & Cnop, M. (2008). The role for endoplasmic reticulum stress in diabetes mellitus. *Endocrine Reviews*, *29*(1), 42–61.
Eizirik, D. L., & Cnop, M. (2010). ER stress in pancreatic beta cells: The thin red line between adaptation and failure. *Science Signaling*, *3*(110), pe7.
El-Assaad, W., Buteau, J., Peyot, M. L., Nolan, C., Roduit, R., Hardy, S., et al. (2003). Saturated fatty acids synergize with elevated glucose to cause pancreatic beta-cell death. *Endocrinology*, *144*(9), 4154–4163.
Fagone, P., & Jackowski, S. (2009). Membrane phospholipid synthesis and endoplasmic reticulum function. *Journal of Lipid Research*, *50*(Suppl), S311–316.
Feltham, R., Bettjeman, B., Budhidarmo, R., Mace, P. D., Shirley, S., Condon, S. M., et al. (2011). Smac mimetics activate the E3 ligase activity of cIAP1 protein by promoting RING domain dimerization. *The Journal of Biological Chemistry*, *286*(19), 17015–17028.
Fonseca, S. G., Fukuma, M., Lipson, K. L., Nguyen, L. X., Allen, J. R., Oka, Y., et al. (2005). WFS1 is a novel component of the unfolded protein response and maintains homeostasis of the endoplasmic reticulum in pancreatic beta-cells. *The Journal of Biological Chemistry*, *280*(47), 39609–39615.
Friedlander, R., Jarosch, E., Urban, J., Volkwein, C., & Sommer, T. (2000). A regulatory link between ER-associated protein degradation and the unfolded-protein response. *Nature Cell Biology*, *2*(7), 379–384.
Fu, H. Y., Okada, K., Liao, Y., Tsukamoto, O., Isomura, T., Asai, M., et al. (2010). Ablation of C/EBP homologous protein attenuates endoplasmic reticulum-mediated apoptosis and cardiac dysfunction induced by pressure overload. *Circulation*, *122*(4), 361–369.
Gardner, B. M., & Walter, P. (2011). Unfolded proteins are Ire1-activating ligands that directly induce the unfolded protein response. *Science*, *333*(6051), 1891–1894.
Giacca, A., Xiao, C., Oprescu, A. I., Carpentier, A. C., & Lewis, G. F. (2011). Lipid induced pancreatic beta-cell dysfunction: Focus on in vivo studies. *American Journal of Physiology, Endocrinology and Metabolism*, *300*(2), E255–E262.
Guest, P. C., Bailyes, E. M., & Hutton, J. C. (1997). Endoplasmic reticulum Ca2+ is important for the proteolytic processing and intracellular transport of proinsulin in the pancreatic beta-cell. *The Biochemical Journal*, *323*(Pt 2), 445–450.
Gyrd-Hansen, M., & Meier, P. (2010). IAPs: From caspase inhibitors to modulators of NF-kappaB, inflammation and cancer. *Nature Reviews Cancer*, *10*(8), 561–574.
Hagman, D. K., Hays, L. B., Parazzoli, S. D., & Poitout, V. (2005). Palmitate inhibits insulin gene expression by altering PDX-1 nuclear localization and reducing MafA expression in isolated rat islets of Langerhans. *The Journal of Biological Chemistry*, *280*(37), 32413–32418.

Hamanaka, R. B., Bobrovnikova-Marjon, E., Ji, X., Liebhaber, S. A., & Diehl, J. A. (2009). PERK-dependent regulation of IAP translation during ER stress. *Oncogene, 28*, 910–920.

Hannun, Y. A., & Obeid, L. M. (2008). Principles of bioactive lipid signalling: Lessons from sphingolipids. *Nature Reviews Molecular Cell Biology, 9*(2), 139–150.

Harding, H. P., Calfon, M., Urano, F., Novoa, I., & Ron, D. (2002). Transcriptional and translational control in the mammalian unfolded protein response. *Annual Review of Cell and Developmental Biology, 18*, 575–599.

Harding, H. P., Zhang, Y., Bertolotti, A., Zeng, H., & Ron, D. (2000). Perk is essential for translational regulation and cell survival during the unfolded protein response. *Molecular Cell, 5*(5), 897–904.

Hattori, T., Ohoka, N., Inoue, Y., Hayashi, H., & Onozaki, K. (2003). C/EBP family transcription factors are degraded by the proteasome but stabilized by forming dimer. *Oncogene, 22*(9), 1273–1280.

Hetz, C. (2012). The unfolded protein response: Controlling cell fate decisions under ER stress and beyond. *Nature Reviews Molecular Cell Biology, 13*(2), 89–102.

Hinds, M. G., Norton, R. S., Vaux, D. L., & Day, C. L. (1999). Solution structure of a baculoviral inhibitor of apoptosis (IAP) repeat. *Natural Structural Biology, 6*(7), 648–651.

Hotamisligil, G. S. (2010). Endoplasmic reticulum stress and the inflammatory basis of metabolic disease. *Cell, 140*(6), 900–917.

Hu, P., Han, Z., Couvillon, A. D., & Exton, J. H. (2004). Critical role of endogenous Akt/IAPs and MEK1/ERK pathways in counteracting endoplasmic reticulum stress-induced cell death. *The Journal of Biological Chemistry, 279*(47), 49420–49429.

Hu, S., & Yang, X. (2003). Cellular inhibitor of apoptosis 1 and 2 are ubiquitin ligases for the apoptosis inducer Smac/DIABLO. *The Journal of Biological Chemistry, 278*(12), 10055–10060.

Huang, C. J., Lin, C. Y., Haataja, L., Gurlo, T., Butler, A. E., Rizza, R. A., et al. (2007). High expression rates of human islet amyloid polypeptide induce endoplasmic reticulum stress mediated beta-cell apoptosis, a characteristic of humans with type 2 but not type 1 diabetes. *Diabetes, 56*(8), 2016–2027.

Hunter, A. M., LaCasse, E. C., & Korneluk, R. G. (2007). The inhibitors of apoptosis (IAPs) as cancer targets. *Apoptosis, 12*(9), 1543–1568.

Igoillo-Esteve, M., Marselli, L., Cunha, D. A., Ladriere, L., Ortis, F., Grieco, F. A., et al. (2010). Palmitate induces a pro-inflammatory response in human pancreatic islets that mimics CCL2 expression by beta cells in type 2 diabetes. *Diabetologia, 53*(7), 1395–1405.

Izumi, T., Yokota-Hashimoto, H., Zhao, S., Wang, J., Halban, P. A., & Takeuchi, T. (2003). Dominant negative pathogenesis by mutant proinsulin in the Akita diabetic mouse. *Diabetes, 52*(2), 409–416.

Jeffrey, K. D., Alejandro, E. U., Luciani, D. S., Kalynyak, T. B., Hu, X., Li, H., et al. (2008). Carboxypeptidase E mediates palmitate-induced beta-cell ER stress and apoptosis. *Proceedings of the National Academy of Sciences of the United States of America, 105*(24), 8452–8457.

Karaskov, E., Scott, C., Zhang, L., Teodoro, T., Ravazzola, M., & Volchuk, A. (2006). Chronic palmitate but not oleate exposure induces endoplasmic reticulum stress, which may contribute to INS-1 pancreatic beta-cell apoptosis. *Endocrinology, 147*(7), 3398–3407.

Kaufman, R. J. (1999). Stress signaling from the lumen of the endoplasmic reticulum: Coordination of gene transcriptional and translational controls. *Genes and Development, 13*(10), 1211–1233.

Kawaguchi, S., & Ng, D. T. (2011). Cell biology. Sensing ER stress. *Science, 333*(6051), 1830–1831.

Kohno, K., Normington, K., Sambrook, J., Gething, M. J., & Mori, K. (1993). The promoter region of the yeast KAR2 (BiP) gene contains a regulatory domain that responds to the presence of unfolded proteins in the endoplasmic reticulum. *Molecular and Cellular Biology, 13*(2), 877–890.

Kusminski, C. M., Shetty, S., Orci, L., Unger, R. H., & Scherer, P. E. (2009). Diabetes and apoptosis: Lipotoxicity. *Apoptosis, 14*(12), 1484–1495.

Lai, E., Teodoro, T., & Volchuk, A. (2007). Endoplasmic reticulum stress: Signaling the unfolded protein response. *Physiology (Bethesda), 22*, 193–201.

Laybutt, D. R., Preston, A. M., Akerfeldt, M. C., Kench, J. G., Busch, A. K., Biankin, A. V., et al. (2007). Endoplasmic reticulum stress contributes to beta cell apoptosis in type 2 diabetes. *Diabetologia, 50*(4), 752–763.

Lei, K., & Davis, R. J. (2003). JNK phosphorylation of Bim-related members of the Bcl2 family induces Bax-dependent apoptosis. *Proceedings of the National Academy of Sciences of the United States of America, 100*(5), 2432–2437.

Li, M., Baumeister, P., Roy, B., Phan, T., Foti, D., Luo, S., et al. (2000). ATF6 as a transcription activator of the endoplasmic reticulum stress element: Thapsigargin stress-induced changes and synergistic interactions with NF-Y and YY1. *Molecular and Cellular Biology, 20*(14), 5096–5106.

Li, X., Yang, Y., & Ashwell, J. D. (2002). TNF-RII and c-IAP1 mediate ubiquitination and degradation of TRAF2. *Nature, 416*(6878), 345–347.

Li, H., Zhu, H., Xu, C. J., & Yuan, J. (1998). Cleavage of BID by caspase 8 mediates the mitochondrial damage in the Fas pathway of apoptosis. *Cell, 94*(4), 491–501.

Lipson, K. L., Fonseca, S. G., Ishigaki, S., Nguyen, L. X., Foss, E., Bortell, R., et al. (2006). Regulation of insulin biosynthesis in pancreatic beta cells by an endoplasmic reticulum-resident protein kinase IRE1. *Cell Metabolism, 4*(3), 245–254.

Liu, F. T., Newland, A. C., & Jia, L. (2003). Bax conformational change is a crucial step for PUMA-mediated apoptosis in human leukemia. *Biochemical and Biophysical Research Communications, 310*(3), 956–962.

Lopez, J., John, S. W., Tenev, T., Rautureau, G. J., Hinds, M. G., Francalanci, F., et al. (2011). CARD-mediated autoinhibition of cIAP1's E3 ligase activity suppresses cell proliferation and migration. *Molecular Cell, 42*(5), 569–583.

Lupi, R., Dotta, F., Marselli, L., Del Guerra, S., Masini, M., Santangelo, C., et al. (2002). Prolonged exposure to free fatty acids has cytostatic and pro-apoptotic effects on human pancreatic islets: Evidence that beta-cell death is caspase mediated, partially dependent on ceramide pathway, and Bcl-2 regulated. *Diabetes, 51*(5), 1437–1442.

Ma, Y., Brewer, J. W., Diehl, J. A., & Hendershot, L. M. (2002). Two distinct stress signaling pathways converge upon the CHOP promoter during the mammalian unfolded protein response. *Journal of Molecular Biology, 318*(5), 1351–1365.

Mace, P. D., Shirley, S., & Day, C. L. (2010). Assembling the building blocks: Structure and function of inhibitor of apoptosis proteins. *Cell Death and Differentiation, 17*(1), 46–53.

Maceyka, M., Harikumar, K. B., Milstien, S., & Spiegel, S. (2012). Sphingosine-1-phosphate signaling and its role in disease. *Trends in Cell Biology, 22*(1), 50–60.

Maechler, P., & Wollheim, C. B. (2001). Mitochondrial function in normal and diabetic beta-cells. *Nature, 414*(6865), 807–812.

Maedler, K., Spinas, G. A., Dyntar, D., Moritz, W., Kaiser, N., & Donath, M. Y. (2001). Distinct effects of saturated and monounsaturated fatty acids on beta-cell turnover and function. *Diabetes, 50*(1), 69–76.

Mandl, J., Meszaros, T., Banhegyi, G., Hunyady, L., & Csala, M. (2009). Endoplasmic reticulum: Nutrient sensor in physiology and pathology. *Trends in Endocrinology and Metabolism, 20*(4), 194–201.

Marciniak, S. J., Yun, C. Y., Oyadomari, S., Novoa, I., Zhang, Y., Jungreis, R., et al. (2004). CHOP induces death by promoting protein synthesis and oxidation in the stressed endoplasmic reticulum. *Genes and Development, 18*(24), 3066–3077.

Martin, S. J. (2001). Dealing the CARDs between life and death. *Trends in Cell Biology, 11*(5), 188–189.
Martinez, S. C., Tanabe, K., Cras-Meneur, C., Abumrad, N. A., Bernal-Mizrachi, E., & Permutt, M. A. (2008). Inhibition of Foxo1 protects pancreatic islet beta-cells against fatty acid and endoplasmic reticulum stress-induced apoptosis. *Diabetes, 57*(4), 846–859.
Matsumoto, M., Minami, M., Takeda, K., Sakao, Y., & Akira, S. (1996). Ectopic expression of CHOP (GADD153) induces apoptosis in M1 myeloblastic leukemia cells. *FEBS Letters, 395*(2–3), 143–147.
McCullough, K. D., Martindale, J. L., Klotz, L. O., Aw, T. Y., & Holbrook, N. J. (2001). Gadd153 sensitizes cells to endoplasmic reticulum stress by down-regulating Bcl2 and perturbing the cellular redox state. *Molecular and Cellular Biology, 21*(4), 1249–1259.
Meusser, B., Hirsch, C., Jarosch, E., & Sommer, T. (2005). ERAD: The long road to destruction. *Nature Cell Biology*, 7(8), 766–772.
Momoi, T. (2004). Caspases involved in ER stress-mediated cell death. *Journal of Chemical Neuroanatomy, 28*(1–2), 101–105.
Morishima, N., Nakanishi, K., Takenouchi, H., Shibata, T., & Yasuhiko, Y. (2002). An endoplasmic reticulum stress-specific caspase cascade in apoptosis. Cytochrome c-independent activation of caspase-9 by caspase-12. *The Journal of Biological Chemistry, 277*(37), 34287–34294.
Nadanaka, S., Yoshida, H., Sato, R., & Mori, K. (2006). Analysis of ATF6 activation in Site-2 protease-deficient Chinese hamster ovary cells. *Cell Structure and Function, 31*(2), 109–116.
Newsholme, P., Keane, D., Welters, H. J., & Morgan, N. G. (2007). Life and death decisions of the pancreatic beta-cell: The role of fatty acids. *Clinical Science (London), 112*(1), 27–42.
Nikawa, J., & Yamashita, S. (1992). IRE1 encodes a putative protein kinase containing a membrane-spanning domain and is required for inositol phototrophy in Saccharomyces cerevisiae. *Molecular Microbiology, 6*(11), 1441–1446.
Nishikawa, S., Brodsky, J. L., & Nakatsukasa, K. (2005). Roles of molecular chaperones in endoplasmic reticulum (ER) quality control and ER-associated degradation (ERAD). *Journal of Biochemistry, 137*(5), 551–555.
Nishitoh, H., Matsuzawa, A., Tobiume, K., Saegusa, K., Takeda, K., Inoue, K., et al. (2002). ASK1 is essential for endoplasmic reticulum stress-induced neuronal cell death triggered by expanded polyglutamine repeats. *Genes and Development, 16*(11), 1345–1355.
Novoa, I., Zhang, Y., Zeng, H., Jungreis, R., Harding, H. P., & Ron, D. (2003). Stress-induced gene expression requires programmed recovery from translational repression. *The EMBO Journal, 22*(5), 1180–1187.
Oda, E., Ohki, R., Murasawa, H., Nemoto, J., Shibue, T., Yamashita, T., et al. (2000). Noxa, a BH3-only member of the Bcl-2 family and candidate mediator of p53-induced apoptosis. *Science, 288*(5468), 1053–1058.
Ohoka, N., Hattori, T., Kitagawa, M., Onozaki, K., & Hayashi, H. (2007). Critical and functional regulation of CHOP (C/EBP homologous protein) through the N-terminal portion. *The Journal of Biological Chemistry, 282*(49), 35687–35694.
Oyadomari, S., Harding, H. P., Zhang, Y., Oyadomari, M., & Ron, D. (2008). Dephosphorylation of translation initiation factor 2 alpha enhances glucose tolerance and attenuates hepatosteatosis in mice. *Cell Metabolism*, 7(6), 520–532.
Oyadomari, S., Koizumi, A., Takeda, K., Gotoh, T., Akira, S., Araki, E., et al. (2002). Targeted disruption of the Chop gene delays endoplasmic reticulum stress-mediated diabetes. *The Journal of Clinical Investigation, 109*(4), 525–532.
Oyadomari, S., & Mori, M. (2004). Roles of CHOP/GADD153 in endoplasmic reticulum stress. *Cell Death and Differentiation, 11*(4), 381–389.
Oyadomari, S., Takeda, K., Takiguchi, M., Gotoh, T., Matsumoto, M., Wada, I., et al. (2001). Nitric oxide-induced apoptosis in pancreatic beta cells is mediated by the

endoplasmic reticulum stress pathway. *Proceedings of the National Academy of Sciences of the United States of America, 98*(19), 10845–10850.

Ozcan, U., Cao, Q., Yilmaz, E., Lee, A. H., Iwakoshi, N. N., Ozdelen, E., et al. (2004). Endoplasmic reticulum stress links obesity, insulin action, and type 2 diabetes. *Science, 306*(5695), 457–461.

Park, S. M., Yoon, J. B., & Lee, T. H. (2004). Receptor interacting protein is ubiquitinated by cellular inhibitor of apoptosis proteins (c-IAP1 and c-IAP2) in vitro. *FEBS Letters, 566*(1–3), 151–156.

Paumen, M. B., Ishida, Y., Muramatsu, M., Yamamoto, M., & Honjo, T. (1997). Inhibition of carnitine palmitoyltransferase I augments sphingolipid synthesis and palmitate-induced apoptosis. *The Journal of Biological Chemistry, 272*(6), 3324–3329.

Poitout, V., Amyot, J., Semache, M., Zarrouki, B., Hagman, D., & Fontes, G. (2010). Glucolipotoxicity of the pancreatic beta cell. *Biochimica et Biophysica Acta, 1801*(3), 289–298.

Prentki, M., & Nolan, C. J. (2006). Islet beta cell failure in type 2 diabetes. *The Journal of Clinical Investigation, 116*(7), 1802–1812.

Prentki, M., Vischer, S., Glennon, M. C., Regazzi, R., Deeney, J. T., & Corkey, B. E. (1992). Malonyl-CoA and long chain acyl-CoA esters as metabolic coupling factors in nutrient-induced insulin secretion. *The Journal of Biological Chemistry, 267*(9), 5802–5810.

Preston, A. M., Gurisik, E., Bartley, C., Laybutt, D. R., & Biden, T. J. (2009). Reduced endoplasmic reticulum (ER)-to-Golgi protein trafficking contributes to ER stress in lipotoxic mouse beta cells by promoting protein overload. *Diabetologia, 52*(11), 2369–2373.

Puthalakath, H., O'Reilly, L. A., Gunn, P., Lee, L., Kelly, P. N., Huntington, N. D., et al. (2007). ER stress triggers apoptosis by activating BH3-only protein Bim. *Cell, 129*(7), 1337–1349.

Qi, Y., Chen, J., Lay, A., Don, A., Vadas, M. A., & Xia, P. (2013). Loss of sphingosine kinase 1 predisposes to the onset of diabetes via promoting pancreatic β-cell death in diet-induced obese mice. *The FASEB Journal, 27*(10), 4294–4304.

Qi, Y., & Xia, P. (2012). Cellular inhibitor of apoptosis protein-1 (cIAP1) plays a critical role in beta-cell survival under endoplasmic reticulum stress: Promoting ubiquitination and degradation of C/EBP homologous protein (CHOP). *The Journal of Biological Chemistry, 287*(38), 32236–32245.

Ramirez-Alcantara, V., LoGuidice, A., & Boelsterli, U. A. (2009). Protection from diclofenac-induced small intestinal injury by the JNK inhibitor SP600125 in a mouse model of NSAID-associated enteropathy. *American Journal of Physiology Gastrointestinal and Liver Physiology, 297*(5), G990–G998.

Rao, R. V., & Bredesen, D. E. (2004). Misfolded proteins, endoplasmic reticulum stress and neurodegeneration. *Current Opinion in Cell Biology, 16*(6), 653–662.

Richly, H., Rape, M., Braun, S., Rumpf, S., Hoege, C., & Jentsch, S. (2005). A series of ubiquitin binding factors connects CDC48/p97 to substrate multiubiquitylation and proteasomal targeting. *Cell, 120*(1), 73–84.

Ron, D., & Walter, P. (2007). Signal integration in the endoplasmic reticulum unfolded protein response. *Nature Reviews Molecular Cell Biology, 8*(7), 519–529.

Rothe, M., Pan, M. G., Henzel, W. J., Ayres, T. M., & Goeddel, D. V. (1995). The TNFR2-TRAF signaling complex contains two novel proteins related to baculoviral inhibitor of apoptosis proteins. *Cell, 83*(7), 1243–1252.

Rothe, M., Wong, S. C., Henzel, W. J., & Goeddel, D. V. (1994). A novel family of putative signal transducers associated with the cytoplasmic domain of the 75 kDa tumor necrosis factor receptor. *Cell, 78*(4), 681–692.

Rotin, D., & Kumar, S. (2009). Physiological functions of the HECT family of ubiquitin ligases. *Nature Reviews Molecular Cell Biology, 10*(6), 398–409.

Rutkowski, D. T., Arnold, S. M., Miller, C. N., Wu, J., Li, J., Gunnison, K. M., et al. (2006). Adaptation to ER stress is mediated by differential stabilities of pro-survival and pro-apoptotic mRNAs and proteins. *PLoS Biology*, *4*(11), e374.

Rutkowski, D. T., & Kaufman, R. J. (2007). That which does not kill me makes me stronger: Adapting to chronic ER stress. *Trends in Biochemical Sciences*, *32*(10), 469–476.

Saleh, M., Mathison, J. C., Wolinski, M. K., Bensinger, S. J., Fitzgerald, P., Droin, N., et al. (2006). Enhanced bacterial clearance and sepsis resistance in caspase-12-deficient mice. *Nature*, *440*(7087), 1064–1068.

Samuel, T., Welsh, K., Lober, T., Togo, S. H., Zapata, J. M., & Reed, J. C. (2006). Distinct BIR domains of cIAP1 mediate binding to and ubiquitination of tumor necrosis factor receptor-associated factor 2 and second mitochondrial activator of caspases. *The Journal of Biological Chemistry*, *281*(2), 1080–1090.

Sanges, D., & Marigo, V. (2006). Cross-talk between two apoptotic pathways activated by endoplasmic reticulum stress: Differential contribution of caspase-12 and AIF. *Apoptosis*, *11*(9), 1629–1641.

Scheuner, D., & Kaufman, R. J. (2008). The unfolded protein response: A pathway that links insulin demand with beta-cell failure and diabetes. *Endocrine Reviews*, *29*(3), 317–333.

Scheuner, D., Song, B., McEwen, E., Liu, C., Laybutt, R., Gillespie, P., et al. (2001). Translational control is required for the unfolded protein response and in vivo glucose homeostasis. *Molecular Cell*, *7*(6), 1165–1176.

Scheuner, D., Vander Mierde, D., Song, B., Flamez, D., Creemers, J. W., Tsukamoto, K., et al. (2005). Control of mRNA translation preserves endoplasmic reticulum function in beta cells and maintains glucose homeostasis. *Nature Medicine*, *11*(7), 757–764.

Schroder, M., & Kaufman, R. J. (2005). ER stress and the unfolded protein response. *Mutation Research*, *569*(1–2), 29–63.

Shi, Y., An, J., Liang, J., Hayes, S. E., Sandusky, G. E., Stramm, L. E., et al. (1999). Characterization of a mutant pancreatic eIF-2alpha kinase, PEK, and co-localization with somatostatin in islet delta cells. *The Journal of Biological Chemistry*, *274*(9), 5723–5730.

Shi, Y., Vattem, K. M., Sood, R., An, J., Liang, J., Stramm, L., et al. (1998). Identification and characterization of pancreatic eukaryotic initiation factor 2 alpha-subunit kinase, PEK, involved in translational control. *Molecular and Cellular Biology*, *18*(12), 7499–7509.

Shimabukuro, M., Higa, M., Zhou, Y. T., Wang, M. Y., Newgard, C. B., & Unger, R. H. (1998). Lipoapoptosis in beta-cells of obese prediabetic fa/fa rats. Role of serine palmitoyltransferase overexpression. *The Journal of Biological Chemistry*, *273*(49), 32487–32490.

Silke, J., Kratina, T., Chu, D., Ekert, P. G., Day, C. L., Pakusch, M., et al. (2005). Determination of cell survival by RING-mediated regulation of inhibitor of apoptosis (IAP) protein abundance. *Proceedings of the National Academy of Sciences of the United States of America*, *102*(45), 16182–16187.

Smith, M. H., Ploegh, H. L., & Weissman, J. S. (2011). Road to ruin: Targeting proteins for degradation in the endoplasmic reticulum. *Science*, *334*(6059), 1086–1090.

Song, B., Scheuner, D., Ron, D., Pennathur, S., & Kaufman, R. J. (2008). Chop deletion reduces oxidative stress, improves beta cell function, and promotes cell survival in multiple mouse models of diabetes. *The Journal of Clinical Investigation*, *118*(10), 3378–3389.

Srinivasula, S. M., & Ashwell, J. D. (2008). IAPs: What's in a name? *Molecular Cell*, *30*(2), 123–135.

Szegezdi, E., Logue, S. E., Gorman, A. M., & Samali, A. (2006). Mediators of endoplasmic reticulum stress-induced apoptosis. *EMBO Reports*, *7*(9), 880–885.

Tabas, I., & Ron, D. (2011). Integrating the mechanisms of apoptosis induced by endoplasmic reticulum stress. *Nature Cell Biology*, *13*(3), 184–190.

Tait, S. W., & Green, D. R. (2010). Mitochondria and cell death: Outer membrane permeabilization and beyond. *Nature Reviews Molecular Cell Biology*, *11*(9), 621–632.

Tan, Y., Dourdin, N., Wu, C., De Veyra, T., Elce, J. S., & Greer, P. A. (2006). Ubiquitous calpains promote caspase-12 and JNK activation during endoplasmic reticulum stress-induced apoptosis. *The Journal of Biological Chemistry*, *281*(23), 16016–16024.

Tang, E. D., Wang, C. Y., Xiong, Y., & Guan, K. L. (2003). A role for NF-kappaB essential modifier/IkappaB kinase-gamma (NEMO/IKKgamma) ubiquitination in the activation of the IkappaB kinase complex by tumor necrosis factor-alpha. *The Journal of Biological Chemistry*, *278*(39), 37297–37305.

Tenev, T., Zachariou, A., Wilson, R., Ditzel, M., & Meier, P. (2005). IAPs are functionally non-equivalent and regulate effector caspases through distinct mechanisms. *Nature Cell Biology*, 7(1), 70–77.

Uren, A. G., Coulson, E. J., & Vaux, D. L. (1998). Conservation of baculovirus inhibitor of apoptosis repeat proteins (BIRPs) in viruses, nematodes, vertebrates and yeasts. *Trends in Biochemical Sciences*, *23*(5), 159–162.

Varfolomeev, E., & Vucic, D. (2008). (Un)expected roles of c-IAPs in apoptotic and NFkappaB signaling pathways. *Cell Cycle*, 7(11), 1511–1521.

Vembar, S. S., & Brodsky, J. L. (2008). One step at a time: Endoplasmic reticulum-associated degradation. *Nature Reviews Molecular Cell Biology*, *9*(12), 944–957.

Veret, J., Coant, N., Gorshkova, I. A., Giussani, P., Fradet, M., Riccitelli, E., et al. (2013). Role of palmitate-induced sphingoid base-1-phosphate biosynthesis in INS-1 beta-cell survival. *Biochimica et Biophysica Acta*, *1831*(2), 251–262.

Wang, X. Z., & Ron, D. (1996). Stress-induced phosphorylation and activation of the transcription factor CHOP (GADD153) by p38 MAP Kinase. *Science*, *272*(5266), 1347–1349.

Warnakulasuriyarachchi, D., Cerquozzi, S., Cheung, H. H., & Holcik, M. (2004). Translational induction of the inhibitor of apoptosis protein HIAP2 during endoplasmic reticulum stress attenuates cell death and is mediated via an inducible internal ribosome entry site element. *The Journal of Biological Chemistry*, *279*(17), 17148–17157.

Woehlbier, U., & Hetz, C. (2011). Modulating stress responses by the UPRosome: A matter of life and death. *Trends in Biochemical Sciences*, *36*(6), 329–337.

Wu, C. J., Conze, D. B., Li, X., Ying, S. X., Hanover, J. A., & Ashwell, J. D. (2005). TNF-alpha induced c-IAP1/TRAF2 complex translocation to a Ubc6-containing compartment and TRAF2 ubiquitination. *The EMBO Journal*, *24*(10), 1886–1898.

Wu, J., & Kaufman, R. J. (2006). From acute ER stress to physiological roles of the Unfolded Protein Response. *Cell Death and Differentiation*, *13*(3), 374–384.

Xia, P., & Wadham, C. (2011). Sphingosine 1-phosphate, a key mediator of the cytokine network: Juxtacrine signaling. *Cytokine and Growth Factor Reviews*, *22*(1), 45–53.

Xu, C., Bailly-Maitre, B., & Reed, J. C. (2005). Endoplasmic reticulum stress: Cell life and death decisions. *The Journal of Clinical Investigation*, *115*(10), 2656 2664.

Xu, L., Zhu, J., Hu, X., Zhu, H., Kim, H. T., LaBaer, J., et al. (2007). c-IAP1 cooperates with Myc by acting as a ubiquitin ligase for Mad1. *Molecular Cell*, *28*(5), 914–922.

Yang, Y., Fang, S., Jensen, J. P., Weissman, A. M., & Ashwell, J. D. (2000). Ubiquitin protein ligase activity of IAPs and their degradation in proteasomes in response to apoptotic stimuli. *Science*, *288*(5467), 874–877.

Ye, J., Rawson, R. B., Komuro, R., Chen, X., Dave, U. P., Prywes, R., et al. (2000). ER stress induces cleavage of membrane-bound ATF6 by the same proteases that process SREBPs. *Molecular Cell*, *6*(6), 1355–1364.

Yoneda, T., Imaizumi, K., Oono, K., Yui, D., Gomi, F., Katayama, T., et al. (2001). Activation of caspase-12, an endoplastic reticulum (ER) resident caspase, through tumor necrosis factor receptor-associated factor 2-dependent mechanism in response to the ER stress. *The Journal of Biological Chemistry*, *276*(17), 13935–13940.

Yoshida, H., Matsui, T., Yamamoto, A., Okada, T., & Mori, K. (2001). XBP1 mRNA is induced by ATF6 and spliced by IRE1 in response to ER stress to produce a highly active transcription factor. *Cell*, *107*(7), 881–891.

Youle, R. J., & Strasser, A. (2008). The BCL-2 protein family: Opposing activities that mediate cell death. *Nature Reviews Molecular Cell Biology*, *9*(1), 47–59.
Yuan, H., Zhang, X., Huang, X., Lu, Y., Tang, W., Man, Y., et al. (2010). NADPH oxidase 2-derived reactive oxygen species mediate FFAs-induced dysfunction and apoptosis of beta-cells via JNK, p38 MAPK and p53 pathways. *PLoS One*, *5*(12), e15726.
Yusta, B., Baggio, L. L., Estall, J. L., Koehler, J. A., Holland, D. P., Li, H., et al. (2006). GLP-1 receptor activation improves beta cell function and survival following induction of endoplasmic reticulum stress. *Cell Metabolism*, *4*(5), 391–406.
Zender, L., Spector, M. S., Xue, W., Flemming, P., Cordon-Cardo, C., Silke, J., et al. (2006). Identification and validation of oncogenes in liver cancer using an integrative oncogenomic approach. *Cell*, *125*(7), 1253–1267.
Zha, J., Harada, H., Yang, E., Jockel, J., & Korsmeyer, S. J. (1996). Serine phosphorylation of death agonist BAD in response to survival factor results in binding to 14-3-3 not BCL-X(L). *Cell*, *87*(4), 619–628.
Zhang, W., Feng, D., Li, Y., Iida, K., McGrath, B., & Cavener, D. R. (2006). PERK EIF2AK3 control of pancreatic beta cell differentiation and proliferation is required for postnatal glucose homeostasis. *Cell Metabolism*, *4*(6), 491–497.
Zhang, P., McGrath, B., Li, S., Frank, A., Zambito, F., Reinert, J., et al. (2002). The PERK eukaryotic initiation factor 2 alpha kinase is required for the development of the skeletal system, postnatal growth, and the function and viability of the pancreas. *Molecular and Cellular Biology*, *22*(11), 3864–3874.
Zhao, Y., Conze, D. B., Hanover, J. A., & Ashwell, J. D. (2007). Tumor necrosis factor receptor 2 signaling induces selective c-IAP1-dependent ASK1 ubiquitination and terminates mitogen-activated protein kinase signaling. *The Journal of Biological Chemistry*, *282*(11), 7777–7782.
Zhou, J., Liu, C. Y., Back, S. H., Clark, R. L., Peisach, D., Xu, Z., et al. (2006). The crystal structure of human IRE1 luminal domain reveals a conserved dimerization interface required for activation of the unfolded protein response. *Proceedings of the National Academy of Sciences of the United States of America*, *103*(39), 14343–14348.
Zhou, Y. P., Pena, J. C., Roe, M. W., Mittal, A., Levisetti, M., Baldwin, A. C., et al. (2000). Overexpression of Bcl-x(L) in beta-cells prevents cell death but impairs mitochondrial signal for insulin secretion. *American Journal of Physiology, Endocrinology and Metabolism*, *278*(2), E340–E351.
Zinszner, H., Kuroda, M., Wang, X., Batchvarova, N., Lightfoot, R. T., Remotti, H., et al. (1998). CHOP is implicated in programmed cell death in response to impaired function of the endoplasmic reticulum. *Genes and Development*, *12*(7), 982–995.

CHAPTER TWELVE

β-Cell Responses to Nitric Oxide

Katarzyna A. Broniowska, Bryndon J. Oleson, John A. Corbett[1]
Department of Biochemistry, Medical College of Wisconsin, Milwaukee, Wisconsin, USA
[1]Corresponding author: e-mail address: jcorbett@mcw.edu

Contents

Abstract

Autoimmune diabetes is characterized by the selective destruction of insulin-secreting β-cells that occurs during an inflammatory reaction in and around pancreatic islets of Langerhans. Cytokines such as interleukin-1, released by activated immune cells, have been shown to inhibit insulin secretion from pancreatic β-cells and cause islet destruction. In response to cytokines, β-cells express inducible nitric oxide synthase and produce micromolar levels of the free radical nitric oxide. Nitric oxide inhibits the mitochondrial oxidation of glucose resulting in an impairment of insulin secretion. Nitric oxide is also responsible for cytokine-mediated DNA damage in β-cells. While nitric oxide mediates the inhibitory and toxic effects of cytokines, it also activates protective pathways that allow β-cells to recover from this damage. This review will focus on the dual role of nitric oxide as a mediator of cytokine-induced damage and the activator of repair mechanisms that protect β-cells from cytokine-mediated injury.

1. INTRODUCTION

Insulin-dependent diabetes mellitus (type-1 diabetes, T1D) is characterized by the selective and autoimmune destruction of insulin-secreting β-cells found in the pancreatic islets of Langerhans. Death of β-cells occurs

Vitamins and Hormones, Volume 95
ISSN 0083-6729
http://dx.doi.org/10.1016/B978-0-12-800174-5.00012-0

during an inflammatory reaction in and around the pancreatic islets. Cytokines, released from infiltrating macrophages and leukocytes, are believed to contribute to the development of diabetes by directly inducing β-cell damage. *In vitro* studies have shown that cytokines mediate β-cell damage via increased expression of inducible nitric oxide synthase (iNOS) and the β-cell production of nitric oxide. This chapter details the responses of β-cells to nitric oxide, with a focus on the characterization of nitric oxide as a mediator of cytokine-induced damage, the mechanisms of β-cell death, and the role of nitric oxide in activating the signaling pathways that facilitate the recovery from cytokine-induced injury.

2. CYTOKINE-INDUCED DAMAGE

The first studies demonstrating that cytokines cause both functional and structural damages to pancreatic islets were published almost 30 years ago. In elegant studies by Mandrup-Poulsen et al. it was observed that treatment of islets with conditioned medium obtained from activated blood mononuclear cells decreased glucose-stimulated insulin secretion, insulin, and glucagon content and caused islet disintegration (Mandrup-Poulsen, Bendtzen, Nielsen, Bendixen, & Nerup, 1985). The primary component of this conditioned medium responsible for islet destruction was identified as interleukin-1 (IL-1) (Bendtzen et al., 1986; Mandrup-Poulsen et al., 1986). These reports were confirmed by studies showing that IL-1 modulates glucose-stimulated insulin secretion from isolated rat islets, with low concentrations stimulating insulin secretion and high concentrations inhibiting insulin secretion in a concentration-dependent manner (Comens, Wolf, Unanue, Lacy, & McDaniel, 1987; Spinas et al., 1986). The inhibitory effects elicited by IL-1 are also time-dependent, with an inhibition of insulin secretion detectable within the first 5–8 h of exposure and maximal inhibitory effect after 18 h (Hughes, Colca, Easom, Turk, & McDaniel, 1990). Prolonged incubation (4–7 days) with cytokines results in complete destruction of islets of Langerhans (Mandrup-Poulsen et al., 1985). The inhibitory effects of IL-1 require ~5 h to develop, and studies have shown that even a brief 1 h pulse with IL-1 is sufficient to inhibit glucose-stimulated insulin secretion several hours later (Hughes et al., 1990). This finding led to the hypothesis that new gene transcription was required to mediate the deleterious effects of IL-1 on islet function. Indeed, an inhibitor of transcription, actinomycin D, administered during a 1 h pulse with IL-1, protected against IL-1-induced inhibition of insulin secretion.

Furthermore, the inhibitory actions of IL-1 require the translation of new proteins, as the addition of cycloheximide, an inhibitor of translation, during the first 8 h after a 1 h pulse with IL-1 also preserved glucose-stimulated insulin secretion (Hughes et al., 1990).

Following the characterization of the inhibitory effects of IL-1 on β-cell function, several studies identified that the resident intraislet macrophages can produce IL-1 in the area surrounding β-cells. The first report examined the activation of islet lymphoid cells as a mechanism responsible for the destruction of islets (Lacy & Finke, 1991). This study showed that prolonged exposure (7 days) to interferon-γ (IFN-γ), which is sufficient to activate islet lymphoid cells, caused the destruction of islets; however, IFN-γ had no effect when lymphoid cells were eliminated by *in vitro* culture at 24 °C (Lacy & Finke, 1991). Based on these observations, Dr. Paul Lacy proposed that cytokines, such as IL-1, may be precipitating factors in T1D pathogenesis, causing initial β-cell damage that leads to antigen release, T-lymphocyte recruitment, and autoimmune destruction of the remaining β-cells (Lacy, 1994). Consistent with the Lacy hypothesis, we showed that treatment of islets with tumor necrosis factor (TNF) and lipopolysaccharide (LPS), conditions that activate macrophages, inhibits glucose-stimulated insulin secretion in intact islets, but not in purified β-cells (Corbett & McDaniel, 1995). Furthermore, treatment of the islets with the IL-1 receptor antagonist protein prevents IFN- and LPS-induced inhibition of insulin secretion, demonstrating that nonendocrine cells within pancreatic islets secrete sufficient amounts of IL-1 to inhibit β-cell function.

The biochemical mechanism by which IL-1 inhibits secretion of insulin relies on the inhibition of mitochondrial oxidation. There is a temporal correlation between inhibition of glucose oxidation to CO_2, decreases in cellular ATP levels, and inhibition of insulin secretion in response to IL-1 (Corbett, Wang, Sweetland, Lancaster, & McDaniel, 1992; Eizirik, 1988). At the same time, glucose utilization through glycolysis is unaffected, demonstrating that the inhibition of glucose oxidation is at the level of mitochondria (Eizirik, 1988). The net effect is a decrease in cellular ATP levels, resulting in an inability to close ATP-sensitive potassium channels, preventing β-cell depolarization, calcium influx, and calcium-dependent insulin secretion.

Taken together, research conducted in the 1980s and early 1990s identified that IL-1, either produced locally in islets or supplied exogenously, causes structural and functional damage to islet β-cells. While it was known that the damaging actions of IL-1 required new gene transcription and protein translation, the cellular mediators of IL-dependent β-cell damage remained unknown.

2.1. Nitric oxide as a mediator of cytokine-induced damage

In the late 1980s, studies from multiple laboratories showed that nitric oxide, a gaseous free radical, was responsible for a diverse set of physiological processes, including endothelial-dependent vessel relaxation (Furchgott & Vanhoutte, 1989; Ignarro, 1990; Moncada, Palmer, & Higgs, 1989), the response of macrophages and neutrophils to endotoxin (Hibbs, Vavrin, & Taintor, 1987), and neurotransmission (Garthwaite, Charles, & Chess-Williams, 1988; Garthwaite, Garthwaite, Palmer, & Moncada, 1989). All these processes required arginine in medium, were inhibited by arginine analogs, and were accompanied by increased accumulation of nitrite in the supernatant. The enzyme, nitric oxide synthase (NOS), generates nitric oxide through the conversion of arginine to nitric oxide and citrulline. Interestingly, the inhibitory effects of cytokines on islets showed a similar dependence on arginine, as isolated rat islets exposed to IL-1 or TNFα in arginine-free medium were protected from cytokine-induced damage (Southern, Schulster, & Green, 1990). Furthermore, the accumulation of nitrite, a stable metabolite of nitric oxide, was observed in the supernatant of islets treated with cytokines, and nitrite accumulation was inhibited by analog of arginine, L-N^G-nitroarginine methyl ester. In the seminal studies in the early 1990s, three groups discovered that nitric oxide production mediated the damaging effects of cytokines on islet function (Corbett, Lancaster, Sweetland, & McDaniel, 1991; Southern et al., 1990; Welsh, Eizirik, Bendtzen, & Sandler, 1991). Nitric oxide was implicated in β-cell dysfunction, as the inhibition of glucose-stimulated insulin secretion from isolated rat and human pancreatic islets and FACS-purified β-cells treated with cytokines was prevented by an inhibitor of NOS, L-N^G-monomethyl arginine (NMMA) (Fig. 12.1) (Corbett et al., 1991; Corbett, Wang, Sweetland et al., 1992). In addition, formation of iron–nitrosyl complex in cytokine-treated rat (IL-1) and human (IL-1, IFN-γ, and TNFα) islets was demonstrated, confirming the generation of nitric oxide in islets and subsequent binding to iron-containing proteins/peptides (Fig. 12.2) (Corbett et al., 1991; Corbett, Sweetland, Wang, Lancaster, & McDaniel, 1993). Welsh et al. showed that the citric acid cycle enzyme, aconitase, which contains 4Fe-4S iron–sulfur cluster, was inhibited in a nitric oxide-dependent manner in IL-1-treated islets, further demonstrating that

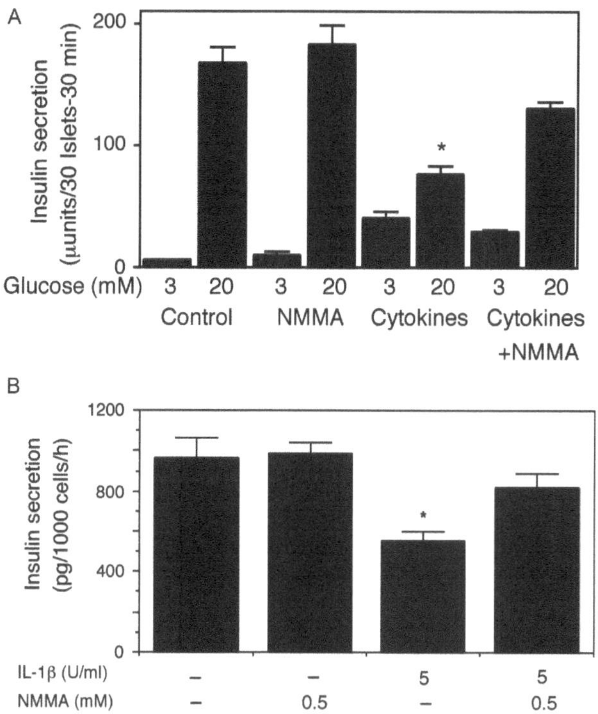

Figure 12.1 (A) Effects of higher cytokine concentrations on glucose-stimulated insulin secretion by human islets. Human islets were pretreated for 24 h in complete CMRL-1066 ± IL-1β at 75 U/ml, 3.5 nM TNF-α, and IFN-γ at 750 U/ml, or cytokines and 0.5 mM NMMA at 37 °C. The islets were washed, and glucose-stimulated insulin secretion was determined. (B) Effects of NMMA and IL-1β on glucose-stimulated insulin secretion by FACS-purified β-cells. β-Cells isolated by FACS purification were pretreated for 18 h at 37 °C in complete CMRL 1066 tissue culture media, or complete CMRL 1066 containing 5 U/ml IL-1β, 0.5 mM NMMA, or both IL-1β and NMMA. After pretreatment, the β-cells were isolated by centrifugation and glucose-stimulated insulin secretion was performed. *Panel (A): This work was originally published in Corbett et al. (1993). Panel (B): This work was originally published in Corbett, Wang, Sweetland et al. (1992).*

nitric oxide was required for the inhibition of mitochondrial oxidation and glucose-stimulated insulin secretion following cytokine exposure (Corbett, Wang, Sweetland, et al., 1992; Welsh et al., 1991). These reports led to a hypothesis that during the development of autoimmune diabetes, cytokine-stimulated production of nitric oxide in islets leads to the inhibition of β-cell function and subsequent β-cell death.

Three different isoforms of NOS were characterized: neuronal NOS (nNOS or NOS1), inducible NOS (iNOS or NOS2), and endothelial

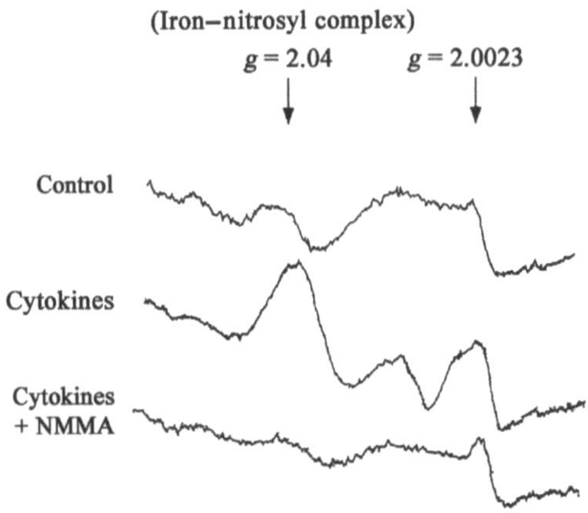

Figure 12.2 Effects of cytokines on iron–nitrosyl complex formation by human islets. Human islets (7000 islets per 8 ml) were treated for 18 h with IL-1β at 75 U/ml, 3.5 nM TNF-α, and IFN-γ at 750 U/ml, or cytokines and 0.5 mM NMMA. The islets were isolated and EPR spectroscopy was done at 77 K. The $g=2.04$ iron–nitrosyl complex and $g=2.0023$ delocalized electron features are as indicated. *This work was originally published in Corbett et al. (1993).*

NOS (eNOS or NOS3). Pancreatic β-cells express nNOS and iNOS, and islet endothelial cells express eNOS (Pollock, Forstermann, Tracey, & Nakane, 1995). Based on reports from multiple groups, nitric oxide, produced by iNOS, was shown to mediate the inhibitory actions of cytokines on β-cell function (Corbett, Wang, Hughes, et al., 1992; Corbett, Wang, Sweetland, et al., 1992; Southern et al., 1990; Welsh et al., 1991). Cytokine treatment stimulated the expression of iNOS in pancreatic β-cells, leading to formation of nitric oxide, which in turn decreased mitochondrial respiration (via aconitase inhibition) and prevented accumulation of ATP. As mentioned before, failure to increase ATP levels prevents β-cell depolarization because ATP-sensitive potassium channels remain open. In the absence of membrane depolarization, there is no calcium influx and insulin is not secreted.

Additionally, pathways responsible for iNOS expression in response to cytokines were elucidated. IL-1 was shown to be sufficient to induce the expression of iNOS in rat islets or rat β-cells (Corbett & McDaniel, 1995; Corbett, Wang, Sweetland, et al., 1992). IFN-γ was shown to prime and potentiate the β-cell response to IL-1 (Cetkovic-Cvrlje & Eizirik, 1994; Heitmeier, Scarim, & Corbett, 1997) and as a result effectively decrease the concentration of IL-1 required to stimulate iNOS expression and nitric oxide production in β-cells. For example, a 50 times lower concentration of IL-1 (0.1 U/ml instead of 5 U/ml) was required to stimulate iNOS expression in rat islets when it was combined with IFN-γ (150 U/ml) (Heitmeier et al., 1997). In fact, due to differences in the iNOS gene promoter between species, there are different requirements between mouse, rat, and human for the minimal cytokine combination that triggers iNOS induction in β-cells. IL-1 alone is sufficient to induce iNOS expression in rat islets, whereas human and mouse tissues require IL-1 and IFN-γ (Corbett et al., 1993; Heitmeier, Scarim, & Corbett, 1999). Transcription of iNOS in response to cytokines is regulated by nuclear factor κB (NF-κB) in case of exposure to IL-1, and interferon regulatory factor 1 and signal transducer and activator of transcription (STAT) 1, when β-cells are additionally exposed to IFN-γ (Eizirik, Flodstrom, Karlsen, & Welsh, 1996; Heitmeier et al., 1999). As previously stated, resident macrophages were identified as an islet cellular source of IL-1 (Corbett & McDaniel, 1995). It has been demonstrated that there are about 10–15 resident macrophages per islet, which upon activation release IL-1 in islets to levels that are sufficient to stimulate β-cell expression of iNOS, production of nitric oxide, and inhibition of insulin secretion (Corbett & McDaniel, 1995). The local production of IL-1 in islets has been observed in rat, mouse, and human islets (Arnush, Heitmeier, et al., 1998; Arnush, Scarim, Heitmeier, Kelly, & Corbett, 1998; Lacy, 1994). These studies have shown that the damaging effects of cytokines, added exogenously to islets, could be reproduced by the endogenous production of IL-1 by activated intraislet macrophages, providing a mechanism by which local cytokine production by immune cells could induce damage to β-cells (Fig. 12.3).

The ability of short exposures to IL-1 to cause damage 18 h later stimulated Comens et al. (1987) to explore whether the actions of cytokines are reversible. The inhibitory actions of 15 h incubation with IL-1 on glucose-stimulated insulin secretion are completely reversible if the cytokine is removed by washing and the islets are cultured for additional 4 days. These original observations were extended to show that recovery from the inhibitory actions of an 18 h treatment with IL-1 on islet secretory functions and aconitase activity can be reduced from 4 days to 8 h, by the addition of a NOS inhibitor without removing IL-1 (Corbett & McDaniel, 1994). The cellular pathways responsible for β-cell recovery from nitric oxide-induced damage will be discussed in the upcoming sections. Interestingly, the recovery from cytokine-induced damage is limited temporarily such that incubations with cytokines for 36 h and longer result in an irreversible inhibition of islet function and islet degeneration (Scarim, Heitmeier,

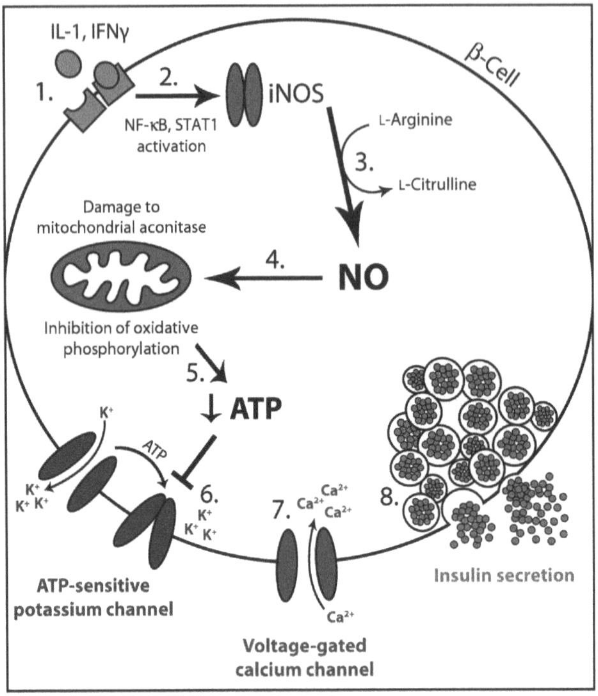

Figure 12.3 The inhibitory effects of nitric oxide on β-cell insulin secretion. Cytokines (IL-1 and IFNγ) bind to their receptors on the β-cell (1) and activate NF-κB and STAT1-signaling cascades, stimulating expression of iNOS (2). iNOS generates micromolar levels of nitric oxide in β-cells via conversion of arginine to nitric oxide and citrulline (3). Nitric oxide mediates the damaging effects of cytokines on β-cells, causing damage to mitochondrial aconitase and resulting in the inhibition of oxidative phosphorylation (4) and a decrease in cellular ATP levels (5). The decrease in ATP prevents closure of ATP-sensitive potassium channels, preventing membrane depolarization (6) and calcium influx (7). The net effect is an inhibition of calcium-dependent secretion of insulin (8). (See the color plate.)

& Corbett, 1997). These reports establish that iNOS and nitric oxide mediate the toxic effects of cytokines on β-cell function. NOS inhibitors prevent cytokine-induced damage, and when added to islets following 18 h incubation with cytokines, NOS inhibitors stimulate the recovery of secretory function and oxidative metabolism, and prevent islet degeneration even in the presence of this cytokine (Scarim et al., 1997).

Similar to the recovery of metabolic function, β-cells maintain the capacity to repair damaged DNA. Cytokines have long been known to induce DNA damage in β-cells (strand breaks) in a nitric oxide-dependent manner (Delaney, Green, Lowe, & Green, 1993; Rosales, Cunningham,

Bone, Green, & Green, 2004). We showed that the addition of NOS inhibitor to rat islets, treated for 24 h with IL-1, or human islets treated with IL-1 + IFN-γ, stimulates the time-dependent repair of damaged DNA that is maximal and complete within 8 h. Following 36 h incubation, cytokines cause irreversible DNA damage in β-cells (Hughes, Chambers, Meares, & Corbett, 2009). Treatment of islets with exogenous nitric oxide donors also results in DNA damage, and removal of these donors by washing away the donor and continued culture results in repair of damage. Similar to the recovery of metabolic functions, the repair of cytokine-induced DNA damage requires the expression of new genes (Hughes, Meares, Chambers, & Corbett, 2009). Although nitric oxide is the mediator of the DNA damage, these findings demonstrate that it is also necessary for the activation of repair pathways, demonstrating that the molecule that causes damage is also a key activator of the recovery or protective pathways in β-cells.

The previous section summarizes the studies investigating the role of iNOS and nitric oxide in cytokine-induced toxicity in pancreatic β-cells. Taken together, these studies demonstrate that (i) cytokine exposure (IL-1 or IL-1 + IFNγ) results in iNOS expression and nitric oxide production; (ii) nitric oxide inhibits metabolic and secretory functions of β-cells and causes DNA damage; and (iii) pancreatic islets can recover from cytokine-induced damage, although this recovery is temporally limited. The reversibility of nitric oxide-induced damage may be especially important physiologically because it allows for restoration of β-cell function after exposure to elevated concentrations of cytokines that may occur during infections.

2.2. Response to cytokines and cellular stress

In the late 1990s, new reports were published that suggested that rodent and human islets differ in their response to cytokines, with human islets being more resistant to cytokine exposure and requiring much higher concentrations of nitric oxide to elicit the damage (Eizirik & Pavlovic, 1997). In addition, studies by Eizirik et al. (1994) suggested that nitric oxide was not a major mediator of cytokine-induced damage in human islets. In these studies, extended incubations of human islets for 6 days with the cytokine combination of IL-1 + IFN-γ + TNFα were reported to inhibit insulin secretion and induce β-cell apoptosis in a nitric oxide-independent manner (Eizirik et al., 1994). Importantly, the experiments were performed using aminoguanidine at concentrations (5 mM) that inhibited insulin secretion by

50% even in the absence of cytokines. Further, the media was replaced multiple times during the 6 days culture of human islets, yet nitric oxide was only measured during the last culture period (days 4–6), or under conditions in which the β-cell no longer produces nitric oxide (Hughes, Chambers, et al., 2009). In addition, studies have shown that cytokine-induced human islet damage is irreversible following a 36 h incubation (Scarim et al., 1997); thus, it is difficult to draw conclusions about the mediator of damage in studies in which the biological effects of cytokines are examined after 6 days of treatment.

A second reason for the observed discrepancies is the induction of cellular stress responses that are often present in human islets. This so-called islet stress seems to occur when islets are isolated and/or transported, and is manifested by elevated expression of heat shock protein 70 (hsp70) (Welsh et al., 1995). Islets that have been stressed do not respond to cytokines and thus are not sensitive to cytokine-induced damage. Under "stress" conditions, hsp70 levels are elevated and IL-1 does not activate NF-κB, and IFN-γ does not activate STAT signaling. In fact, it is possible to make rat islets insensitive to cytokine-induced damage by exposing them to elevated temperature for 1 h (Scarim, Heitmeier, & Corbett, 1998). This prevents NF-κB nuclear localization and subsequent expression of iNOS in response to IL-1. Importantly, hsp70 is only a marker of stress and does not play a key role in blocking cytokine signaling, as depletion of hsp70 does not relieve the stress-induced inhibition of cytokine signaling (Weber, Scarim, & Corbett, 2003). Unfortunately, very few studies evaluate the levels of hsp70 in islet preparations. Similar to the heat shock response, activation of the unfolded protein response (UPR) results in the attenuation of cytokine-dependent signaling in β-cells (Weber, Chambers, Bensch, Scarim, & Corbett, 2004). Under conditions that stimulate endoplasmatic reticulum (ER) stress, the UPR is activated, and one effect of this cellular response is the inhibition of IL-1- and IFNγ-dependent signaling (Weber et al., 2004).

Overall, we do not believe that there is a difference in the response to cytokines between human and rodent islets when one examines how experiments have been performed and the potential role of "islet stress" in confounding the interpretation of the data. Human islets not subjected to stress respond to IL-1 and IFN-γ stimulation by expressing iNOS, which results in the production of nitric oxide and nitric oxide-dependent inhibition of mitochondrial aconitase activity, insulin secretion, protein translation, and DNA damage (Steer, Scarim, Chambers, & Corbett, 2006). Overall, IL-1 and IFN-γ are minimal cytokine combination required for induction of iNOS in both rodent and human tissues. In further studies, the expression of hsp70 in human islets may be a useful marker that could provide an index for whether human islet preparations will be responsive to cytokines. This evaluation would avoid the misinterpretation of the results that may be due to elevated levels of islet stress.

3. MECHANISMS OF NITRIC OXIDE-INDUCED β-CELL DEATH: APOPTOSIS OR NECROSIS?

Following the seminal studies that identified nitric oxide as the mediator of cytokine-induced damage in β-cells (Corbett et al., 1991; Southern et al., 1990; Welsh et al., 1991), studies have focused on elucidating the mechanisms by which β-cell death occurs after cytokine exposure. Currently, there is debate about the type of death that β-cells undergo as a result of cytokine and nitric oxide treatment, with reports of β-cells dying by either necrosis or apoptosis (Padgett, Broniowska, Hansen, Corbett, & Tse, 2013). Apoptosis is classically defined as a regulated mode of cell death occurring in the absence of inflammation, while necrosis is considered an unregulated process in which the loss of membrane integrity and the release of cellular contents result in inflammation. The following sections will highlight studies aimed at determining mechanisms of β-cell death, discuss the ability of β-cells to recover from nitric oxide-induced damage, and review the cellular mechanisms that participate in the determination of β-cell fate.

3.1. Apoptosis

Though the literature supports evidence for both β-cell apoptosis and necrosis, the majority of studies have focused on apoptosis as the type of cell death β-cells undergo following cytokine exposure (Cnop et al., 2005; Eizirik & Mandrup-Poulsen, 2001; Mandrup-Poulsen, 2001). Cytokine-induced apoptosis in β-cells appears to occur via the intrinsic mitochondrial pathway (Gurzov & Eizirik, 2011; Thomas & Kay, 2011). Cytokine treatment of β-cells causes upregulation of the proapoptotic BH3-only family of Bcl-2 proteins, including p53-upregtulated mediator of apoptosis (PUMA), Bcl-2-interacting mediator of cell death (BIM), BH3-interacting domain death agonist, Bcl-2 antagonist of cell death, and death protein 5 (Grunnet et al., 2009; Gurzov et al., 2010; McKenzie et al., 2010; Mehmeti, Lenzen, & Lortz, 2011). The family of BH3-only proteins promotes apoptosis via two possible mechanisms. The first mechanism involves binding of

BH3-only proteins to antiapoptotic proteins such as Bcl-2, a Bcl-2-like protein (Bcl-Xl), and myeloid cell leukemia sequence-1 (Willis et al., 2007). The result is inhibition of these antiapoptotic proteins and liberation of the proapoptotic proteins, Bcl-2-antagonist/killer-1 (BAK), and Bcl-2-associated X protein (BAX). Additional studies suggest that some BH3-only proteins, such as PUMA and BIM, promote apoptosis through direct activation of BAK and BAX (Kuwana et al., 2005). Liberation of BAK and BAX induces permeabilization of the mitochondrial outer membrane, resulting in the release of mitochondrial proteins such as cytochrome *c* (Youle & Strasser, 2008). Once released, cytochrome *c* binds to apoptotic protease-activating factor 1 (APAF-1), leading to apoptosome formation, caspase-9 activation, and cell death (Riedl & Salvesen, 2007). Many groups have examined the involvement of these components of the intrinsic apoptotic pathway in cytokine-induced β-cell death. Treatment of human islets with a BAX inhibitor was found to attenuate cytokine-induced caspase-3 cleavage and apoptosis (Grunnet et al., 2009). Studies examining the role of Bcl-2 in β-cell apoptosis demonstrate that overexpression of Bcl-2 in β-cells protects from cytokine-induced apoptosis (Iwahashi et al., 1996; Liu et al., 1996), though others have reported that Bcl-2 overexpression has no effect on the incidence of cytokine-induced apoptosis (Barbu, Akusjarvi, & Welsh, 2002; Hughes, Chambers, et al., 2009; Tran, Chen, Newgard, & Hohmeier, 2003). Furthermore, studies in the spontaneously diabetic NOD mouse show that while Bcl-2 overexpression attenuates β-cell apoptosis, it does not prevent autoimmune destruction of pancreatic islets and progression to diabetes (Allison et al., 2000).

A number of proteins upstream of the intrinsic apoptotic pathway have been implicated in mediating cytokine-induced apoptosis in the β-cell. Inhibition of the mitogen-activated protein kinases, c-Jun N-terminal kinase (JNK), extracellular signal-regulated kinase, and p38 mitogen-activated protein kinase (p38) attenuates cytokine-induced apoptosis in β-cells (Bonny et al., 2000; Pavlovic, Andersen, Mandrup-Poulsen, & Eizirik, 2000; Saldeen, Lee, & Welsh, 2001). In contrast, a protective role for JNK in β-cell recovery from nitric oxide- and cytokine-mediated β-cell damage has also been discovered (Hughes, Meares, et al., 2009; Scarim, Nishimoto, Weber, & Corbett, 2003). Nitric oxide also decreases the phosphorylation (activation) of protein kinase B (Akt), a known inhibitor of apoptosis (Storling et al., 2005).

One proposed mechanism of cytokine- and nitric oxide-induced β-cell apoptosis is the prolonged occurrence of ER stress and activation of a terminal UPR (Eizirik, Cardozo, & Cnop, 2008; Oyadomari et al., 2001). The UPR is activated in response to ER stress to restore homeostatic function (Papa, 2012). UPR signaling is transduced by three signaling "arms": inositol-requiring enzyme 1a, protein kinase regulated by RNA/ER-like kinase, and activating transcription factor-4 (ATF-4) (Schroder & Kaufman, 2005). IL-1 stimulates a nitric oxide-dependent activation of the UPR in β-cells, observed by an increase in UPR markers including C/EBP homologous protein (CHOP), ATF-4, growth arrest and DNA damage-inducible protein (GADD34), splicing of X-box binding protein, and phosphorylation of eukaryotic translation initiation factor 2 subunit alpha (Chambers et al., 2008). An additional mechanism proposed to be involved in cytokine-induced ER stress is through nitric oxide-dependent downregulation of sarcoendoplasmic reticulum pump Ca^{2+} ATPase 2b, which causes a depletion of Ca^{2+} stores in the ER (Cardozo et al., 2005). CHOP has been implicated as a primary mediator of ER stress-induced death in β-cells, as islets isolated from $CHOP^{-/-}$ mice are protected from nitric oxide- and cytokine-induced death (Oyadomari et al., 2001). Additionally, insulinoma cells overexpressing the ER chaperone, immunoglobulin heavy chain-binding protein (BiP), have decreased CHOP expression, and necrosis and apoptosis following cytokine exposure is attenuated in these cells (Wang et al., 2007). However, other studies have suggested that depletion of CHOP or overexpression of BiP has no effect on cytokine-induced β-cell death (Akerfeldt et al., 2008). Furthermore, cytokine-induced death is not potentiated in mouse embryonic fibroblasts in which each arm of the UPR has been selectively knocked down or in insulinoma cells expressing mutants of each of the ER stress transducers, suggesting that nitric oxide-induced activation of the UPR may not be a mediator of β-cell death (Chambers et al., 2008).

3.2. Necrosis

In contrast to reports that cytokines induce β-cell apoptosis, several studies report that β-cell death occurs by necrosis. Nitric oxide stimulates release of high mobility group box 1 protein (Steer et al., 2006) and cyclophilin A (Tamura et al., 2011), biomarkers of necrotic cell death (Christofferson & Yuan, 2010; Raucci, Palumbo, & Bianchi, 2007). Additionally, studies have shown that inhibition of caspase-3 does not modify cytokine-induced death in β-cells; however, it prevents death in β-cells treated with the apoptotic agent camptothecin (Steer et al., 2006). Furthermore, knockdown of the proapoptotic BAX and BAK in insulinoma

INS832/13 cells has no effect on cytokine-induced death, and overexpression of the antiapoptotic Akt protects from cell death induced by apoptotic agents, but does not attenuate cytokine-induced β-cell death (Collier, Fueger, Hohmeier, & Newgard, 2006). Collier et al. (2011) more recently demonstrated that siRNA knockdown of APAF-1 or caspase-9, components of the apoptosome, did not protect against cytokine-induced β-cell death, though death by apoptotic agents was attenuated. This group has also shown that the metabolic profile induced by cytokine treatment of INS832/13 cells is distinct from that induced by apoptotic agents, suggesting that cytokine-induced death may occur by a nonapoptotic mechanism (Collier et al., 2011). While the above findings suggest that cytokine- and nitric oxide-induced β-cell death does not occur via classical apoptosis, others have suggested that both forms of cell death occur and share a common pathway (Saldeen, 2000).

While the role of nitric oxide as the mediator of cytokine-induced β-cell damage is well documented, very few current studies consider the role of nitric oxide when examining the signaling mechanisms regulating cytokine-induced death. This is unfortunate, as there is compelling evidence for nitric oxide as the mediator of cytokine-induced β-cell death. Liu et al. (2000) found that while cytokine treatment of mouse islets for 6 days results in an 88% decrease in viability, islets from iNOS knockout mice are completely protected from cytokine-induced death. Furthermore, transgenic mice expressing iNOS cDNA under control of the insulin promoter develop diabetes, and administration of an iNOS inhibitor delays or prevents diabetes induction in these animals (Takamura et al., 1998).

4. RECOVERY FROM NITRIC OXIDE-INDUCED DAMAGE

As previously mentioned, β-cells exposed to nitric oxide experience an inhibition of insulin secretion, mitochondrial aconitase activity, and protein synthesis; the induction of DNA damage; and subsequent death. However, β-cells possess a limited capacity to recover from nitric oxide-induced damage if the source of nitric oxide is removed before the damage becomes too extensive. For example, inhibition of iNOS following 18 h IL-1 treatment of rat islets, and continued culture of islets (without removing the cytokine from the media), allows for the time-dependent recovery of insulin secretion that is maximal and complete 8 h after NMMA addition (Corbett & McDaniel, 1994). This recovery process is not limited to insulin secretion, as β-cells recover oxidative metabolism, protein synthesis, and repair DNA damage in a similar time-dependent manner (Corbett & McDaniel, 1994; Rosales et al., 2004; Scarim et al., 1997). This ability to repair and recover from cytokine-mediated damage is lost as the length of cytokine exposure is extended. Exposure of β-cells to cytokines for 36 h and longer results in irreversible damage and inhibition of β-cell function (Hughes, Chambers, et al., 2009; Scarim et al., 1997). Ultimately, this inability to repair and recover from nitric oxide-induced damage is temporally associated with a commitment of β-cells to death (Hughes, Chambers, et al., 2009; Scarim et al., 1997).

The discordance in observations regarding β-cell apoptosis and necrosis could be explained by this limited ability of β-cells to recover from nitric oxide-induced damage. Short exposures of β-cells to cytokines may cause a necrotic process that shifts to an apoptotic response as cytokine exposure persists and damage becomes too extensive to repair. In this process, the rate of nitric oxide production during cytokine stimulation of β-cells is a potential mechanism controlling when apoptosis occurs. Nitric oxide is produced at a high rate following short exposures to cytokines (0–24 h IL-1), but this rate decreases by sixfold during longer exposures (36 h) to IL-1 (Hughes, Chambers, et al., 2009). Importantly, nitric oxide is an effective inhibitor of caspase activity, through direct *S*-nitrosation of the active site cysteine (Kim, Talanian, & Billiar, 1997; Li, Billiar, Talanian, & Kim, 1997; Mohr, Zech, Lapetina, & Brune, 1997). Therefore, apoptosis would not be possible under conditions of high nitric oxide production due to caspase inhibition, and only when the rate of nitric oxide decreases could apoptosis occur. Although caspase-3 activity is not increased in rat islets after 36 h exposure to IL-1, it is activated as evidenced by increased cleavage of procaspase-3 to caspase-3. However, the residual nitric oxide that is produced following this 36 h cytokine exposure is sufficient to attenuate caspase 3 activity. The addition of an iNOS inhibitor following the 36 h IL-1 incubation, and continued culture for eight additional hours, results in a 2.5-fold increase in caspase-3 activity (Hughes, Chambers, et al., 2009). Associated with this increase in caspase-3 activity is irreversible inhibition of β-cell function, oxidative metabolism, and DNA damage (Hughes, Chambers, et al., 2009; Scarim et al., 1997). Consistent with these observations, many of the studies that report necrotic β-cell death have examined β-cell viability after shorter treatment with cytokines (24 h and less) while β-cells reported to die by apoptosis have often been exposed to cytokines for longer periods of time (36 h and longer). These variations in the length of cytokine exposure, as well as assay design and cell types examined, may ultimately explain the disparity in observations regarding the mechanism of cytokine- and nitric oxide-induced β-cell death.

Recent studies have identified several key mechanisms involved in the regulation of β-cell recovery following nitric oxide-induced damage. AMP-activated protein kinase (AMPK), the master energy sensor of the cell, is one regulator of the β-cell response to nitric oxide. AMPK is rapidly activated by nitric oxide produced in response to cytokines or administered using chemical donors. AMPK participates in the recovery of aconitase activity and cell survival, as overexpression of dominant-negative AMPK mutants in β-cells increases apoptosis and attenuates the recovery of aconitase activity following nitric oxide-induced damage (Meares et al., 2009). The activation of AMPK by nitric oxide occurs by unique mechanisms, as the canonical activators of AMPK (TAK1, LKB1, CamKK) do not participate in this process. Instead, nitric oxide-stimulated AMPK activation requires the RNase domain of IRE1α (Meares et al., 2009). As IRE1α is one of the three arms of the UPR (Bonny et al., 2000), regulation of AMPK activation following nitric oxide treatment may serve as a mechanistic link between the ER stress responses and the regulation of metabolism.

In contrast to reports that JNK promotes β-cell apoptosis following cytokine treatment, JNK has also been implicated in the recovery from nitric oxide-induced damage (Hughes, Meares, et al., 2009; Scarim et al., 2003). JNK is rapidly activated by nitric oxide, and inhibition of JNK prevents recovery of mitochondrial aconitase. Furthermore, JNK is required for nitric oxide-induced expression of growth arrest and DNA damage 45α (GADD45α), an essential participant in the repair of DNA damage following cytokine treatment of islets (Hughes, Meares, et al., 2009; Scarim et al., 2003). JNK may play a dual role in β-cells exposed to cytokines, with early activation of JNK eliciting a protective pathway and late activation of JNK-stimulating apoptotic cascades when nitric oxide-induced damage becomes too extensive. Interestingly, the JNK-GADD45α DNA repair pathway activated by nitric oxide occurs independently of p53, which is classically required for GADD45α expression and DNA repair following oxidative DNA damage (Hughes, Meares, et al., 2009).

The transcription factor Forkhead box protein O1 (FOXO1) is a transcription factor that can regulate both survival and death-signaling pathways (Huang & Tindall, 2007). Treatment of β-cells with nitric oxide (generated endogenously by iNOS or added exogenously using nitric oxide donors) results in the rapid nuclear translocation of FOXO1. Once in the nucleus, the acetylation status of FOXO1 appears to determine whether a transcriptional program promoting recovery or death is activated (Hughes, Meares, Hansen, & Corbett, 2011). FOXO1 participates in the recovery from nitric oxide-induced damage, as GADD45α expression and DNA repair are both attenuated in β-cells transfected with a dominant-negative mutant of FOXO1 (Hughes et al., 2011). In contrast, when in the acetylated state (potentially due to decreased SIRT1 activity or the increased activity of a histone acetyltransferase (HAT) such as p300), FOXO1 is proposed to activate a transcriptional death program featuring increased expression of proapoptotic genes such as p53-upregulated mediator of apoptosis (PUMA) (Giannakou & Partridge, 2004). The NAD^+-dependent deacetylase SIRT1 is one regulator of FOXO1, deacetylating FOXO1 and directing the expression of protective and recovery genes (Giannakou & Partridge, 2004). In INS832/13 cells, SIRT1 activation with resveratrol potentiates nitric oxide-induced GADD45α expression and strongly enhances the rate of DNA repair following nitric oxide-induced DNA damage (Hughes et al., 2011). Additionally, SIRT1 overexpression has been shown to attenuate cytokine-induced β-cell death (Lee et al., 2009). In contrast, inhibition of SIRT1 prevents the repair of DNA damage and leads to an increase in PUMA expression and FOXO1-dependent apoptosis following IL-1 treatment of INS832/13 cells (Hughes et al., 2011). A proposed model of the dual role of FOXO1 and other cellular mechanisms in the regulation of β-cell fate in response to cytokines is shown in Fig. 12.4. When nitric oxide-induced damage is reversible (0–24 h of IL-1 treatment), deacetylated FOXO1 is proposed to promote pathways that are responsible for protection and recovery of β-cells. As the damage becomes too extensive (36 h and longer exposure to IL-1), acetylated FOXO1 accumulates and initiates a proapoptotic pathway (Fig. 12.4). Taken together, the cellular mechanisms controlling nuclear localization of FOXO1 and its acetylation status may be key regulators of the β-cell responses to nitric oxide. Additional studies are necessary to identify the mechanisms by which nitric oxide regulates SIRT1 and FOXO1, and how this regulation determines β-cell fate following IL-1 exposure.

5. CONCLUSIONS

In this chapter, we discussed the responses of β-cells to nitric oxide, starting from the original discovery that this free radical is responsible for

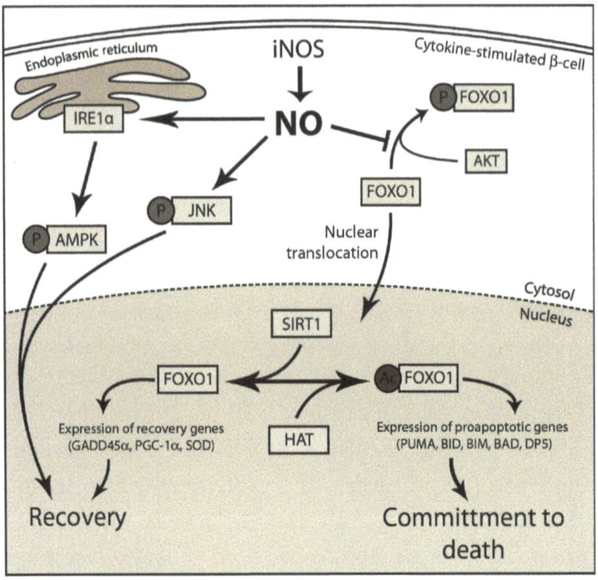

Figure 12.4 Cellular mechanisms that control the β-cell responses to nitric oxide. Cytokines stimulate iNOS expression in β-cells, resulting in the production of micromolar levels of nitric oxide. Nitric oxide stimulates nuclear translocation of FOXO1. Once in the nucleus, FOXO1 can direct the expression of recovery genes or proapoptotic genes. The acetylation state of FOXO1 dictates which transcriptional program is activated. SIRT1-mediated deacetylation of FOXO1 promotes β-cell recovery, while acetylation of FOXO1 by a HAT (such as p300) activates a death cascade. AMPK and JNK are also rapidly activated by nitric oxide and participate in β-cell recovery. (See the color plate.)

mediating the effects of cytokines on β-cell function and viability. More recently, emphasis was focused on how nitric oxide controls signal transduction and gene expression to determine if β-cells survive or die following cytokine exposure. The proposed model for how nitric oxide controls responses of β-cells following cytokine treatment is shown in Fig. 12.4. Cytokines stimulate expression of iNOS and subsequent production of nitric oxide in pancreatic β-cells. Nitric oxide stimulates the nuclear localization of FOXO1, and once in the nucleus, FOXO1 directs transcriptional program that leads either to recovery (expression of GADD 45α) or to apoptosis (expression of PUMA). AMPK and JNK are activated by nitric oxide, and they facilitate the recovery from nitric oxide-induced damage.

Multiple studies indicate that nitric oxide is the primary regulator controlling β-cell response to cytokines. While nitric oxide can directly inhibit oxidative metabolism and cause DNA damage, it can also affect the activity of multiple proteins, including FOXO1 and JNK. There are many unanswered questions concerning the delicate balance between protective and death pathways regulated by nitric oxide in β-cells. How does nitric oxide influence the activity of SIRT1? What are the factors influencing the cellular localization of FOXO1? While we have learned many details regarding the actions of cytokines in controlling β-cell function, there is still much to be uncovered. Although the past 30 years have been highly productive, it is hoped that in the next 30 years we will gain a more complete understanding of mechanisms that drive β-cell failure in T1D and how nitric oxide controls death and survival of pancreatic β-cells.

REFERENCES

Akerfeldt, M. C., Howes, J., Chan, J. Y., Stevens, V. A., Boubenna, N., McGuire, H. M., et al. (2008). Cytokine-induced beta-cell death is independent of endoplasmic reticulum stress signaling. *Diabetes*, *57*(11), 3034–3044.

Allison, J., Thomas, H., Beck, D., Brady, J. L., Lew, A. M., Elefanty, A., et al. (2000). Transgenic overexpression of human Bcl-2 in islet beta cells inhibits apoptosis but does not prevent autoimmune destruction. *International Immunology*, *12*(1), 9–17.

Arnush, M., Heitmeier, M. R., Scarim, A. L., Marino, M. H., Manning, P. T., & Corbett, J. A. (1998). IL-1 produced and released endogenously within human islets inhibits beta cell function. *Journal of Clinical Investigation*, *102*(3), 516–526.

Arnush, M., Scarim, A. L., Heitmeier, M. R., Kelly, C. B., & Corbett, J. A. (1998). Potential role of resident islet macrophage activation in the initiation of autoimmune diabetes. *Journal of Immunology*, *160*(6), 2684–2691.

Barbu, A. R., Akusjarvi, G., & Welsh, N. (2002). Adenoviral-induced islet cell cytotoxicity is not counteracted by Bcl-2 overexpression. *Molecular Medicine*, *8*(11), 733–741.

Bendtzen, K., Mandrup-Poulsen, T., Nerup, J., Nielsen, J. H., Dinarello, C. A., & Svenson, M. (1986). Cytotoxicity of human pI 7 interleukin-1 for pancreatic islets of Langerhans. *Science*, *232*(4757), 1545–1547.

Bonny, C., Oberson, A., Steinmann, M., Schorderet, D. F., Nicod, P., & Waeber, G. (2000). IB1 reduces cytokine-induced apoptosis of insulin-secreting cells. *Journal of Biological Chemistry*, *275*(22), 16466–16472.

Cardozo, A. K., Ortis, F., Storling, J., Feng, Y. M., Rasschaert, J., Tonnesen, M., et al. (2005). Cytokines downregulate the sarcoendoplasmic reticulum pump Ca2+ ATPase 2b and deplete endoplasmic reticulum Ca2+, leading to induction of endoplasmic reticulum stress in pancreatic beta-cells. *Diabetes*, *54*(2), 452–461.

Cetkovic-Cvrlje, M., & Eizirik, D. L. (1994). TNF-alpha and IFN-gamma potentiate the deleterious effects of IL-1 beta on mouse pancreatic islets mainly via generation of nitric oxide. *Cytokine*, *6*(4), 399–406.

Chambers, K. T., Unverferth, J. A., Weber, S. M., Wek, R. C., Urano, F., & Corbett, J. A. (2008). The role of nitric oxide and the unfolded protein response in cytokine-induced beta-cell death. *Diabetes*, *57*(1), 124–132.

Christofferson, D. E., & Yuan, J. (2010). Cyclophilin A release as a biomarker of necrotic cell death. *Cell Death and Differentiation*, *17*(12), 1942–1943.

Cnop, M., Welsh, N., Jonas, J. C., Jorns, A., Lenzen, S., & Eizirik, D. L. (2005). Mechanisms of pancreatic beta-cell death in type 1 and type 2 diabetes: Many differences, few similarities. *Diabetes*, *54*(Suppl. 2), S97–S107.

Collier, J. J., Burke, S. J., Eisenhauer, M. E., Lu, D., Sapp, R. C., Frydman, C. J., et al. (2011). Pancreatic beta-cell death in response to pro-inflammatory cytokines is distinct from genuine apoptosis. *PloS One*, *6*(7), e22485.
Collier, J. J., Fueger, P. T., Hohmeier, H. E., & Newgard, C. B. (2006). Pro- and anti-apoptotic proteins regulate apoptosis but do not protect against cytokine-mediated cytotoxicity in rat islets and beta-cell lines. *Diabetes*, *55*(5), 1398–1406.
Comens, P. G., Wolf, B. A., Unanue, E. R., Lacy, P. E., & McDaniel, M. L. (1987). Interleukin 1 is potent modulator of insulin secretion from isolated rat islets of Langerhans. *Diabetes*, *36*(8), 963–970.
Corbett, J. A., Lancaster, J. R., Jr., Sweetland, M. A., & McDaniel, M. L. (1991). Interleukin-1 beta-induced formation of EPR-detectable iron-nitrosyl complexes in islets of Langerhans. Role of nitric oxide in interleukin-1 beta-induced inhibition of insulin secretion. *Journal of Biological Chemistry*, *266*(32), 21351–21354.
Corbett, J. A., & McDaniel, M. L. (1994). Reversibility of interleukin-1 beta-induced islet destruction and dysfunction by the inhibition of nitric oxide synthase. *Biochemical Journal*, *299*(Pt. 3), 719–724.
Corbett, J. A., & McDaniel, M. L. (1995). Intraislet release of interleukin 1 inhibits beta cell function by inducing beta cell expression of inducible nitric oxide synthase. *Journal of Experimental Medicine*, *181*(2), 559–568.
Corbett, J. A., Sweetland, M. A., Wang, J. L., Lancaster, J. R., Jr., & McDaniel, M. L. (1993). Nitric oxide mediates cytokine-induced inhibition of insulin secretion by human islets of Langerhans. *Proceedings of the National Academy of Sciences of the United States of America*, *90*(5), 1731–1735.
Corbett, J. A., Wang, J. L., Hughes, J. H., Wolf, B. A., Sweetland, M. A., Lancaster, J. R., Jr., et al. (1992). Nitric oxide and cyclic GMP formation induced by interleukin 1 beta in islets of Langerhans. Evidence for an effector role of nitric oxide in islet dysfunction. *Biochemical Journal*, *287*(Pt. 1), 229–235.
Corbett, J. A., Wang, J. L., Sweetland, M. A., Lancaster, J. R., Jr., & McDaniel, M. L. (1992). Interleukin 1 beta induces the formation of nitric oxide by beta-cells purified from rodent islets of Langerhans. Evidence for the beta-cell as a source and site of action of nitric oxide. *Journal of Clinical Investigation*, *90*(6), 2384–2391.
Delaney, C. A., Green, M. H., Lowe, J. E., & Green, I. C. (1993). Endogenous nitric oxide induced by interleukin-1 beta in rat islets of Langerhans and HIT-T15 cells causes significant DNA damage as measured by the 'comet' assay. *FEBS Letters*, *333*(3), 291–295.
Eizirik, D. L. (1988). Interleukin-1 induced impairment in pancreatic islet oxidative metabolism of glucose is potentiated by tumor necrosis factor. *Acta Endocrinologica*, *119*(3), 321–325.
Eizirik, D. L., Cardozo, A. K., & Cnop, M. (2008). The role for endoplasmic reticulum stress in diabetes mellitus. *Endocrine Reviews*, *29*(1), 42–61.
Eizirik, D. L., Flodstrom, M., Karlsen, A. E., & Welsh, N. (1996). The harmony of the spheres: Inducible nitric oxide synthase and related genes in pancreatic beta cells. *Diabetologia*, *39*(8), 875–890.
Eizirik, D. L., & Mandrup-Poulsen, T. (2001). A choice of death—The signal-transduction of immune-mediated beta-cell apoptosis. *Diabetologia*, *44*(12), 2115–2133 [erratum appears in Diabetologia. 2002 Jun;45(6):936.].
Eizirik, D. L., & Pavlovic, D. (1997). Is there a role for nitric oxide in beta-cell dysfunction and damage in IDDM? *Diabetes/Metabolism Reviews*, *13*(4), 293–307.
Eizirik, D. L., Sandler, S., Welsh, N., Cetkovic-Cvrlje, M., Nieman, A., Geller, D. A., et al. (1994). Cytokines suppress human islet function irrespective of their effects on nitric oxide generation. *Journal of Clinical Investigation*, *93*(5), 1968–1974.
Furchgott, R. F., & Vanhoutte, P. M. (1989). Endothelium-derived relaxing and contracting factors. *FASEB Journal*, *3*(9), 2007–2018.

Garthwaite, J., Charles, S. L., & Chess-Williams, R. (1988). Endothelium-derived relaxing factor release on activation of NMDA receptors suggests role as intercellular messenger in the brain. *Nature, 336*(6197), 385–388.
Garthwaite, J., Garthwaite, G., Palmer, R. M., & Moncada, S. (1989). NMDA receptor activation induces nitric oxide synthesis from arginine in rat brain slices. *European Journal of Pharmacology, 172*(4–5), 413–416.
Giannakou, M. E., & Partridge, L. (2004). The interaction between FOXO and SIRT1: Tipping the balance towards survival. *Trends in Cell Biology, 14*(8), 408–412.
Grunnet, L. G., Aikin, R., Tonnesen, M. F., Paraskevas, S., Blaabjerg, L., Storling, J., et al. (2009). Proinflammatory cytokines activate the intrinsic apoptotic pathway in beta-cells. *Diabetes, 58*(8), 1807–1815.
Gurzov, E. N., & Eizirik, D. L. (2011). Bcl-2 proteins in diabetes: Mitochondrial pathways of beta-cell death and dysfunction. *Trends in Cell Biology, 21*(7), 424–431.
Gurzov, E. N., Germano, C. M., Cunha, D. A., Ortis, F., Vanderwinden, J. M., Marchetti, P., et al. (2010). p53 up-regulated modulator of apoptosis (PUMA) activation contributes to pancreatic beta-cell apoptosis induced by proinflammatory cytokines and endoplasmic reticulum stress. *Journal of Biological Chemistry, 285*(26), 19910–19920.
Heitmeier, M. R., Scarim, A. L., & Corbett, J. A. (1997). Interferon-gamma increases the sensitivity of islets of Langerhans for inducible nitric-oxide synthase expression induced by interleukin 1. *Journal of Biological Chemistry, 272*(21), 13697–13704.
Heitmeier, M. R., Scarim, A. L., & Corbett, J. A. (1999). Prolonged STAT1 activation is associated with interferon-gamma priming for interleukin-1-induced inducible nitric-oxide synthase expression by islets of Langerhans. *Journal of Biological Chemistry, 274*(41), 29266–29273.
Hibbs, J. B., Jr., Vavrin, Z., & Taintor, R. R. (1987). L-arginine is required for expression of the activated macrophage effector mechanism causing selective metabolic inhibition in target cells. *Journal of Immunology, 138*(2), 550–565.
Huang, H., & Tindall, D. J. (2007). Dynamic FoxO transcription factors. *Journal of Cell Science, 120*(Pt. 15), 2479–2487.
Hughes, K. J., Chambers, K. T., Meares, G. P., & Corbett, J. A. (2009). Nitric oxides mediates a shift from early necrosis to late apoptosis in cytokine-treated beta-cells that is associated with irreversible DNA damage. *American Journal of Physiology. Endocrinology and Metabolism, 297*(5), E1187–E1196.
Hughes, J. H., Colca, J. R., Easom, R. A., Turk, J., & McDaniel, M. L. (1990). Interleukin 1 inhibits insulin secretion from isolated rat pancreatic islets by a process that requires gene transcription and mRNA translation. *Journal of Clinical Investigation, 86*(3), 856–863.
Hughes, K. J., Meares, G. P., Chambers, K. T., & Corbett, J. A. (2009). Repair of nitric oxide-damaged DNA in beta-cells requires JNK-dependent GADD45alpha expression. *Journal of Biological Chemistry, 284*(40), 27402–27408.
Hughes, K. J., Meares, G. P., Hansen, P. A., & Corbett, J. A. (2011). FoxO1 and SIRT1 regulate beta-cell responses to nitric oxide. *Journal of Biological Chemistry, 286*(10), 8338–8348.
Ignarro, L. J. (1990). Nitric oxide: A novel signal transduction mechanism for transcellular communication. *Hypertension, 16*(5), 477–483.
Iwahashi, H., Hanafusa, T., Eguchi, Y., Nakajima, H., Miyagawa, J., Itoh, N., et al. (1996). Cytokine-induced apoptotic cell death in a mouse pancreatic beta-cell line: Inhibition by Bcl-2. *Diabetologia, 39*(5), 530–536.
Kim, Y. M., Talanian, R. V., & Billiar, T. R. (1997). Nitric oxide inhibits apoptosis by preventing increases in caspase-3-like activity via two distinct mechanisms. *Journal of Biological Chemistry, 272*(49), 31138–31148.
Kuwana, T., Bouchier-Hayes, L., Chipuk, J. E., Bonzon, C., Sullivan, B. A., Green, D. R., et al. (2005). BH3 domains of BH3-only proteins differentially regulate Bax-mediated

mitochondrial membrane permeabilization both directly and indirectly. *Molecular Cell, 17*(4), 525–535.

Lacy, P. E. (1994). The intraislet macrophage and type I diabetes. *Mount Sinai Journal of Medicine, 61*(2), 170–174.

Lacy, P. E., & Finke, E. H. (1991). Activation of intraislet lymphoid cells causes destruction of islet cells. *American Journal of Pathology, 138*(5), 1183–1190.

Lee, J. H., Song, M. Y., Song, E. K., Kim, E. K., Moon, W. S., Han, M. K., et al. (2009). Overexpression of SIRT1 protects pancreatic beta-cells against cytokine toxicity by suppressing the nuclear factor-kappaB signaling pathway. *Diabetes, 58*(2), 344–351.

Li, J., Billiar, T. R., Talanian, R. V., & Kim, Y. M. (1997). Nitric oxide reversibly inhibits seven members of the caspase family via S-nitrosylation. *Biochemical and Biophysical Research Communications, 240*(2), 419–424.

Liu, D., Pavlovic, D., Chen, M. C., Flodstrom, M., Sandler, S., & Eizirik, D. L. (2000). Cytokines induce apoptosis in beta-cells isolated from mice lacking the inducible isoform of nitric oxide synthase (iNOS$^{-/-}$). *Diabetes, 49*(7), 1116–1122.

Liu, Y., Rabinovitch, A., Suarez-Pinzon, W., Muhkerjee, B., Brownlee, M., Edelstein, D., et al. (1996). Expression of the bcl-2 gene from a defective HSV-1 amplicon vector protects pancreatic beta-cells from apoptosis. *Human Gene Therapy*, 7(14), 1719–1726.

Mandrup-Poulsen, T. (2001). Beta-cell apoptosis: Stimuli and signaling. *Diabetes, 50*(Suppl. 1), S58–S63.

Mandrup-Poulsen, T., Bendtzen, K., Nerup, J., Dinarello, C. A., Svenson, M., & Nielsen, J. H. (1986). Affinity-purified human interleukin I is cytotoxic to isolated islets of Langerhans. *Diabetologia, 29*(1), 63–67.

Mandrup-Poulsen, T., Bendtzen, K., Nielsen, J. H., Bendixen, G., & Nerup, J. (1985). Cytokines cause functional and structural damage to isolated islets of Langerhans. *Allergy, 40*(6), 424–429.

McKenzie, M. D., Jamieson, E., Jansen, E. S., Scott, C. L., Huang, D. C., Bouillet, P., et al. (2010). Glucose induces pancreatic islet cell apoptosis that requires the BH3-only proteins Bim and Puma and multi-BH domain protein Bax. *Diabetes, 59*(3), 644–652.

Meares, G., Hughes, K., Jaimes, K., Salvatori, A., Rhodes, C., & Corbett, J. (2009). AMP-activated protein kinase attenuates nitric oxide induced beta-cell death. *Journal of Biological Chemistry, 285*, 3191–3200.

Mehmeti, I., Lenzen, S., & Lortz, S. (2011). Modulation of Bcl-2-related protein expression in pancreatic beta cells by pro-inflammatory cytokines and its dependence on the antioxidative defense status. *Molecular and Cellular Endocrinology, 332*(1–2), 88–96.

Mohr, S., Zech, B., Lapetina, E. G., & Brune, B. (1997). Inhibition of caspase-3 by S-nitrosation and oxidation caused by nitric oxide. *Biochemical and Biophysical Research Communications, 238*(2), 387–391.

Moncada, S., Palmer, R. M., & Higgs, E. A. (1989). The biological significance of nitric oxide formation from L-arginine. *Biochemical Society Transactions, 17*(4), 642–644.

Oyadomari, S., Takeda, K., Takiguchi, M., Gotoh, T., Matsumoto, M., Wada, I., et al. (2001). Nitric oxide-induced apoptosis in pancreatic beta cells is mediated by the endoplasmic reticulum stress pathway. *Proceedings of the National Academy of Sciences of the United States of America, 98*(19), 10845–10850.

Padgett, L. E., Broniowska, K. A., Hansen, P. A., Corbett, J. A., & Tse, H. M. (2013). The role of reactive oxygen species and proinflammatory cytokines in type 1 diabetes pathogenesis. *Annals of the New York Academy of Sciences, 1281*, 16–35.

Papa, F. R. (2012). Endoplasmic reticulum stress, pancreatic beta-cell degeneration, and diabetes. *Cold Spring Harbor Perspectives in Medicine, 2*(9), a007666.

Pavlovic, D., Andersen, N. A., Mandrup-Poulsen, T., & Eizirik, D. L. (2000). Activation of extracellular signal-regulated kinase (ERK)1/2 contributes to cytokine-induced apoptosis in purified rat pancreatic beta-cells. *European Cytokine Network, 11*(2), 267–274.

Pollock, J. S., Forstermann, U., Tracey, W. R., & Nakane, M. (1995). Nitric oxide synthase isozymes antibodies. *Histochemical Journal, 27*(10), 738–744.

Raucci, A., Palumbo, R., & Bianchi, M. E. (2007). HMGB1: A signal of necrosis. *Autoimmunity, 40*(4), 285–289.

Riedl, S. J., & Salvesen, G. S. (2007). The apoptosome: Signalling platform of cell death. *Nature Reviews. Molecular Cell Biology, 8*(5), 405–413.

Rosales, A. L., Cunningham, J. M., Bone, A. J., Green, I. C., & Green, M. H. (2004). Repair of cytokine-induced DNA damage in cultured rat islets of Langerhans. *Free Radical Research, 38*(7), 665–674.

Saldeen, J. (2000). Cytokines induce both necrosis and apoptosis via a common Bcl-2-inhibitable pathway in rat insulin-producing cells. *Endocrinology, 141*(6), 2003–2010.

Saldeen, J., Lee, J. C., & Welsh, N. (2001). Role of p38 mitogen-activated protein kinase (p38 MAPK) in cytokine-induced rat islet cell apoptosis. *Biochemical Pharmacology, 61*(12), 1561–1569.

Scarim, A. L., Heitmeier, M. R., & Corbett, J. A. (1997). Irreversible inhibition of metabolic function and islet destruction after a 36-hour exposure to interleukin-1beta. *Endocrinology, 138*(12), 5301–5307.

Scarim, A. L., Heitmeier, M. R., & Corbett, J. A. (1998). Heat shock inhibits cytokine-induced nitric oxide synthase expression by rat and human islets. *Endocrinology, 139*(12), 5050–5057.

Scarim, A. L., Nishimoto, S. Y., Weber, S. M., & Corbett, J. A. (2003). Role for c-Jun N-terminal kinase in beta-cell recovery from nitric oxide-mediated damage. *Endocrinology, 144*(8), 3415–3422.

Schroder, M., & Kaufman, R. J. (2005). The mammalian unfolded protein response. *Annual Review of Biochemistry, 74*, 739–789.

Southern, C., Schulster, D., & Green, I. C. (1990). Inhibition of insulin secretion by interleukin-1 beta and tumour necrosis factor-alpha via an L-arginine-dependent nitric oxide generating mechanism. *FEBS Letters, 276*(1–2), 42–44.

Spinas, G. A., Mandrup-Poulsen, T., Molvig, J., Baek, L., Bendtzen, K., Dinarello, C. A., et al. (1986). Low concentrations of interleukin-1 stimulate and high concentrations inhibit insulin release from isolated rat islets of Langerhans. *Acta Endocrinologica, 113*(4), 551–558.

Steer, S. A., Scarim, A. L., Chambers, K. T., & Corbett, J. A. (2006). Interleukin-1 stimulates beta-cell necrosis and release of the immunological adjuvant HMGB1. *PLoS Medicine, 3*(2), e17.

Storling, J., Binzer, J., Andersson, A. K., Zullig, R. A., Tonnesen, M., Lehmann, R., et al. (2005). Nitric oxide contributes to cytokine-induced apoptosis in pancreatic beta cells via potentiation of JNK activity and inhibition of Akt. *Diabetologia, 48*(10), 2039–2050.

Takamura, T., Kato, I., Kimura, N., Nakazawa, T., Yonekura, H., Takasawa, S., et al. (1998). Transgenic mice overexpressing type 2 nitric-oxide synthase in pancreatic beta cells develop insulin-dependent diabetes without insulitis. *Journal of Biological Chemistry, 273*(5), 2493–2496.

Tamura, Y., Chiba, Y., Tanioka, T., Shimizu, N., Shinozaki, S., Yamada, M., et al. (2011). NO donor induces Nec-1-inhibitable, but RIP1-independent, necrotic cell death in pancreatic beta-cells. *FEBS Letters, 585*(19), 3058–3064.

Thomas, H. E., & Kay, T. W. (2011). Intracellular pathways of pancreatic beta-cell apoptosis in type 1 diabetes. *Diabetes/Metabolism Research and Reviews, 27*(8), 790–796.

Tran, V. V., Chen, G., Newgard, C. B., & Hohmeier, H. E. (2003). Discrete and complementary mechanisms of protection of beta-cells against cytokine-induced and oxidative damage achieved by bcl-2 overexpression and a cytokine selection strategy. *Diabetes, 52*(6), 1423–1432.

Wang, M., Zhao, X. R., Wang, P., Li, L., Dai, Y., Huang, H., et al. (2007). Glucose regulated proteins 78 protects insulinoma cells (NIT-1) from death induced by streptozotocin, cytokines or cytotoxic T lymphocytes. *International Journal of Biochemistry and Cell Biology, 39*(11), 2076–2082.

Weber, S. M., Chambers, K. T., Bensch, K. G., Scarim, A. L., & Corbett, J. A. (2004). PPARgamma ligands induce ER stress in pancreatic beta-cells: ER stress activation results in attenuation of cytokine signaling. *American Journal of Physiology. Endocrinology and Metabolism, 287*(6), E1171–E1177.

Weber, S. M., Scarim, A. L., & Corbett, J. A. (2003). Inhibition of IFN-gamma -induced STAT1 activation by 15- deoxy-Delta 12,14-prostaglandin J2. *American Journal of Physiology Endocrinology and Metabolism, 284*(5), E883–E891.

Welsh, N., Eizirik, D. L., Bendtzen, K., & Sandler, S. (1991). Interleukin-1 beta-induced nitric oxide production in isolated rat pancreatic islets requires gene transcription and may lead to inhibition of the Krebs cycle enzyme aconitase. *Endocrinology, 129*(6), 3167–3173.

Welsh, N., Margulis, B., Borg, L. A., Wiklund, H. J., Saldeen, J., Flodstrom, M., et al. (1995). Differences in the expression of heat-shock proteins and antioxidant enzymes between human and rodent pancreatic islets: Implications for the pathogenesis of insulin-dependent diabetes mellitus. *Molecular Medicine, 1*(7), 806–820.

Willis, S. N., Fletcher, J. I., Kaufmann, T., van Delft, M. F., Chen, L., Czabotar, P. E., et al. (2007). Apoptosis initiated when BH3 ligands engage multiple Bcl-2 homologs, not Bax or Bak. *Science, 315*(5813), 856–859.

Youle, R. J., & Strasser, A. (2008). The BCL-2 protein family: Opposing activities that mediate cell death. *Nature Reviews. Molecular Cell Biology, 9*(1), 47–59.

CHAPTER THIRTEEN

Activated Protein C and Its Potential Applications in Prevention of Islet β-Cell Damage and Diabetes

Meilang Xue[1], Christopher J. Jackson

Sutton Arthritis Research Laboratories, Kolling Institute of Medical Research, The University of Sydney at Royal North Shore Hospital, St Leonards, New South Wales, Australia

[1]Corresponding author: e-mail address: meilang.xue@sydney.edu.au

Contents

Abstract

Activated protein C (APC) is derived from its precursor, protein C (PC). Originally thought to be synthesized exclusively by the liver, recent reports have shown that PC is also produced by many other cells including pancreatic islet β cells. APC functions as a physiological anticoagulant with anti-inflammatory, anti-apoptotic, and barrier-stabilizing properties. APC exerts its protective effects via an intriguing mechanism requiring combinations of endothelial PC receptor, protease-activated receptors, epidermal growth factor receptor, Tie2 or CD11b, depending on cell types. Diabetes is a chronic condition resulted from the body's inability to produce and/or properly use insulin. The prevalence of diabetes has risen dramatically and has become one of the major causes of

Vitamins and Hormones, Volume 95
ISSN 0083-6729
http://dx.doi.org/10.1016/B978-0-12-800174-5.00013-2

premature mortality and morbidity worldwide. Diabetes prevention is an ideal approach to reduce this burden. Type 1 and type 2 diabetes are the major forms of diabetes mellitus, and both are characterized by an autoimmune response, intraislet inflammation, β-cell apoptosis, and progressive β-cell loss. Protecting β-cell from damage is critical in both prevention and treatment of diabetes. Recent *in vitro* and animal studies show that APC's strong anti-inflammatory and anti-apoptotic properties are beneficial in preventing β-cell destruction and diabetes in the NOD mouse model of type 1 diabetes. Future preventive and therapeutic uses of APC in diabetes look very promising.

1. INTRODUCTION

Protein C (PC), a vitamin K-dependent glycoprotein, is synthesized mostly in the liver and secreted into the blood plasma as a zymogen. PC is converted to its activated form (APC) when thrombin binds to thrombomodulin at the endothelial surface. This conversion is augmented by endothelial PC receptor (EPCR). APC plays an important role in the regulation of blood coagulation. The importance of APC as an anticoagulant is reflected by the findings that deficiencies in PC result in severe familial disorders of thrombosis. Replenishment of PC/APC in patients with systemic or local hypercoagulation can reverse the abnormality. Independent of anticoagulation, APC exerts a broad range of cytoprotective actions including inhibition of inflammation, prevention of cell apoptosis, stimulation of cell proliferation, and stabilization of endothelial and epithelia barrier function. These protective properties of APC are mediated by binding to its receptors and subsequent initiation of cellular signaling. A number of receptors have been identified to mediate APC's functions, including EPCR, protease-activated receptor (PAR)-1, PAR-2, and PAR-3, epidermal growth factor receptor (EGFR), Tie2, CD11b, β_1 and β_3 integrins, and apolipoprotein E receptor 2 (ApoER2).

Diabetes is a group of metabolic diseases in which a person has high blood glucose resulting from either inadequate insulin production or improper response to insulin, or both. Diabetes incidence is increasing rapidly and expected to rise further due to the aging population. Diabetes and its associated complications, such as kidney failure, heart disease, and stroke, have become the major causes of premature mortality and morbidity and will lead to a serious health crisis to many countries. At present there is no cure for diabetes. Diabetes prevention is an alternative strategy now receiving priority to reduce this burden. Type 1 and type 2 diabetes are the major forms of diabetes mellitus and both forms are inflammatory diseases with progressive β-cell loss by apoptosis (Donath & Shoelson, 2011; Eizirik, Colli, & Ortis, 2009). In this chapter, we provide a review of APC's functions and EPCR.

2. PROTEIN C AND ACTIVATED PROTEIN C

PC was first discovered by Johan Stenflo in 1976 from bovine plasma (Esmon, Stenflo, & Suttie, 1976). Charles Esmon and colleagues discovered a few years later that its activated form was a natural anticoagulant. Human PC gene (*PROC*) is positioned at Ch2q13–14; the genomic sequence is approximately 10,802 bp long and consists of nine exons (1790 bp), eight of which encode the protein (Foster, Yoshitake, & Davie, 1985; Plutzky, Hoskins, Long, & Crabtree, 1986). PC precursor consists of 461 amino acids. Posttranslational modifications include β-hydroxylation at Asp71, N-linked glycosylation at residues 97, 248, 313, and 329 and γ-carboxylation of nine glutamic acid residues which forms the Gla domain at the amino terminus. Mature human PC is a 62-kD protein and consists of 419 amino acids as a two-chain (heavy and light chains), disulfide-linked protein with four major moieties: (i) Gla domain, (ii) two epidermal growth factor-like regions, (iii) small activation peptide, and (iv) active serine protease domain (Griffin, 2002).

2.1. PC activation

PC is synthesized mostly in the liver and secreted into the blood plasma and circulates at 70 nM as an inactive zymogen with a half-life of 6–16 h, and its activated form APC at 40 pM with a half-life of 10–40 min (Gruber & Griffin, 1992). PC is activated by thrombin, the only currently known PC activator of physiologic relevance. When thrombin binds to thrombomodulin at the endothelial surface, it cleaves the activation peptide between Arg 12 and Leu 13 of the heavy chain and converts PC to its activated form (Griffin, 2002; Fig. 13.1). This conversion is augmented by EPCR (Fukudome & Esmon, 1994; Stearns-Kurosawa, Kurosawa, Mollica, Ferrell, & Esmon, 1996). Blocking the PC–EPCR interaction results in more than 80% decrease in circulating APC level generated in response to thrombin infusion (Taylor, Peer, Lockhart, Ferrell, & Esmon, 2001). In addition, Salem, Broze, Miletich, & Majerus (1983) have demonstrated that factor (F)Va can also promote thrombin-catalyzed PC activation, and the rate of this activation is no more than 10% that obtained with

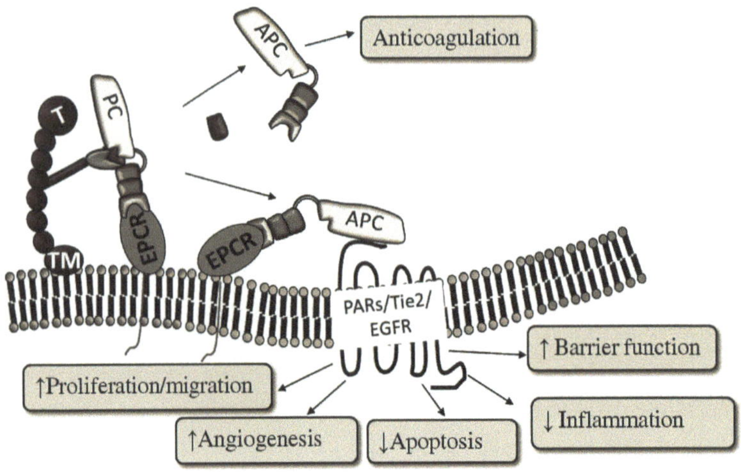

Figure 13.1 PC activation and cytoprotective function of APC mediated by EPCR. On the endothelial surface, EPCR binds and positions PC to allow it to bind thrombin (T) and thrombomodulin (TM) complex which enhances PC activation by thrombin. APC can exert its anticoagulant activity either as bound or in free form. Beneficial cytoprotective activities of APC require the cellular receptors EPCR and PARs and subsequent activation of Tie2/EGFR. These activities include the suppression of inflammation and cell apoptosis and the stimulation of cell proliferation, angiogenesis, and barrier function. (For color version of this figure, the reader is referred to the online version of this chapter.)

thrombomodulin. After activation, APC can dissociate from EPCR to exert its anticoagulant activity, or be retained on EPCR to exert multiple direct cellular activities as shown in Fig. 13.1.

2.2. Anticoagulation

Coagulation factors FVa and FVIIIa are two key factors in control of the coagulation cascade. APC cleaves at arginine 506, 306, and 679 in FVa and at arginine 336 and 562 in FVIIIa (Castoldi & Rosing, 2010), leading to the loss of binding affinity (and hence of cofactor activity) for FXa. For the full expression of anticoagulant activity, APC requires the plasma cofactors: protein S, FV, FVIII, calcium ions, and phospholipids. In the presence of its cofactor, protein S, APC inhibits thrombin generation by degrading the coagulation factors Va and VIIIa and promotes fibrinolysis by preventing inhibition of plasminogen conversion to plasmin. The importance of APC as an anticoagulant is reflected by the findings that deficiencies in PC result in severe familial disorders of thrombosis (Baker & Bick, 1999). Replenishment of PC/APC in patients with systemic or local hypercoagulation can reverse the abnormality.

2.3. PC deficiency

Familial PC deficiency was first associated with thrombosis in 1981 (Griffin, Evatt, Zimmerman, Kleiss, & Wideman, 1981). The prevalence of mild (heterozygous) PC deficiency in the general population is estimated at 1/200-500 (Tait et al., 1995), and this has been associated with a mild increased risk of venous thrombosis (Bertina, Broekmans, Van Der Linden, & Mertens, 1982; Dahlback, 2008; Goldenberg & Manco-Johnson, 2008). Only a small proportion of these individuals have a clinical significant disorder, which may also be associated with co-inheritance of additional thrombotic risk factors (Bertina et al., 1994; Dahlback, 2008; Goldenberg & Manco-Johnson, 2008). Severe (homozygous) PC deficiency is rare and usually associated with a severe prothrombotic diathesis. The clinical presentation is that of acute disseminated intravascular coagulation and hemorrhagic skin necrosis (Goldenberg & Manco-Johnson, 2008). Neonatal purpura fulminans is a rare, life-threatening condition of PC deficiency; the management includes an acute phase of replacement therapy with fresh frozen plasma or PC concentrate and a maintenance therapy that includes anticoagulation with warfarin or low molecular weight heparin (Chalmers et al., 2011; Price, Ledingham, Krumpel, & Chan, 2011). In addition to causing recurrent thrombotic disease, PC deficiency is also associated with both nonrecurrent and recurrent first, second, and third trimester miscarriages, intrauterine fetal death, intrauterine growth retardation, placental abruption and preeclampsia (Sugiura, 2005), high fetal loss and perinatal mortality (Chalmers et al., 2011), liver fibrogenesis (Anstee, Dhar, & Thursz, 2011), and hypercoagulability in calciphylaxis (Harris & Cropley, 2011). The risk of thrombotic occlusion following arterial revascularization in patients with an identified thrombophilia defect appears to be almost three times that of patients with no evidence of a thrombophilia defect (Vig et al., 2004).

Mice with a designed total genetic deficiency in PC (*PC−/−*) have severe perinatal consumptive coagulopathy in the brain and liver and do not survive beyond 24 h after delivery (Jalbert et al., 1998). In contrast, mice with only partial PC deficiency (expressing 1–18% of normal PC levels) can survive beyond birth, but they can develop thrombosis and inflammation (Lay, Liang, Rosen, & Castellino, 2005). The onset and severity of these phenotypes are strongly dependent on the levels of plasma PC. Mice with a severe deficiency in PC (1–3% of normal PC levels) display prothrombotic and proinflammatory phenotypes and compromized maternal reproductive capabilities (Lay et al., 2005). $PC+/^{-}$ mice ($63\% \pm 5\%$ of normal PC levels) do not display abnormal phenotype, however, in response to endotoxin challenge, plasma levels of proinflammatory cytokines, tumor necrosis factor-α (TNF-α), interleukin-6 (IL-6), and IL-1β are significantly higher (Levi et al., 2003).

2.4. Cytoprotective function of APC

In addition to anticoagulation, APC exerts a broad range of cytoprotective actions including inhibition of inflammation, prevention of cell apoptosis, stimulation of cell proliferation, and stabilization of endothelial and epithelial barrier function. Many of the antiinflammatory properties of APC are mediated through its specific receptor, EPCR (5), as discussed below.

2.4.1 Suppression of inflammation

Independent of its effect on coagulation, APC possesses strong anti-inflammatory properties. During acute inflammation, plasma APC levels are diminished (Liaw et al., 2004), and inflammatory cytokines such as IL-1β and TNF-α, as well as endotoxin, can inhibit thrombomodulin and EPCR expression, which further reduces the ability of endothelial cells to generate APC. A thrombomodulin mutation, which impairs APC generation, results in uncontrolled lung inflammation during murine tuberculosis (Weijer, Wieland, Florquin, & Van Der Poll, 2005). In several experimental models, including asthma, sepsis, ischemia–reperfusion injury, intestinal inflammation, and type 1 diabetes, in which the conversion of PC into APC is impaired or endogenous PC/APC level is low, administration of recombinant human (rh)APC consistently inhibits inflammatory cytokine production, leukocyte activation and infiltration (Elphick et al., 2009; Galley, El Sakka, Webster, Lowes, & Cuthbertson, 2008; Murakami et al., 1997; Nick et al., 2004; Xue, Dervish, Harrison, Fulcher, & Jackson, 2012). In central venous sinus thrombosis, APC protects the microvasculature by decreasing inflammatory cell recruitment (Nagai et al., 2010). Systemic APC treatment prevents the lethal effects of *Escherichia coli* in animal models of sepsis and significantly reduces endotoxin-induced pulmonary vascular injury by suppressing inflammation (Kerschen et al., 2007, 2010; Taylor et al., 1987, 2000); displays a potent antiinflammatory and neuroprotective effect in a murine model of focal ischemic stroke (Shibata et al., 2001); significantly reduces leukocyte rolling and adhesion to the mesenteric vessels and prevents leukocyte influx in a model of intestinal ischemia–reperfusion injury (Isobe, Okajima, Harada, Liu, & Okabe, 2004; Mizutani, Okajima, Uchiba, & Noguchi, 2000). Intratracheal administration of APC inhibits bleomycin-induced lung fibrosis in mice (Tanaka et al., 2008) and inhalation of APC suppresses endotoxin-induced pulmonary inflammation in mice (Slofstra et al., 2006). Topical administration of APC promotes cutaneous wound healing in both mouse and rat models partly by inhibition of inflammation (Jackson et al., 2005; Julovi et al., 2011). The involvement of APC in the inflammatory response is further demonstrated in transgenic mice in which the circulating levels of PC are an important marker of acute inflammatory responses (Lay, Donahue, Tsai, & Castellino, 2007). The genetic dosing of PC strongly correlates with survival outcomes following endotoxin LPS challenge in these mice. Reconstitution of low-PC mice with rhAPC improves hypotension and extends survival after LPS challenge (Xu, Ji, Zhang, Drake, & Esmon, 2009).

The antiinflammatory properties of APC are associated with a decrease in proinflammatory cytokines, a reduction in leukocyte recruitment, and suppression in the activation of nuclear factor (NF)-κB (Esmon, 2004a, 2012; Okajima, 2004). APC inhibits the adhesion, activation, and migration of neutrophils, monocytes, and lymphocytes both *in vitro* and *in vivo* (Elphick et al., 2009; Esmon, 2004a; Galley et al., 2008; Isobe et al., 2004; Mizutani et al., 2000; Murakami et al., 1997; Nick et al., 2004; Xue et al., 2012). In mouse experimental model of cerebral venous sinus thrombosis, APC decreases inflammatory cell recruitment to protect the microvasculature (Nagai et al., 2010). In endotoxemia and sepsis models, APC controls leukocyte recruitment during inflammation and improves survival to reduce the mortality of endotoxemia in mice (Frommhold et al., 2011; Kerschen et al., 2010). In NOD mice, APC inhibits T cells and macrophage infiltration, stimulates T regulatory cells (Tregs), and prevents the onset and development of diabetes (Xue et al., 2012). APC prevents both vascular leakage and accumulation of activated leukocytes to the mouse peritoneal cavity elicited by polyphosphate (Bae, Lee, & Rezaie, 2012). The infusion of APC attenuates the inflammatory response during systemic hypoxia by inhibition of leukocyte adherence, emigration, and venular permeability (Bartolome, Wood, Casillan, Simpson, & O'brien-Ladner, 2008). Neutrophil migration *in vitro* toward serum or IL-8 is significantly inhibited by pretreatment with APC (Slofstra et al., 2006).

The inhibitory role of APC on leukocyte recruitment could be mediated by suppression of adhesion molecules and cytokines/chemokines. For example, APC inhibits the synthesis of intercellular adhesion molecule (ICAM) and monocyte chemotactic protein (MCP)-1 (Franscini et al., 2004) as well as suppressing the expression of ICAM-1, vascular cell adhesion protein (VCAM)-1, and IL-8 induced by TNF-α in human dermal microvascular endothelial cells (Pina-Canseco Mdel et al., 2012) and monocytes (Xue, March, Sambrook, Fukudome, & Jackson, 2007). APC treatment of human neutrophils results in a decreased IL-6 expression which is responsible for the reduced chemotaxis (Galley et al., 2008). In monocytes, APC selectively inhibits inflammatory cytokine production while maintaining phagocytosis to combat invading pathogens and adherence capabilities, thereby promoting antimicrobial properties while limiting tissue damage (Stephenson, Toltl, Beaudin, & Liaw, 2006). Monocytes treated with APC decrease the release of tissue factor (Toltl, Beaudin, & Liaw, 2008), TNF-α (Grey et al., 1994), IL-1β, IL-6, IL-8 (Stephenson et al., 2006), and interferon (INF)γ (Pereira, Schaer, Bachli, Kurrer, & Schoedon, 2008). In Sprague-Dawley rats, APC treatment attenuates INFγ and IL-1β and preserves renal function in sepsis (Keller, Moore, Evans, Mckillop, & Huynh, 2011). APC also significantly reduces the deterioration of the mesenteric microcirculation and systemic IL-1β-release caused by endotoxin challenge during experimental endotoxemia in rats (Lehmann et al., 2008).

In addition to suppressing inflammatory cytokines, APC selectively upregulates antiinflammatory cytokine production. For example, APC increases IL-10, which subsequently reduces tissue factor in LPS-challenged blood monocytes (Toltl et al., 2008). In mouse spleen cells, APC dose dependently increases expression of transforming growth factor-β1 and IL-2, two cytokines that are required for the development, maintenance, and function of immunosuppressive Tregs (Xue et al., 2012).

One of the major mechanisms that augment inflammation is mediated through NF-κB activation and nuclear translocation from the cytosol (Joyce & Grinnell, 2002; White et al., 2000). NF-κB is a signaling molecule that controls the expression of a wide range of inflammatory genes including TNF-α, IL-1β, and cell adhesion molecules that are associated with diseases ranging from inflammation to cancer (Li & Verma, 2002). Direct inhibition of NF-κB is sufficient to block symptoms of many inflammatory diseases; so, these inhibitors have potential therapeutic value (Calzado, Bacher, & Schmitz, 2007; Li & Verma, 2002). APC directly suppresses the expression and activation of NF-κB in unstimulated and stimulated monocytes (White et al., 2000; Xue, March, Sambrook, Fukudome, & Jackson, 2007; Yuksel, Okajima, Uchiba, Horiuchi, & Okabe, 2002), keratinocytes (Xue, Thompson, Kelso, & Jackson, 2004), and endothelial cells (Franscini et al., 2004). APC also suppresses inflammation *in vivo* by inhibition of

NF-κB (Cheng et al., 2006) and exerts a cardioprotective function in ischemic/reperfusion injury partly through modulation of NF-κB signaling pathway (Wang, Yang, Rezaie, & Li, 2011). APC can reduce the synthesis of NF-κB components, p50 and p52 subunits, in endothelial cells (Joyce, Gelbert, Ciaccia, Dehoff, & Grinnell, 2001; Joyce & Grinnell, 2002), decrease NF-κB nuclear translocation (White et al., 2000), and reduce degradation of the NF-κB inhibitor, IκBα (Toltl, Austin, & Liaw, 2011).

APC has the ability to upregulate and activate matrix metalloproteinase (MMP)-2 in endothelial cells and skin keratinocytes (Nguyen, Arkell, & Jackson, 2000; Xue et al., 2004), an MMP with antiinflammatory properties (Itoh et al., 2002; Mcquibban et al., 2002) and to suppress MMP-9 (Cheng et al., 2006; Xue, March, Sambrook, & Jackson, 2007), an MMP associated with many inflammatory conditions (Itoh et al., 2002; Ram, Sherer, & Shoenfeld, 2006). APC colocalizes with MMP-2 in the synovial fluid and lining layer of the synovial joint (Buisson-Legendre, Smith, March, & Jackson, 2004). In rheumatoid arthritic (RA) synovial fibroblasts and RA monocytes, APC simultaneously upregulates MMP-2 activity and inhibits MMP-9 (Xue, March, Sambrook, & Jackson, 2007). In addition to the degradation of extracellular matrix, these two MMPs regulate inflammation by processing cytokines/chemokines with MMP-9 having stimulatory and MMP-2 having inhibitory effects on inflammation both *in vitro* and *in vivo* (Gearing et al., 1994; Itoh et al., 2002; Mcquibban et al., 2000). In RA, MMP-9 positively correlates with disease progression and severity (Gruber et al., 1996).

Together these activities constitute the major mechanisms by which APC suppresses inflammation *in vitro* and *in vivo*.

2.4.2 Promotion of cell proliferation and inhibition of cell apoptosis

APC induces cell proliferation in cultured human umbilical vein endothelial cells (HUVEC) (Uchiba et al., 2004), smooth muscle cells (Bretschneider et al., 2007), skin epidermal keratinocytes (Xue et al., 2004), neural stem and progenitor cells (Guo et al., 2013; Thiyagarajan, Fernandez, Lane, Griffin, & Zlokovic, 2008), neuroblasts (Petraglia, Marky, Walker, Thiyagarajan, & Zlokovic, 2010), osteoblasts (Kurata et al., 2010), and sheep tenocytes (Xue et al., 2009). These promoting effects of APC are likely via modulation of MAP kinase activity (Guo et al., 2013; Kurata et al., 2010; Thiyagarajan et al., 2008; Uchiba et al., 2004; Xue et al., 2004), a family of highly conserved serine/threonine protein kinases that regulate cell survival/apoptosis, differentiation, and enhance DNA synthesis to stimulate cell growth (Bretschneider et al., 2007).

Consistent with the stimulatory effects on cell growth, APC displays strong antiapoptotic properties. APC prevents keratinocyte and endothelial apoptosis (Xue et al., 2010, 2004), protects against glucose-induced podocyte apoptosis (Isermann et al., 2007), and prevents vascular endothelial cells from apoptosis triggered by sera from malaria and sepsis patients (Hemmer et al., 2011). APC-dependent antiapoptotic activity is associated with improved survival in sepsis in human and in various animal models (Cheng et al., 2003; Hotchkiss et al., 2000; Joyce et al., 2001; Liu et al., 2004; Mosnier & Griffin, 2003; Yen et al., 2013). APC prolongs the lifespan of *in vivo* circulating monocytes by inhibition of spontaneous monocyte apoptosis to increase phagocytosis of invading pathogens during infection (Joyce & Grinnell, 2002) and protects mouse cortical neurons from *N*-methyl-D-aspartate and staurosporine excitotoxicity-induced apoptosis in mice (Guo et al., 2004).

APC protects cells from apoptosis by regulation of caspase activation, DNA degradation, and induction of antiapoptotic mediators (Cheng et al., 2003; Joyce et al., 2001; Liu et al., 2004; Mosnier & Griffin, 2003). APC decreases sepsis-induced apoptosis resulting from increased p21 and p53 proteins in mice (Sakar, Vatansever, Sepit, Ozbilgin, & Yorgancioglu, 2007) and exerts an antiapoptotic effect via diminishing caspase-3 activity in monocytes (Stephenson et al., 2006; Toltl et al., 2011), human skin keratinocytes (Xue et al., 2004), and HUVEC (Seol, Lee, Jackson, Sambrook, & Park, 2011; Xue et al., 2010). APC prevents glucose-induced apoptosis in endothelial cells and podocytes by preventing the glucose-dependent induction of Bax and reduction of Bcl-2 modulation of caspase activation (Isermann et al., 2007). In stressed human brain endothelial cells, APC reduces the amounts of p53 protein and mRNA and maintains levels of protective Bcl-2 protein, thereby blocking the apoptotic pathway (Cheng et al., 2003). APC can reduce ischemia-induced cytotoxicity via blocking the activation of caspase-3, -8, and -9 both *in vitro* and *in vivo* (Du et al., 2011).

2.4.3 Barrier stabilization

The endothelium, a thin layer of cells that lines the interior surface of blood vessels and lymphatic vessels, acts as a semi-selective barrier between the vessel lumen and surrounding tissue, controlling the transfer of molecules and leukocytes into and out of the bloodstream. Breakdown of this barrier increases the permeability of the endothelial monolayer, leading to tissue edema and is a key pathogenic factor in inflammatory disorders, such as sepsis, cancer, RA, cardiovascular diseases, and diabetes (Van Zonneveld, De Boer, Van Der Veer, & Rabelink, 2010; Villasenor & Cleaver, 2012; Zanone, Favaro, & Camussi, 2008). APC enhances endothelial barrier integrity via regulation of cytoskeleton rearrangement, tight junction protein production/redistribution, and stabilization and angiopoietin/Tie2 axis (Feistritzer & Riewald, 2005; Finigan et al., 2005; Minhas, Xue, Fukudome, & Jackson, 2010; Xue et al., 2010).

Tie2 and its activating ligand angiopoietin (Ang)-1 are required for vascular remodeling and vessel integrity. They play key roles in development and maintenance of the vascular system and potently inhibit vascular leakage and suppress endothelial apoptosis and vessel regression (Makinde & Agrawal, 2008; Peters, 2004; Salmon et al., 2009). Tie2 belongs to the receptor tyrosine kinase family and functions as a receptor for Ang1 and Ang2. While Ang1 is a Tie2 agonist, Ang2 acts as an antagonist on endothelium, by inhibiting Ang1-induced Tie2 activation (Hansen, Singh, Tahir, & Brindle, 2010). In confluent cells, Ang1 induces Tie2 translocation to cell–cell contacts to form homotypic Tie2–Tie2 trans-associated complexes, leading to inhibition of paracellular permeability (Fukuhara et al., 2008). APC significantly upregulates gene and protein expression of Tie2 and Ang1 in a dose- and time-dependent manner in HUVEC, while it markedly inhibits Ang2 (Minhas et al., 2010). HUVEC permeability, measured using Evans blue dye transfer, is significantly reduced in the presence of APC and, in concordance, the tight-junction-associated protein, zona occludens (ZO)-1, is upregulated and localized peripherally around cells, compared to control (Minhas et al., 2010). HUVEC transfected with PCsiRNA display reduced levels of Ang1 and Tie2 and elevated Ang2, resulting in an increase in endothelial permeability (Xue et al., 2010). In addition, PC siRNA causes diffuse distribution of Tie2 and ZO-1, while APC relocates Tie2 and ZO-1 to the peripheral cell–cell contact borders of HUVEC. This concurs with the report showing that trans-association of Tie2 contributes to maintenance of vascular quiescence by enhancing endothelial survival and integrity (Fukuhara et al., 2008).

The inner lining of quiescent capillary blood vessels consists of a continuous barrier of vascular endothelium surrounded by a basement membrane. Type IV collagen is the major component of the vascular basement membrane structure and provides stability to the blood vessel. APC stimulates type IV collagen production by HUVEC, which is localized pericellularly, indicative of a basement membrane protein. In addition, endogenous PC is associated with MMP-2 expression and activation by HUVEC (Xue et al.,

2010). MMP-2 is one of the major proteases responsible for basement membrane turnover. In endothelial cells, recombinant APC upregulates the activity of MMP-2 (Nguyen et al., 2000). The protective effect of endogenous PC/APC on endothelial cells may be mediated via Angs, ZO-1, collagen type IV, and MMP-2. Barrier stabilization is more effective when APC is derived endogenously and functions in an autocrine manner, than when the source of APC is exogenous (Feistritzer, Schuepbach, et al., 2006). Comparable barrier-protective effects by exogenous APC required a fourfold higher concentration of APC generated on the endothelial cell surface.

APC also enhances sphingosine-1-phosphate (S1P) production, which signals through its G-protein-coupled receptor to stabilize the cytoskeleton and reduce endothelial permeability (Feistritzer & Riewald, 2005; Finigan et al., 2005). In lung endothelial cells, APC treatment transactivates S1P1 and results in endothelial cell cytoskeletal rearrangement and barrier protection. Targeted silencing of S1P1 expression using siRNA significantly reduces APC-mediated barrier protection against thrombin (Finigan et al., 2005). Similarly, in HUVEC, siRNA that targets sphingosine kinase-1 or S1P receptor-1 blocks APC's protective signaling (Feistritzer & Riewald, 2005). Endogenous APC limits cancer cell extravasation through S1P1 receptor 1-mediated VE-cadherin-dependent vascular barrier enhancement (Van Sluis et al., 2009).

Recent studies have shed light on a new role of the PC system in controlling epithelial permeability. The primary function of the epithelial layer is to constitute a tight, highly selective barrier to protect areas of the body that come into contact with the external environment, so they are mostly found in skin and the gastrointestinal tract and are essential for survival (Kirschner & Brandner, 2012). Epithelial barrier function is mainly mediated by tight junctions. Loss of proper epithelial barrier function in the gut may lead to intestinal inflammation. The epithelial expression of PC and EPCR is downregulated in patients with inflammatory bowel disease (D'alessio, Genua, & Vetrano, 2012; Marchiando, Graham, & Turner, 2010; Vetrano et al., 2011). APC inhibits intestinal permeability by regulating tight junction molecules and promoting mucosal healing (Vetrano et al., 2011). PC severe deficient mice, expressing only 3% of normal PC level, develop spontaneous intestinal inflammation and are prone to severe experimental colitis with a spontaneous elevated production of inflammatory cytokines and increased intestinal permeability. Structural analysis of epithelial tight junction molecules revealed that lack of PC leads to decreased junctional adhesion molecule (JAM)-A and claudin-3 expression and an altered pattern of ZO-1 expression (Vetrano et al., 2011). *In vitro*, treatment of epithelial cells with APC leads to protection of tight junction disruption induced by TNF-α, and *in vivo*, topical treatment with APC causes mucosal healing and amelioration of colitis (Vetrano et al., 2011). In addition, APC reduces the thrombin-induced disruption of alveolar epithelial barrier integrity via decreasing epithelial permeability, cell stiffening, cell contraction, and enhancing ZO-1 aggregates at cell–cell interface (Puig et al., 2013).

The barrier-protective effect of APC is also relevant to skin epidermal keratinocytes (Xue et al., 2011). Keratinocytes play a critical role in maintaining epidermal barrier function. Disruption of this barrier function is responsible for many skin disorders, such as psoriasis and atopic dermatitis (Koster, 2009). The barrier properties of skin epidermis are largely dependent on the function and integrity of the tight junctions (occludins, claudins, and JAMs) between keratinocytes (Proksch, Brandner, & Jensen, 2008; Proksch & Brasch, 2012; Vandenbroucke, Mehta, Minshall, & Malik, 2008). Deregulation of these junction proteins perturbs this barrier (Proksch et al., 2008; Proksch & Brasch, 2012). For example, deficiency of claudin-1 results in epidermal water loss and, ultimately, the neonatal death of mice (Furuse et al., 2002).

In response to APC treatment, Tie2 is rapidly activated within 30 min on keratinocyte monolayers, and relocated to cell–cell contacts, the expression of junction proteins, ZO-1, claudin-1, and VE-cadherin, are also increased. Inhibition of Tie2 by its peptide inhibitor or siRNA abolishes the barrier-protective effect of APC. Interestingly, APC does not activate Tie2 through its major ligand, Ang-1, but instead acted by binding to endothelial PC receptor, cleaving PAR-1 and transactivating EGFR. Furthermore, when activation of Akt, but not ERK, is inhibited, the barrier-protective effect of APC on keratinocytes is abolished. Thus, APC activates Tie2, via a mechanism requiring, in sequential order, the receptors, EPCR, PAR-1, and EGFR, which selectively enhances the PI3K/Akt signaling to enhance junctional complexes and reduce keratinocyte monolayer permeability (Xue et al., 2011).

2.5. APC cellular signaling

2.5.1 EPCR and PAR-1

EPCR is a type I transmembrane protein that shares homology with the major histocompatibility class 1/CD1 family of proteins. It is the first receptor identified on endothelial cells and binds PC and APC with a similar affinity (Fukudome & Esmon, 1994). Originally thought to be expressed exclusively on endothelial cells, EPCR was subsequently found on many types of cells including various leukocytes such as neutrophils, monocytes (Esmon, 2004b), the basal layer of epidermis and cultured keratinocytes (Xue, Campbell, Sambrook, Fukudome, & Jackson, 2005), synovial lining cells (Xue, March, Sambrook, Fukudome, et al., 2007), smooth muscle cells (Bretschneider et al., 2007), and murine $CD8^{+}$ conventional dendritic cells (Kerschen et al., 2010). EPCR is an established murine hematopoietic stem cell marker (Balazs, Fabian, Esmon, & Mulligan, 2006). In addition, high EPCR-expressing cells are observed in basal-like tumors in breast cancer (Park et al., 2010).

As a receptor, EPCR mediates many cytoprotective properties of APC, including the antiapoptotic, anti-inflammatory, and barrier-protective functions (Bouwens & Mosnier, 2012; Esmon, 2004b). In addition, EPCR itself is a central player in the convergent pathways of homeostasis and inflammation (Esmon, 2004b). For example, overexpression of EPCR protects transgenic mice from endotoxin-induced injury (Li, Zheng, Gu, Hunter, et al., 2005), and EPCR is essential for normal embryonic development as deletion of the EPCR gene in mice is lethal by embryonic day (E) 10 (Gu et al., 2002; Li, Zheng, Gu, Ferrell, et al., 2005).

After binding to EPCR, APC can cleave PAR-1 to promote its cytoprotective actions in endothelial cells (Riewald, Petrovan, Donner, Mueller, & Ruf, 2002) and keratinocytes (Xue et al., 2005). PARs are members of the G-protein-coupled receptor superfamily whose cellular responses are driven through various G-protein and non-G-protein pathways, resulting in a diverse array of physiologic outputs (Coughlin, 2000). PARs are expressed on nearly all cell types in the blood vessel wall and blood, the notable exception being red blood cells (Leger, Covic, & Kuliopulos, 2006). The four known PARs are activated via proteolytic cleavage by a wide range of proteases that results in an intramolecular tethered ligand that triggers activation of a G protein and subsequent intracellular signaling. Thrombin activates PAR-1, PAR-3, and PAR-4, whereas other serine proteases activate PAR-2. Recently, MMP-1 (Trivedi et al., 2009) and MMP-13 (Jaffre, Friedman, Hu, Mackman, & Blaxall, 2012) have been found to cleave and activate PAR-1. These data indicate that selective proteolytic activation of PAR-1 by MMPs may be important to the evolution of many disease processes, including atherosclerosis, sepsis, heart failure, and cancer. Thrombin activation of PAR-1 promotes platelet aggregation, shape change, adhesion, cell proliferation, increases vascular permeability, activates NF-κB, increases inflammatory cytokine/chemokine production, and leukocyte activation and migration via G_q, G_i, and $G_{12/13}$ pathways (Soh, Dores, Chen, & Trejo, 2010; Trejo, 2003), all of which promote an inflammatory response. Activation of PAR-1 by thrombin also results in Ras homolog gene family member A (RhoA) activation, disassembly of adherens junctions, and disruption of the endothelial barrier. However, when APC cleaves PAR-1, its actions are directly opposite to that of thrombin in being antiinflammatory and stabilizing barrier integrity. Activation of PAR-1 by APC results in β-arrestin-dependent recruitment of disheveled-2 scaffold which activates Ras-related C3 botulinum toxin substrate 1 (Rac1) and endothelial barrier protection. Depletion of β-arrestin expression leads to the loss of APC-induced Rac1 activation but not of thrombin-stimulated RhoA signaling. APC fails to protect against thrombin-induced endothelial barrier permeability in cells deficient in β-arrestin expression (Soh & Trejo, 2011). Bae, Yang, Manithody, and Rezaie (2007) have shown that EPCR is associated with caveolin-1 in lipid rafts in endothelial cells. When APC binds to EPCR in the lipid raft, caveolin-1 is replaced with PAR-1 which couples with the pertussis toxin sensitive G_i protein to initiate a protective signaling pathway. In contrast, when thrombin cleaves PAR-1 outside the lipid raft signaling occurs via G_q and/or $G_{12/13}$ which exert inflammatory effects. Interestingly, if EPCR is occupied on the lipid raft, even thrombin, can induce activation of the G_i protein and mimic the protective effects of APC (Bae et al., 2007). Mosnier, Sinha, Burnier, Bouwens, and Griffin (2012) further reveal that the biased agonism of PAR-1 by APC is caused by noncanonical cleavage at Arg46 and by thrombin at Arg41. APC cleavage of PAR-1 at Arg46 results in the activation of Akt and glycogen synthase kinase 3β, Rac 1 and barrier stabilization effects on endothelial cells. A synthetic peptide, which mimics APC's action on PAR-1, stimulates protective signaling in endothelial cells (Mosnier et al., 2012).

2.5.2 EGFR and Tie-2

In normal epidermis, EGFR is important for autocrine growth of this renewing tissue, suppression of terminal differentiation, promotion of cell survival, and regulation of cell migration during epidermal morphogenesis. In wounded skin, EGFR is momentarily upregulated and is a major contributor to the proliferative and migratory aspects of wound reepithelialization. EGFR is able to regulate cell adhesion, expression of matrix degrading proteinases, and cell migration to provide a vital contribution to the migratory and invasive potential of keratinocytes (Hudson & Mccawley, 1998). EPCR and activated EGFR are colocalized in basal and suprabasal keratinocytes in the epidermis, which is identical to PC/APC localization in skin epidermis (Xue, Campbell, & Jackson, 2007). When keratinocytes are stimulated with APC, the expression and activation of EGFR are markedly increased, and conversely, when cells are treated with PC siRNA, EGFR activation is inhibited by more than 50% (Xue, Campbell, & Jackson, 2007). APC exerts the barrier-protective effect on keratinocytes via binding to EPCR, cleaving PAR-1, and trans-activating EGFR followed by transactivation of Tie2 (Xue et al., 2011). Similarly, APC requires three receptors, the EPCR, PAR-1, and Tie2, to perform its barrier stabilization functions on endothelial cells (Minhas et al., 2010). In MDA-MB-231 cells, APC engages EPCR, PAR-1, and EGFR to increase the invasiveness of these cells (Gramling, Beaulieu, & Church, 2010). In human lymphocytes, APC stimulates phosphorylation of EGFR to arrest directed migration of these cells (Feistritzer, Mosheimer, et al., 2006).

2.5.3 Other receptors

2.5.3.1 CD11

On macrophages, the antiinflammatory activity of APC is dependent on integrin CD11b/CD18, but not on EPCR. Genetic inactivation of CD11b, PAR-1, or sphingosine kinase-1, but not EPCR, abolishes the ability of APC to suppress the macrophage inflammatory response *in vitro*. APC administration reduces the mortality of wild-type mice, but not CD11b-deficient mice in a LPS-induced mouse model of lethal endotoxemia. These data reveal that CD11b is required for suppression of the endotoxin-induced macrophage inflammatory response and EPCR-independent antiinflammatory effects of APC (Cao et al., 2010).

2.5.3.2 ApoER2

Using human monocytic-like U937 cells, Yang et al. (2009) find that receptor-associated protein (RAP) inhibits APC-induced phosphorylation of adaptor protein disabled-1 (Dab1), Akt and glycogen synthase kinase 3β, whereas anti-EPCR or anti-PAR-1 blocking antibodies did not. Knocking down ApoER2 by siRNA ablates APC-induced Dab1 activation, suggesting that RAP-sensitive APC-induced signaling requires ApoER2 (Yang et al., 2009). In surface plasmon resonance equilibrium binding studies, APC binds to soluble (s) ApoER2 and purified ectodomains of the receptors ApoER2 with high affinity (White et al., 2008). RAP blocks APC binding to sApoER2 but not to sEPCR, and suppresses binding of U937 cells to immobilized APC. APC's ability to inhibit endotoxin-induced tissue factor procoagulant activity of U937 cells is abolished by RAP blocking (Yang et al., 2009). These findings indicate that APC may directly promote cell signaling in these cells by binding to ApoER2.

2.5.3.3 PAR-2

APC was originally found to activate PAR-2 (Riewald et al., 2002); however, no known function was resolved. Our recent study indicates that APC acts through both PAR-1 and PAR-2 to activate Akt and to increase keratinocyte proliferation and yet APC-induced murine wound healing depends only on PAR-2 activity (Julovi et al., 2011).

2.5.3.4 PAR-3

In podocytes, APC inhibits apoptosis through proteolytic activation of PAR-3 and independent of EPCR. Genetic deletion of PAR-3 impairs the nephroprotective effect of APC, demonstrating the crucial role of PAR-3 for APC-dependent podocyte protection (Madhusudhan et al., 2012). APC-ameliorated diabetic nephropathy is achieved via PAR-1 and PAR-3 by inhibiting the expression of redox-regulating protein $p66^{Shc}$ in podocytes (Bock et al., 2013). By using different anti-PAR blocking antibodies and mice with single PAR-1, PAR-3, or PAR-4 deletion, direct neuronal protective effects of APC *in vitro* and *in vivo* have also been found to require PAR-1 and PAR-3 (Guo et al., 2004).

2.5.3.5 β_1 and β_3 integrins

Elphick et al. (2009) demonstrate that rhAPC inhibits neutrophil adhesion and migration on extracellular matrix proteins by directly binding to β_1 and β_3 integrins on the neutrophil surface both *in vitro* and *in vivo*. This action of APC does not require EPCR (Elphick et al., 2009).

3. PANCREAS AND PANCREATIC ISLET β-CELL FUNCTION

3.1. Pancreas and pancreatic islet β-cells

The pancreas is a dual-function glandular organ, having features of both endocrine and exocrine, which regulate metabolic homeostasis via two parallel functions. The exocrine secretes pancreatic juices into the gastrointestinal tract for digestion of food, and the endocrine produces hormones, such as insulin and glucagon, into the bloodstream to control blood glucose levels. The exocrine (90% pancreas) is comprised of grape-like clusters of trapezoid shaped exocrine acinar cells located at the tips of a branching, ramifying network of ducts. Embedded within this abundant exocrine tissue are scattered spheroid groups of endocrine cells (10% pancreas), termed the "Islets of Langerhans" by the German pathologist Paul Langerhans, who first identified them in 1869. A human pancreas contains approximately one million islets that range in size from a few cells to a few hundred cells each. Islets consist of five principal endocrine lineages by their secretion: β cells (70%) produce insulin and amylin (decrease glucose in blood), α cells (20%) secrete glucagon (increase glucose in blood), δ cells (10%) secrete somatostatin (regulates/stops α and β cells), PP cells or gamma cells (2%) producing pancreatic polypeptide, and ghrelin-producing epsilon cells (Brissova et al., 2005; Elayat, El-Naggar, & Tahir, 1995). The islet of Langerhans plays an imperative role in glucose metabolism and regulation of blood glucose concentration. Maintaining proper blood glucose levels is crucial to the functioning of key organs including the brain, liver, and kidney. It has been recognized that the cytoarchitecture of pancreatic islets differs between species (Brissova et al., 2005; Cabrera et al., 2006). In rodents, β cells make up the bulk of the islet, with α cells and other endocrine cell types forming a mantle around the islet periphery. In humans, this organization is less clear. Human islets display α and β cells in close relationship with each other throughout the cluster, and α cells are found within the islet core. It has been proposed that human islets may consist of many smaller "rodent-like" endocrine aggregates or of folded "plates" of α and β cells lined by blood vessels (Bosco et al., 2010). Nevertheless, in all vertebrates, endocrine cells of mature islets release their hormone contents into dense networks of tightly associated capillaries, which connect them to the rest of the body.

The pancreatic islet is one of the most vascularized organs, having a blood perfusion of about 10% of that of the whole pancreas, despite representing only 1% of the gland. The islet capillaries show about 10 times more fenestrations than those within the exocrine tissue and are highly permeable. Besides providing oxygen and nutrients to the endocrine cells, islet endothelium is crucial in fine-tuning blood glucose sensing and regulation, and to behave as an active "gatekeeper" in the control of leukocyte recruitment into the islets, adopting an activated phenotype during autoimmune insulitis in type 1 diabetes (Villasenor & Cleaver, 2012; Zanone et al., 2008).

3.2. Islet β-cell damage

Once the pancreas or pancreatic insulin-producing β cells are damaged or destroyed, the patient loses the ability to produce sufficient insulin, resulting in diseases which require permanent insulin therapy. The main types of pancreatic diseases associated β-cell damage are type 1 diabetes (also known as Juvenile Diabetes) and type 2 diabetes.

Cell damage/death can be regulated via apoptosis, autophagy, necrosis, senescence, and mitotic catastrophe (Sasi, Hwang, Jaboin, Csiki, & Lu, 2009). Pancreatic β-cells damage is mainly mediated via two independent pathways: necrosis and apoptosis. Apoptosis is the dominant form of β-cell death. During apoptosis, cells first shrink and their nuclei condense, and then they disintegrate into well-enclosed apoptotic bodies. The process of apoptosis has a critical role for the survival of an organism and is functionally conserved in all higher eukaryotes. Impairment of normal apoptosis can lead to cancer or autoimmune diseases (Favaloro, Allocati, Graziano, Di Ilio, & De Laurenzi, 2012; Norbury & Hickson, 2001). The alternative to apoptotic cell death is necrosis, which is considered to be a toxic process where the cell is a passive victim and follows an energy-independent mode of death. During necrosis, cells first swell and then the plasma membrane collapses and cells are rapidly lysed (Majno & Joris, 1995). Necrosis is caused by factors external to the cell or tissue, such as infection, toxins, or trauma that result in the loss of cell membrane integrity and an uncontrolled release of products of cell death into the intracellular space (Sasi et al., 2009). Necrosis usually evokes powerful inflammatory response (Proskuryakov, Konoplyannikov, & Gabai, 2003).

Apoptosis can be initiated by extrinsic and intrinsic signaling pathways. Extrinsic apoptosis indicates a form of death induced by extracellular signals that result in the binding of ligands such as Fas ligand (FasL), TRAIL/Apo2L, and TNF-α, or agonistic monoclonal antibodies, to specific transmembrane receptors, collectively known as death receptors (DRs) belonging to the TNF superfamily (Locksley, Killeen, & Lenardo, 2001). The intrinsic signaling pathway is activated by a diverse array of non-receptor-mediated stimuli that lead to permeabilization of the outer mitochondrial membrane and some proteins, such as cytochrome c, which are released from the intermembrane space of mitochondria (Tait & Green, 2010). These stimuli include UV- and γ-irradiation, chemotherapeutic drugs, hypoxia, hyperthermia, viral infections, free radicals, and the removal of certain growth factors, hormones, and cytokines (Cory & Adams, 2002; Saelens et al., 2004). This pathway is regulated by pro- and antiapoptotic Bcl-2 superfamily proteins (Cory & Adams, 2002).

The extrinsic and intrinsic pathways both end at the execution phase, initiated by the activation of the execution caspases. Execution caspases activate cytoplasmic endonuclease and proteases that degrade DNA and nuclear and cytoskeletal proteins, ultimately cause the morphological and biochemical changes seen in apoptotic cells (Slee, Adrain, & Martin, 2001). Execution caspases are activated by initiator caspases. The main initiator caspases are caspase-2, -8, -9, and -10, whereas caspase-3 and to a lesser extent caspase-6 and -7 serve as effector or execution caspases in mammals (Degterev, Boyce, & Yuan, 2003; Kumar, 2007; Slee et al., 2001). Cross talk between the extrinsic and intrinsic pathways occurs through caspase-8-mediated cleavage of Bcl-2 homology 3-interacting domain death agonist (Tait & Green, 2010).

In addition to the extrinsic and the intrinsic caspase-dependent pathway, cytotoxic T lymphocytes are also able to exert their cytotoxic effects on cells via perforin/granzyme-mediated caspase-independent pathway with a subsequent exophytic release of serine proteases granzyme A and granzyme B from cytoplasmic granules (Anthony, Andrews, Watt, Trapani, & Smyth, 2010; Brunner et al., 2003; Voskoboinik, Dunstone, Baran, Whisstock, & Trapani, 2010). Granzyme A cleaves DNA molecules in the nucleus and leads to cellular apoptosis (Nakajima, Park, & Henkart, 1995). Granzyme B induces mostly caspase-dependent apoptosis (Zhou, 2010).

3.3. β-Cell damage and diabetes

Type 1 and type 2 diabetes are characterized by intraislet expression of inflammatory mediators, triggering a final common pathway of β-cell apoptosis, progressive β-cell loss, and diabetes. Pancreatic β-cell death by apoptosis contributes significantly to both forms of diabetes (Cnop et al., 2005; Johnson & Luciani, 2010).

The destruction of β cells in type 1 diabetes in humans and in autoimmune diabetes in the NOD mouse model is a consequence of chronic islet inflammation in the pancreas (Bettini & Vignali, 2011). Type 1 diabetes has two distinct phases: sub-clinical, when mononuclear cells infiltrate the islets (insulitis) selectively destroying β cells, and clinical, when most β cells have been destroyed leading to inadequate insulin production and hyperglycemia (Bluestone, Herold, & Eisenbarth, 2010). Apoptosis studies in NOD mouse model of type 1 diabetes demonstrate that β-cell destruction is mediated by autoreactive T cells (Adorini, Gregori, & Harrison, 2002; Bluestone et al., 2010), and $CD8^+$ T lymphocytes are considered as final effectors for type 1 diabetes (Christianson, Shultz, & Leiter, 1993). $CD4^+$ and $CD8^+$ T cells can transfer diabetes from recent diabetic mice to young, irradiated NOD mice or NOD.SCID mice (Adorini et al., 2002; Bluestone et al., 2010).

Autoreactive effector $CD8^+$ T lymphocytes that recognize β-cell-derived antigens can be detected in humans (Coppieters et al., 2012; Velthuis et al., 2010).

Autoreactive T cells are normally held in check by a variety of Tregs. Prototypic $CD4^+CD25^+$ Tregs are programmed by the forkhead box transcription factor (FoxP3) (Sakaguchi, Yamaguchi, Nomura, & Ono, 2008). The critical role of FoxP3 is illustrated by its natural mutation in scurfy mice and in humans with immune dysregulation polyendocrinopathy enteropathy, X-linked (IPEX) syndrome, which leads to multiorgan-specific autoimmune disease in infancy (Ochs, Ziegler, & Torgerson, 2005). Tregs suppress differentiation of islet-reactive $CD8^+$ T cells to cytotoxic T cells (Green, Gorelik, Mcgregor, Tran, & Flavell, 2003) and protect against diabetes development in the NOD mouse (Salomon et al., 2000).

In the course of insulitis, other cell types including B cells, macrophages, dendritic cells, and NK cells are also present in the pancreatic infiltrate and can contribute to β-cell destruction (Bending, Zaccone, & Cooke, 2012; Cai, 2012). In addition, β cells can also be damaged by granzymes and perforin released from $CD8^+$ cytotoxic T cells and by soluble mediators such as cytokines and reactive oxygen molecules and oxygen-free radicals released from activated macrophages in the islets (Bettini & Vignali, 2011).

There is a progressive deterioration in β-cell function and mass in type 2 diabetes. The reduction in β-cell mass is attributable to accelerated apoptosis. The major factors for progressive loss of β-cell function and mass in type 2 diabetes are glucotoxicity, lipotoxicity, proinflammatory cytokines, leptin, and islet cell amyloid (Wajchenberg, 2007). Glucotoxicity may greatly contribute to the pathogenesis of type 2 diabetes. Regular physiological stimulation by glucose plays a crucial role in the maintenance of the β-cell-differentiated phenotype. In contrast, prolonged or repeated exposure to elevated glucose concentrations induced β-cell overstimulation, oxidative stress, excessive unfolded protein response activation, and loss of differentiation in the alteration of the β-cell phenotype, inflammation, amyloidogenesis, protein glycation, hypoxia, excessive formation of reactive oxygen, and reactive nitrogen species, ultimately leading to apoptosis related to oxidative stress (Bensellam, Laybutt, & Jonas, 2012; Kohnert, Freyse, & Salzsieder, 2012).

As death effector molecules, *in vivo* as well as *in vitro* studies support a role for perforin/granzyme, Fas/FasL, TRAIL/TRAIL receptors, proinflammatory cytokines, and free radicals in β-cell killing. Among the regulators of apoptosis, NF-κB has emerged as a master switch of cytokine-induced β-cell dysfunction and death (Kim & Lee, 2009). Conditional and specific NF-κB blockade protects pancreatic β cells from diabetogenic agents (Eldor et al., 2006). Induction of NF-κB and its downstream genes by TNF-α and IL-1β has a proapoptotic role in pancreatic β cells (Ortis et al., 2008). Thus, β-cell-specific activation of NF-κB is a key event in the progressive loss of β cells in diabetes. Inhibition of this process could be a potential effective strategy for β-cell protection (Melloul, 2008).

Collectively, killing β cells resulting in diabetes occurs through a range of redundant and compensatory mechanisms including necrotic cell death, mitochondrial-mediated, caspase-dependent, and caspase-independent apoptosis (Campbell et al., 2008; Lightfoot, Chen, & Mathews, 2011) as shown in Fig. 13.2.

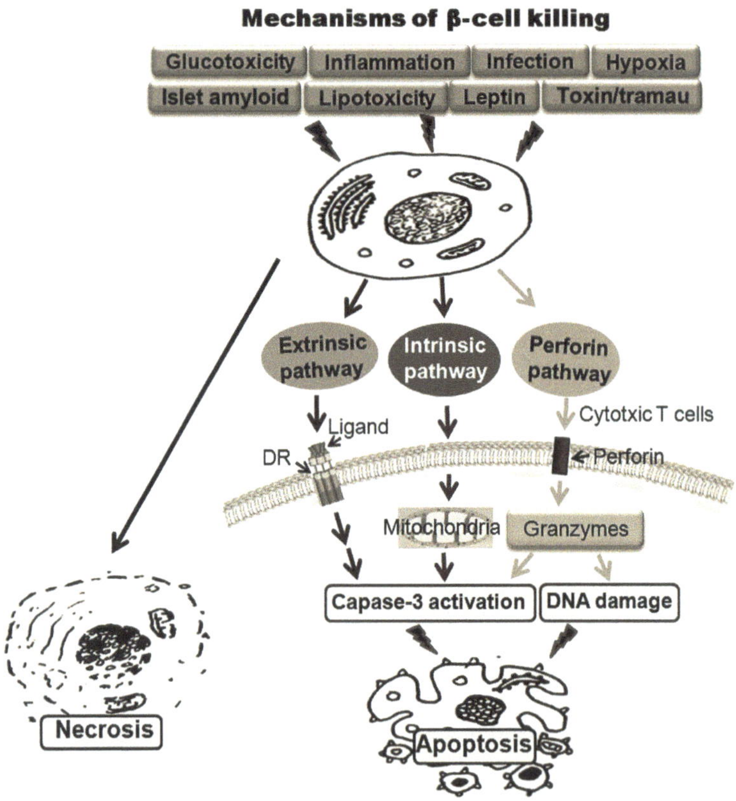

Figure 13.2 Mechanisms of β-cell killing. β Cells are damaged mainly by necrosis and apoptosis with the latter being the dominant form of β-cell death. β-Cell apoptosis is regulated by extrinsic, intrinsic, and perforin pathways. DR, death receptor. (For color version of this figure, the reader is referred to the online version of this chapter.)

Once the β cells are destroyed, the patient loses the ability to make insulin and must rely on insulin injection therapy. Given the complications associated with long-term administration of insulin and difficulties in maintaining optimal levels of blood glucose, alternative therapies are being sought. Replacement of the β cells by transplantation of islet cells is a radical but promising therapy for human diabetes (Ablamunits, Sherry, Kushner, & Herold, 2007; Dominguez-Bendala, Inverardi, & Ricordi, 2012). Its clinical impact remains limited by early islet destruction mediated by prothrombotic and innate inflammatory responses elicited upon transplantation. Apoptotic β-cell death appears to be central in islet graft rejection. The control of alloimmunity and/or autoimmunity to prevent β-cell death will also be of utmost importance when using allogeneic or syngeneic β cells generated to replace lost β cells in humans in future therapy (Baiu, Merriam, & Odorico, 2011).

Mechanistic insights into the control of pancreatic β-cell apoptosis are therefore important for the prevention and treatment of diabetes (Johnson & Luciani, 2010). In addition, therapies capable of stimulating β-cell regeneration in the absence of active autoimmune destruction are urgently needed (Ablamunits et al., 2007). Resolving the critical molecular and cell death mechanism(s) in diabetes will allow for the development of targeted therapies toward the prevention of diabetes and protection of pancreatic islet grafts.

4. APC AND β-CELL PRESERVATION IN DIABETES

APC's strong anti-inflammatory, antiapoptotic, and barrier-stabilizing properties appear to be beneficial in preventing destruction of islet cells in diabetes as discussed below.

4.1. APC preserves islet mass after transplantation

Inflammation and autoimmunity play an important role in the destruction of pancreatic islet β cells in diabetes of both animal models and humans. Murine (m)APC therapy significantly reduces loss of functional islet mass after intraportal transplantation in diabetic mice (Contreras et al., 2004). Animals given mAPC exhibit better glucose control, higher glucose disposal rates, and higher arginine-stimulated acute insulin release. These effects are associated with reduced plasma proinsulin, intrahepatic fibrin deposition, and islet apoptosis early after the transplant. *In vitro* and *in vivo* data demonstrate that mAPC treatment is associated with significant reductions in proinflammatory cytokine release and in endothelial cell activation and dysfunction inherent to pancreatic islet transplantation (Contreras et al., 2004). Instant blood-mediated inflammatory reaction (IBMIR) occurs when islets are exposed to blood and manifests clinically as portal vein thrombosis and graft failure. rhAPC monotherapy prevents IBMIR in a dose-dependent manner, preserving islet integrity while maintaining platelet and leukocyte counts, fibrinogen and coagulation factor levels (Akima et al., 2009). Liposomal formulations of thrombomodulin, which generates APC, improve the engraftment of allogeneic islets through a reduction in local thrombotic and inflammatory processes (Cui et al., 2009). These studies suggest that APC therapy may enhance the therapeutic efficacy of islet transplantation or β-cell replacement in diabetic patients.

4.2. APC prevents type 1 diabetes in NOD mice

The NOD mouse model is believed to best reflect the mechanisms of the disease pathogenesis in the human type 1 diabetes. Both the antigens and their sequence of appearance are similar in NOD and human diabetes. Moreover, the kinetics of the disease in NOD is analogous to human type 1 diabetes (Delovitch & Singh, 1997). Our recent data show a novel effect of APC to prevent development of autoimmune diabetes in NOD mice. APC treatment for 5 weeks reduces diabetes incidence by approximately 50%. When treatment is extended to 10 weeks, only 8% of mice develop diabetes by 26 weeks of age, whereas 70% control mice are diabetic (Xue et al., 2012). APC appears to act by directly inhibiting β-cell apoptosis, dampening inflammation, and suppressing the autoimmune response by increasing the frequency and function of Tregs (Xue et al., 2012).

4.2.1 APC stimulates growth and inhibits apoptosis of pancreatic islet cells

βTC3 cells are a mouse islet β-cell line. These cells express both PC/APC and its receptor, EPCR (Fig. 13.3A). When βTC3 cells are pretreated with APC, proliferation is dose-dependently increased (Fig. 13.3B), while apoptosis under control or TNF-α-stimulated conditions is reduced (Fig. 13.3C). The protective effect of APC on βTC3 apoptosis is abolished when cells are pretreated with the blocking antibody to mouse EPCR, RCR16 (Fig. 13.3C).

4.2.2 APC reduces inflammation and increases EPCR and PC/APC expression in islet cells

Pancreata from control diabetic mice exhibit almost complete islet loss, associated with massive infiltration by leukocytes. In the nondiabetic control

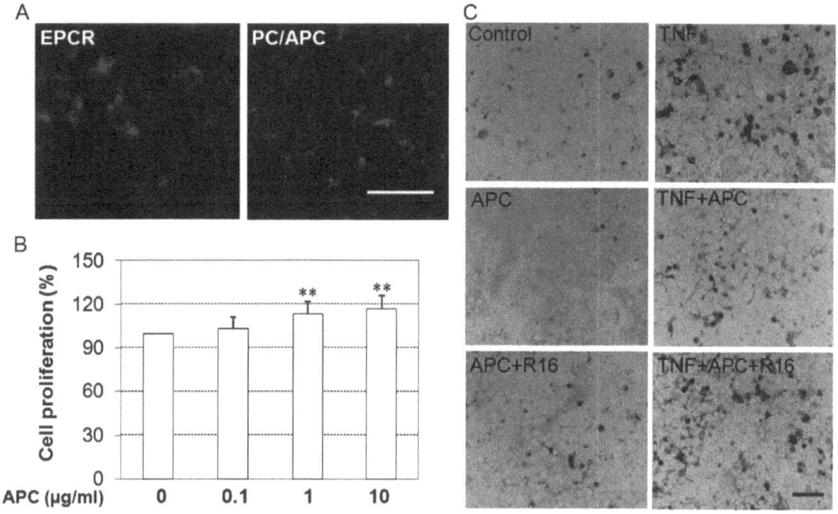

Figure 13.3 APC stimulates proliferation and inhibits apoptosis of βTC3 cells. (A) Immunostaining of EPCR and PC/APC on βTC3 cells and counterstained with DAPI. Images were merged with Image J. (B and C) Cells were incubated in serum-free medium and treated with (B) APC and proliferation measured at 48 h using the MTT assay or (C) no test agent (control), APC (10 μg/ml), TNF (100 ng/ml), or APC plus TNF at the presence or absence of EPCR-blocking antibody R16 (10 μg/ml). After 24 h, apoptosis was detected using an *in situ* cell death detection kit (Roche Diagnostics). Scale bar: 50 μm. $^{*}P<0.05$, $^{**}P<0.01$. (For color version of this figure, the reader is referred to the online version of this chapter.)

NOD mice, inflammatory cells typically comprise >50% of islet volume, and insulin expression is weak and restricted to the central regions of islets (Xue et al., 2012). In APC-treated NOD mice, however, inflammatory cells comprised <10% islet volume on average and islets stained strongly for insulin (Xue et al., 2012). *In vitro*, APC inhibits MCP-1-stimulated macrophage and $CD4^{+}$ T-cell migration, two critical inflammatory cells in the killing of β cells, by 50% and 40%, respectively (Xue et al., 2012).

PC/APC and EPCR are expressed in islet and ductal cells from BALB/c mice (Fig. 13.4A). In contrast, NOD mice, with the BALB/c background, which spontaneously develop diabetes, express considerably less PC/APC and EPCR (Fig. 13.4A). APC treatment stimulates the expression of PC/APC and EPCR in NOD mouse islet cells (Fig. 13.4A), and serum APC activity at week 25, 10 weeks after the final APC treatment, is also significantly increased (Fig. 13.4B). Interestingly, plasma levels of PC/APC are significantly lower in the type 1 diabetic patients than in the control subjects (Gruden et al., 1997; Vukovich & Schernthaner, 1986). PC levels show a significant negative correlation with the blood glucose levels (Vukovich &

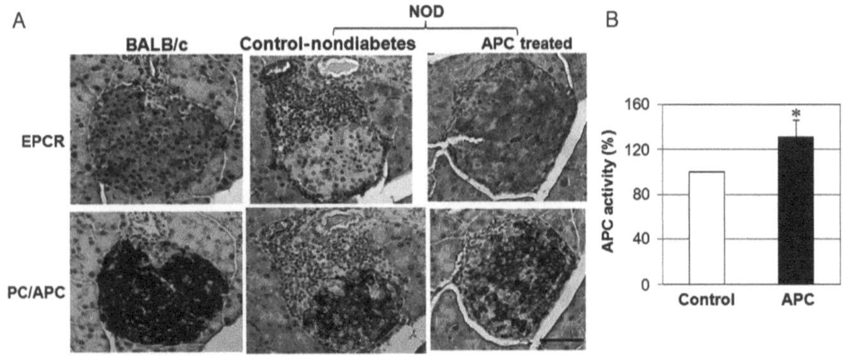

Figure 13.4 APC increases the expression of EPCR/PC/APC in islet cells and APC activity in sera from NOD mice. NOD mice were treated with APC (2 mg/kg) or PBS (control) for 10 weeks from 6 until 15 weeks of age. Pancreata or sera were collected from NOD mice at 26 weeks of age. (A) Immunostaining of EPCR and PC/APC in pancreatic islets from nondiabetic mice. BALB/c mice (no treatment) at the same age served as positive controls. (B) APC activity in sera of NOD mice measured by Spectrozyme assay and expressed as percentage of control. Data are expressed as mean ± SEM ($n=6$, each serum sample was pooled from two mice). Scale bar: 100 μm. $^{*}P<0.05$. (For color version of this figure, the reader is referred to the online version of this chapter.)

Schernthaner, 1986), while the level of soluble EPCR, which retains its affinity for, but inhibits activity of APC, is elevated (Wu et al., 2000). Loss of thrombomodulin-dependent APC formation interrupts cross talk between the vascular compartment and podocytes, causing glomerular apoptosis and diabetic nephropathy and maintaining high APC levels during long-term diabetes protects against diabetic nephropathy (Isermann et al., 2007).

4.2.3 *APC promotes differentiation of Tregs and inhibits T-cell proliferation* in vitro

Tregs hold an important check point for auto-immunoreactive T cells. The frequency of Tregs is increased in the spleens, pancreatic islets, and draining pancreatic lymph nodes of NOD mice treated with APC. The suppressive capacity of these Tregs on the proliferation of $CD4^{+}CD25^{-}$ T cells is greater than Tregs from control mice (Xue et al., 2012). *In vitro*, APC also significantly increases the expression of FoxP3 protein (Xue et al., 2012).

Considering that APC is thought to have a biological half-life of ~20 min (Gruber & Griffin, 1992), it is noteworthy that its protective effect in preventing diabetes persists for at least 10 weeks after the last treatment. This suggests that APC treatment between 6 and 16 weeks of age permanently ameliorates the autoimmune process leading to β-cell destruction.

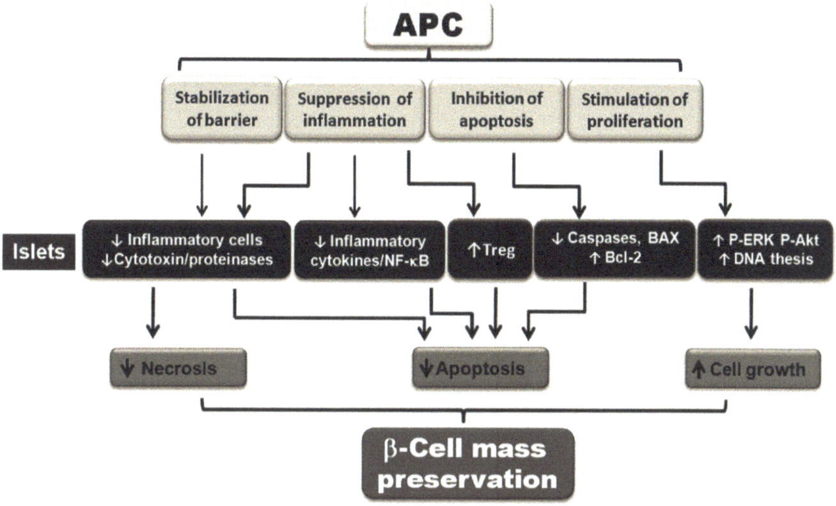

Figure 13.5 The protective role of APC on islet β cells. (For color version of this figure, the reader is referred to the online version of this chapter.)

This long-term effect could be explained by APC's ability to promote the number and function of Tregs and directly suppress T-cell activation and proliferation, and by promoting endogenous PC/APC (Xue et al., 2012). The protective role of APC on islet β cell is summarized in Fig. 13.5. Although APC can prevent diabetes in NOD mice, it is unable to reverse overt diabetes (Xue et al., 2012). This may be due to dosing issues or the fact that most islet β cells are irreversibly destroyed in overt diabetes.

Type 2 diabetes is the most common form of diabetes in humans, and growing evidence indicates that inflammation and β-cell damage are central to the development and progression of this form of diabetes (Donath & Shoelson, 2011). Since live β cells are present in type 2 diabetic patients, it is feasible that APC's beneficial effects can also be extended to type 2 diabetes.

5. CONCLUSIONS

Over the last 30 years, diabetes has evolved to become one of the major contemporary causes of premature mortality and morbidity worldwide, accounting for at least 10% of total health-care expenditure in many countries (Shaw, Sicree, & Zimmet, 2010). Between 2010 and 2030, there will be a 69% increase in numbers of adults with diabetes in developing countries and a 20% increase in developed countries (Shaw et al., 2010).

The total number of excess deaths attributable to diabetes worldwide is estimated to be 3.96 million in the age group 20–79 years, 6.8% of global (all ages) mortality. Diabetes prevention is urgently required to reduce this burden (Roglic & Unwin, 2010). In type 1 diabetes, it has been established that β-cell death is a major pathogenic component. Recent discoveries in human genetics have revealed that genes important for β-cell survival, proliferation, and function are also involved in type 2 diabetes. These findings point to the importance of developing therapies able to preserve or restore depleted numbers of β cells to physiologically sufficient levels to maintain metabolic control for type 1 and type 2 diabetes. Current evidence shows that impaired β-cell function and possibly β-cell mass may be reversible, particularly at early stages of the disease where the limiting threshold for reversibility of decreased β-cell mass has probably not been passed (Wajchenberg, 2007).

Advanced information on genetic and serologic markers has increased our ability to identify individuals at risk. Combining both immunological and metabolic strategies, the current opinion is that type 1 diabetes progression can be predicted with 80–100% accuracy within 5- and 10-year follow-up, respectively (Xu et al., 2010; Ziegler & Nepom, 2010). Novel biochemical risk factors for type 2 diabetes are also emerging (Sattar, 2012). These recent research discoveries emphasize the importance of finding therapies that prevent diabetes.

Recombinant human APC was the first drug approved by the FDA for the treatment of severe sepsis. However, efficacy was questionable, and safety is not ideal, with bleeding occurring in some patients, especially those who had recent surgery. Nonetheless, APC is reported to be beneficial and safe in clinical trials for chronic wound healing (Whitmont et al., 2008; Wijewardena, Vandervord, Lajevardi, Vandervord, & Jackson, 2011), acute lung injury (Cornet et al., 2013), and solid organ transplantation (Funk, Palma Vargas, Tuttle-Newhall, & Moretti, 2011). Furthermore, a modified APC, containing 405 amino acid residues, 3K3A-APC, is designed to possess significantly reduced anticoagulant activity (<10%) while maintaining full cytoprotective properties (Mosnier, Yang, & Griffin, 2007). Based on the anticoagulant profiles, the risk for APC-induced bleeding in clinical trials of 3K3A-APC is greatly reduced relative to wild-type APC which makes this new drug a feasible therapy for ischemic stroke patients (Williams, Zlokovic, Griffin, Pryor, & Davis, 2012). In a separate approach to increase APC availability to β cells, a novel biomolecular strategy, which immobilizes recombinant thrombomodulin on islet surfaces through streptavidin–biotin interactions, results in a nearly threefold increase in the catalytic capacity of islets to generate APC (Wilson et al., 2010).

Taken together, with new discoveries enabling diabetes predictable and new technologies engineering APC with minimized anticoagulant activity and maximized anti-inflammatory and antiapoptotic properties, APC holds a remarkable promise to prevent diabetes, although further preclinical data are required before translation to the bedside.

REFERENCES

Ablamunits, V., Sherry, N. A., Kushner, J. A., & Herold, K. C. (2007). Autoimmunity and beta cell regeneration in mouse and human type 1 diabetes: The peace is not enough. *Annals of the New York Academy of Sciences*, *1103*, 19–32.

Adorini, L., Gregori, S., & Harrison, L. C. (2002). Understanding autoimmune diabetes: Insights from mouse models. *Trends in Molecular Medicine*, *8*, 31–38.

Akima, S., Hawthorne, W. J., Favaloro, E., Patel, A., Blyth, K., Mudaliar, Y., et al. (2009). Tirofiban and activated protein C synergistically inhibit the instant blood mediated inflammatory reaction (IBMIR) from allogeneic islet cells exposure to human blood. *American Journal of Transplantation*, *9*, 1533–1540.

Anstee, Q. M., Dhar, A., & Thursz, M. R. (2011). The role of hypercoagulability in liver fibrogenesis. *Clinics and Research in Hepatology and Gastroenterology*, *35*, 526–533.

Anthony, D. A., Andrews, D. M., Watt, S. V., Trapani, J. A., & Smyth, M. J. (2010). Functional dissection of the granzyme family: Cell death and inflammation. *Immunological Reviews*, *235*, 73–92.

Bae, J. S., Lee, W., & Rezaie, A. R. (2012). Polyphosphate elicits pro-inflammatory responses that are counteracted by activated protein C in both cellular and animal models. *Journal of Thrombosis and Haemostasis*, *10*, 1145–1151.

Bae, J. S., Yang, L., Manithody, C., & Rezaie, A. R. (2007). The ligand occupancy of endothelial protein C receptor switches the protease-activated receptor 1-dependent signaling specificity of thrombin from a permeability-enhancing to a barrier-protective response in endothelial cells. *Blood*, *110*, 3909–3916.

Baiu, D., Merriam, F., & Odorico, J. (2011). Potential pathways to restore beta-cell mass: Pluripotent stem cells, reprogramming, and endogenous regeneration. *Current Diabetes Reports*, *11*, 392–401.

Baker, W. F., Jr., & Bick, R. L. (1999). Treatment of hereditary and acquired thrombophilic disorders. *Seminars in Thrombosis and Hemostasis*, *25*, 387–406.

Balazs, A. B., Fabian, A. J., Esmon, C. T., & Mulligan, R. C. (2006). Endothelial protein C receptor (CD201) explicitly identifies hematopoietic stem cells in murine bone marrow. *Blood*, *107*, 2317–2321.

Bartolome, S., Wood, J. G., Casillan, A. J., Simpson, S. Q., & O'brien-Ladner, A. R. (2008). Activated protein C attenuates microvascular injury during systemic hypoxia. *Shock*, *29*, 384–387.

Bending, D., Zaccone, P., & Cooke, A. (2012). Inflammation and type one diabetes. *International Immunology*, *24*, 339–346.

Bensellam, M., Laybutt, D. R., & Jonas, J. C. (2012). The molecular mechanisms of pancreatic beta-cell glucotoxicity: Recent findings and future research directions. *Molecular and Cellular Endocrinology*, *364*, 1–27.

Bertina, R. M., Broekmans, A. W., Van Der Linden, I. K., & Mertens, K. (1982). Protein C deficiency in a Dutch family with thrombotic disease. *Thrombosis and Hemostasis*, *48*, 1–5.

Bertina, R. M., Koeleman, B. P., Koster, T., Rosendaal, F. R., Dirven, R. J., De Ronde, H., et al. (1994). Mutation in blood coagulation factor V associated with resistance to activated protein C. *Nature*, *369*, 64–67.

Bettini, M., & Vignali, D. A. (2011). T cell-driven initiation and propagation of autoimmune diabetes. *Current Opinion in Immunology*, *23*, 754–760.

Bluestone, J. A., Herold, K., & Eisenbarth, G. (2010). Genetics, pathogenesis and clinical interventions in type 1 diabetes. *Nature*, *464*, 1293–1300.

Bock, F., Shahzad, K., Wang, H., Stoyanov, S., Wolter, J., Dong, W., et al. (2013). Activated protein C ameliorates diabetic nephropathy by epigenetically inhibiting the redox enzyme p66Shc. *Proceedings of the National Academy of Sciences of the United States of America*, *110*, 648–653.

Bosco, D., Armanet, M., Morel, P., Niclauss, N., Sgroi, A., Muller, Y. D., et al. (2010). Unique arrangement of alpha- and beta-cells in human islets of Langerhans. *Diabetes*, *59*, 1202–1210.

Bouwens, E. A., & Mosnier, L. O. (2012). EPCR encryption induces cellular APC resistance. *Blood*, *119*, 2703–2705.

Bretschneider, E., Uzonyi, B., Weber, A. A., Fischer, J. W., Pape, R., Lotzer, K., et al. (2007). Human vascular smooth muscle cells express functionally active endothelial cell protein C receptor. *Circulation Research*, *100*, 255–262.

Brissova, M., Fowler, M. J., Nicholson, W. E., Chu, A., Hirshberg, B., Harlan, D. M., et al. (2005). Assessment of human pancreatic islet architecture and composition by laser scanning confocal microscopy. *The Journal of Histochemistry and Cytochemistry*, *53*, 1087–1097.

Brunner, T., Wasem, C., Torgler, R., Cima, I., Jakob, S., & Corazza, N. (2003). Fas (CD95/Apo-1) ligand regulation in T cell homeostasis, cell-mediated cytotoxicity and immune pathology. *Seminars in Immunology*, *15*, 167–176.

Buisson-Legendre, N., Smith, S., March, L., & Jackson, C. (2004). Elevation of activated protein C in synovial joints in rheumatoid arthritis and its correlation with matrix metalloproteinase 2. *Arthritis and Rheumatism*, *50*, 2151–2156.

Cabrera, O., Berman, D. M., Kenyon, N. S., Ricordi, C., Berggren, P. O., & Caicedo, A. (2006). The unique cytoarchitecture of human pancreatic islets has implications for islet cell function. *Proceedings of the National Academy of Sciences of the United States of America*, *103*, 2334–2339.

Cai, D. (2012). One step from prediabetes to diabetes: Hypothalamic inflammation? *Endocrinology*, *153*, 1010–1013.

Calzado, M. A., Bacher, S., & Schmitz, M. L. (2007). NF-kappaB inhibitors for the treatment of inflammatory diseases and cancer. *Current Medicinal Chemistry*, *14*, 367–376.

Campbell, P. D., Estella, E., Dudek, N. L., Jhala, G., Thomas, H. E., Kay, T. W., et al. (2008). Cytotoxic T-lymphocyte-mediated killing of human pancreatic islet cells in vitro. *Human Immunology*, *69*, 543–551.

Cao, C., Gao, Y., Li, Y., Antalis, T. M., Castellino, F. J., & Zhang, L. (2010). The efficacy of activated protein C in murine endotoxemia is dependent on integrin CD11b. *The Journal of Clinical Investigation*, *120*, 1971–1980.

Castoldi, E., & Rosing, J. (2010). APC resistance: Biological basis and acquired influences. *Journal of Thrombosis and Haemostasis*, *8*, 445–453.

Chalmers, E., Cooper, P., Forman, K., Grimley, C., Khair, K., Minford, A., et al. (2011). Purpura fulminans: Recognition, diagnosis and management. *Archives of Disease in Childhood*, *96*, 1066–1071.

Cheng, T., Liu, D., Griffin, J. H., Fernandez, J. A., Castellino, F., Rosen, E. D., et al. (2003). Activated protein C blocks p53-mediated apoptosis in ischemic human brain endothelium and is neuroprotective. *Nature Medicine*, *9*, 338–342.

Cheng, T., Petraglia, A. L., Li, Z., Thiyagarajan, M., Zhong, Z., Wu, Z., et al. (2006). Activated protein C inhibits tissue plasminogen activator-induced brain hemorrhage. *Nature Medicine*, *12*, 1278–1285.

Christianson, S. W., Shultz, L. D., & Leiter, E. H. (1993). Adoptive transfer of diabetes into immunodeficient NOD-scid/scid mice. Relative contributions of CD4+ and CD8+ T-cells from diabetic versus prediabetic NOD.NON-Thy-1a donors. *Diabetes, 42*, 44–55.

Cnop, M., Welsh, N., Jonas, J. C., Jorns, A., Lenzen, S., & Eizirik, D. L. (2005). Mechanisms of pancreatic beta-cell death in type 1 and type 2 diabetes: Many differences, few similarities. *Diabetes, 54*(Suppl. 2), S97–S107.

Contreras, J. L., Eckstein, C., Smyth, C. A., Bilbao, G., Vilatoba, M., Ringland, S. E., et al. (2004). Activated protein C preserves functional islet mass after intraportal transplantation: A novel link between endothelial cell activation, thrombosis, inflammation, and islet cell death. *Diabetes, 53*, 2804–2814.

Coppieters, K. T., Dotta, F., Amirian, N., Campbell, P. D., Kay, T. W., Atkinson, M. A., et al. (2012). Demonstration of islet-autoreactive CD8 T cells in insulitic lesions from recent onset and long-term type 1 diabetes patients. *Journal of Experimental Medicine, 209*, 51–60.

Cornet, A. D., Hofstra, J. J., Vlaar, A. P., Tuinman, P. R., Levi, M., Girbes, A. R., et al. (2013). Activated protein C attenuates pulmonary coagulopathy in patients with acute respiratory distress syndrome. *Journal of Thrombosis and Haemostasis, 11*, 894–901.

Cory, S., & Adams, J. M. (2002). The Bcl2 family: Regulators of the cellular life-or-death switch. *Nature Reviews. Cancer, 2*, 647–656.

Coughlin, S. R. (2000). Thrombin signalling and protease-activated receptors. *Nature, 407*, 258–264.

Cui, W., Wilson, J. T., Wen, J., Angsana, J., Qu, Z., Haller, C. A., et al. (2009). Thrombomodulin improves early outcomes after intraportal islet transplantation. *American Journal of Transplantation, 9*, 1308–1316.

Dahlback, B. (2008). Advances in understanding pathogenic mechanisms of thrombophilic disorders. *Blood, 112*, 19–27.

D'alessio, S., Genua, M., & Vetrano, S. (2012). The protein C pathway in intestinal barrier function: Challenging the hemostasis paradigm. *Annals of the New York Academy of Sciences, 1258*, 78–85.

Degterev, A., Boyce, M., & Yuan, J. (2003). A decade of caspases. *Oncogene, 22*, 8543–8567.

Delovitch, T. L., & Singh, B. (1997). The nonobese diabetic mouse as a model of autoimmune diabetes: Immune dysregulation gets the NOD. *Immunity, 7*, 727–738.

Dominguez-Bendala, J., Inverardi, L., & Ricordi, C. (2012). Regeneration of pancreatic beta-cell mass for the treatment of diabetes. *Expert Opinion on Biological Therapy, 12*, 731–741.

Donath, M. Y., & Shoelson, S. E. (2011). Type 2 diabetes as an inflammatory disease. *Nature Review Immunology, 11*, 98–107.

Du, Z. J., Yamamoto, T., Ueda, T., Suzuki, M., Tano, Y., & Kamei, M. (2011). Activated protein C rescues the retina from ischemia-induced cell death. *Investigative Ophthalmology & Visual Science, 52*, 987–993.

Eizirik, D. L., Colli, M. L., & Ortis, F. (2009). The role of inflammation in insulitis and [beta]-cell loss in type 1 diabetes. *Nature Reviews. Endocrinology, 5*, 219–226.

Elayat, A. A., El-Naggar, M. M., & Tahir, M. (1995). An immunocytochemical and morphometric study of the rat pancreatic islets. *Journal of Anatomy, 186*(Pt 3), 629–637.

Eldor, R., Yeffet, A., Baum, K., Doviner, V., Amar, D., Ben-Neriah, Y., et al. (2006). Conditional and specific NF-kappaB blockade protects pancreatic beta cells from diabetogenic agents. *Proceedings of the National Academy of Sciences of the United States of America, 103*, 5072–5077.

Elphick, G. F., Sarangi, P. P., Hyun, Y. M., Hollenbaugh, J. A., Ayala, A., Biffl, W. L., et al. (2009). Recombinant human activated protein C inhibits integrin-mediated neutrophil migration. *Blood, 113*, 4078–4085.

Esmon, C. T. (2004a). Crosstalk between inflammation and thrombosis. *Maturitas, 47*, 305–314.

Esmon, C. T. (2004b). Structure and functions of the endothelial cell protein C receptor. *Critical Care Medicine, 32*, S298–S301.

Esmon, C. T. (2012). Protein C anticoagulant system—Anti-inflammatory effects. *Seminars in Immunopathology, 34*, 127–132.

Esmon, C. T., Stenflo, J., & Suttie, J. W. (1976). A new vitamin K-dependent protein. A phospholipid-binding zymogen of a serine esterase. *Journal of Biological Chemistry, 251*, 3052–3056.

Favaloro, B., Allocati, N., Graziano, V., Di Ilio, C., & De Laurenzi, V. (2012). Role of apoptosis in disease. *Aging (Albany NY), 4*, 330–349.

Feistritzer, C., Mosheimer, B. A., Sturn, D. H., Riewald, M., Patsch, J. R., & Wiedermann, C. J. (2006). Endothelial protein C receptor-dependent inhibition of migration of human lymphocytes by protein C involves epidermal growth factor receptor. *Journal of Immunology, 176*, 1019–1025.

Feistritzer, C., & Riewald, M. (2005). Endothelial barrier protection by activated protein C through PAR1-dependent sphingosine 1-phosphate receptor-1 crossactivation. *Blood, 105*, 3178–3184.

Feistritzer, C., Schuepbach, R. A., Mosnier, L. O., Bush, L. A., Di, C. E., Griffin, J. H., et al. (2006). Protective signaling by activated protein C is mechanistically linked to protein C activation on endothelial cells. *Journal of Biological Chemistry, 281*, 20077–20084.

Finigan, J. H., Dudek, S. M., Singleton, P. A., Chiang, E. T., Jacobson, J. R., Camp, S. M., et al. (2005). Activated protein C mediates novel lung endothelial barrier enhancement: Role of sphingosine 1-phosphate receptor transactivation. *Journal of Biological Chemistry, 280*, 17286–17293.

Foster, D. C., Yoshitake, S., & Davie, E. W. (1985). The nucleotide sequence of the gene for human protein C. *Proceedings of the National Academy of Sciences of the United States of America, 82*, 4673–4677.

Franscini, N., Bachli, E. B., Blau, N., Leikauf, M. S., Schaffner, A., & Schoedon, G. (2004). Gene expression profiling of inflamed human endothelial cells and influence of activated protein C. *Circulation, 110*, 2903–2909.

Frommhold, D., Tschada, J., Braach, N., Buschmann, K., Doerner, A., Pflaum, J., et al. (2011). Protein C concentrate controls leukocyte recruitment during inflammation and improves survival during endotoxemia after efficient in vivo activation. *American Journal of Pathology, 179*, 2637–2650.

Fukudome, K., & Esmon, C. T. (1994). Identification, cloning, and regulation of a novel endothelial cell protein c activated protein c receptor. *Journal of Biological Chemistry, 269*, 26486–26491.

Fukuhara, S., Sako, K., Minami, T., Noda, K., Kim, H. Z., Kodama, T., et al. (2008). Differential function of Tie2 at cell-cell contacts and cell-substratum contacts regulated by angiopoietin-1. *Nature Cell Biology, 10*, 513–526.

Funk, D. J., Palma Vargas, J., Tuttle-Newhall, J., & Moretti, E. W. (2011). The use of recombinant human activated protein C (drotrecogin alpha) in solid organ transplant recipients: Case series and review of the literature. *Transplant Infectious Disease, 13*, 592–597.

Furuse, M., Hata, M., Furuse, K., Yoshida, Y., Haratake, A., Sugitani, Y., et al. (2002). Claudin-based tight junctions are crucial for the mammalian epidermal barrier: A lesson from claudin-1-deficient mice. *Journal of Cell Biology, 156*, 1099–1111.

Galley, H. F., El Sakka, N. E., Webster, N. R., Lowes, D. A., & Cuthbertson, B. H. (2008). Activated protein C inhibits chemotaxis and interleukin-6 release by human neutrophils without affecting other neutrophil functions. *British Journal of Anaesthesia, 100*, 815–819.

Gearing, A. J., Beckett, P., Christodoulou, M., Churchill, M., Clements, J., Davidson, A. H., et al. (1994). Processing of tumour necrosis factor-alpha precursor by metalloproteinases. *Nature, 370*, 555–557.

Goldenberg, N. A., & Manco-Johnson, M. J. (2008). Protein C deficiency. *Haemophilia, 14*, 1214–1221.

Gramling, M. W., Beaulieu, L. M., & Church, F. C. (2010). Activated protein C enhances cell motility of endothelial cells and MDA-MB-231 breast cancer cells by intracellular signal transduction. *Experimental Cell Research, 316*, 314–328.

Green, E. A., Gorelik, L., Mcgregor, C. M., Tran, E. H., & Flavell, R. A. (2003). CD4+CD25+ T regulatory cells control anti-islet CD8+ T cells through TGF-beta-TGF-beta receptor interactions in type 1 diabetes. *Proceedings of the National Academy of Sciences of the United States of America, 100*, 10878–10883.

Grey, S. T., Tsuchida, A., Hau, H., Orthner, C. L., Salem, H. H., & Hancock, W. W. (1994). Selective inhibitory effects of the anticoagulant activated protein C on the responses of human mononuclear phagocytes to LPS, IFN-gamma, or phorbol ester. *Journal of Immunology, 153*, 3664–3672.

Griffin, J. H. (2002). Stabilization of protein complexes by introduction cysteine residues and the formation of disulfide bonds (p. 98), Vol. 2002-US19017. Patent Number: 2002103024. US.

Griffin, J. H., Evatt, B., Zimmerman, T. S., Kleiss, A. J., & Wideman, C. (1981). Deficiency of protein C in congenital thrombotic disease. *The Journal of Clinical Investigation, 68*, 1370–1373.

Gruber, A., & Griffin, J. H. (1992). Direct detection of activated protein C in blood from human subjects. *Blood, 79*, 2340–2348.

Gruber, B. L., Sorbi, D., French, D. L., Marchese, R. R. J., Nuovo, G. J., Kew, R. R., et al. (1996). Markedly elevated serum mmp-9 (gelatinase b) levels in rheumatoid arthritis—A potentially useful laboratory marker. *Clinical Immunology and Immunopathology, 78*, 161–171.

Gruden, G., Olivetti, C., Cavallo-Perin, P., Bazzan, M., Stella, S., Tamponi, G., et al. (1997). Activated protein C resistance in type I diabetes. *Diabetes Care, 20*, 424–425.

Gu, J. M., Crawley, J. T. B., Ferrell, G., Zhang, F., Li, W., Esmon, N. L., et al. (2002). Disruption of the endothelial cell protein C receptor gene in mice causes placental thrombosis and early embryonic lethality. *Journal of Biological Chemistry, 277*, 43335–43343.

Guo, H., Liu, D., Gelbard, H., Cheng, T., Insalaco, R., Fernandez, J. A., et al. (2004). Activated protein C prevents neuronal apoptosis via protease activated receptors 1 and 3. *Neuron, 41*, 563–572.

Guo, H., Zhao, Z., Yang, Q., Wang, M., Bell, R. D., Wang, S., et al. (2013). An activated protein C snalog stimulates neuronal production by human neural progenitor cells via a PAR1-PAR3-S1PR1-Akt pathway. *Journal of Neuroscience, 33*, 6181–6190.

Hansen, T. M., Singh, H., Tahir, T. A., & Brindle, N. P. (2010). Effects of angiopoietins-1 and -2 on the receptor tyrosine kinase Tie2 are differentially regulated at the endothelial cell surface. *Cellular Signalling, 22*, 527–532.

Harris, R. J., & Cropley, T. G. (2011). Possible role of hypercoagulability in calciphylaxis: Review of the literature. *Journal of the American Academy of Dermatology, 64*, 405–412.

Hemmer, C. J., Lobermann, M., Unverricht, M., Vogt, A., Krause, R., & Reisinger, E. C. (2011). Activated protein C protects vascular endothelial cells from apoptosis in malaria and in sepsis. *Tropical Medicine & International Health, 16*, 906–913.

Hotchkiss, R. S., Chang, K. C., Swanson, P. E., Tinsley, K. W., Hui, J. J., Klender, P., et al. (2000). Caspase inhibitors improve survival in sepsis: A critical role of the lymphocyte. *Nature Immunology, 1*, 496–501.

Hudson, L. G., & Mccawley, L. J. (1998). Contributions of the epidermal growth factor receptor to keratinocyte motility. *Microscopy Research and Technique, 43*, 444–455.

Isermann, B., Vinnikov, I. A., Madhusudhan, T., Herzog, S., Kashif, M., Blautzik, J., et al. (2007). Activated protein C protects against diabetic nephropathy by inhibiting endothelial and podocyte apoptosis. *Nature Medicine, 13*, 1349–1358.

Isobe, H., Okajima, K., Harada, N., Liu, W., & Okabe, H. (2004). Activated protein C reduces stress-induced gastric mucosal injury in rats by inhibiting the endothelial cell injury. *Journal of Thrombosis and Haemostasis, 2*, 313–320.

Itoh, T., Matsuda, H., Tanioka, M., Kuwabara, K., Itohara, S., & Suzuki, R. (2002). The role of matrix metalloproteinase-2 and matrix metalloproteinase-9 in antibody-induced arthritis. *Journal of Immunology, 169*, 2643–2647.

Jackson, C. J., Xue, M., Thompson, P., Davey, R. A., Whitmont, K., Smith, S., et al. (2005). Activated protein C prevents inflammation yet stimulates angiogenesis to promote cutaneous wound healing. *Wound Repair and Regeneration, 13*, 284–294.

Jaffre, F., Friedman, A. E., Hu, Z., Mackman, N., & Blaxall, B. C. (2012). Beta-adrenergic receptor stimulation transactivates protease-activated receptor 1 via matrix metalloproteinase 13 in cardiac cells. *Circulation, 125*, 2993–3003.

Jalbert, L. R., Rosen, E. D., Moons, L., Chan, J. C., Carmeliet, P., Collen, D., et al. (1998). Inactivation of the gene for anticoagulant protein C causes lethal perinatal consumptive coagulopathy in mice. *Journal of Clininal Investigation, 102*, 1481–1488.

Johnson, J. D., & Luciani, D. S. (2010). Mechanisms of pancreatic beta-cell apoptosis in diabetes and its therapies. *Advances in Experimental Medicine and Biology, 654*, 447–462.

Joyce, D. E., Gelbert, L., Ciaccia, A., Dehoff, B., & Grinnell, B. W. (2001). Gene expression profile of antithrombotic protein c defines new mechanisms modulating inflammation and apoptosis. *Journal of Biological Chemistry, 276*, 11199–11203.

Joyce, D. E., & Grinnell, B. W. (2002). Recombinant human activated protein C attenuates the inflammatory response in endothelium and monocytes by modulating nuclear factor-kappaB. *Critical Care Medicine, 30*, S288–S293.

Julovi, S. M., Xue, M., Dervish, S., Sambrook, P. N., March, L., & Jackson, C. J. (2011). Protease activated receptor-2 mediates activated protein C-induced cutaneous wound healing via inhibition of p38. *American Journal of Pathology, 179*, 2233–2242.

Keller, S. A., Moore, C. C., Evans, S. L., Mckillop, I. H., & Huynh, T. (2011). Activated protein C alters inflammation and protects renal function in sepsis. *Journal of Surgical Research, 168*, e103–e109.

Kerschen, E. J., Fernandez, J. A., Cooley, B. C., Yang, X. V., Sood, R., Mosnier, L. O., et al. (2007). Endotoxemia and sepsis mortality reduction by non-anticoagulant activated protein C. *Journal of Experimental Medicine, 204*, 2439–2448.

Kerschen, E., Hernandez, I., Zogg, M., Jia, S., Hessner, M. J., Fernandez, J. A., et al. (2010). Activated protein C targets CD8 + dendritic cells to reduce the mortality of endotoxemia in mice. *The Journal of Clinical Investigation, 120*, 3167–3178.

Kim, K. A., & Lee, M. S. (2009). Recent progress in research on beta-cell apoptosis by cytokines. *Frontiers in Bioscience, 14*, 657–664.

Kirschner, N., & Brandner, J. M. (2012). Barriers and more: Functions of tight junction proteins in the skin. *Annals of the New York Academy of Sciences, 1257*, 158–166.

Kohnert, K. D., Freyse, E. J., & Salzsieder, E. (2012). Glycaemic variability and pancreatic beta-cell dysfunction. *Current Diabetes Reviews, 8*, 345–354.

Koster, M. I. (2009). Making an epidermis. *Annals of the New York Academy of Sciences, 1170*, 7–10.

Kumar, S. (2007). Caspase function in programmed cell death. *Cell Death and Differentiation, 14*, 32–43.

Kurata, T., Hayashi, T., Yoshikawa, T., Okamoto, T., Yoshida, K., Iino, T., et al. (2010). Activated protein C stimulates osteoblast proliferation via endothelial protein C receptor. *Thrombosis Research, 125*, 184–191.

Lay, A. J., Donahue, D., Tsai, M. J., & Castellino, F. J. (2007). Acute inflammation is exacerbated in mice genetically predisposed to a severe protein C deficiency. *Blood, 109*, 1984–1991.

Lay, A. J., Liang, Z., Rosen, E. D., & Castellino, F. J. (2005). Mice with a severe deficiency in protein C display prothrombotic and proinflammatory phenotypes and compromised maternal reproductive capabilities. *The Journal of Clinical Investigation, 115*, 1552–1561.

Leger, A. J., Covic, L., & Kuliopulos, A. (2006). Protease-activated receptors in cardiovascular diseases. *Circulation, 114*, 1070–1077.

Lehmann, C., Scheibe, R., Schade, M., Meissner, K., Grundling, M., Usichenko, T., et al. (2008). Effects of activated protein C on the mesenteric microcirculation and cytokine release during experimental endotoxemia. *Canadian Journal of Anesthesia, 55*, 155–162.

Levi, M., Dorffler-Melly, J., Reitsma, P., Buller, H., Florquin, S., Van Der Poll, T., et al. (2003). Aggravation of endotoxin-induced disseminated intravascular coagulation and cytokine activation in heterozygous protein-C-deficient mice. *Blood, 101*, 4823–4827.

Li, Q., & Verma, I. M. (2002). NF-kappaB regulation in the immune system. *Nature Reviews. Immunology, 2*, 725–734.

Li, W., Zheng, X., Gu, J. M., Ferrell, G. L., Brady, M., Esmon, N. L., et al. (2005). Extraembryonic expression of EPCR is essential for embryonic viability. *Blood, 106*, 2716–2722.

Li, W., Zheng, X., Gu, J., Hunter, J., Ferrell, G. L., Lupu, F., et al. (2005). Overexpressing endothelial cell protein C receptor alters the hemostatic balance and protects mice from endotoxin. *Journal of Thrombosis and Haemostasis, 3*, 1351–1359.

Liaw, P. C., Esmon, C. T., Kahnamoui, K., Schmidt, S., Kahnamoui, S., Ferrell, G., et al. (2004). Patients with severe sepsis vary markedly in their ability to generate activate protein C. *Blood, 104*, 3958–3964.

Lightfoot, Y. L., Chen, J., & Mathews, C. E. (2011). Role of the mitochondria in immune-mediated apoptotic death of the human pancreatic beta cell line betaLox5. *PLoS One, 6*, e20617.

Liu, D., Cheng, T., Guo, H., Fernandez, J. A., Griffin, J. H., Song, X., et al. (2004). Tissue plasminogen activator neurovascular toxicity is controlled by activated protein C. *Nature Medicine, 10*, 1379–1383.

Locksley, R. M., Killeen, N., & Lenardo, M. J. (2001). The TNF and TNF receptor superfamilies: Integrating mammalian biology. *Cell, 104*, 487–501.

Madhusudhan, T., Wang, H., Straub, B. K., Grone, E., Zhou, Q., Shahzad, K., et al. (2012). Cytoprotective signaling by activated protein C requires protease-activated receptor-3 in podocytes. *Blood, 119*, 874–883.

Majno, G., & Joris, I. (1995). Apoptosis, oncosis, and necrosis. An overview of cell death. *American Journal of Pathology, 146*, 3–15.

Makinde, T., & Agrawal, D. K. (2008). Intra and extravascular transmembrane signalling of angiopoietin-1-Tie2 receptor in health and disease. *Journal of Cellular and Molecular Medicine, 12*, 810–828.

Marchiando, A. M., Graham, W. V., & Turner, J. R. (2010). Epithelial barriers in homeostasis and disease. *Annual Review of Pathology, 5*, 119–144.

Mcquibban, G. A., Gong, J. H., Tam, E. M., Mcculloch, C. A., Clark-Lewis, I., & Overall, C. M. (2000). Inflammation dampened by gelatinase A cleavage of monocyte chemoattractant protein-3. *Science, 289*, 1202–1206.

Mcquibban, G. A., Gong, J. H., Wong, J. P., Wallace, J. L., Clark-Lewis, I., & Overall, C. M. (2002). Matrix metalloproteinase processing of monocyte chemoattractant proteins generates CC chemokine receptor antagonists with anti-inflammatory properties in vivo. *Blood, 100*, 1160–1167.

Melloul, D. (2008). Role of NF-kappaB in beta-cell death. *Biochemical Society Transactions, 36*, 334–339.

Minhas, N., Xue, M., Fukudome, K., & Jackson, C. J. (2010). Activated protein C utilizes the angiopoietin/Tie2 axis to promote endothelial barrier function. *FASEB Journal, 24*, 873–881.

Mizutani, A., Okajima, K., Uchiba, M., & Noguchi, T. (2000). Activated protein C reduces ischemia/reperfusion-induced renal injury in rats by inhibiting leukocyte activation. *Blood, 95*, 3781–3787.

Mosnier, L. O., & Griffin, J. H. (2003). Inhibition of staurosporine-induced apoptosis of endothelial cells by activated protein C requires protease-activated receptor-1 and endothelial cell protein C receptor. *Biochemical Journal, 373*, 65–70.

Mosnier, L. O., Sinha, R. K., Burnier, L., Bouwens, E. A., & Griffin, J. H. (2012). Biased agonism of protease-activated receptor 1 by activated protein C caused by noncanonical cleavage at Arg46. *Blood, 120*, 5237–5246.

Mosnier, L. O., Yang, X. V., & Griffin, J. H. (2007). Activated protein C mutant with minimal anticoagulant activity, normal cytoprotective activity, and preservation of thrombin activable fibrinolysis inhibitor-dependent cytoprotective functions. *Journal of Biological Chemistry, 282*, 33022–33033.

Murakami, K., Okajima, K., Uchiba, M., Johno, M., Nakagaki, T., Okabe, H., et al. (1997). Activated protein C prevents LPS-induced pulmonary vascular injury by inhibiting cytokine production. *American Journal of Physiology, 272*, L197–L202.

Nagai, M., Yilmaz, C. E., Kirchhofer, D., Esmon, C. T., Mackman, N., & Granger, D. N. (2010). Role of coagulation factors in cerebral venous sinus and cerebral microvascular thrombosis. *Neurosurgery, 66*, 560–565, discussion 565–566.

Nakajima, H., Park, H. L., & Henkart, P. A. (1995). Synergistic roles of granzymes A and B in mediating target cell death by rat basophilic leukemia mast cell tumors also expressing cytolysin/perforin. *Journal of Experimental Medicine, 181*, 1037–1046.

Nguyen, M., Arkell, J., & Jackson, C. J. (2000). Activated protein C directly activates human endothelial gelatinase A. *Journal of Biological Chemistry, 275*, 9095–9098.

Nick, J. A., Coldren, C. D., Geraci, M. W., Poch, K. R., Fouty, B. W., O'brien, J., et al. (2004). Recombinant human activated protein C reduces human endotoxin-induced pulmonary inflammation via inhibition of neutrophil chemotaxis. *Blood, 104*, 3878–3885.

Norbury, C. J., & Hickson, I. D. (2001). Cellular responses to DNA damage. *Annual Review of Pharmacology and Toxicology, 41*, 367–401.

Ochs, H. D., Ziegler, S. F., & Torgerson, T. R. (2005). FOXP3 acts as a rheostat of the immune response. *Immunology Review, 203*, 156–164.

Okajima, K. (2004). Regulation of inflammatory responses by activated protein C: The molecular mechanism(s) and therapeutic implications. *Clinical Chemistry and Laboratory Medicine, 42*, 132–141.

Ortis, F., Pirot, P., Naamane, N., Kreins, A. Y., Rasschaert, J., Moore, F., et al. (2008). Induction of nuclear factor-kappaB and its downstream genes by TNF-alpha and IL-1beta has a pro-apoptotic role in pancreatic beta cells. *Diabetologia, 51*, 1213–1225.

Park, S. Y., Lee, H. E., Li, H., Shipitsin, M., Gelman, R., & Polyak, K. (2010). Heterogeneity for stem cell-related markers according to tumor subtype and histologic stage in breast cancer. *Clinical Cancer Research, 16*, 876–887.

Pereira, C., Schaer, D. J., Bachli, E. B., Kurrer, M. O., & Schoedon, G. (2008). Wnt5A/CaMKII signaling contributes to the inflammatory response of macrophages and is a target for the antiinflammatory action of activated protein C and interleukin-10. *Arteriosclerosis, Thrombosis, and Vascular Biology, 28*, 504–510.

Peters, K. G. (2004). Functional significance of Tie2 signaling in the adult vasculature. *Recent Progress in Hormone Research, 59*, 51–71.

Petraglia, A. L., Marky, A. H., Walker, C., Thiyagarajan, M., & Zlokovic, B. V. (2010). Activated protein C is neuroprotective and mediates new blood vessel formation and neurogenesis after controlled cortical impact. *Neurosurgery, 66*, 165–171.

Pina-Canseco Mdel, S., Paez-Arenas, A., Masso, F., Perez-Campos, E., Martinez-Cruz, R., Hernandez-Cruz, P., et al. (2012). Protein C activation peptide inhibits the expression of ICAM-1, VCAM-1, and interleukin-8 induced by TNF-alpha in human dermal microvascular endothelial cells. *Folia Histochemica et Cytobiologica*, *50*, 407–413.

Plutzky, J., Hoskins, J. A., Long, G. L., & Crabtree, G. R. (1986). Evolution and organization of the human protein C gene. *Proceedings of the National Academy of Sciences of the United States of America*, *83*, 546–550.

Price, V. E., Ledingham, D. L., Krumpel, A., & Chan, A. K. (2011). Diagnosis and management of neonatal purpura fulminans. *Seminars in Fetal & Neonatal Medicine*, *16*, 318–322.

Proksch, E., Brandner, J. M., & Jensen, J. M. (2008). The skin: An indispensable barrier. *Experimental Dermatology*, *17*, 1063–1072.

Proksch, E., & Brasch, J. (2012). Abnormal epidermal barrier in the pathogenesis of contact dermatitis. *Clinical Dermatology*, *30*, 335–344.

Proskuryakov, S. Y., Konoplyannikov, A. G., & Gabai, V. L. (2003). Necrosis: A specific form of programmed cell death? *Experimental Cell Research*, *283*, 1–16.

Puig, F., Fuster, G., Adda, M., Blanch, L., Farre, R., Navajas, D., et al. (2013). Barrier-protective effects of activated protein C in human alveolar epithelial cells. *PLoS One*, *8*, e56965.

Ram, M., Sherer, Y., & Shoenfeld, Y. (2006). Matrix metalloproteinase-9 and autoimmune diseases. *Journal of Clinical Immunology*, *26*, 299–307.

Riewald, M., Petrovan, R. J., Donner, A., Mueller, B. M., & Ruf, W. (2002). Activation of endothelial cell protease activated receptor 1 by the protein C pathway. *Science*, *296*, 1880–1882.

Roglic, G., & Unwin, N. (2010). Mortality attributable to diabetes: Estimates for the year 2010. *Diabetes Research and Clinical Practice*, *87*, 15–19.

Saelens, X., Festjens, N., Vande Walle, L., Van Gurp, M., Van Loo, G., & Vandenabeele, P. (2004). Toxic proteins released from mitochondria in cell death. *Oncogene*, *23*, 2861–2874.

Sakaguchi, S., Yamaguchi, T., Nomura, T., & Ono, M. (2008). Regulatory T cells and immune tolerance. *Cell*, *133*, 775–787.

Sakar, A., Vatansever, S., Sepit, L., Ozbilgin, K., & Yorgancioglu, A. (2007). Effect of recombinant human activated protein C on apoptosis-related proteins. *European Journal of Histochemistry*, *51*, 103–109.

Salem, H. H., Broze, G. J., Miletich, J. P., & Majerus, P. W. (1983). Human coagulation factor Va is a cofactor for the activation of protein C. *Proceedings of the National Academy of Sciences of the United States of America*, *80*, 1584–1588.

Salmon, A. H. J., Neal, C. R., Sage, L. M., Glass, C. A., Harper, S. J., & Bates, D. O. (2009). Angiopoietin-1 alters microvascular permeability coefficients in vivo via modification of endothelial glycocalyx. *Cardiovascular Research*, *83*, 24–33.

Salomon, B., Lenschow, D. J., Rhee, L., Ashourian, N., Singh, B., Sharpe, A., et al. (2000). B7/CD28 costimulation is essential for the homeostasis of the CD4+CD25+ immunoregulatory T cells that control autoimmune diabetes. *Immunity*, *12*, 431–440.

Sasi, N., Hwang, M., Jaboin, J., Csiki, I., & Lu, B. (2009). Regulated cell death pathways: New twists in modulation of BCL2 family function. *Molecular Cancer Therapeutics*, *8*, 1421–1429.

Sattar, N. (2012). Biomarkers for diabetes prediction, pathogenesis or pharmacotherapy guidance? Past, present and future possibilities. *Diabetic Medicine*, *29*, 5–13.

Seol, J. W., Lee, Y. J., Jackson, C. J., Sambrook, P. N., & Park, S. Y. (2011). Activated protein C inhibits bisphosphonate-induced endothelial cell death via the endothelial protein C receptor and nuclear factor-kappaB pathways. *International Journal of Molecular Medicine*, *27*, 835–840.

Shaw, J. E., Sicree, R. A., & Zimmet, P. Z. (2010). Global estimates of the prevalence of diabetes for 2010 and 2030. *Diabetes Research and Clinical Practice*, *87*, 4–14.

Shibata, M., Kumar, S. R., Amar, A., Fernandez, J. A., Hofman, F., Griffin, J. H., et al. (2001). Anti-inflammatory, antithrombotic, and neuroprotective effects of activated protein C in a murine model of focal ischemic stroke. *Circulation, 103*, 1799–1805.

Slee, E. A., Adrain, C., & Martin, S. J. (2001). Executioner caspase-3, -6, and -7 perform distinct, non-redundant roles during the demolition phase of apoptosis. *Journal of Biological Chemistry, 276*, 7320–7326.

Slofstra, S. H., Groot, A. P., Maris, N. A., Reitsma, P. H., Cate, H. T., & Spek, C. A. (2006). Inhalation of activated protein C inhibits endotoxin-induced pulmonary inflammation in mice independent of neutrophil recruitment. *British Journal of Pharmacology, 149*, 740–746.

Soh, U. J., Dores, M. R., Chen, B., & Trejo, J. (2010). Signal transduction by protease-activated receptors. *British Journal of Pharmacology, 160*, 191–203.

Soh, U. J., & Trejo, J. (2011). Activated protein C promotes protease-activated receptor-1 cytoprotective signaling through beta-arrestin and dishevelled-2 scaffolds. *Proceedings of the National Academy of Sciences of the United States of America, 108*, E1372–E1380.

Stearns-Kurosawa, D. J., Kurosawa, S., Mollica, J. S., Ferrell, G. L., & Esmon, C. T. (1996). The endothelial cell protein C receptor augments protein C activation by the thrombin-thrombomodulin complex. *Proceedings of the National Academy of Sciences of the United States of America, 93*, 10212–10216.

Stephenson, D. A., Toltl, L. J., Beaudin, S., & Liaw, P. C. (2006). Modulation of monocyte function by activated protein C, a natural anticoagulant. *The Journal of Immunology, 177*, 2115–2122.

Sugiura, M. (2005). Pregnancy and delivery in protein C-deficiency. *Current Drug Targets, 6*, 577–583.

Tait, S. W., & Green, D. R. (2010). Mitochondria and cell death: Outer membrane permeabilization and beyond. *Nature Reviews. Molecular Cell Biology, 11*, 621–632.

Tait, R. C., Walker, I. D., Reitsma, P. H., Islam, S. I., Mccall, F., Poort, S. R., et al. (1995). Prevalence of protein C deficiency in the healthy population. *Thrombosis and Haemostasis, 73*, 87–93.

Tanaka, A., Minoguchi, K., Chen, X., Oda, N., Yokoe, T., Yamamoto, Y., et al. (2008). Activated protein C attenuates leukocyte elastase-induced lung injury in mice. *Shock, 30*, 153–158.

Taylor, F. B., Jr., Chang, A., Esmon, C. T., D'angelo, A., Vigano-D'angelo, S., & Blick, K. E. (1987). Protein C prevents the coagulopathic and lethal effects of Escherichia coli infusion in the baboon. *The Journal of Clinical Investigation, 79*, 918–925.

Taylor, F. B., Peer, G. T., Lockhart, M. S., Ferrell, G., & Esmon, C. T. (2001). Endothelial cell protein C receptor plays an important role in protein C activation in vivo. *Blood, 97*, 1685–1688.

Taylor, F. B., Jr., Stearns-Kurosawa, D. J., Kurosawa, S., Ferrell, G., Chang, A. C., Laszik, Z., et al. (2000). The endothelial cell protein C receptor aids in host defense against Escherichia coli sepsis. *Blood, 95*, 1680–1686.

Thiyagarajan, M., Fernandez, J. A., Lane, S. M., Griffin, J. H., & Zlokovic, B. V. (2008). Activated protein C promotes neovascularization and neurogenesis in postischemic brain via protease-activated receptor 1. *Journal of Neuroscience, 28*, 12788–12797.

Toltl, L. J., Austin, R. C., & Liaw, P. C. (2011). Activated protein C modulates inflammation, apoptosis and tissue factor procoagulant activity by regulating endoplasmic reticulum calcium depletion in blood monocytes. *Journal of Thrombosis and Haemostasis, 9*, 582–592.

Toltl, L. J., Beaudin, S., & Liaw, P. C. (2008). Activated protein C up-regulates IL-10 and inhibits tissue factor in blood monocytes. *Journal of Immunology, 181*, 2165–2173.

Trejo, J. (2003). Protease-activated receptors: New concepts in regulation of G protein-coupled receptor signaling and trafficking. *Journal of Pharmacology and Experimental Therapeutics, 307*, 437–442.

Trivedi, V., Boire, A., Tchernychev, B., Kaneider, N. C., Leger, A. J., O'callaghan, K., et al. (2009). Platelet matrix metalloprotease-1 mediates thrombogenesis by activating PAR1 at a cryptic ligand site. *Cell, 137*, 332–343.

Uchiba, M., Okajima, K., Oike, Y., Ito, Y., Fukudome, K., Isobe, H., et al. (2004). Activated protein C induces endothelial cell proliferation by mitogen-activated protein kinase activation in vitro and angiogenesis in vivo. *Circulation Research, 95*, 34–41.

Van Sluis, G. L., Niers, T. M., Esmon, C. T., Tigchelaar, W., Richel, D. J., Buller, H. R., et al. (2009). Endogenous activated protein C limits cancer cell extravasation through sphingosine-1-phosphate receptor 1-mediated vascular endothelial barrier enhancement. *Blood, 114*, 1968–1973.

Van Zonneveld, A. J., De Boer, H. C., Van Der Veer, E. P., & Rabelink, T. J. (2010). Inflammation, vascular injury and repair in rheumatoid arthritis. *Annals of the Rheumatic Diseases, 69*, i57–i60.

Vandenbroucke, E., Mehta, D., Minshall, R., & Malik, A. B. (2008). Regulation of endothelial junctional permeability. *Annals of the New York Academy of Sciences, 1123*, 134–145.

Velthuis, J. H., Unger, W. W., Abreu, J. R., Duinkerken, G., Franken, K., Peakman, M., et al. (2010). Simultaneous detection of circulating autoreactive CD8+ T-cells specific for different islet cell-associated epitopes using combinatorial MHC multimers. *Diabetes, 59*, 1721–1730.

Vetrano, S., Ploplis, V. A., Sala, E., Sandoval-Cooper, M., Donahue, D. L., Correale, C., et al. (2011). Unexpected role of anticoagulant protein C in controlling epithelial barrier integrity and intestinal inflammation. *Proceedings of the National Academy of Sciences of the United States of America, 108*, 19830–19835.

Vig, S., Chitolie, A., Sleight, S., Bevan, D., Dormandy, J., Thompson, M. M., et al. (2004). Prevalence and risk of thrombophilia defects in vascular patients. *European Journal of Vascular and Endovascular Surgery, 28*, 124–131.

Villasenor, A., & Cleaver, O. (2012). Crosstalk between the developing pancreas and its blood vessels: An evolving dialog. *Seminars in Cell and Developmental Biology, 23*, 685–692.

Voskoboinik, I., Dunstone, M. A., Baran, K., Whisstock, J. C., & Trapani, J. A. (2010). Perforin: Structure, function, and role in human immunopathology. *Immunology Review, 235*, 35–54.

Vukovich, T. C., & Schernthaner, G. (1986). Decreased protein C levels in patients with insulin-dependent type I diabetes mellitus. *Diabetes, 35*, 617–619.

Wajchenberg, B. L. (2007). Beta-cell failure in diabetes and preservation by clinical treatment. *Endocrine Reviews, 28*, 187–218.

Wang, J., Yang, L., Rezaie, A. R., & Li, J. (2011). Activated protein C protects against myocardial ischemic/reperfusion injury through AMP-activated protein kinase signaling. *Journal of Thrombosis and Haemostasis, 9*, 1308–1317.

Weijer, S., Wieland, C. W., Florquin, S., & Van Der Poll, T. (2005). A thrombomodulin mutation that impairs activated protein C generation results in uncontrolled lung inflammation during murine tuberculosis. *Blood, 106*, 2761–2768.

White, T. C., Berny, M. A., Tucker, E. I., Urbanus, R. T., De Groot, P. G., Fernandez, J. A., et al. (2008). Protein C supports platelet binding and activation under flow: Role of glycoprotein Ib and apolipoprotein E receptor 2. *Journal of Thrombosis and Haemostasis, 6*, 995–1002.

White, B., Schmidt, M., Murphy, C., Livingstone, W., O'toole, D., Lawler, M., et al. (2000). Activated protein C inhibits lipopolysaccharide-induced nuclear translocation of nuclear factor kappaB (NF-kappaB) and tumour necrosis factor alpha (TNF-alpha) production in the THP-1 monocytic cell line. *British Journal of Haematology, 110*, 130–134.

Whitmont, K., Reid, I., Tritton, S., March, L., Xue, M., Lee, M., et al. (2008). Treatment of chronic leg ulcers with topical activated protein C. *Archives of Dermatology, 144*, 1479–1483.

Wijewardena, A., Vandervord, E., Lajevardi, S. S., Vandervord, J., & Jackson, C. J. (2011). Combination of activated protein C and topical negative pressure rapidly regenerates granulation tissue over exposed bone to heal recalcitrant orthopedic wounds. *The International Journal of Lower Extremity Wounds, 10*, 146–151.

Williams, P. D., Zlokovic, B. V., Griffin, J. H., Pryor, K. E., & Davis, T. P. (2012). Preclinical safety and pharmacokinetic profile of 3K3A-APC, a novel, modified activated protein C for ischemic stroke. *Current Pharmaceutical Design, 18*, 4215–4222.

Wilson, J. T., Haller, C. A., Qu, Z., Cui, W., Urlam, M. K., & Chaikof, E. L. (2010). Biomolecular surface engineering of pancreatic islets with thrombomodulin. *Acta Biomaterialia, 6*, 1895–1903.

Wu, J., Zhou, Z., Ye, S., Dai, H., Ma, L., Xu, X., et al. (2000). Detection of soluble endothelial protein C receptor (sEPCR) in patients with CHD, DM and SLE. *Zhonghua Xue Ye Xue Za Zhi, 21*, 472–474.

Xu, J., Ji, Y., Zhang, X., Drake, M., & Esmon, C. T. (2009). Endogenous activated protein C signaling is critical to protection of mice from lipopolysaccaride-induced septic shock. *Journal of Thrombosis and Haemostasis*, 7, 851–856.

Xu, P., Wu, Y., Zhu, Y., Dagne, G., Johnson, G., Cuthbertson, D., et al. (2010). Prognostic performance of metabolic indexes in predicting onset of type 1 diabetes. *Diabetes Care, 33*, 2508–2513.

Xue, M., Campbell, D., & Jackson, C. J. (2007). Protein C is an autocrine growth factor for human skin keratinocytes. *Journal of Biological Chemistry, 282*, 13610–13616.

Xue, M., Campbell, D., Sambrook, P. N., Fukudome, K., & Jackson, C. J. (2005). Endothelial protein C receptor and protease-activated receptor-1 mediate induction of a wound-healing phenotype in human keratinocytes by activated protein C. *Journal of Investigative Dermatology, 125*, 1279–1285.

Xue, M., Chow, S. O., Dervish, S., Chan, Y. K., Julovi, S. M., & Jackson, C. J. (2011). Activated protein C enhances human keratinocyte barrier integrity via sequential activation of epidermal growth factor receptor and Tie2. *Journal of Biological Chemistry, 286*, 6742–6750.

Xue, M., Dervish, S., Harrison, L. C., Fulcher, G., & Jackson, C. J. (2012). Activated protein C inhibits pancreatic islet inflammation, stimulates T regulatory cells and prevents diabetes in NOD mice. *Journal of Biological Chemistry, 287*, 16356–16364.

Xue, M., March, L., Sambrook, P. N., Fukudome, F., & Jackson, C. J. (2007). Endothelial protein C receptor is over-expressed in rheumatoid arthritic (RA) synovium and mediates the anti-inflammatory effects of activated protein C in RA monocytes. *Annals of the Rheumatic Diseases, 66*, 1574–1580.

Xue, M., March, L., Sambrook, P. N., & Jackson, C. J. (2007). Differential regulation of matrix metalloproteinase 2 and matrix metalloproteinase 9 by activated protein C: Relevance to inflammation in rheumatoid arthritis. *Arthritis Rheumtism, 56*, 2864–2874.

Xue, M., Minhas, N., Chow, S. O., Dervish, S., Sambrook, P. N., March, L., et al. (2010). Endogenous protein C is essential for the functional integrity of human endothelial cells. *Cellular and Molecular Life Sciences, 67*, 1537–1546.

Xue, M., Smith, M. M., Little, C. B., Sambrook, P., March, L., & Jackson, C. J. (2009). Activated protein C mediates a healing phenotype in cultured tenocytes. *Journal of Cellular and Molecular Medicine, 13*, 749–757.

Xue, M., Thompson, P., Kelso, I., & Jackson, C. (2004). Activated protein C stimulates proliferation, migration and wound closure, inhibits apoptosis and upregulates MMP-2 activity in cultured human keratinocytes. *Experimental Cell Research, 299*, 119–127.

Yang, X. V., Banerjee, Y., Fernandez, J. A., Deguchi, H., Xu, X., Mosnier, L. O., et al. (2009). Activated protein C ligation of ApoER2 (LRP8) causes Dab1-dependent signaling in U937 cells. *Proceedings of the National Academy of Sciences of the United States of America, 106*, 274–279.

Yen, Y. T., Yang, H. R., Lo, H. C., Hsieh, Y. C., Tsai, S. C., Hong, C. W., et al. (2013). Enhancing autophagy with activated protein C and rapamycin protects against sepsis-induced acute lung injury. *Surgery*, *153*, 689–698.

Yuksel, M., Okajima, K., Uchiba, M., Horiuchi, S., & Okabe, H. (2002). Activated protein C inhibits lipopolysaccharide-induced tumor necrosis factor-alpha production by inhibiting activation of both nuclear factor-kappa B and activator protein-1 in human monocytes. *Thrombosis and Haemostasis*, *88*, 267–273.

Zanone, M. M., Favaro, E., & Camussi, G. (2008). From endothelial to beta cells: Insights into pancreatic islet microendothelium. *Current Diabetes Reviews*, *4*, 1–9.

Zhou, F. (2010). Expression of multiple granzymes by cytotoxic T lymphocyte implies that they activate diverse apoptotic pathways in target cells. *International Reviews of Immunology*, *29*, 38–55.

Ziegler, A. G., & Nepom, G. T. (2010). Prediction and pathogenesis in type 1 diabetes. *Immunity*, *32*, 468–478.

CHAPTER FOURTEEN

Zinc and Its Transporters, Pancreatic β-Cells, and Insulin Metabolism

Liping Huang[*,†,1]
[*]United States Department of Agriculture/Agricultural Research Service/Western Human Nutrition Research Center, Obesity and Metabolism Research Unit, Davis, California, USA
[†]Department of Nutrition, University of California Davis, Davis, California, USA
[1]Corresponding author: e-mail address: liping.huang@ars.usda.gov

Contents

Abstract

Zinc is an essential trace metal for life. Two families of zinc transporters, SLC30A (ZNT) and SLC39A (ZIP) are required for maintaining cellular zinc homeostasis. ZNTs function to decrease cytoplasmic zinc concentrations whereas ZIPs do the opposite. Expression of zinc transporters can be tissue/cell-type specific or ubiquitous. Zinc transporters that are limited in tissue/cell distributions usually perform specialized tasks to satisfy biological processes in a given cell. For example, ZNT8 is mainly expressed in β-cells and functions to deliver zinc into granules for insulin maturation and secretion. Many other zinc

Vitamins and Hormones, Volume 95
ISSN 0083-6729
http://dx.doi.org/10.1016/B978-0-12-800174-5.00014-4

transporters are also expressed in β-cells. Defects in these zinc transporters have been associated with abnormalities in insulin synthesis, maturation, and secretion and subsequent glucose metabolism. This review focuses on the specific roles of zinc and its transporters in insulin metabolism and describes the current knowledge of the function of zinc transporters in β-cell health in animal knockout mouse models with respect to diabetes development in humans.

1. INTRODUCTION

Zinc is an essential trace metal for the development and growth of humans and animals (Prasad, Miale, Farid, Sandstead, & Schulert, 1963; Todd, Elvehjem, & Hart, 1934). Zinc ions play vital roles in almost all aspects of metabolism and biological processes as they are required for activities of hundreds of metalloenzymes and zinc-finger proteins that are involved in regulation of gene transcription (Fraústo da Silva & Williams, 2001). Dietary zinc deficiency in humans and in experimental animals is associated with stunted growth, poor appetite, dermatitis, alopecia, hypogonadism, and impaired immune function (Prasad, 1985; Prasad et al., 1963). Zinc deficiency caused by autosomal recessive disorders has been described in humans (acrodermatitis enteropathica, AE) and mice (*lethal milk*, *lm*) (Dickie, 1969; Moynahan, 1974; Piletz and Ganschow, 1978b). AE and *lm* are similar in that affected individuals or mice show clinical features of dietary zinc deficiency. Nevertheless, AE and *lm* are two different genetic disorders. AE is a result of a defect in intestinal absorption of zinc (Wang, Zhou, Kuo, Zemansky, & Gitschier, 2002). Zinc deficiency appears soon after birth in bottle-fed AE infants (Eckhert, Sloan, Duncan, & Hurley, 1977). For those AE infants who are breast-fed, zinc deficiency manifests after weaning. *lm* results from a defect in zinc deposition from mammary glands into the milk of an affected dam (Huang and Gitschier, 1997). Suckling pups of *lm* dams suffer from zinc deficiency (Piletz and Ganschow, 1978a). Both forms of zinc deficiency are lethal for the affected infants and for the pups that are nursed on affected dams unless therapeutic zinc supplementations are given, demonstrating a vital role of zinc in development and growth in early life.

In humans and animals, dietary zinc is absorbed through the intestinal epithelium into the bloodstream where the metal is delivered to tissues or cells for uptake (Dufner-Beattie, Wang, et al., 2003; Geiser, Venken, De Lisle, & Andrews, 2012; Wang et al., 2002). Body zinc homeostasis is tightly regulated in a narrow range largely through regulation of synthesis and activities of zinc transporters and metallothioneins (MTs). Two families of zinc transporters (SLC30A/ZNT and SLC39A/ZIP) have been identified in humans and animals (Huang & Tepaamorndech, 2013; Jeong & Eide, 2013). The SLC30A/ZNT family contains 10 members, while the SLC39A/ZIP family has 14 members. Members in each family share similar topological protein structures. For example, ZNT proteins are predicted to have six transmembrane (TM) domains and a histidine-rich loop between TM4 and TM5 except for ZNT5 which contains additional TM domains at the N-terminal end of the protein. Both N- and C-terminal ends of ZNT proteins are localized intracellularly, facing the cytosol. While ZIP proteins have eight predicted TMs and a histidine-rich loop between TM3 and TM4 with two ends facing either the extracellular space or the lumen of an organelle in the cell. ZNT proteins function to transport zinc out of the cell or to sequester cytoplasmic zinc into cellular compartments when zinc is replete or in excess whereas ZIP proteins function to bring zinc into the cytosol from either the extracellular space or the intracellular storage compartment when zinc is depleted. The expression and activities of ZNT and ZIP proteins are precisely regulated at multiple levels including transcription, posttranscription, translation, and posttranslation in response to environmental cues.

Other important players in maintaining cellular zinc homeostasis are the MTs, a group of small cysteine-rich proteins that can tightly bind to heavy metal ions which protect cells from toxic heavy metals (Kagi & Schaffer, 1988). The expression of MTs is greatly induced when cells are exposed to heavy metals, such as zinc. Increased cytoplasmic zinc levels trigger MTF1, a metal regulatory transcription factor 1, to translocate into the nucleus. In the nucleus, MTF1 is able to bind the metal response elements (MREs) in the promoter regions of the *MT* genes (Radtke et al., 1993) and induces gene transcription. Together, ZNTs, ZIPs, and MTs act in a concert to regulate cellular zinc homeostasis in a tissue- or cell-type-specific manner.

2. ZINC AND ITS TRANSPORTERS IN INSULIN SYNTHESIS AND SECRETION IN PANCREATIC β-CELLS

The pancreas contains high levels of zinc in both exocrine and endocrine cells (Sondergaard, Stoltenberg, Doering, Flyvbjerg, & Rungby, 2006). Zinc is required for many digestive enzymes secreted from pancreatic acinar cells that assist the digestion and absorption of nutrients in the small intestine (Wildman & Medeiros, 2000). Zinc secretion via pancreatic juice also serves a crucial route for excretion of excess endogenous zinc to maintain body zinc homeostasis (Krebs, 2000). This review section focuses on endocrine function of the pancreatic β-cell and the roles of zinc and its transporters in insulin synthesis, processing, and secretion.

Insulin, a peptide hormone secreted from pancreatic β-cells in response to increasing blood glucose levels, stimulates glucose uptake, glycogenesis, glycolysis, and lipogenesis in insulin-sensitive peripheral tissues (Haataja et al., 2013; Le Roith & Zick, 2001). In pancreatic β-cells, zinc is required for insulin crystallization by facilitating the formation of dense core granules (Dunn, 2005). Therefore, it is not surprising that, in pancreatic β-cells, zinc is most associated with secretory granules where insulin is localized (Vinkenborg, Nicolson, Bellomo, Koay, Rutter, & Merkx, 2009). Insulin is transcribed from the insulin genes, and zinc has been shown to positively influence insulin gene transcription (Huang, Yan, & Kirschke, 2010). Increase in cellular zinc accumulation in rat β-cells by overexpression of mouse ZnT7 stimulates Mtf1 to bind the MREs in the promoter regions of the insulin genes which enhances insulin transcription (Fig. 14.1). Insulin mRNAs are then translated into a single peptide known as preproinsulin that is processed to proinsulin by removal of a signal peptide from the preproinsulin (Patzelt et al., 1978). A C-peptide is then removed by endopeptidases creating an insulin peptide in which two disulfide bonds link A-chain and B-chain of the insulin peptide together. These endopeptidases including prohormone convertases (PC1 and PC2) and exoprotease carboxypeptidase E are zinc-dependent enzymes (Davidson, Rhodes, & Hutton, 1988; Smeekens et al., 1992). The process of proinsulin to insulin starts in the Golgi apparatus and continues in the secretory granules (Haataja et al., 2013). Inadequate zinc supply to these enzymes along the secretory pathway can have negative impact on proinsulin conversion into insulin leading to a high release of proinsulin into the blood upon glucose stimulation (Haataja et al., 2013). Recent studies have suggested that ZnT8 is associated with the availability of zinc for these insulin processing enzymes. In mice deficient for *Znt8*, granular zinc content is low in the β-cell, which negatively affects activities of proinsulin processing enzymes, leading to an increased proinsulin to insulin ratio in the blood (Wijesekara et al., 2010). Consistent with the finding in the mouse *Znt8* knockout models, human subjects who carry a risk allele (R325) of ZNT8 are more likely to have increased proinsulin to insulin ratio during OGTT (oral glucose tolerance test), suggesting an impaired proinsulin conversion in the human

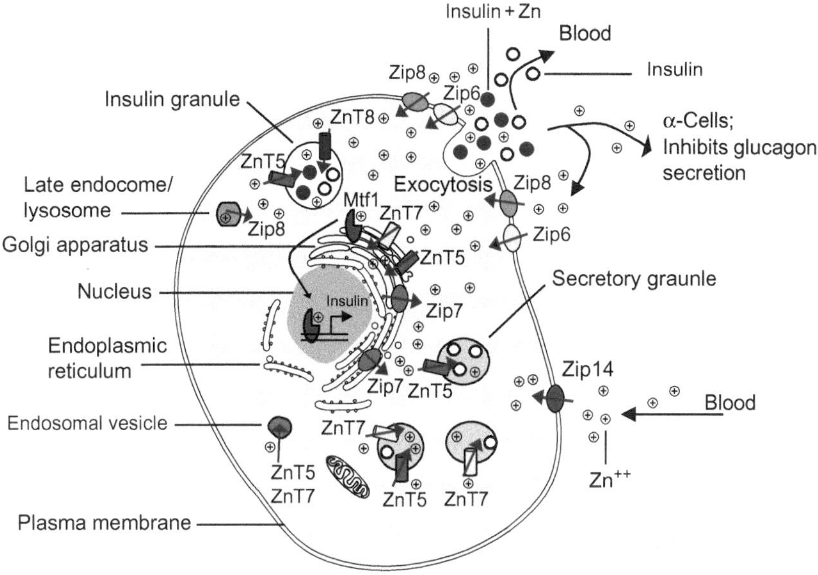

Figure 14.1 Cellular localization of expressed zinc transporters in the pancreatic β-cell. Exocytosis of insulin upon glucose stimulation is shown. Organelles of the cell are labeled. Zn ions (Zn^{++}) are also labeled. Arrows indicate the direction of translocation of zinc ions across the membrane by zinc transporters. Only the zinc transporters that are reported to be expressed in the β-cell are shown. Also shown is the nuclear translocation of zinc-bound Mtf1 to the insulin promoter and subsequent transcription stimulation. (For color version of this figure, the reader is referred to the online version of this chapter.)

β-cell (Kirchhoff et al., 2008). Processed insulin is subsequently packaged with zinc ions inside secretory granules forming crystallized structures before secretion (Dunn, 2005). When blood glucose levels increase, for example, after a meal, β-cells are stimulated and insulin is secreted into intraislet periportal circulation via exocytosis (Fig. 14.1). Zinc is secreted along with insulin during exocytosis and then released from insulin. The dissociated zinc ions can be either recycled back into the β-cell or act on pancreatic α-cells to inhibit glucagon secretion (Franklin, Gromada, Gjinovci, Theander, & Wollheim, 2005). Together, both insulin and glucagon control the blood glucose level in a normal range. Thus, it is clear that zinc is an essential element required for insulin synthesis, processing, and maturation as well as glucose homeostasis.

According to the EST (expressed sequence tag) expression profiles (human and mouse/rat databases), most zinc transporters are expressed in the pancreas (http://www.ncbi.nlm.nih.gov/UniGene). However, the expression profiles of many ZNTs and ZIPs in pancreatic β-cells have not been elucidated (Tables 14.1 and 14.2). Up to date, eight zinc transporters, *ZnT3*, *ZnT5*(*ZNT5*), *ZnT7*, *ZnT8* (*ZNT8*), *Zip6*, *Zip7*, *Zip8*, and *Zip14* have been reported expressing in pancreatic β-cells in rodents and/or humans (Tables 14.1 and 14.2).

ZnT3 expression is mostly restricted to synaptic vesicles of the central nervous system (Cole, Wenzel, Kafer, Schwartzkroin, & Palmiter, 1999). However, *Znt3* mRNA is also detected in vesicles of the mouse testis and rat insulin-secreting β-cells (INS-1E) (Palmiter, Cole, Quaife, & Findley, 1996; Smidt et al., 2009). siRNA-mediated knockdown *Znt3* in INS-1E cells decreases insulin secretion (Petersen, Smidt, Magnusson, Moore, Egefjord, & Rungby, 2011). The negative effect of ZnT3 deficiency on insulin metabolism is also displayed in *Znt3* knockout mice. It was shown that *Znt3* KO mice were more prone to β-cell destruction induced by streptozotocin (a toxin to the pancreatic β-cell) (Smidt et al., 2009).

ZnT5 (ZNT5) and ZnT7 are widely expressed in the body and are localized on the membrane of the Golgi apparatus and cytoplasmic vesicles of the

Table 14.1 Expression of SLC30A family members in pancreatic β-cells

Official symbol	Other name	Expression in the pancreas	Expression in β-cells	Cellular localization
SLC30A1	ZNT1	Detected[a–c]	ND	ND
SLC30A2	ZNT2	Not detected[a–c]	–	–
SLC30A3	ZNT3	Detected[b]	Detected[b]	Vesicles[b]
SLC30A4	ZNT4	Detected[a]	ND	ND
SLC30A5	ZNT5	Detected[b]	Detected[b]	Vesicles[b]
SLC30A6	ZNT6	Detected[a–c]	ND	ND
SLC30A7	ZNT7	Detected[b]	Detected[b]	Golgi[b], vesicles[b]
SLC30A8	ZNT8	Detected[a,b]	Detected[a,b]	Granules[a,b]
SLC30A9	ZNT9	Detected[a–c]	ND	ND
SLC30A10	ZNT10	Not detected[a–c]	–	–

[a]Human.
[b]Rodent.
[c]Data from EST expression profiles (mouse, rat, and human databases; http://www.ncbi.nlm.nih.gov/UniGene).
ND, not determined.

Table 14.2 Expression of SLC39 family members in pancreatic β-cells

Official symbol	Other name	Expression in the pancreas	Expression in β-cells	Cellular localization
SLC39A1	ZIP1	Detected[a,b]	ND	ND
SLC39A2	ZIP2	Not detected[a–c]	–	–
SLC39A3	ZIP3	Detected[c]	ND	ND
SLC39A4	ZIP4	Detected[a,b] Not detected[c]	Not detected[c]	–
SLC39A5	ZIP5	Not detected[c]	Not detected[c]	–
SLC39A6	ZIP6	Detected[a–c]	Detected[c]	Predicted on cell surface
SLC39A7	ZIP7	Detected[c]	Detected[c]	Intracellular
SLC39A8	ZIP8	Detected[a–c]	Detected[c]	Predicted on cell surface, intracellular
SLC39A9	ZIP9	Detected[a–c]	ND	ND
SLC39A10	ZIP10	Detected[a–c]	ND	ND
SLC39A11	ZIP11	Detected[a–c]	ND	ND
SLC39A12	ZIP12	Not detected[a–c]	–	–
SLC39A13	ZIP13	Detected[a,b]	ND	ND
SLC39A14	ZIP14	Detected[c]	Detected[c]	Cell surface, intracellular

[a]Human.
[b]Data from EST expression profiles (mouse, rat, and human databases; http://www.ncbi.nlm.nih.gov/UniGene).
[c]Rodent.
ND, not determined.

cell. The main function of ZnT5 and ZnT7 is to sequester cytoplasmic zinc into the Golgi apparatus and secretory vesicles for zinc-dependent enzymes/proteins or for zinc storage in these compartments (Fig. 14.1; Kambe et al., 2002; Kirschke and Huang, 2003; Suzuki et al., 2005). ZnT5 and ZnT7 have been shown to work together to supply zinc to alkaline phosphatases (ALPs) in the early secretory pathway in chicken DT40 cells (Suzuki et al., 2005). In regard to insulin metabolism in pancreatic β-cells, ZnT7 has been shown to positively regulate insulin gene expression in rat β-cells. Upregulation of insulin gene transcription by ZnT7 is followed by increased insulin protein synthesis and subsequent insulin secretion (Huang et al., 2010).

Interestingly, β-cells overexpressing ZnT7 synthesize and secrete high amounts of insulin at the basal level. Glucose-stimulated insulin secretion is also increased in these cells due to a high basal insulin level (Huang et al., 2010). Human ZNT5 resides on the membrane of the secretory granules of β-cells (Kambe et al., 2002). However, the role of ZnT5 in insulin synthesis, processing, and secretion has not elucidated both *in vitro* and *in vivo*. More experiments are needed to determine the importance of ZnT5 in regulation of zinc homeostasis in β-cells and to understand whether or not ZnT5 and ZnT7 work together in maintenance of zinc levels in the secretory pathway of the β-cell.

ZnT8 is largely restricted in pancreatic β-cells (Chimienti, Devergnas, Favier, & Seve, 2004). It is mainly detected on the membrane of secretory granules where insulin resides and is responsible for delivery of zinc into these insulin-containing granules for insulin maturation and storage (Wijesekara et al., 2010). Deficiency of ZnT8 (mouse models) or an allelic change of ZNT8 (R325, humans) reduces zinc accumulation in the secretory granules which subsequently affects insulin processing and crystallization leading to a reduced glucose-induced insulin secretion and then hyperglycemia and diabetes.

Zip6, *Zip7*, and *Zip8* are widely expressed in organs/tissues (http://www.ncbi.nlm.nih.gov/UniGene). Zip6 and Zip8 proteins have been shown to localize on the cytoplasmic membrane in many cell types to facilitate zinc uptake while Zip7 protein mainly resides on the membrane of the endoplasmic reticulum (ER) and/or the Golgi apparatus in the cell (Huang, Kirschke, Zhang, & Yu, 2005; Suzuki & Endo, 2002; Taylor, Morgan, Johnson, & Nicholson, 2004) to facilitate zinc release from intracellular zinc stores to the cytoplasmic compartment (Huang et al., 2005; Taylor, Hiscox, Nicholson, Hogstrand, & Kille, 2012). Localization of ZIP8 to the lysosomal compartment has been demonstrated in human T cells (Aydemir, Liuzzi, McClellan, & Cousins, 2009). It is known that during glucose stimulation, cytoplasmic zinc concentration is greatly elevated (Bellomo, Meur, & Rutter, 2011; Bensellam, Van Lommel, Overbergh, Schuit, & Jonas, 2009) accompanied by a reduction in compartmental zinc stores (Zalewski et al., 1994). The expression of *Zip6*, *Zip7*, and *Zip8* mRNAs in β-cells is upregulated by glucose stimulation. Therefore, it is suggested that the elevated labile cytoplasmic zinc concentration in the β-cell after glucose stimulation is largely mediated by Zip6, Zip7, and Zip8 proteins (Bellomo et al., 2011). It is also plausible that both Zip6 and Zip8 may facilitate zinc recycling during insulin secretion after glucose stimulation (Fig. 14.1).

Zip14 expression is abundantly detected in bone, liver, and acinar cells in the pancreas (Aydemir, Sitren, & Cousins, 2012; Hojyo et al., 2011). It is localized on the cytoplasmic membrane for zinc uptake into the cell (Hojyo et al., 2011). Zip14 is also expressed in pancreatic β-cells overlapping with insulin (Aydemir et al., 2012). Mice deficient for *Zip14* have abnormal glucose metabolism in addition to the disorders of bone growth, body weight gain, and iron metabolism (Aydemir et al., 2012; Hojyo et al., 2011; Nam et al., 2013). *Zip14* KO mice have enlarged islets and increased β-cell mass in the pancreas. Moreover, ZnT8 and insulin expression is increased in the β-cell of *Zip14* KO mice (Aydemir et al., 2012). As the result, the KO mice suffer from hypoglycemia and hyperinsulinemia. The underlying mechanism of generalized islet hypertrophy and β-cell hyperplasia in the *Zip14* KO pancreas is not yet clear. However, there are some clues that may explain the β-cell hyperplasia. Studies have shown that Zip14 controls G-protein-coupled receptor-mediated signaling pathways in response to endocrine cues (Hojyo et al., 2011). In chondrocytes, Zip14 is involved in regulation of enzymatic activities of cyclic nucleotide phosphodiesterases (PDEs), a group of enzymes that degrade second messenger molecules cAMP and cGMP. Zip14 functions to repress PDE enzymatic activities to maintain the basal level of cAMP in chondrocytes (Hojyo et al., 2011). Indeed, mice deficient for *Zip14* have low basal cAMP levels in the growth plate as well as in purified primary chondrocytes. Decreased basal cAMP levels in chondrocytes can lead to low activity of PTH1R (parathyroid hormone receptor)-cAMP-CREB (cAMP response element-binding protein) signaling resulting in hypertrophy of growth plates (Hojyo et al., 2011) as PTH (parathyroid hormone)-PTH1R signaling is required for suppression of hypertrophy of the growth plate (Guo, Chung, Yang, Karsenty, Bringhurst, & Kronenberg, 2006). One may speculate that similar abnormalities in signaling pathways may exist in the pancreatic β-cell leading to islet hypertrophy in *Zip14* KO mice.

Taken together, Zip6, Zip8, and Zip14 may work together to acquire zinc ions including those delivered through the blood as well as those released from insulin hexamers in the intraislet periportal region into β-cells whereas Zip7 as well as Zip8 may function to release stored zinc into the cytoplasmic compartment to maintain cellular zinc homeostasis during insulin maturation and secretion. Zip7 and Zip8 may also be involved in activations of zinc signaling pathways that regulate apoptosis and cell survival during β-cell development (Aydemir, Liuzzi, McClellan, & Cousins, 2009; Taylor, Hiscox, Nicholson, Hogstrand, & Kille, 2012; Fig. 14.1).

3. ZINC TRANSPORTERS AND THEIR PHYSIOLOGICAL ROLES AND CONTRIBUTIONS TO INSULIN METABOLISM AND GLUCOSE HOMEOSTASIS: STUDIES IN MOUSE KNOCKOUT MODELS OF ZINC TRANSPORTERS

3.1. Slc30a1/ZnT1

ZnT1 is a ubiquitously expressed zinc exporter, contributing to the removal of excess zinc ions from the cytoplasm of the cell to the extracellular space when cellular zinc levels increase (Palmiter & Findley, 1995). ZnT1 is also implicated in dietary zinc absorption in the gut (Wang, Wu, & Zhou, 2009). It is, therefore, not surprising to observe that mice deficient for *Znt1* are embryonic lethal (Andrews et al., 2004). This lethality of the null mutation of *Znt1* in the embryonic development cannot be rescued by manipulating dietary zinc intake in pregnant female mice. Although male mice heterozygous for *Znt1* appear normal, female heterozygous *Znt1* mice fed low zinc diets during pregnancy tend to produce developmentally retarded embryos (Andrews, Wang, Dey, & Palmiter, 2004). *Znt1* mRNA is detected in the mouse pancreas, and its expression is downregulated by dietary zinc deficiency (Guo, Lichten, Ryu, Liuzzi, Wang, & Cousins, 2010). However, the *Znt1* mRNA expression is restricted to the exocrine acinar cells in the pancreas. Little to no ZnT1, both at mRNA and protein levels, is detected in the endocrine cells of the pancreas including β-cells isolated from mice fed either the normal diet or low zinc diet (Liuzzi, Bobo, Lichten, Samuelson, & Cousins, 2004). No data regarding to insulin synthesis and secretion have been reported in *Znt1* knockout mice.

3.2. Slc30a3/ZnT3

The expression of ZnT3 is largely restricted on the membrane of specialized vesicles, such as synaptic vesicles of zinc-enriched neurons (Wenzel, Cole, Born, Schwartzkroin, & Palmiter, 1997) and vesicles of pancreatic β-cells (Smidt et al., 2009). ZnT3 concentrates zinc ions in glutamatergic synapses in the hippocampus and cortex which can be released into the synaptic cleft along with other neurotransmitters upon neuronal activity (Cole et al., 1999; Linkous et al., 2008). Downregulation of ZnT3 expression has been shown to attenuate insulin expression and secretion in INS-1E cells (Petersen et al., 2011; Smidt et al., 2009). Based on the expression pattern of *Znt3* and its function, one might reasonably expect that a null mutation of *Znt3* would cause abnormality of brain function and insulin metabolism. Indeed, *Znt3* KO mice show signs of brain malfunction, such as age-dependent learning deficit and memory loss (Adlard, Parncutt, Finkelstein, & Bush, 2010; Martel, Hevi, Kane-Goldsmith, & Shumyatsky, 2011), even though they grow and reproduce normally and have normal sensorimotor functions (Cole, Martyanova, & Palmiter, 2001; Cole et al., 1999). Abnormal insulin secretion and glucose metabolism have not been observed in *Znt3* KO mice; however, the KO mice are sensitive to streptozotocin-induced insulin deficiency (Smidt et al., 2009), indicating that ZnT3 works together with other zinc transporters to maintain intracellular as well as intravesicular zinc levels and to support normal insulin metabolism in pancreatic β-cells.

3.3. Slc30a4/ZnT4

Znt4 expression is detected in many tissues and cell types including mammary epithelial cells and pancreatic β-cells (Huang & Gitschier, 1997; Liuzzi, Blanchard, & Cousins, 2000; Murgia, Vespignani, Cerase, Nobili, & Perozzi, 1999). ZnT4 expression is greatly induced during lactation in mice (Huang & Gitschier, 1997; Liuzzi, Bobo, Cui, McMahon, & Cousins, 2003). It is, therefore, not surprising that lactating *lm* dams that carry a defective *Znt4* gene have reduced zinc levels in their milk (Ackland & Mercer, 1992; Dickie, 1969; Huang & Gitschier, 1997; Lee, Shay, & Cousins, 1992; Piletz & Ganschow, 1978b). Pups of any genotype suckled on homozygous *lm* dams die of zinc deficiency before weaning. However, pups can be rescued by administration of zinc to them or by fostering them on normal dams (Erway and Grider Jr., 1984). ZnT4 is also implicated in maintaining whole body zinc homeostasis in middle- or late-adulthood age evident by the fact that *lm* mice fed normal rodent diets suffer from zinc deficiency around 8 months of age. Although ZnT4 is detected in insulin-expressing INS-1E cells, the functional significance of ZnT4 in insulin secretion and glucose metabolism has not been demonstrated in the null mutant of *Znt4* (Sondergaard et al., 2005).

3.4. Slc30a5/ZnT5

Znt5 is widely expressed in mouse tissues with high abundance in heart, smooth muscle, liver, small intestine, and lung (Jackson, Helston, McKay, O'Neill, Mathers, & Ford, 2007). It appears to transport cytoplasmic zinc into vesicular compartments of secretory cells including pancreatic β-cells

(Kambe et al., 2002; Suzuki et al., 2005). *Znt5* KO mice grow poorly in terms of body size and body weight. They have a hunched back. The bone density is reduced due to a defect in osteoblast maturation to the osteocyte. Body fat accumulation is reduced resulting in a lean body mass. Male *Znt5* KO mice suffer from sudden death due to cardiac arrhythmia between ages 15 and 40 weeks. Electrocardiography suggests that *Znt5* KO mice undergo a complete AV block and sinus bradycardia just before or at the time of death (Inoue et al., 2002). Human *ZNT5* is highly expressed in pancreatic β-cells and is detected to co-reside with insulin in the granules, indicating ZNT5 may play a role in insulin secretion (Kambe et al., 2002). However, the exact physiological role of ZNT5 in insulin synthesis and secretion in pancreatic β-cells has not been elucidated in humans and in animal models.

3.5. Slc30a7/ZnT7

Znt7 is detected in many mouse tissues (Kirschke & Huang, 2003). The physiological function of ZnT7 has been illustrated using *Znt7* KO mice (Huang, Yu, Kirschke, Gertz, & Lloyd, 2007). *Znt7* KO mice grow slower than the wild-type (WT) controls. They accumulate less body fat resulting in a lean phenotype. The slow growth of *Znt7* KO mice cannot be stimulated by feeding the KO mice with a zinc supplemental diet. In addition, *Znt7* KO mice have low serum zinc levels as well as low zinc contents in many tissues, such as liver, intestine, kidney, and bone (Huang, Yu, Kirschke, Gertz, & Lloyd, 2007).

An interesting finding in *Znt7* KO mice is that the male KO mice are prone to develop glucose intolerance (Huang et al., 2007). This impaired glucose metabolism can partly be explained by the reduced circulating insulin levels in the male *Znt7* KO mice (Huang, Kirschke, Lay, Levy, Lamirande, & Zhang, 2012). Another interesting finding is that male *Znt7* KO mice are susceptible to diet-induced glucose intolerance and insulin resistance. It is known that long-term feeding of a high-fat diet induces insulin resistance leading to glucose intolerance and type 2 diabetes in C57BL/6 mice (Surwit, Kuhn, Cochrane, McCubbin, & Feinglos, 1988). Indeed, both male *Znt7* KO and control mice develop hyperglycemia and insulin resistance after 12 weeks on a high-fat diet (HF, 45% kcal) (Huang et al., 2012). However, hyperglycemia and insulin resistance are much more severe in male *Znt7* KO mice than the control. Nonfasting serum glucose level is significantly high in *Znt7* KO mice fed the HF diet. Conversely, blood insulin level is low in these KO mice, indicating inadequacy of insulin secretion. It was shown that decreased insulin sensitivity in male *Znt7* KO mice fed the HF diet was partly because of decreased insulin-stimulated Irs and Akt phosphorylation and decreased Akt activity in the skeletal muscle (Huang et al., 2012). In addition, reduced secretion of insulin-sensitizing adipokines from adipocytes, such as leptin, in *Znt7* KO mice may also contribute to insulin resistance observed in these mice as circulating levels of leptin are correlated to body fat stores and glucose homeostasis (Huang et al., 2007; Margetic, Gazzola, Pegg, & Hill, 2002; Rosen & Spiegelman, 2006; Zhang, Proenca, Maffei, Barone, Leopold, & Friedman, 1994). Taken together, a combination of decreased insulin secretion and increased insulin resistance accounts for postprandial hyperglycemia and type 2 diabetes-like symptoms observed in male *Znt7* KO mice.

While male *Znt7* KO mice display abnormalities in insulin and glucose metabolism and insulin sensitivity, female *Znt7* KO mice are resistant to high-fat diet-induced obesity and insulin resistance. Fasting and nonfasting glucose and insulin levels in female *Znt7* KO mice fed the HF diet are comparable to that in the control. Glucose and insulin tolerances are normal in female *Znt7* KO mice, while circulating lipid levels as demonstrated by fasting serum triglycerides are 50% of the normal value in female *Znt7* KO mice fed the high diet (Huang et al., 2012). Thus, it is clear that ZnT7 plays an important role in regulation of lipid metabolism and lipid accumulation in the adipose tissue as both male and female KO mice have a generalized decrease in adipose tissue mass and female KO mice show low levels of circulating triglycerides.

3.6. Slc30a8/ZnT8

ZnT8 is predominantly expressed on the membrane of insulin-containing granules of pancreatic β-cells. It supplies zinc ions to insulin for its maturation and crystallization in insulin-containing vesicles and granules before secretion (Chimienti et al., 2004). Due to its restricted tissue distribution, *Znt8*-null mice (both global and β-cell-specific *Znt8* KO) have phenotypes mainly associated with β-cell functions. *Znt8* KO mice have significantly low zinc content in the secretory granules of β-cells. Numbers of insulin-containing granules are considerably reduced in the β-cell of *Znt8* KO mice, while numbers of atypical granules are increased in the cell. Insulin crystallization in the secretory granules is attenuated by the null mutation of *Znt8*. As a result, *Znt8* KO mice exhibit low fasting blood insulin levels and low glucose-induced insulin secretion, and the KO mice are glucose intolerant (Nicolson et al., 2009; Pound et al., 2009). The null mutations of *Znt8* (both global and β-cell specific) in mice seem to have no effect on the islet size and number, β-cell mass, and β-cell to α-cell ratio in the islet as well as total insulin content in the islet (Nicolson et al., 2009; Pound et al., 2009; Wijesekara et al., 2010). Exocytosis of insulin-containing secretory granules in terms of the number of granules attached to the plasma membrane, glucose-induced membrane depolarization, ATP-sensitive K^+ current, and depolarization-induced Ca^{2+} currents is normal in the β-cells isolated from *Znt8* KO mice (Nicolson et al., 2009).

It is interesting to note that although ZnT8 is mainly expressed, if not exclusively, in β-cells, the physiological impact of the *Znt8*-null mutation on β-cell function and whole body glucose metabolism varies in mice with global or β-cell-specific knockout. Generally speaking, whole body *Znt8* KO mice fed a regular rodent diet show slower glucose clearance after a glucose load. Insulin crystallization in secretory granules in the β-cell of *Znt8* KO mice is affected leading to a decreased glucose-induced insulin secretion. However, it seems that glucose-induced insulin secretion as well as the basal insulin secretion in the islet of global *Znt8* KO mice improves with age (>12 weeks of age), even though insulin crystallization remains poor in the β-cell (Nicolson et al., 2009; Pound et al., 2009). This suggests that other zinc transporter's activities, likely ZnT5 and/or ZnT7, may compensate for the loss of *Znt8* in the β-cell. Although β-cells isolated from β-cell-specific *Znt8* (*Znt8*B) KO mice have similar defects as those in the β-cells isolated from global *Znt8* KO mice (see above) (Wijesekara et al., 2010), the impact of the β-cell-specific *Znt8*-null mutation on insulin secretion is limited. While *Znt8*B KO mice are glucose intolerant during OGTT, their fasting blood glucose and insulin levels as well as glucose-induced insulin secretion during OGTT are normal. Peripheral insulin sensitivity is also normal in *Znt8*B KO mice (Wijesekara et al., 2010). Moreover, glucagon secretion from α-cells of the islet is not disturbed in *Znt8*B KO mice. So what is the cause of impaired glucose tolerance observed in *Znt8*B KO mice? The answer may lie in the impairment of the processing of proinsulin to mature insulin which leads to an increased proinsulin to insulin ratio in the blood (Wijesekara et al., 2010). This increased proinsulin to insulin ratio is also observed in human subjects who carry the risk allele (R325) of ZNT8 (Kirchhoff et al., 2008).

The discrepancy between the global *Znt8* KO and *Znt8*B KO on whole body glucose handling becomes apparent when both types of *Znt8* KO mice are under metabolic stress (Hardy et al., 2012). When male global *Znt8* KO mice fed a high-fat diet (45%kcal) for 17 weeks, they gain much more weight than the control and become obese. They develop severe insulin resistance evident by increased fasting glucose and insulin levels accompanied by increased islet numbers and sizes as well as β-cell mass in the islet of the pancreas. On the other hand, *Znt8*B KO mice (both the constitutive and inducible *Znt8*-null mutations) fed the same high-fat diet are resistant to weight gain after 17 weeks of feeding. Insulin resistance is not observed in *Znt8*B KO mice. These mice have normal fasting glucose level, but their fasting blood insulin concentrations are low compared to the control. In the pancreas of *Znt8*B KO mice, the islet size is reduced as well as the β-cell mass in the islet. Nevertheless, the numbers of the islet in the pancreas is normal in *Znt8*B KO mice.

Both global and β-cell-specific *Znt8* KO mice display impaired glucose tolerance after a glucose load. It is hypothesized that the glucose impairment in global *Znt8* KO mice is largely due to severe insulin resistance, whereas in *Znt8*B KO mice, it is due to inadequate insulin secretion from the pancreas. It is worth to note, in global *Znt8* KO mice, β-cell compensation to the diet-induced insulin resistance is more robust compared to the control. Fasting blood insulin level is approximately four times more than the control. Yet, they show poor glucose control. One possible explanation for this physiological β-cell compensation is the reduced mature insulin level in the circulation in *Znt8* KO mice due to a defect in the processing of insulin which positively feedbacks to upregulate the islet number and size as well as β-cell mass in the islet. The same defect in the insulin processing is also observed in the β-cell of *Znt8*B KO mice. However, β-cell compensation is not evident in the islet of *Znt8*B KO mice. Taken together, these data clearly suggest that expression of ZnT8 in β-cells play a major role in insulin processing, maturation, and secretion. However, ZnT8 expressed in other endocrine cells (albeit in low levels relative to β-cells), such as glucagon-secreting α-cells and pancreatic polypeptide-secreting PP cells in the islet, thyroglobulin-secreting cells in the thyroid gland, and cortex of the adrenal gland where corticosteroid hormone is synthesized and secreted, may also be involved in whole body glucose homeostasis (Murgia, Devirgiliis, Mancini, Donadel, Zalewski, & Perozzi, 2009; Nicolson et al., 2009).

The pancreatic α-cells synthesize and secrete glucagon, a counterregulatory hormone of insulin (Unger & Orci, 1981b). Glucagon functions to maintain blood glucose homeostasis during hypoglycemia (Unger & Orci, 1981a; Unger & Orci, 1981b). ZnT8 is expressed in α-cells in low abundance. The impact of the *Znt8*-null mutation on glucagon secretion and whole body glucose homeostasis in mice has been revealed by studying α-cell-specific *Znt8* KO mice (Wijesekara et al., 2010). Surprisingly, mice without ZnT8 expressed in α-cells are normal, without defects in pancreatic glucagon secretion and in body glucose metabolism, suggesting that ZnT8 is dispensable for the α-cell function. This conclusion is further supported by the observations of normal pancreatic glucagon secretion and a normal level of circulating glucagon in global *Znt8* KO mice (Hardy, Serino, Wijesekara, Chimienti, & Wheeler, 2011; Hardy et al., 2012).

3.7. Slc39a1, Slc39a2, and Slc39a3/Zip1, Zip2, and Zip3

Among the 14 members of the SLC39A family of zinc transporters, Zip1, Zip2, and Zip3 are the most conserved and related (Dufner-Beattie, Langmade, Wang, Eide, & Andrews, 2003). In mice, these genes can be coexpressed in tissues, such as the liver and the lamina propria in the intestinal tract. But they are also expressed in a cell-type-specific manner (Dufner-Beattie, Huang, Geiser, Xu, & Andrews, 2006; Dufner-Beattie, Langmade et al., 2003; Peters et al., 2007). Targeted knockout of *Zip2* or *Zip3* in mice has no apparent negative effects on mouse development as well as body zinc homeostasis when the KO mice are zinc replete (Dufner-Beattie, Huang, Geiser, Xu, & Andrews, 2005; Peters et al., 2007). On the other hand, when the KO mice are zinc depleted such as from inadequate dietary zinc intake, they display poor adaptations to zinc deficiency. It is interesting to note that mice with double (*Zip1* and *Zip3*) or triple (*Zip1*, *Zip2*, and *Zip3*) null mutations grow as well as the WT mice if adequate zinc is given in the diet, suggesting that these three *Zip* genes are dispensable for body zinc homeostasis in mice when zinc is replete (Dufner-Beattie et al., 2006; Kambe, Geiser, Lahner, Salt, & Andrews, 2008). Although Zip3 expression is detected in the islet of the mouse pancreas (Dufner-Beattie et al., 2006), its physiological role in insulin and glucose metabolism has not been elucidated.

3.8. Slc39a4/Zip4

AE is a recessive human disorder due to a defect in dietary zinc uptake leading to zinc deficiency. Symptoms of zinc deficiency, such as alopecia, eczematous dermatitis, and diarrhea, appear soon in bottle-fed AE newborns and in weaning AE infants from breastfeeding. The disease is lethal unless babies are given a large dose of exogenous zinc for life. Mutations in the human *ZIP4* gene are responsible for AE. *ZIP4* mRNA and protein are predominantly expressed in the enterocytes of the small intestine in both humans and mice. Therefore, mouse *Zip4* knockout mice were created to understand the physiological function of *Zip4*. Unlike the human AE fetus who can reach full-term and be born alive, globally knocking out *Zip4* in mice is embryonic lethal. On the other hand, weaning mice with tamoxifen-induced enterocyte-specific *Zip4* knockout can survive a few weeks without dietary zinc supplementation, and they present phenotypes similar to that of AE patients (Geiser et al., 2012). Although human *ZIP4* is detected in pancreatic cancer cells (Li et al., 2007), *Zip4* is not expressed in the mouse pancreas (Dufner-Beattie, Wang, Kuo, Gitschier, Eide, & Andrews, 2003).

3.9. Slc39a13/Zip13

Mice deficient for *Zip13* have defects in skeletal and connective tissue development reminiscent of a human genetic disorder, the spondylocheiro dysplastic Ehlers–Danlos syndrome (SCD-EDS) (Fukada et al., 2008; Giunta et al., 2008). Patients with SCD-EDS present short stature and skeletal and connective tissue abnormalities (Fukada et al., 2008; Giunta et al., 2008). Mutations in the human *ZIP13* gene were found responsible for this genetic disorder (Giunta et al., 2008). It has been demonstrated that ZIP13 functions to release labile zinc from vesicular stores in the cell, a function similar to the ZIP7 protein which releases stored zinc from the Golgi apparatus (Huang et al., 2005; Jeong et al., 2012). Mice with a null mutation of *Zip13* display stunted growth, osteopenia, hunched back, reduced bone mass and length, craniofacial abnormality among other disorders in skin and cartilage formation. Nevertheless, defects in insulin and glucose metabolism have not been reported in *Zip13* KO mice as well as in humans with SCD-EDS (Fukada et al., 2008).

3.10. Slc39a14/Zip14

Mice deficient for *Zip14* exhibit abnormalities in bone development, energy balance, and endocrine hormone production as well as iron metabolism (Aydemir et al., 2012; Aydemir et al., 2012; Hojyo et al., 2011; Nam et al., 2013). Zinc absorption is significantly decreased in *Zip14* KO mice. As the result, the KO mice have less zinc in tissues such as liver and bone (Aydemir et al., 2012). On the other hand, *Zip14* KO mice absorb more iron (Aydemir et al., 2012; Nam et al., 2013) resulting in high liver nonheme iron content. Enhanced hepatic iron uptake and stores are thought to be due to upregulation of *Dmt1*, *Tfr-1*, and *ferritin* expression (Aydemir et al., 2012).

Zip14 KO mice are small and growth retarded with wry neck due to abnormal bone development and decreased circulating growth hormone and insulin-like growth factor (Hojyo et al., 2011). Despite slow growth, *Zip14* KO mice accumulate more body fat (~5%) than the control mice. As expected, genes that are involved in lipogenesis, such as *Glut2*, *Srebp-1c*, and *Fasn* are upregulated because of enhanced activity of the insulin signaling pathway in *Zip14* KO mice (Aydemir et al., 2012). Interestingly, *Zip14* KO mice are hypoglycemic and develop hyperinsulinemia (Aydemir et al., 2012). Fasting gluconeogenesis is decreased in the liver of *Zip14* KO mice (Hojyo et al., 2011). In line with hyperinsulinemia, *Zip14* KO mice exhibit enlarged islets with increased cell mass in the pancreas accompanied by elevated ZnT8 and insulin expression in the β-cell (Aydemir et al., 2012). In conclusion, the abnormalities of insulin, glucose, and lipid metabolism in *Zip14* KO mice are likely the result of an enhanced production/secretion of insulin in the pancreatic β-cell of the KO mice. The phenotypes shown in *Zip14* KO mice are consistent with the expression pattern of *Zip14*, suggesting that *Zip14* is indispensable for zinc homeostasis in tissues and cells which includes bone, pituitary gland, liver, white fat, and pancreatic β-cells.

4. ZINC AND ITS TRANSPORTERS IN THE DEVELOPMENT OF DIABETES IN HUMANS

Zinc is required for insulin crystallization, storage, and secretion in the secretory granules of pancreatic β-cells. Delivery of zinc into the insulin-containing granules is largely accomplished by the ZNT8 protein. Studies have shown that the expression of *ZnT8* is reduced in the islets of diabetic mouse models, such as *db/db* and *Akita* mice (Tamaki, Fujitani, Uchida, Hirose, Kawamori, & Watada, 2009). The involvement of human ZNT8 in insulin and glucose metabolism and type 2 diabetes (T2D) is revealed by several whole genome association studies (Saxena et al., 2007; Scott et al., 2007; Sladek et al., 2007). These studies discovered that the R325W allele of ZNT8 (dbSNP ID: rs1326663) is a risk factor of T2D in human subjects. Individuals carrying the R325 risk allele of ZNT8 have low basal and glucose-stimulated insulin secretion (Cauchi et al., 2008; Staiger et al., 2007). The R325 allele carriers are also likely to have abnormal glucose tolerance during OGTT (Kirchhoff et al., 2008). Moreover, it has been shown that the R325 allele has a negative impact on the first phase insulin release during glucose challenge which is consistent with the function of ZNT8 in insulin maturation and crystallization (Boesgaard et al.,

2008). The pathogenic impact of the R325 allele on T2D development is more obvious in renal allograft patients who carry two R325 alleles. These patients are more likely to develop posttransplantation diabetes than the patients who carry two W325 alleles of ZNT8 (Kang et al., 2008).

ZNT8 is also a major autoantigen in development of autoimmunity against pancreatic β-cells leading to type 1 diabetes (T1D) in children and young adults (Wenzlau et al., 2007). A high amount of ZNT8 autoantibodies are frequently detected in the early stage of T1D. With disease progression, ZNT8 autoantibody titers drop significantly. Multiple epitopes in ZNT8 contribute to the development of autoimmunity against β-cells. However, a majority of ZNT8 autoantibodies (~80%) react with the epitopes in the C-terminal end of the ZNT8 protein (Achenbach et al., 2009; Wenzlau et al., 2007). Moreover, the epitope containing R325 is a major determinant for the ZNT8 autoimmunity (Wenzlau et al., 2007). Nevertheless, the risk allele R325 of ZNT8 is a predominant allele in human populations. The highest carrier rate of the R325 allele (92–99%) is found in Africans and their descendants (Lewis et al., 2008; Palmer et al., 2008), followed by Hispanic Americans at 95% (Palmer et al., 2008) and European Caucasians and Asians at 80–90% (Horikawa et al., 2008; Staiger et al., 2007). The impact of this risk allele on T2D development varies among racial/ethnic groups. Caucasians and Asians carrying the R325 allele have a higher risk for developing T2D (Cauchi et al., 2008; Ng et al., 2008) than Africans and Hispanic Americans carrying the same risk allele, indicating other genetic factors can affect the phenotypic expression of the risk allele of ZNT8 in human populations (Lewis et al., 2008; Palmer et al., 2008).

5. CONCLUSIONS AND FUTURE DIRECTIONS

Zinc transporter knockout studies in mice have provided direct evidence for a relationship between zinc and insulin metabolism in the pancreatic β-cell. Zinc uptake by Zip proteins (Zip6, Zip8, and Zip14) and subsequent sequestration into cytoplasmic secretory vesicles by ZnT proteins (ZnT3, ZnT5/ZnT7, and ZnT8) are critical for insulin synthesis, maturation, and secretion in β-cells. An abnormal cellular zinc level in the β-cell can have adverse biological and pathological impacts on humans. Individuals who carry the R325 allele of ZNT8 have a high risk for malfunction of β-cells due to autoimmunity or insulin maturation and secretion leading to insulin insufficiency and hyperglycemia. As for diabetes prevention and treatment in humans, detecting the R325 SNP for ZNT8 in adults as well as monitoring autoantibodies against ZNT8 in children and young adults may become effective tools to increase the odds to identify at-risk individuals. Dietary and physical training recommendations can then be provided to these at-risk individuals before disease develops. Or a therapeutic intervention can be provided for children whose autoantibodies against ZNT8 are positive (De Grijse et al., 2010). The physiological impacts of SNPs in other zinc transporters that are expressed in the pancreatic β-cell (ZNT3, ZNT5, ZNT7, ZIP6, ZIP7, ZIP8, and ZIP14) remain largely unknown. Screening of SNPs in these zinc transporters for their association with T2D is needed, especially for these individuals who carry the R325 allele of ZNT8. The compounding effect of R325 of ZNT8 and SNP changes in other zinc transporters may exist in individuals, which would place them at high risk for development of diabetes.

ACKNOWLEDGMENTS

We thank Dr. Sean Adams and Catherine Kirschke of the Western Human Nutrition Research Center for the support and critical reading of the manuscript. This work is supported by the United States Department of Agriculture, ARS Projects 5306-515-30-016-00D and 5306-515-20-006-00D. USDA is an equal opportunity provider and employer.

REFERENCES

Achenbach, P., Lampasona, V., Landherr, U., Koczwara, K., Krause, S., Grallert, H., et al. (2009). Autoantibodies to zinc transporter 8 and SLC30A8 genotype stratify type 1 diabetes risk. *Diabetologia, 52*, 1881–1888.

Ackland, M. L., & Mercer, J. F. (1992). The murine mutation, lethal milk, results in production of zinc-deficient milk. *The Journal of Nutrition, 122*, 1214–1218.

Adlard, P. A., Parncutt, J. M., Finkelstein, D. I., & Bush, A. I. (2010). Cognitive loss in zinc transporter-3 knock-out mice: A phenocopy for the synaptic and memory deficits of Alzheimer's disease? *The Journal of Neuroscience, 30*, 1631–1636.

Andrews, G. K., Wang, H., Dey, S. K., & Palmiter, R. D. (2004). Mouse zinc transporter 1 gene provides an essential function during early embryonic development. *Genesis, 40*, 74–81.

Aydemir, T. B., Chang, S. M., Guthrie, G. J., Maki, A. B., Ryu, M. S., Karabiyik, A., et al. (2012). Zinc transporter ZIP14 functions in hepatic zinc, iron and glucose homeostasis during the innate immune response (endotoxemia). *PLoS One*, 7, e48679.

Aydemir, T. B., Liuzzi, J. P., McClellan, S., & Cousins, R. J. (2009). Zinc transporter ZIP8 (SLC39A8) and zinc influence IFN-gamma expression in activated human T cells. *Journal of Leukocyte Biology, 86*, 337–348.

Aydemir, T. B., Sitren, H. S., & Cousins, R. J. (2012). The zinc transporter Zip14 influences c-Met phosphorylation and hepatocyte proliferation during liver regeneration in mice. *Gastroenterology, 142*, 1536–1546.

Bellomo, E. A., Meur, G., & Rutter, G. A. (2011). Glucose regulates free cytosolic Zn(2)(+) concentration, Slc39 (ZiP), and metallothionein gene expression in primary pancreatic islet beta-cells. *The Journal of Biological Chemistry, 286*, 25778–25789.

Bensellam, M., Van Lommel, L., Overbergh, L., Schuit, F. C., & Jonas, J. C. (2009). Cluster analysis of rat pancreatic islet gene mRNA levels after culture in low-, intermediate- and high-glucose concentrations. *Diabetologia*, *52*, 463–476.

Boesgaard, T. W., Zilinskaite, J., Vanttinen, M., Laakso, M., Jansson, P. A., Hammarstedt, A., et al. (2008). The common SLC30A8 Arg325Trp variant is associated with reduced first-phase insulin release in 846 non-diabetic offspring of type 2 diabetes patients—The EUGENE2 study. *Diabetologia*, *51*, 816–820.

Cauchi, S., Proenca, C., Choquet, H., Gaget, S., De Graeve, F., Marre, M., et al. (2008). Analysis of novel risk loci for type 2 diabetes in a general French population: The D.E.S.I.R. study. *Journal of Molecular Medicine*, *86*, 341–348.

Chimienti, F., Devergnas, S., Favier, A., & Seve, M. (2004). Identification and cloning of a beta-cell-specific zinc transporter, ZnT-8, localized into insulin secretory granules. *Diabetes*, *53*, 2330–2337.

Cole, T. B., Martyanova, A., & Palmiter, R. D. (2001). Removing zinc from synaptic vesicles does not impair spatial learning, memory, or sensorimotor functions in the mouse. *Brain Research*, *891*, 253–265.

Cole, T. B., Wenzel, H. J., Kafer, K. E., Schwartzkroin, P. A., & Palmiter, R. D. (1999). Elimination of zinc from synaptic vesicles in the intact mouse brain by disruption of the ZnT3 gene. *Proceedings of the National Academy of Sciences of the United States of America*, *96*, 1716–1721.

Davidson, H. W., Rhodes, C. J., & Hutton, J. C. (1988). Intraorganellar calcium and pH control proinsulin cleavage in the pancreatic beta cell via two distinct site-specific endopeptidases. *Nature*, *333*, 93–96.

De Grijse, J., Asanghanwa, M., Nouthe, B., Albrecher, N., Goubert, P., Vermeulen, I., et al. (2010). Predictive power of screening for antibodies against insulinoma-associated protein 2 beta (IA-2beta) and zinc transporter-8 to select first-degree relatives of type 1 diabetic patients with risk of rapid progression to clinical onset of the disease: Implications for prevention trials. *Diabetologia*, *53*, 517–524.

Dickie, M. M. (1969). lm. *Mouse News Letter*, *41*, 30–31.

Dufner-Beattie, J., Huang, Z. L., Geiser, J., Xu, W., & Andrews, G. K. (2005). Generation and characterization of mice lacking the zinc uptake transporter ZIP3. *Molecular and Cellular Biology*, *25*, 5607–5615.

Dufner-Beattie, J., Huang, Z. L., Geiser, J., Xu, W., & Andrews, G. K. (2006). Mouse ZIP1 and ZIP3 genes together are essential for adaptation to dietary zinc deficiency during pregnancy. *Genesis*, *44*, 239–251.

Dufner-Beattie, J., Langmade, S. J., Wang, F., Eide, D., & Andrews, G. K. (2003). Structure, function, and regulation of a subfamily of mouse zinc transporter genes. *The Journal of Biological Chemistry*, *278*, 50142–50150.

Dufner-Beattie, J., Wang, F., Kuo, Y. M., Gitschier, J., Eide, D., & Andrews, G. K. (2003). The acrodermatitis enteropathica gene ZIP4 encodes a tissue-specific, zinc-regulated zinc transporter in mice. *The Journal of Biological Chemistry*, *278*, 33474–33481.

Dunn, M. F. (2005). Zinc-ligand interactions modulate assembly and stability of the insulin hexamer—A review. *Biometals*, *18*, 295–303.

Eckhert, C. D., Sloan, M. V., Duncan, J. R., & Hurley, L. S. (1977). Zinc binding: A difference between human and bovine milk. *Science*, *195*, 789–790.

Erway, L. C., & Grider, A., Jr. (1984). Zinc metabolism in lethal-milk mice. Otolith, lactation, and aging effects. *Journal of Heredity*, *75*, 480–484.

Franklin, I., Gromada, J., Gjinovci, A., Theander, S., & Wollheim, C. B. (2005). Beta-cell secretory products activate alpha-cell ATP-dependent potassium channels to inhibit glucagon release. *Diabetes*, *54*, 1808–1815.

Fraústo da Silva, J. J. R., & Williams, R. J. P. (2001). *The biological chemistry of the elements: The inorganic chemistry of life* (2nd ed.). Oxford, NY: Oxford University Press.

Fukada, T., Civic, N., Furuichi, T., Shimoda, S., Mishima, K., Higashiyama, H., et al. (2008). The zinc transporter SLC39A13/ZIP13 is required for connective tissue development; its involvement in BMP/TGF-beta signaling pathways. *PLoS One*, *3*, e3642.

Geiser, J., Venken, K. J., De Lisle, R. C., & Andrews, G. K. (2012). A mouse model of acrodermatitis enteropathica: Loss of intestine zinc transporter ZIP4 (Slc39a4) disrupts the stem cell niche and intestine integrity. *PLoS Genetics*, *8*, e1002766.

Giunta, C., Elcioglu, N. H., Albrecht, B., Eich, G., Chambaz, C., Janecke, A. R., et al. (2008). Spondylocheiro dysplastic form of the Ehlers-Danlos syndrome—An autosomal-recessive entity caused by mutations in the zinc transporter gene SLC39A13. *American Journal of Human Genetics*, *82*, 1290–1305.

Guo, J., Chung, U. I., Yang, D., Karsenty, G., Bringhurst, F. R., & Kronenberg, H. M. (2006). PTH/PTHrP receptor delays chondrocyte hypertrophy via both Runx2-dependent and -independent pathways. *Developmental Biology*, *292*, 116–128.

Guo, L., Lichten, L. A., Ryu, M. S., Liuzzi, J. P., Wang, F., & Cousins, R. J. (2010). STAT5-glucocorticoid receptor interaction and MTF-1 regulate the expression of ZnT2 (Slc30a2) in pancreatic acinar cells. *Proceedings of the National Academy of Sciences of the United States of America*, *107*, 2818–2823.

Haataja, L., Snapp, E., Wright, J., Liu, M., Hardy, A. B., Wheeler, M. B., et al. (2013). Proinsulin intermolecular interactions during secretory trafficking in pancreatic beta cells. *The Journal of Biological Chemistry*, *288*, 1896–1906.

Hardy, A. B., Serino, A. S., Wijesekara, N., Chimienti, F., & Wheeler, M. B. (2011). Regulation of glucagon secretion by zinc: Lessons from the beta cell-specific Znt8 knockout mouse model. *Diabetes, Obesity & Metabolism*, *13*(Suppl 1), 112–117.

Hardy, A. B., Wijesekara, N., Genkin, I., Prentice, K. J., Bhattacharjee, A., Kong, D., et al. (2012). Effects of high-fat diet feeding on Znt8-null mice: Differences between beta-cell and global knockout of Znt8. *American Journal of Physiology - Endocrinology and Metabolism*, *302*, E1084–E1096.

Hojyo, S., Fukada, T., Shimoda, S., Ohashi, W., Bin, B. H., Koseki, H., et al. (2011). The zinc transporter SLC39A14/ZIP14 controls G-protein coupled receptor-mediated signaling required for systemic growth. *PloS One*, *6*, e18059.

Horikawa, Y., Miyake, K., Yasuda, K., Enya, M., Hirota, Y., Yamagata, K., et al. (2008). Replication of genome-wide association studies of type 2 diabetes susceptibility in Japan. *The Journal of Clinical Endocrinology and Metabolism*, *93*, 3136–3141.

Huang, L. P., & Gitschier, J. (1997). A novel gene involved in zinc transport is deficient in the lethal milk mouse. *Nature Genetics*, *17*, 292–297.

Huang, L., Kirschke, C. P., Lay, Y. A., Levy, L. B., Lamirande, D. E., & Zhang, P. H. (2012). Znt7-null mice are more susceptible to diet-induced glucose intolerance and insulin resistance. *The Journal of Biological Chemistry*, *287*, 33883–33896.

Huang, L., Kirschke, C. P., Zhang, Y., & Yu, Y. Y. (2005). The ZIP7 gene (Slc39a7) encodes a zinc transporter involved in zinc homeostasis of the Golgi apparatus. *The Journal of Biological Chemistry*, *280*, 15456–15463.

Huang, L., & Tepaamorndech, S. (2013). The SLC30 family of zinc transporters—A review of current understanding of their biological and pathophysiological roles. *Molecular Aspects of Medicine*, *34*, 548–560.

Huang, L., Yan, M., & Kirschke, C. P. (2010). Over-expression of ZnT7 increases insulin synthesis and secretion in pancreatic beta-cells by promoting insulin gene transcription. *Experimental Cell Research*, *316*, 2630–2643.

Huang, L., Yu, Y. Y., Kirschke, C. P., Gertz, E. R., & Lloyd, K. K. (2007). Znt7 (Slc30a7)-deficient mice display reduced body zinc status and body fat accumulation. *The Journal of Biological Chemistry*, *282*, 37053–37063.

Inoue, K., Matsuda, K., Itoh, M., Kawaguchi, H., Tomoike, H., Aoyagi, T., et al. (2002). Osteopenia and male-specific sudden cardiac death in mice lacking a zinc transporter gene, Znt5. *Human Molecular Genetics*, *11*, 1775–1784.

Jackson, K. A., Helston, R. M., McKay, J. A., O'Neill, E. D., Mathers, J. C., & Ford, D. (2007). Splice variants of the human zinc transporter ZnT5 (SLC30A5) are differentially localized and regulated by zinc through transcription and mRNA stability. *The Journal of Biological Chemistry, 282*, 10423–10431.

Jeong, J., & Eide, D. J. (2013). The SLC39 family of zinc transporters. *Molecular Aspects of Medicine, 34*, 612–619.

Jeong, J., Walker, J. M., Wang, F., Park, J. G., Palmer, A. E., Giunta, C., et al. (2012). Promotion of vesicular zinc efflux by ZIP13 and its implications for spondylocheiro dysplastic Ehlers-Danlos syndrome. *Proceedings of the National Academy of Sciences of the United States of America, 109*, E3530–E3538.

Kagi, J. H., & Schaffer, A. (1988). Biochemistry of metallothionein. *Biochemistry, 27*, 8509–8515.

Kambe, T., Geiser, J., Lahner, B., Salt, D. E., & Andrews, G. K. (2008). Slc39a1 to 3 (subfamily II) Zip genes in mice have unique cell-specific functions during adaptation to zinc deficiency. *American Journal of Physiology - Regulatory, Integrative and Comparative Physiology, 294*, R1474–R1481.

Kambe, T., Narita, H., Yamaguchi-Iwai, Y., Hirose, J., Amano, T., Sugiura, N., et al. (2002). Cloning and characterization of a novel mammalian zinc transporter, zinc transporter 5, abundantly expressed in pancreatic beta cells. *The Journal of Biological Chemistry, 277*, 19049–19055.

Kang, E. S., Kim, M. S., Kim, Y. S., Kim, C. H., Han, S. J., Chun, S. W., et al. (2008). A polymorphism in the zinc transporter gene SLC30A8 confers resistance against posttransplantation diabetes mellitus in renal allograft recipients. *Diabetes, 57*, 1043–1047.

Kirchhoff, K., Machicao, F., Haupt, A., Schafer, S. A., Tschritter, O., Staiger, H., et al. (2008). Polymorphisms in the TCF7L2, CDKAL1 and SLC30A8 genes are associated with impaired proinsulin conversion. *Diabetologia, 51*, 597–601.

Kirschke, C. P., & Huang, L. (2003). ZnT7, a novel mammalian zinc transporter, accumulates zinc in the Golgi apparatus. *The Journal of Biological Chemistry, 278*, 4096–4102.

Krebs, N. F. (2000). Overview of zinc absorption and excretion in the human gastrointestinal tract. *The Journal of Nutrition, 130*, 1374S–1377S.

Lee, D. Y., Shay, N. F., & Cousins, R. J. (1992). Altered zinc metabolism occurs in murine lethal milk syndrome. *The Journal of Nutrition, 122*, 2233–2238.

Le Roith, D., & Zick, Y. (2001). Recent advances in our understanding of insulin action and insulin resistance. *Diabetes Care, 24*, 588–597.

Lewis, J. P., Palmer, N. D., Hicks, P. J., Sale, M. M., Langefeld, C. D., Freedman, B. I., et al. (2008). Association analysis in African Americans of European-derived type 2 diabetes single nucleotide polymorphisms from whole-genome association studies. *Diabetes, 57*, 2220–2225.

Li, M., Zhang, Y., Liu, Z., Bharadwaj, U., Wang, H., Wang, X., et al. (2007). Aberrant expression of zinc transporter ZIP4 (SLC39A4) significantly contributes to human pancreatic cancer pathogenesis and progression. *Proceedings of the National Academy of Sciences of the United States of America, 104*, 18636–18641.

Linkous, D. H., Flinn, J. M., Koh, J. Y., Lanzirotti, A., Bertsch, P. M., Jones, B. F., et al. (2008). Evidence that the ZNT3 protein controls the total amount of elemental zinc in synaptic vesicles. *The Journal of Histochemistry and Cytochemistry, 56*, 3–6.

Liuzzi, J. P., Blanchard, R. K., & Cousins, R. J. (2000). Differential regulation of zinc transporter 1, 2, and 4 mRNA expression by dietary zinc in rates. *The Journal of Nutrition, 131*, 46–52.

Liuzzi, J. P., Bobo, J. A., Cui, L., McMahon, R. J., & Cousins, R. J. (2003). Zinc transporters 1, 2 and 4 are differentially expressed and localized in rats during pregnancy and lactation. *The Journal of Nutrition, 133*, 342–351.

Liuzzi, J. P., Bobo, J. A., Lichten, L. A., Samuelson, D. A., & Cousins, R. J. (2004). Responsive transporter genes within the murine intestinal-pancreatic axis form a basis of zinc

homeostasis. *Proceedings of the National Academy of Sciences of the United States of America, 101*, 14355–14360.
Margetic, S., Gazzola, C., Pegg, G. G., & Hill, R. A. (2002). Leptin: A review of its peripheral actions and interactions. *International Journal of Obesity and Related Metabolic Disorders, 26*, 1407–1433.
Martel, G., Hevi, C., Kane-Goldsmith, N., & Shumyatsky, G. P. (2011). Zinc transporter ZnT3 is involved in memory dependent on the hippocampus and perirhinal cortex. *Behavioural Brain Research, 223*, 233–238.
Moynahan, E. J. (1974). Letter: Acrodermatitis enteropathica: A lethal inherited human zinc-deficiency disorder. *Lancet, 2*, 399–400.
Murgia, C., Devirgiliis, C., Mancini, E., Donadel, G., Zalewski, P., & Perozzi, G. (2009). Diabetes-linked zinc transporter ZnT8 is a homodimeric protein expressed by distinct rodent endocrine cell types in the pancreas and other glands. *Nutrition, Metabolism, and Cardiovascular Diseases, 19*, 431–439.
Murgia, C., Vespignani, I., Cerase, J., Nobili, F., & Perozzi, G. (1999). Cloning, expression, and vesicular localization of zinc transporter Dri 27/ZnT4 in intestinal tissue and cells. *The American Journal of Physiology, 277*, G1231–G1239.
Nam, H., Wang, C. Y., Zhang, L., Zhang, W., Hojyo, S., Fukada, T., et al. (2013). ZIP14 and DMT1 in the liver, pancreas, and heart are differentially regulated by iron deficiency and overload: Implications for tissue iron uptake in iron-related disorders. *Haematologica, 98*, 1049–1057.
Ng, M. C., Park, K. S., Oh, B., Tam, C. H., Cho, Y. M., Shin, H. D., et al. (2008). Implication of genetic variants near TCF7L2, SLC30A8, HHEX, CDKAL1, CDKN2A/B, IGF2BP2, and FTO in type 2 diabetes and obesity in 6,719 Asians. *Diabetes, 57*, 2226–2233.
Nicolson, T. J., Bellomo, E. A., Wijesekara, N., Loder, M. K., Baldwin, J. M., Gyulkhandanyan, A. V., et al. (2009). Insulin storage and glucose homeostasis in mice null for the granule zinc transporter ZnT8 and studies of the type 2 diabetes-associated variants. *Diabetes, 58*, 2070–2083.
Palmer, N. D., Goodarzi, M. O., Langefeld, C. D., Ziegler, J., Norris, J. M., Haffner, S. M., et al. (2008). Quantitative trait analysis of type 2 diabetes susceptibility loci identified from whole genome association studies in the Insulin Resistance Atherosclerosis Family Study. *Diabetes, 57*, 1093–1100.
Palmiter, R. D., Cole, T. B., Quaife, C. J., & Findley, S. D. (1996). ZnT-3, a putative transporter of zinc into synaptic vesicles. *Proceedings of the National Academy of Sciences of the United States of America, 93*, 14934–14939.
Palmiter, R. D., & Findley, S. D. (1995). Cloning and functional-characterization of a mammalian zinc transporter that confers resistance to zinc. *The EMBO Journal, 14*, 639–649.
Patzelt, C., Labrecque, A. D., Duguid, J. R., Carroll, R. J., Keim, P. S., Heinrikson, R. L., et al. (1978). Detection and kinetic behavior of preproinsulin in pancreatic islets. *Proceedings of the National Academy of Sciences of the United States of America, 75*, 1260–1264.
Peters, J. L., Dufner-Beattie, J., Xu, W., Geiser, J., Lahner, B., Salt, D. E., et al. (2007). Targeting of the mouse Slc39a2 (Zip2) gene reveals highly cell-specific patterns of expression, and unique functions in zinc, iron, and calcium homeostasis. *Genesis, 45*, 339–352.
Petersen, A. B., Smidt, K., Magnusson, N. E., Moore, F., Egefjord, L., & Rungby, J. (2011). siRNA-mediated knock-down of ZnT3 and ZnT8 affects production and secretion of insulin and apoptosis in INS-1E cells. *Acta Pathologica, Microbiologica et Immunologica Scandinavica, 119*, 93–102.
Piletz, J. A., & Ganschow, R. E. (1978a). Lethal milk mutation results in dietary zinc deficiency in nursing mice. *The American Journal of Clinical Nutrition, 31*, 560–562.

Piletz, J. E., & Ganschow, R. E. (1978b). Zinc deficiency in murine milk underlies expression of the lethal milk (lm) mutation. *Science*, *199*, 181–183.
Pound, L. D., Sarkar, S. A., Benninger, R. K., Wang, Y., Suwanichkul, A., Shadoan, M. K., et al. (2009). Deletion of the mouse Slc30a8 gene encoding zinc transporter-8 results in impaired insulin secretion. *The Biochemical Journal*, *421*, 371–376.
Prasad, A. S. (1985). Clinical manifestations of zinc deficiency. *Annual Review of Nutrition*, *5*, 341–363.
Prasad, A. S., Miale, A., Jr., Farid, Z., Sandstead, H. H., & Schulert, A. R. (1963). Zinc metabolism in patients with the syndrome of iron deficiency anemia, hepatosplenomegaly, dwarfism, and hypognadism. *The Journal of Laboratory and Clinical Medicine*, *61*, 537–549.
Radtke, F., Heuchel, R., Georgiev, O., Hergersberg, M., Gariglio, M., Dembic, Z., et al. (1993). Cloned transcription factor MTF-1 activates the mouse metallothionein I promoter. *The EMBO Journal*, *12*, 1355–1362.
Rosen, E. D., & Spiegelman, B. M. (2006). Adipocytes as regulators of energy balance and glucose homeostasis. *Nature*, *444*, 847–853.
Saxena, R., Voight, B. F., Lyssenko, V., Burtt, N. P., de Bakker, P. I., Chen, H., et al. (2007). Genome-wide association analysis identifies loci for type 2 diabetes and triglyceride levels. *Science*, *316*, 1331–1336.
Scott, L. J., Mohlke, K. L., Bonnycastle, L. L., Willer, C. J., Li, Y., Duren, W. L., et al. (2007). A genome-wide association study of type 2 diabetes in Finns detects multiple susceptibility variants. *Science*, *316*, 1341–1345.
Sladek, R., Rocheleau, G., Rung, J., Dina, C., Shen, L., Serre, D., et al. (2007). A genome-wide association study identifies novel risk loci for type 2 diabetes. *Nature*, *445*, 881–885.
Smeekens, S. P., Montag, A. G., Thomas, G., Albiges-Rizo, C., Carroll, R., Benig, M., et al. (1992). Proinsulin processing by the subtilisin-related proprotein convertases furin, PC2, and PC3. *Proceedings of the National Academy of Sciences of the United States of America*, *89*, 8822–8826.
Smidt, K., Jessen, N., Petersen, A. B., Larsen, A., Magnusson, N., Jeppesen, J. B., et al. (2009). SLC30A3 responds to glucose- and zinc variations in beta-cells and is critical for insulin production and in vivo glucose-metabolism during beta-cell stress. *PloS One*, *4*, e5684.
Sondergaard, L. G., Brock, B., Stoltenberg, M., Flyvbjerg, A., Schmitz, O., Smidt, K., et al. (2005). Zinc fluxes during acute and chronic exposure of INS-1E cells to increasing glucose levels. *Hormone and Metabolic Research*, *37*, 133–139.
Sondergaard, L. G., Stoltenberg, M., Doering, P., Flyvbjerg, A., & Rungby, J. (2006). Zinc ions in the endocrine and exocrine pancreas of zinc deficient rats. *Histology and Histopathology*, *21*, 619 625.
Staiger, H., Machicao, F., Stefan, N., Tschritter, O., Thamer, C., Kantartzis, K., et al. (2007). Polymorphisms within novel risk loci for type 2 diabetes determine beta-cell function. *PloS One*, *2*, e832.
Surwit, R. S., Kuhn, C. M., Cochrane, C., McCubbin, J. A., & Feinglos, M. N. (1988). Diet-induced type II diabetes in C57BL/6 J mice. *Diabetes*, *37*, 1163–1167.
Suzuki, A., & Endo, T. (2002). Ermelin, an endoplasmic reticulum transmembrane protein, contains the novel HELP domain conserved in eukaryotes. *Gene*, *284*, 31–40.
Suzuki, T., Ishihara, K., Migaki, H., Ishihara, K., Nagao, M., Yamaguchi-Iwai, Y., et al. (2005). Two different zinc transport complexes of cation diffusion facilitator proteins localized in the secretory pathway operate to activate alkaline phosphatases in vertebrate cells. *The Journal of Biological Chemistry*, *280*, 30956–30962.
Tamaki, M., Fujitani, Y., Uchida, T., Hirose, T., Kawamori, R., & Watada, H. (2009). Downregulation of ZnT8 expression in pancreatic beta-cells of diabetic mice. *Islets*, *1*, 124–128.

Taylor, K. M., Hiscox, S., Nicholson, R. I., Hogstrand, C., & Kille, P. (2012). Protein kinase CK2 triggers cytosolic zinc signaling pathways by phosphorylation of zinc channel ZIP7. *Science Signaling*, *5*, ra11.

Taylor, K. M., Morgan, H. E., Johnson, A., & Nicholson, R. I. (2004). Structure-function analysis of HKE4, a member of the new LIV-1 subfamily of zinc transporters. *The Biochemical Journal*, *377*, 131–139.

Todd, W. R., Elvehjem, C. A., & Hart, B. B. (1934). Zinc in the nutrition of the rats. *American Journal of Physiology*, *107*, 146–156.

Unger, R. H., & Orci, L. (1981a). Glucagon and the A cell: Physiology and pathophysiology (first two parts). *The New England Journal of Medicine*, *304*, 1518–1524.

Unger, R. H., & Orci, L. (1981b). Glucagon and the A cell: Physiology and pathophysiology (second of two parts). *The New England Journal of Medicine*, *304*, 1575–1580.

Vinkenborg, J. L., Nicolson, T. J., Bellomo, E. A., Koay, M. S., Rutter, G. A., & Merkx, M. (2009). Genetically encoded FRET sensors to monitor intracellular Zn2+ homeostasis. *Nature Methods*, *6*, 737–740.

Wang, X., Wu, Y., & Zhou, B. (2009). Dietary zinc absorption is mediated by ZnT1 in Drosophila melanogaster. *FASEB Journal*, *23*, 2650–2661.

Wang, K., Zhou, B., Kuo, Y. M., Zemansky, J., & Gitschier, J. (2002). A novel member of a zinc transporter family is defective in acrodermatitis enteropathica. *American Journal of Human Genetics*, *71*, 66–73.

Wenzel, H. J., Cole, T. B., Born, D. E., Schwartzkroin, P. A., & Palmiter, R. D. (1997). Ultrastructural localization of zinc transporter-3 (ZnT-3) to synaptic vesicle membranes within mossy fiber boutons in the hippocampus of mouse and monkey. *Proceedings of the National Academy of Sciences of the United States of America*, *94*, 12676–12681.

Wenzlau, J. M., Juhl, K., Yu, L., Moua, O., Sarkar, S. A., Gottlieb, P., et al. (2007). The cation efflux transporter ZnT8 (Slc30A8) is a major autoantigen in human type 1 diabetes. *Proceedings of the National Academy of Sciences of the United States of America*, *104*, 17040–17045.

Wijesekara, N., Dai, F. F., Hardy, A. B., Giglou, P. R., Bhattacharjee, A., Koshkin, V., et al. (2010). Beta cell-specific Znt8 deletion in mice causes marked defects in insulin processing, crystallisation and secretion. *Diabetologia*, *53*, 1656–1668.

Wildman, R. E. C., & Medeiros, D. M. (2000). *Advanced human nutrition*. Boca Raton, FL: CRC Press.

Zalewski, P. D., Millard, S. H., Forbes, I. J., Kapaniris, O., Slavotinek, A., Betts, W. H., et al. (1994). Video image analysis of labile zinc in viable pancreatic islet cells using a specific fluorescent probe for zinc. *The Journal of Histochemistry and Cytochemistry*, *42*, 877–884.

Zhang, Y., Proenca, R., Maffei, M., Barone, M., Leopold, L., & Friedman, J. M. (1994). Positional cloning of the mouse obese gene and its human homologue. *Nature*, *372*, 425–432.

CHAPTER FIFTEEN

The NOTCH Pathway in β-Cell Growth and Differentiation

Yael Bar, Shimon Efrat[1]
Department of Human Molecular Genetics and Biochemistry, Sackler School of Medicine, Tel Aviv University, Tel Aviv, Israel
[1]Corresponding author: e-mail address: sefrat@post.tau.ac.il

Contents

Abstract

Beta-cell replacement represents the optimal therapy for type 1 diabetes. Efforts to manipulate β-cell proliferation and differentiation could be advanced by a better understanding of the normal pathways regulating β-cell development and renewal. NOTCH signaling is a highly conserved pathway which plays a central role in pancreas development. Cell-lineage tracing has revealed the reactivation of the NOTCH pathway in adult human β cells cultured under conditions which induce cell proliferation and dedifferentiation. Inhibition of NOTCH signaling in dedifferentiated cells following *ex vivo* expansion has been shown to promote restoration of the β-cell phenotype. This approach may increase the availability of functional β cells for transplantation.

1. INTRODUCTION

Beta-cell replacement by regeneration or transplantation represents the optimal therapy for type 1 diabetes. Both approaches rely on understanding of the normal pathways regulating β-cell development and homeostasis. Efforts to stimulate β-cell regeneration by replication of the patient's residual β cells or neogenesis from pancreas stem cells, as well as to reprogram other cell types *in vivo* or *ex vivo* into β cells, differentiate pluripotent stem cells into

Vitamins and Hormones, Volume 95
ISSN 0083-6729
http://dx.doi.org/10.1016/B978-0-12-800174-5.00015-6

insulin-producing cells, or expand cadaver donor islet cells in culture, all attempt to manipulate key pathways which regulate cell proliferation and differentiation, and could be greatly advanced by a better understanding of these mechanisms.

NOTCH signaling is an evolutionarily conserved pathway which plays a central role in embryonic development, as well as in renewal of many adult cell types. This signaling pathway, which was first studied in neurons, controls cell fate through local cell-to-cell interactions in a broad spectrum of tissues and processes. Signals exchanged between neighboring cells through the NOTCH receptor promote or suppress cell proliferation, cell death, acquisition of specific cell fates, or activation of differentiation programs. NOTCH signals are often used to select between two cell fates in a process termed lateral inhibition, in which a cell adopting a particular fate inhibits development of the same fate in its immediate neighbors (Artavanis-Tsakonas, Rand, & Lake, 1999; Kopan & Ilagan, 2009). Aberrant gain or loss of NOTCH pathway components has been directly linked to multiple human disorders, including developmental syndromes (Gridley, 2003), adult-onset diseases (Louvi, Arboleda-Velasquez, & Artavanis-Tsakonas, 2006), and cancer (van Es et al., 2005; Weng et al., 2004).

The NOTCH signaling cascade is highly conserved and found in organisms as diverse as worms and humans (Guruharsha, Kankel, & Artavanis-Tsakonas, 2012; Fig. 15.1). Mammals encode four NOTCH receptors (NOTCH1–4), which are bound by five ligands (DLL1, 3, and 4, and JAG1 and 2). Newly synthesized NOTCH receptors are proteolytically cleaved in the Golgi during their transport to the cell surface. This cleavage generates a heterodimeric receptor consisting of an extracellular subunit (N^{EC}), and a transmembrane domain linked to the cytoplasmic subunit (N^{TM}). NOTCH signaling is initiated by ligand–receptor interaction between neighboring cells, leading to two successive proteolytic cleavages of the receptor. These liberate the intracellular domain of NOTCH receptors (NICD), which subsequently traffics to the nucleus and heterodimerizes with the DNA-binding transcription factor CSL (also known as Suppressor of Hairless in Drosophila, and RBP-JK in mouse) to form a short-lived nuclear transcription complex. Once bound to CSL, NICD recruits other coactivators to activate expression of downstream target genes. Members of the Hairy Enhancer of Split (*Hes*) or Hairy-Related (*Hey* or *Hrt*) genes have been identified as key NOTCH target genes in many tissues (Gordon, Arnett, & Blacklow, 2008; Kopan & Ilagan, 2009). Among them, *Hes1* encodes a basic helix-loop-helix (bHLH) protein which acts as a

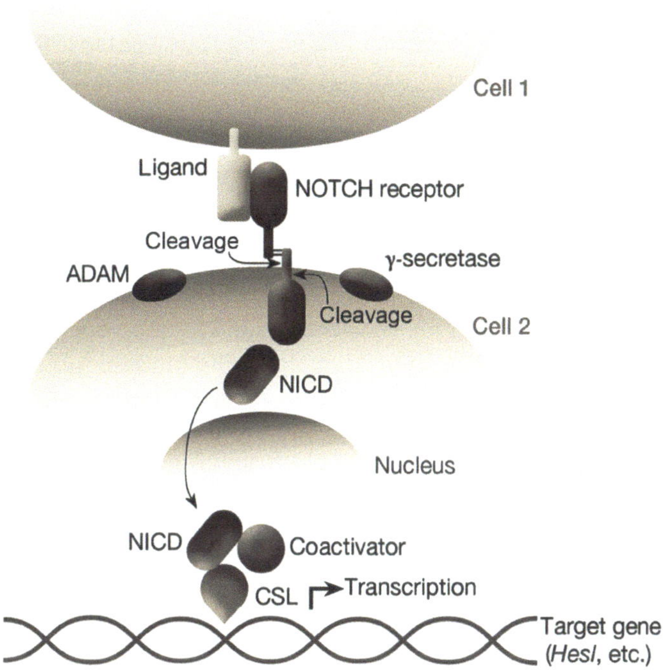

Figure 15.1 The NOTCH pathway. NOTCH signaling is triggered by ligands expressed on the surface of neighboring cells. Upon ligand binding, NOTCH receptors undergo successive proteolytic cleavages by an ADAM family protease and γ-secretase. The released NOTCH intracellular domain (NICD) translocates to the nucleus and associates with CSL and additional coactivators to form a transcription activation complex at target genes, such as *Hes1*. (See the color plate.)

transcriptional repressor. HES1 plays an essential role in the development of many organs, including the pancreas, by regulating progenitor cell expansion and binary cell fate decisions (Kageyama, Ohtsuka, & Kobayashi, 2007).

2. ROLE OF THE NOTCH PATHWAY IN PANCREAS DEVELOPMENT

During embryonic development, pancreatic cells (endocrine, exocrine, and duct) originate from common multipotent proliferating progenitor cells expressing the factors PDX1, NKX6.1, PTF1a, and SOX9. These cells form the pancreatic bud that can be first detected on E9.5 of embryonic development in mice (Gu, Dubauskaite, & Melton, 2002; Kawaguchi et al., 2002). Expression of the bHLH factor NGN3 in these precursor cells promotes their differentiation into all four endocrine cell types (Apelqvist et al., 1999; Gu et al., 2002; Jensen et al., 2000), while expression of the bHLH factor PTF1a promotes differentiation toward the exocrine lineage. The NOTCH signaling pathway plays a central role during this process. Expression of NOTCH receptors (NOTCH1–3), ligands (JAG-1, JAG-2, DLL-1, and DLL-3), and targets (HES1) has been observed in undifferentiated cells within the embryonic mouse pancreas but not in terminally differentiated endocrine cells in the fetal or adult pancreas (Jensen et al., 2000, 2005; Lammert, Brown, & Melton, 2000). In fetal mouse pancreas, HES1 inhibits *Ngn3* gene expression by direct binding to its promoter (Jensen, Pedersen, et al., 2000). In addition, HES1 regulates the cell cycle by inhibiting expression of genes encoding the cyclin kinase inhibitors p27 and p57 (Georgia, Soliz, Li, Zhang, & Bhushan, 2006; Murata et al., 2005). p57 is known to mediate the exit of the precursor cells from the cell cycle and the switch into their differentiation program. HES1 directly binds the promoter *of CDKN1C*, the gene encoding p57, thereby maintaining precursor cell proliferation (Georgia et al., 2006). Some evidence suggests that HES1 may also inhibit *Ins* gene expression (Hald et al., 2003). *Hes1* gene knockout in mice leads to upregulation of *Ngn3* and severe pancreatic hypoplasia, caused by insufficient expansion of the progenitor cell pool prior to differentiation (Jensen, Pedersen, et al., 2000). Similar defects are observed following inactivation of *Dll1*, encoding a NOTCH ligand, and *Rbp-jk*, encoding the NICD transactivation partner, and by overexpression of NGN3 or NOTCH3, which antagonizes NOTCH1 action (Apelqvist et al., 1999; Fujikura et al., 2006). As expected, forced expression of NOTCH1 inhibits pancreas cell differentiation (Hald et al., 2003; Murtaugh, Stanger, Kwan, & Melton, 2003). Together, these data suggest that the major roll of the NOTCH–HES1 pathway is stimulation of pancreatic progenitor cell replication and prevention of premature endocrine differentiation. In this manner, the NOTCH system helps maintain a sufficient pool of progenitor cells for generation of a normal-size organ.

Recently, findings have provided new insights into the involvement of the NOTCH pathway in mouse pancreas development, indicating different effects in early and late developmental stages. In early pancreatic development (E9.5–E10.5), the NOTCH pathway components and PTF1a are uniformly expressed in pancreatic progenitor cells. At this stage, NOTCH signaling acts through HES1 to prevent NGN3 expression and maintain PTF1a expression. PTF1a itself is directly needed for expression of the NOTCH ligand DLL1, thereby closing a positive feedback loop. In this way, NOTCH signaling uniformly prevents endocrine differentiation of early progenitor cells (Ahnfelt-Ronne et al., 2012). Interestingly, in late pancreatic development (E12.5), NOTCH signaling acts in a concentration-dependent manner. High NOTCH expression activates HES1 and SOX9 expression, resulting in generation of pancreatic duct cells. Low NOTCH expression activates SOX9 but not HES1, resulting in NGN3 activation and endocrine differentiation (Shih et al., 2012).

3. EVIDENCE FOR REACTIVATION OF THE NOTCH PATHWAY IN ADULT PANCREATIC CELLS

The NOTCH pathway components are not normally expressed in adult terminally differentiated murine pancreatic cells (Esni et al., 2004; Jensen, Pedersen, et al., 2000). Unlike in pancreatic progenitor cells, NICD overexpression (Murtaugh et al., 2003) or *Rbp-jk* inactivation (Fujikura et al., 2006) in fully differentiated β cells does not cause an obvious phenotype. These studies suggest that cells undergoing endocrine differentiation lose their responsiveness to NOTCH signaling. Nevertheless, there are reports of reactivation of the NOTCH pathway in adult pancreatic cells. The NOTCH receptors and ligands are frequently expressed in human pancreatic tumor cells (Miyamoto et al., 2003). NOTCH1, NOTCH2, HES1, JAG2, and low levels of DLL1 are also detected in the pancreatic exocrine epithelium during mouse acinar cell regeneration following experimental pancreatitis (Jensen et al., 2005). In addition, Rooman et al. (2006) reported that isolated rat exocrine cells which were induced to proliferate in culture showed elevated expression of NOTCH pathway genes, including *Notch1–2* and *Hes1*, in parallel to reduced expression of differentiated exocrine cell markers. The same group reported a method for generation of insulin-expressing cells from cultured exocrine rat cells by differentiation-inducing factors (Baeyens et al., 2005), and showed that the conversion of adult acinar cells into β-like cells is negatively regulated by NOTCH1 signaling. Inhibition of NOTCH1 signaling significantly improved β-cell neoformation, with approximately 30% of acinar cells converted into β cells, compared to only 10% with differentiation factors alone (Baeyens et al., 2009). In all these cases (pancreatic neoplasia, exocrine regeneration, and adult exocrine cell metaplasia in culture), cell replication and dedifferentiation are associated with NOTCH pathway reactivation (Jensen et al., 2005; Miyamoto et al., 2003; Rooman et al., 2006). Moreover, several NOTCH receptors and ligands, as well as the NOTCH target gene *Hes1*, were upregulated in dedifferentiated adult rat β cells following exposure to cytokines (Darville & Eizirik, 2006). Bouckenooghe et al. have shown that *HES1* gene expression was upregulated in cultured sorted human β cells, while expression of β-cell differentiation markers was downregulated (Bouckenooghe et al., 2005). Using cell-lineage tracing, our group has documented the activation of the NOTCH pathway in cultured adult human β cells, under conditions which induce cell proliferation and dedifferentiation.

4. EFFECT OF THE NOTCH PATHWAY ON PROLIFERATION, DEDIFFERENTIATION, AND REDIFFERENTIATION OF CULTURED HUMAN β-CELL-DERIVED CELLS

In vitro expansion of adult human β cells from cadaver donors holds the promise of generating an abundant source of insulin-producing cells for transplantation. However, expansion of adult human β cells *in vitro* is associated with loss of the β-cell phenotype (Beattie, Cirulli, Lopez, & Hayek, 1997; Beattie et al., 1999; Gershengorn et al., 2004; Hayek et al., 1995; Ouziel-Yahalom et al., 2006; Parnaud et al., 2008), which could reflect β-cell dedifferentiation, or β-cell death accompanied by expansion of cells from a non-β-cell origin in the islet cell culture. Using a lineage-tracing approach, we demonstrated that ~40% of cells proliferating in these cultures are β-cell-derived (BCD) cells (Russ, Bar, Ravassard, & Efrat, 2008). This approach is based on infection of primary islet cells with a mixture of two lentivirus vectors 1 day following seeding in culture, one of them expressing a Cre recombinase-estrogen receptor fusion protein under the insulin promoter (RIP-Cre/ER), and the other a reporter cassette, in which the cytomegalovirus promoter is separated from an enhanced green fluorescent protein (eGFP) gene by a loxP-flanked stop region (Fig. 15.2). Only β cells infected by both viruses and treated with tamoxifen express Cre protein and

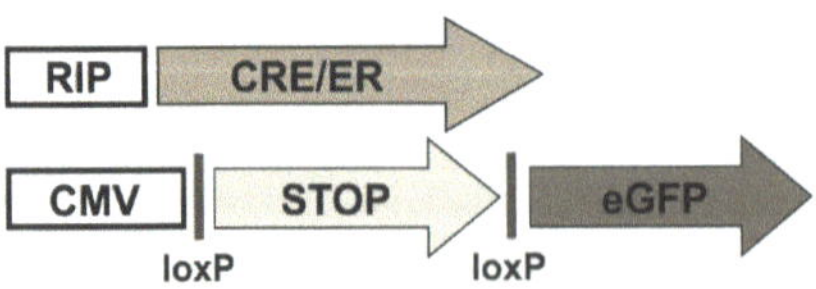

Figure 15.2 β-cell-specific labeling system. Schematic representation of the two lentivirus vectors used for β-cell-lineage tracing. *Reproduced from Russ, Ravassard, Kerr-Conte, Pattou, and Efrat (2009).* (See the color plate.)

translocate it into the nucleus, leading to removal of the floxed DNA fragment in the reporter construct and activation of eGFP expression. Residual insulin expression in β cells during the initial days in culture provides a sufficient window of time for RIP-Cre/ER expression and eGFP activation.

Analyses of expression of NOTCH pathway components in the labeled cells revealed upregulation of *NOTCH1–3* and *HES1* transcripts. In contrast, *NOTCH4*, *DELTA1*, and *JAG2* transcripts were downregulated. Upregulation of the NOTCH pathway correlated with cell dedifferentiation, as manifested by a great decrease in insulin transcripts, and cell entrance into the cell cycle, as manifested by downregulation of p57 transcripts and an increase in Ki67 staining (Bar, Russ, Knoller, Ouziel-Yahalom, & Efrat, 2008). Immunostaining demonstrated a negative correlation between the presence of HES1 or NICD in the nucleus, and insulin expression, in $eGFP^+$ cells, which marked their origin from β cells (Fig. 15.3). These *in situ* analyses also detected a positive correlation between p57 and insulin expression, confirming the view that β-cell replication involves dedifferentiation.

The key role of HES1 in these events was revealed by inhibiting its upregulation using shRNA. In cells infected with *HES1* shRNA at culture initiation, the decrease in p57 was prevented (Bar et al., 2008) and cell proliferation was greatly reduced, as jugged by staining for BrdU incorporation. In addition, staining for Ki67 in $eGFP^+$ cells demonstrated a lower replication rate among BCD cells. While cell dedifferentiation was not completely prevented, it was significantly inhibited, compared with cells in which HES1 upregulation was not repressed. This was manifested by higher levels of insulin transcripts, as well as transcripts encoding β-cell transcription factors (Bar et al., 2008). In agreement with the higher insulin mRNA levels, insulin immunostaining detected a significantly higher number of insulin-positive cells in cultures expressing HES1 shRNA, compared with those treated with the control virus. The fraction of insulin-positive cells among $eGFP^+$ cells was also higher in the presence of *HES1* shRNA, indicating that fewer β cells underwent dedifferentiation. These findings suggest that partial cell dedifferentiation is independent of HES1 activity and cell replication; however, induction of advanced dedifferentiation and cell replication requires HES1 upregulation. This interpretation is supported by the finding that the bulk of decrease in insulin mRNA occurs during the first week in culture (Bar et al., 2008), which precedes the peak in *HES1* mRNA levels. It is therefore possible that loss of the bulk of insulin content is a precondition for β-cell entrance into cell cycle *in vitro*.

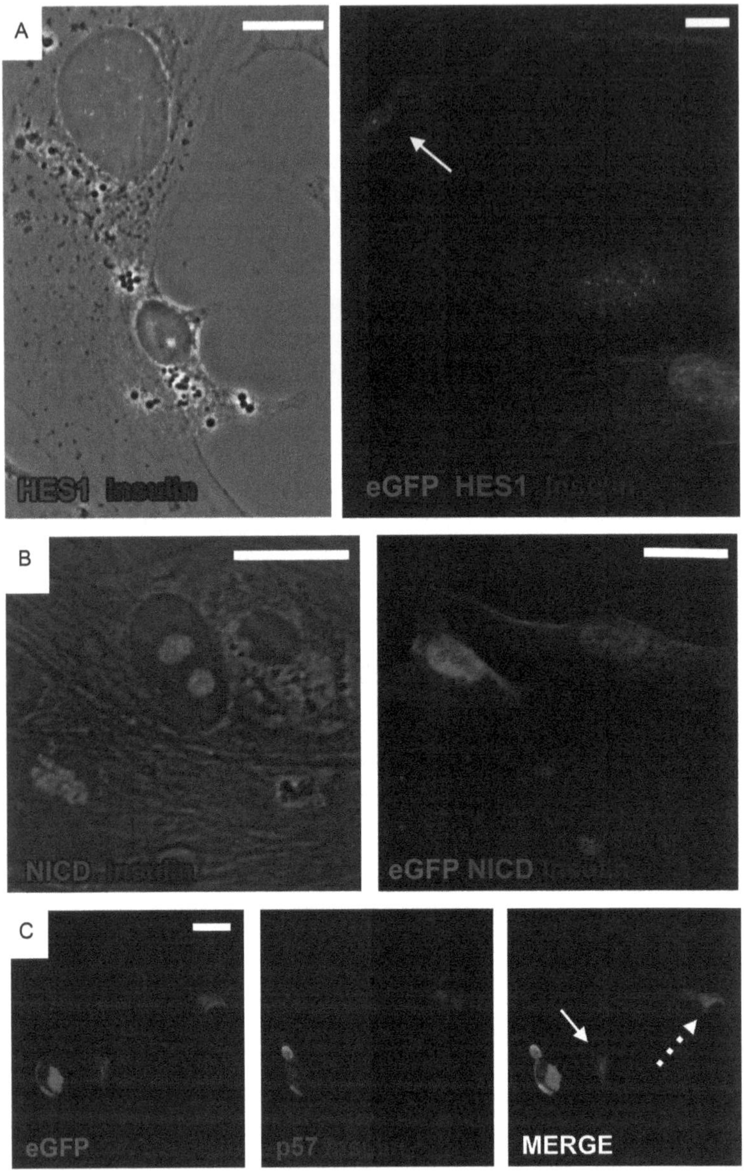

Figure 15.3 Notch pathway activation in BCD cells. (A, B) Immunofluorescence analysis of islet cells (left panels) and eGFP^{+} cells derived from β cells following 10 days in culture (right panels). The left panels are merged with phase contrast images. Arrow points to a β cell that still expresses insulin and is not labeled for HES1. eGFP is detected in both cytoplasm and nucleus. (C) Immunofluorescence analysis of eGFP^{+} cells derived from β cells following 10 days in culture. Solid arrow points to an eGFP^{+} cell that has lost both insulin and p57 expression; dashed arrow points to an eGFP^{+} β cell that maintains both insulin and p57 expression. Bar = 20 μm. *Reproduced from Bar et al. (2008).* (See the color plate.)

Given the fact that upregulation of the NOTCH pathway in islet cell cultures followed cell dissociation into single cells, it is unlikely that it was triggered by a cell-associated ligand, as required by the lateral inhibition model (Apelqvist et al., 1999). Rather, it is possible that this pathway is activated in response to soluble serum components, as was demonstrated in a number of cultured cell types (Hirata et al., 2002). This possibility is supported by our findings of decreased expression of NOTCH ligands in islet cell cultures concomitantly with HES1 upregulation (Bar et al., 2008). The wave of HES1 upregulation peaked within the first 2 weeks of culture and was downregulated thereafter (Bar et al., 2008). Nevertheless, the effects of HES1 were not reversed, as manifested by continuous replication of cells derived from dedifferentiated β cells for up to 16 population doublings (Ouziel-Yahalom et al., 2006; Russ et al., 2008). The levels of p57 and insulin transcripts did not rebound thereafter, suggesting that their reinduction requires other signals, in addition to the decrease in the inhibitory effect of HES1. This finding suggests a transient role of HES1 upregulation that is limited to the initial adaptation of islet cells to culture, after which cell replication may continue in the presence of the low HES1 levels found in nonreplicating cells. These findings emphasize the role of components of the NOTCH pathway in the transition of quiescent β cells into a dedifferentiated, proliferative state *in vitro*. Our findings demonstrate a negative correlation between replication and maintenance of differentiated function in cultured β cells, suggesting that significant cell expansion inevitably involves dedifferentiation, and will require the development of methods for cell redifferentiation following expansion.

Given the role of the NOTCH pathway in adaptation of BCD cells to proliferation in culture, we investigated a possible effect of inhibition of the NOTCH pathway following cell expansion, as part of a treatment aimed at inducing BCD cell redifferentiation into functional insulin-producing cells. Our findings demonstrate that inhibition of the NOTCH pathway by *HES1* shRNA is sufficient for induction of partial BCD cell redifferentiation following significant expansion *in vitro*. Redifferentiation is manifested by activation of insulin expression, as well as expression of transcription factors required for insulin gene transcription (Fig. 15.4; Bar et al., 2012). *HES1* inhibition also induces expression of the cell cycle inhibitors p57 and p27 and growth arrest. However, growth arrest alone is insufficient for induction of redifferentiation, as evidenced by the finding that p57 overexpression in expanded islet cells did not lead by itself to cell redifferentiation. Using the lineage-tracing system, we showed that these changes occurred specifically

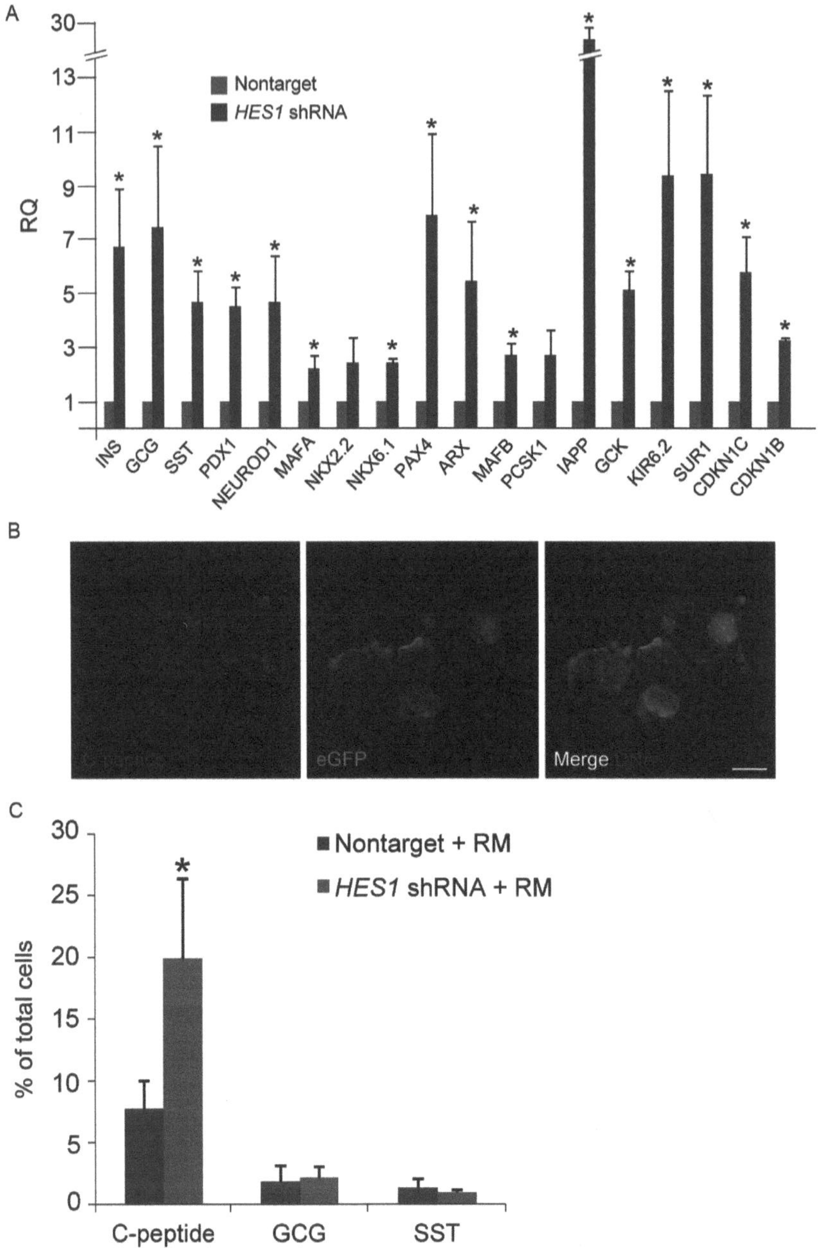

Figure 15.4 Effects of NOTCH pathway inhibition on BCD cell redifferentiation *in vitro*. (A) qPCR analyses of cultured islet cells at passage 4, 9 days following infection with *HES1* shRNA or nontarget viruses. RQ, relative quantification compared to nontarget virus. Values are mean ± SE ($n=3$–4 donors). Asterisks mark significant changes ($p<0.01$). (B) Coimmunofluorescence analysis for C-peptide and eGFP in labeled islet cells infected at passage 5 with *HES1* shRNA, and seeded 2 days later in medium with soluble differentiation factors (redifferentiation medium, RM) for 4 days. Bar = 10 μm. (C) Quantitation of 2000 cells in each group in the experiment in (B). Values are mean ± SE ($n=3$ donors). No hormone-positive cells were found in untreated cells. Asterisk marks significant difference ($p<0.05$). *Reproduced from Bar et al. (2012).* (See the color plate.)

in BCD ($eGFP^+$) cells, and therefore represent *bona fide* redifferentiation, rather than *de novo* differentiation of another cell type present in the heterogeneous expanded islet cell population (Fig. 15.4). We have recently shown that dedifferentiated BCD cells can be redifferentiated into insulin-producing cells by a combination of soluble factors (25 mM D-glucose, 10 mM nicotinamide, 8 nM exendin-4, and 8 nM activin A) in serum-free medium, under conditions which promote cell aggregation (Russ et al., 2011). Combination of this treatment with inhibition of the NOTCH pathway by *HES1* shRNA produced a synergistic effect, resulting in higher levels of β-cell gene transcripts and doubling of the fraction of redifferentiated BCD cells, from 25% with soluble factors alone to 50% (Fig. 15.4). Furthermore, treatment with *HES1* shRNA alone is sufficient for priming BCD cells for further differentiation *in vivo* into functional β-like cells, which are capable of restoring euglycemia in hyperglycemic mice (Fig. 15.5).

These findings are summarized in the model in Fig. 15.6. Human islet cells are likely induced to replicate in culture following tissue dissociation and exposure to growth factors present in the growth medium. The loss

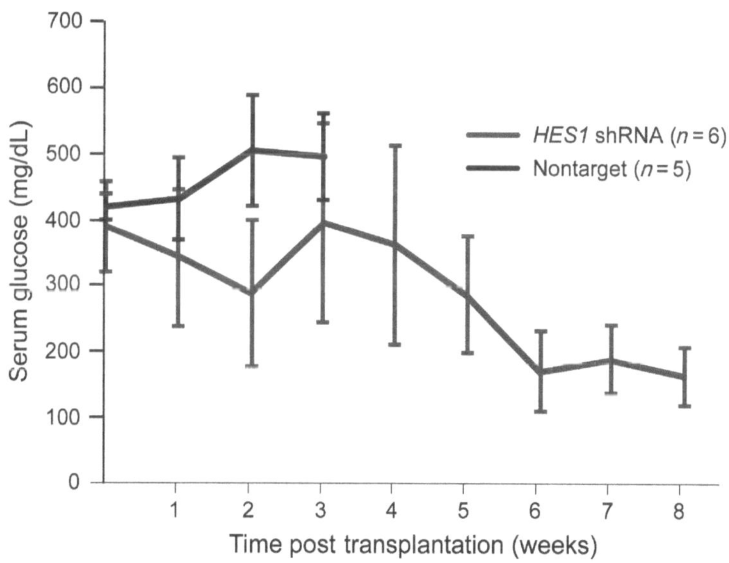

Figure 15.5 Effects of NOTCH pathway inhibition on BCD cell redifferentiation *in vivo*. Changes in blood glucose levels in immunodeficient mice made diabetic by treatment with streptozotocin and transplanted with 2×10^6 expanded islet cells infected at passage 5 with *HES1* shRNA or nontarget virus. Values are mean ± SE. *Reproduced from Bar et al. (2012).* (See the color plate.)

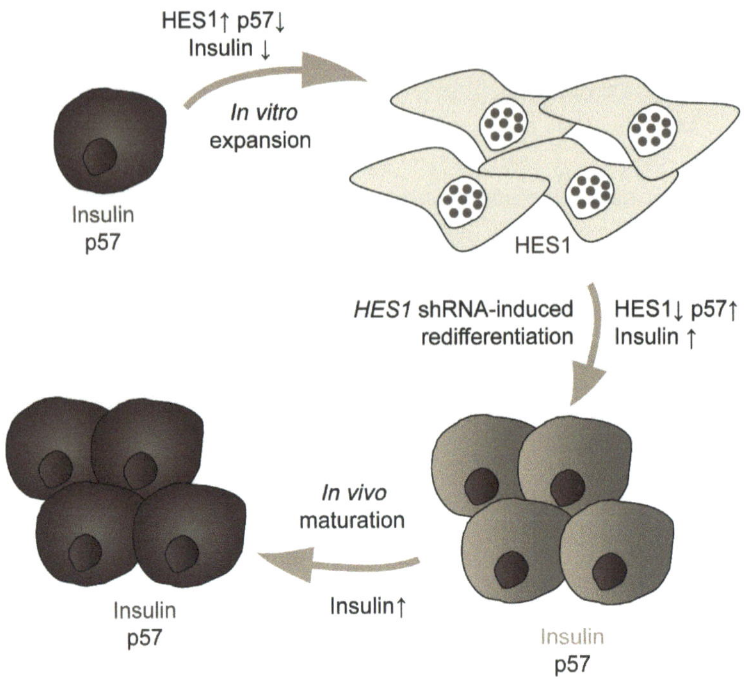

Figure 15.6 Model of HES1 involvement in proliferation, dedifferentiation, and redifferentiation of cultured human BCD cells. *Reproduced from Bar et al. (2012).* (See the color plate.)

of normal cell–cell and cell–matrix contacts following islet isolation and dissociation likely leads to profound changes in gene expression in cultured β cells, and plays a key role in their dedifferentiation and induction of replication. These changes include activation of the NOTCH pathway, downregulation of insulin and cell cycle inhibitor expression, and activation of cell replication. Following significant cell expansion in culture, *HES1* shRNA can induce BCD cell redifferentiation, which is manifested in reactivation of insulin and cell cycle inhibitor expression. Redifferentiated cells are capable of further maturation *in vivo* into functional β-like cells.

This work offers a novel way for generation of an abundant source of insulin-expressing cells for transplantation into diabetes patients. Cells from single donors can be expanded in culture, redifferentiated by manipulating the NOTCH pathway and exposure to a cocktail of soluble factors, and transplanted into multiple recipients, given efficient methods for preventing allograft rejection and recurring autoimmunity.

ACKNOWLEDGMENTS

This work was supported by the Israel Science Foundation and the Juvenile Diabetes Research Foundation.

REFERENCES

Ahnfelt-Ronne, J., Jorgensen, M. C., Klinck, R., Jensen, J. N., Fuchtbauer, E. M., Deering, T., et al. (2012). Ptf1a-mediated control of Dll1 reveals an alternative to the lateral inhibition mechanism. *Development, 139*(1), 33–45.

Apelqvist, A., Li, H., Sommer, L., Beatus, P., Anderson, D. J., Honjo, T., et al. (1999). Notch signalling controls pancreatic cell differentiation. *Nature, 400*(6747), 877–881.

Artavanis-Tsakonas, S., Rand, M. D., & Lake, R. J. (1999). Notch signaling: Cell fate control and signal integration in development. *Science, 284*(5415), 770–776.

Baeyens, L., Bonne, S., Bos, T., Rooman, I., Peleman, C., Lahoutte, T., et al. (2009). Notch signaling as gatekeeper of rat acinar-to-beta-cell conversion in vitro. *Gastroenterology, 136*(5), 1750–1760.

Baeyens, L., De Breuck, S., Lardon, J., Mfopou, J. K., Rooman, I., & Bouwens, L. (2005). In vitro generation of insulin-producing beta cells from adult exocrine pancreatic cells. *Diabetologia, 48*(1), 49–57.

Bar, Y., Russ, H. A., Knoller, S., Ouziel-Yahalom, L., & Efrat, S. (2008). HES-1 is involved in adaptation of adult human beta-cells to proliferation in vitro. *Diabetes, 57*(9), 2413–2420.

Bar, Y., Russ, H. A., Sintov, E., Anker-Kitai, L., Knoller, S., & Efrat, S. (2012). Redifferentiation of expanded human pancreatic beta-cell-derived cells by inhibition of the NOTCH pathway. *The Journal of Biological Chemistry, 287*(21), 17269–17280.

Beattie, G. M., Cirulli, V., Lopez, A. D., & Hayek, A. (1997). Ex vivo expansion of human pancreatic endocrine cells. *The Journal of Clinical Endocrinology and Metabolism, 82*(6), 1852–1856.

Beattie, G. M., Itkin Ansari, P., Cirulli, V., Leibowitz, G., Lopez, A. D., Bossie, S., et al. (1999). Sustained proliferation of PDX-1+ cells derived from human islets. *Diabetes, 48*(5), 1013–1019.

Bouckenooghe, T., Vandewalle, B., Moerman, E., Danze, P. M., Lukowiak, B., Muharram, G., et al. (2005). Expression of progenitor cell markers during expansion of sorted human pancreatic beta cells. *Gene Expression, 12*(2), 83–98.

Darville, M. I., & Eizirik, D. L. (2006). Notch signaling: A mediator of beta-cell de-differentiation in diabetes? *Biochemical and Biophysical Research Communications, 339*(4), 1063–1068.

Esni, F., Ghosh, B., Biankin, A. V., Lin, J. W., Albert, M. A., Yu, X., et al. (2004). Notch inhibits Ptf1 function and acinar cell differentiation in developing mouse and zebrafish pancreas. *Development, 131*(17), 4213–4224.

Fujikura, J., Hosoda, K., Iwakura, H., Tomita, T., Noguchi, M., Masuzaki, H., et al. (2006). Notch/Rbp-j signaling prevents premature endocrine and ductal cell differentiation in the pancreas. *Cell Metabolism, 3*(1), 59–65.

Georgia, S., Soliz, R., Li, M., Zhang, P., & Bhushan, A. (2006). p57 and Hes1 coordinate cell cycle exit with self-renewal of pancreatic progenitors. *Developmental Biology, 298*(1), 22–31.

Gershengorn, M. C., Hardikar, A. A., Wei, C., Geras-Raaka, E., Marcus-Samuels, B., & Raaka, B. M. (2004). Epithelial-to-mesenchymal transition generates proliferative human islet precursor cells. *Science, 306*(5705), 2261–2264.

Gordon, W. R., Arnett, K. L., & Blacklow, S. C. (2008). The molecular logic of Notch signaling—A structural and biochemical perspective. *Journal of Cell Science, 121*(Pt. 19), 3109–3119.
Gridley, T. (2003). Notch signaling and inherited disease syndromes. *Human Molecular Genetics, 12*(Spec No 1), R9–R13.
Gu, G., Dubauskaite, J., & Melton, D. A. (2002). Direct evidence for the pancreatic lineage: NGN3+ cells are islet progenitors and are distinct from duct progenitors. *Development, 129*(10), 2447–2457.
Guruharsha, K. G., Kankel, M. W., & Artavanis-Tsakonas, S. (2012). The Notch signalling system: Recent insights into the complexity of a conserved pathway. *Nature Reviews. Genetics, 13*(9), 654–666.
Hald, J., Hjorth, J. P., German, M. S., Madsen, O. D., Serup, P., & Jensen, J. (2003). Activated Notch1 prevents differentiation of pancreatic acinar cells and attenuate endocrine development. *Developmental Biology, 260*(2), 426–437.
Hayek, A., Beattie, G. M., Cirulli, V., Lopez, A. D., Ricordi, C., & Rubin, J. S. (1995). Growth factor/matrix-induced proliferation of human adult beta-cells. *Diabetes, 44*(12), 1458–1460.
Hirata, H., Yoshiura, S., Ohtsuka, T., Bessho, Y., Harada, T., Yoshikawa, K., et al. (2002). Oscillatory expression of the bHLH factor Hes1 regulated by a negative feedback loop. *Science, 298*(5594), 840–843.
Jensen, J. N., Cameron, E., Garay, M. V., Starkey, T. W., Gianani, R., & Jensen, J. (2005). Recapitulation of elements of embryonic development in adult mouse pancreatic regeneration. *Gastroenterology, 128*(3), 728–741.
Jensen, J., Heller, R. S., Funder-Nielsen, T., Pedersen, E. E., Lindsell, C., Weinmaster, G., et al. (2000). Independent development of pancreatic alpha- and beta-cells from neurogenin3-expressing precursors: A role for the notch pathway in repression of premature differentiation. *Diabetes, 49*(2), 163–176.
Jensen, J., Pedersen, E. E., Galante, P., Hald, J., Heller, R. S., Ishibashi, M., et al. (2000). Control of endodermal endocrine development by Hes-1. *Nature Genetics, 24*(1), 36–44.
Kageyama, R., Ohtsuka, T., & Kobayashi, T. (2007). The Hes gene family: Repressors and oscillators that orchestrate embryogenesis. *Development, 134*(7), 1243–1251.
Kawaguchi, Y., Cooper, B., Gannon, M., Ray, M., MacDonald, R. J., & Wright, C. V. (2002). The role of the transcriptional regulator Ptf1a in converting intestinal to pancreatic progenitors. *Nature Genetics, 32*(1), 128–134.
Kopan, R., & Ilagan, M. X. (2009). The canonical Notch signaling pathway: Unfolding the activation mechanism. *Cell, 137*(2), 216–233.
Lammert, E., Brown, J., & Melton, D. A. (2000). Notch gene expression during pancreatic organogenesis. *Mechanisms of Development, 94*(1–2), 199–203.
Louvi, A., Arboleda-Velasquez, J. F., & Artavanis-Tsakonas, S. (2006). CADASIL: A critical look at a Notch disease. *Developmental Neuroscience, 28*(1–2), 5–12.
Miyamoto, Y., Maitra, A., Ghosh, B., Zechner, U., Argani, P., Iacobuzio-Donahue, C. A., et al. (2003). Notch mediates TGF alpha-induced changes in epithelial differentiation during pancreatic tumorigenesis. *Cancer Cell, 3*(6), 565–576.
Murata, K., Hattori, M., Hirai, N., Shinozuka, Y., Hirata, H., Kageyama, R., et al. (2005). Hes1 directly controls cell proliferation through the transcriptional repression of p27Kip1. *Molecular and Cellular Biology, 25*(10), 4262–4271.
Murtaugh, L. C., Stanger, B. Z., Kwan, K. M., & Melton, D. A. (2003). Notch signaling controls multiple steps of pancreatic differentiation. *Proceedings of the National Academy of Sciences of the United States of America, 100*(25), 14920–14925.
Ouziel-Yahalom, L., Zalzman, M., Anker-Kitai, L., Knoller, S., Bar, Y., Glandt, M., et al. (2006). Expansion and redifferentiation of adult human pancreatic islet cells. *Biochemical and Biophysical Research Communications, 341*(2), 291–298.

Parnaud, G., Bosco, D., Berney, T., Pattou, F., Kerr-Conte, J., Donath, M. Y., et al. (2008). Proliferation of sorted human and rat beta cells. *Diabetologia, 51*(1), 91–100.

Rooman, I., De Medts, N., Baeyens, L., Lardon, J., De Breuck, S., Heimberg, H., et al. (2006). Expression of the Notch signaling pathway and effect on exocrine cell proliferation in adult rat pancreas. *The American Journal of Pathology, 169*(4), 1206–1214.

Russ, H. A., Bar, Y., Ravassard, P., & Efrat, S. (2008). In vitro proliferation of cells derived from adult human beta-cells revealed by cell-lineage tracing. *Diabetes, 57*(6), 1575–1583.

Russ, H. A., Ravassard, P., Kerr-Conte, J., Pattou, F., & Efrat, S. (2009). Epithelial-mesenchymal transition in cells expanded in vitro from lineage-traced adult human pancreatic beta cells. *PLoS One, 4*, e6417.

Russ, H. A., Sintov, E., Anker-Kitai, L., Friedman, O., Lenz, A., Toren, G., et al. (2011). Insulin-producing cells generated from dedifferentiated human pancreatic beta cells expanded in vitro. *PLoS One, 6*(9), e25566.

Shih, H. P., Kopp, J. L., Sandhu, M., Dubois, C. L., Seymour, P. A., Grapin-Botton, A., et al. (2012). A Notch-dependent molecular circuitry initiates pancreatic endocrine and ductal cell differentiation. *Development, 139*(14), 2488–2499.

van Es, J. H., van Gijn, M. E., Riccio, O., van den Born, M., Vooijs, M., Begthel, H., et al. (2005). Notch/gamma-secretase inhibition turns proliferative cells in intestinal crypts and adenomas into goblet cells. *Nature, 435*(7044), 959–963.

Weng, A. P., Ferrando, A. A., Lee, W., Morris, J. P. t., Silverman, L. B., Sanchez-Irizarry, C., et al. (2004). Activating mutations of NOTCH1 in human T cell acute lymphoblastic leukemia. *Science, 306*(5694), 269–271.

CHAPTER SIXTEEN

Roles of HNF1α and HNF4α in Pancreatic β-Cells: Lessons from a Monogenic Form of Diabetes (MODY)

Kazuya Yamagata[1]
Department of Medical Biochemistry, Faculty of Life Sciences, Kumamoto University, Kumamoto, Japan
[1]Corresponding author: e-mail address: k-yamaga@kumamoto-u.ac.jp

Contents

Abstract

Mutations in the genes encoding hepatocyte nuclear factor (HNF)1α and HNF4α cause a monogenic form of diabetes mellitus known as maturity-onset diabetes of the young (MODY). The primary cause of MODY is an impairment of glucose-stimulated insulin secretion by pancreatic β-cells, indicating the important roles of HNF1α and HNF4α in β-cells. Large scale genetic studies have clarified that the common variants of *HNF1α* and *HNF4α* genes are also associated with type 2 diabetes, suggesting that they are involved in the pathogenesis of both diseases. Recent experimental studies revealed that HNF1α controls both β-cell function and growth by regulating target genes such as glucose transporter 2, pyruvate kinase, collectrin, hepatocyte growth factor activator, and HNF4α. In contrast, HNF4α mainly regulates the function of β-cells. Although direct target genes of HNF4α in β-cells are largely unknown, we recently identified Anks4b as a novel target of HNF4α that regulates β-cell susceptibility to endoplasmic reticulum stress. Studies of MODY have led to a better understanding of the molecular mechanism of glucose-stimulated insulin secretion by pancreatic β-cells.

Vitamins and Hormones, Volume 95
ISSN 0083-6729
http://dx.doi.org/10.1016/B978-0-12-800174-5.00016-8

1. INTRODUCTION

Diabetes mellitus is a heterogeneous group of disorders characterized by high blood glucose levels. Although multiple genetic factors contribute to its development, it is estimated that about 1–2% of all cases of diabetes constitutes the monogenic form known as maturity-onset diabetes of the young (MODY) (Fajans & Bell, 2011; Tattersall, 1974). MODY is characterized by an autosomal dominant inheritance, an early age of onset (frequently during childhood or adolescence), and a primary defect of pancreatic β-cell function. In contrast to most common type 2 diabetes, MODY is not usually associated with obesity.

MODY can result from mutations in any of at least 13 different genes that encode the glycolytic enzyme glucokinase (MODY2) (Vionnet et al., 1992), the transcription factors hepatocyte nuclear factor (HNF)4α (MODY1) (Yamagata, Furuta, et al., 1996), HNF1α (MODY3) (Yamagata, Oda, et al., 1996), HNF1β (MODY5) (Horikawa et al., 1997), insulin promoter factor-1 (IPF-1) (MODY4) (Stoffers, Ferrer, Clarke, & Habener, 1997), neurogenic differentiation 1 (NeuroD1) (MODY6) (Malecki et al., 1999), kruppel-like factor 11 (KLF11) (MODY7) (Neve et al., 2005), paired box gene 4 (PAX4) (MODY9) (Plengvidhya et al., 2007) and B-lymphocyte-specific tyrosine kinase (BLK) (MODY11) (Borowiec et al., 2009), the carboxyl ester lipase (CEL) (MODY8) (Raeder et al., 2006), insulin (MODY10) (Edghill et al., 2008), and the components of the ATP-sensitive potassium (K_{ATP}) channel: sulfonylurea receptor 1 (SUR1) (MODY12) (Bowman et al., 2012) and Kir6.2 (MODY13) (Bonnefond et al., 2012).

In the majority of populations, mutations in the *HNF1A* gene (MODY3) are the most common cause of MODY (Hattersley & Pearson, 2006). This transcription factor was initially identified as liver enriched, and its critical role in pancreatic β-cells was not recognized before MODY3 cloning. Interestingly, *HNF4α/MODY1* is one of the direct target genes of HNF1α in pancreatic β-cells (Boj, Parrizas, Maestro, & Ferrer, 2001; Thomas et al., 2001), indicating that these two MODY transcription factors are functionally related. In this chapter, I focus on the importance of HNF1α and HNF4α in β-cell function.

2. CLINICAL FEATURES OF HNF1α DIABETES (MODY3)

In 1996, we identified that heterozygous mutations in the gene encoding HNF1α cause MODY3 by positional cloning (Yamagata, Oda, et al., 1996). HNF1α belongs to a subclass of the homeodomain family and is expressed in the liver, pancreas, kidney, and intestine (Frain et al., 1989; Mendel & Crabtree, 1991). Both endocrine cells (glucagon-positive, insulin-positive, somatostatin-positive, and pancreatic polypeptide cells) and exocrine cells in the pancreas express HNF1α from the developmental stage (Nammo et al., 2002). HNF1α has an N-terminal dimerization domain, a DNA-binding domain with POU-like and homeodomain-like motifs, and a C-terminal transactivation domain. Mutations associated with diabetes have been found in all regions of the *HNF1A* gene (Fig. 16.1).

The main clinical characteristics of HNF1α diabetes are impaired insulin secretion by pancreatic β-cells, with decreased insulin secretion in response to high glucose evident in HNF1α-mutated prediabetic subjects (Byrne et al., 1996). Although *Hnf1a* (−/−) knockout mice exhibit hepatic

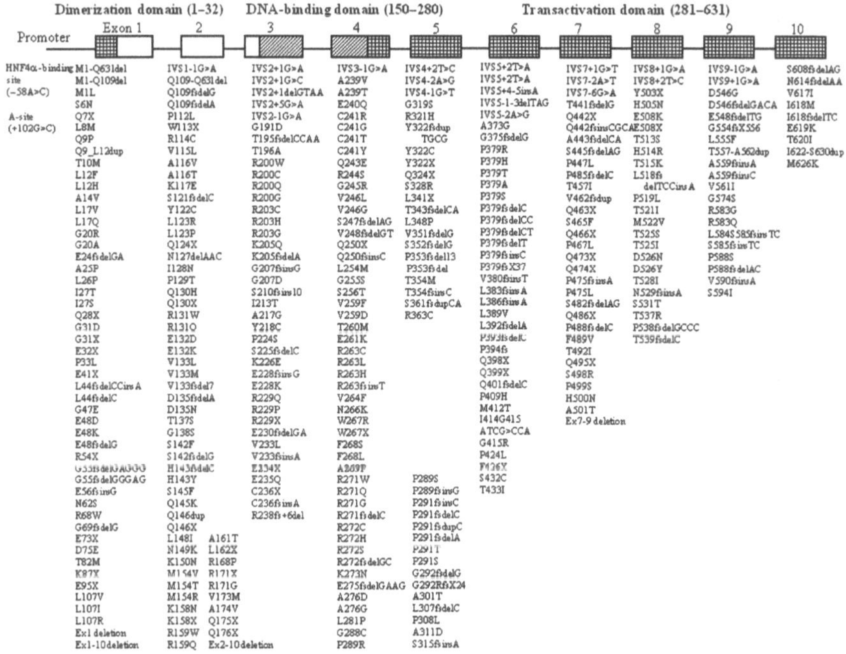

Figure 16.1 Reported mutations in the human *HNF1A* gene (Awa et al., 2011; Bazalová et al., 2010; Bellanné-Chantelot et al., 2008; Buchbinder et al., 2011; Cappelli et al., 2009; Carette et al., 2010; Conn et al., 2009; Eide et al., 2008; Ellard & Colclough, 2006, Ellard et al., 2007; Forlani et al., 2010; Jesić et al., 2008; Karges et al., 2007; Kooptiwut et al., 2009; Kyithar et al., 2011; Lopez et al., 2011; Lorini et al., 2009; Maraschin et al., 2008; Plengvidhya et al., 2009; Radha et al., 2009; Stanescu, Hughes, Kaplan, Stanley, & De León, 2012; Toaima et al., 2005; Yamagata, Furuta, et al., 1996; Yorifuji et al., 2012). Mutations are shown by commonly used nomenclature.

dysfunction, phenylketonuria, and renal Fanconi syndrome (Pontoglio et al., 1996), MODY3 patients show no liver or kidney abnormalities (Iwasaki et al., 1998). Obesity and insulin resistance are important clinical features of common type 2 diabetes, but the majority of HNF1α diabetic patients are not obese.

Disease penetrance is high and patients with *HNF1A* gene mutations usually develop diabetes between the ages of 10 and 30, showing a rapid deterioration of glycemia with age (Frayling et al., 2001). In keeping with the rapid worsening of their glucose levels, they sometimes suffer severe diabetic microvascular and macrovascular complications (Isomaa et al., 1998). Although most HNF1α diabetic patients are recommended to receive sulfonylurea treatment (Pearson et al., 2003), our experience indicates that the insulin secretion capacities of MODY3 patients are often very low, especially in Japanese cases (Yoshiuchi et al., 1999). Thus, if necessary, insulin therapy should be selected according to the insulin secretion capacity of each patient.

Mutations of the *HNF1A* gene have also been identified in subjects with type 2 diabetes. For example, G319S is a missense mutation in the transactivation domain that reduces transactivation activity by nearly 50% and is found in about 40% of Canadian Oji-Cree Indians with type 2 diabetes (Triggs-Raine et al., 2002). Furthermore, recent large-scale genetic studies identified that the common genetic variants in the *HNF1A* gene are associated with type 2 diabetes (Voight et al., 2010), suggesting that HNF1α may be involved in β-cell dysfunction in common type 2 diabetes. In this regard, understanding of the role of HNF1α in β-cells would provide an insight into the pathophysiology of type 2 diabetes as well as MODY.

HNF1β is a homeodomain-containing transcription factor that is structurally related to HNF1α, but the clinical features of HNF1β diabetes (MODY5) are very different from those of HNF1α diabetes. Mutations in the *HNF1B* gene cause renal cystic disease, cholestatic jaundice, and pancreatic hypoplasia in addition to diabetes mellitus (Bellanné-Chantelot et al., 2004; Horikawa et al., 1997).

3. FUNCTIONAL REGULATION OF β-CELLS BY HNF1α

To understand the role of HNF1α in pancreatic β-cells, it is necessary to identify the full spectrum of genes regulated by this factor. We and others have demonstrated that *Slc2a2* (encoding glucose transporter 2 (GLUT2)), *Pklr* (encoding liver pyruvate kinase (PKL)), *Tmem27* (encoding collectrin),

Hgfac (encoding hepatocyte growth factor (HGF) activator), and *Hnf4a* (encoding HNF4α/MODY1) are direct targets of HNF1α in β-cells (Akpinar, Kuwajima, Krützfeldt, & Stoffel, 2005; Boj et al., 2001; Fukui et al., 2005; Ohki et al., 2012; Párrizas et al., 2001; Shih et al., 2001; Thomas et al., 2001; Wang, Maechler, Hagenfeldt, & Wollheim, 1998; Yamagata et al., 1998).

HNF1α can activate *Slc2a2* and *Pklr* genes by binding to their promoter sequences. GLUT2 is a low-affinity, high-capacity glucose transporter in pancreatic β-cells that facilitates the translocation of glucose across the plasma membrane, while PKL is a rate-limiting glycolytic enzyme expressed in β-cells. Collectrin, originally cloned as a kidney-specific gene, is a type I transmembrane protein homologous to the C-terminal of angiotensin-converting enzyme-related carboxypeptidase (ACE2) (Zhang et al., 2001). We found that collectrin is highly expressed in pancreatic β-cells and is a direct target of HNF1α (Fukui et al., 2005). In addition, we clarified that collectrin controls insulin exocytosis by soluble NSF attachment protein receptor (SNARE) complex formation with snapin (Fukui et al., 2005; Yamagata et al., 2007). HNF4α regulates HNF1α transcription in hepatocytes (Kuo et al., 1992), but HNF1α conversely transactivates the expression of HNF4α in pancreatic β-cells, indicating that *HNF4α/MODY1* is a direct target gene of HNF1α in β-cells (Boj et al., 2001; Thomas et al., 2001). Thus, impaired insulin secretion in HNF1α diabetes might be associated, at least in part, with the decreased expression of *SLC2A2, PKLR, TMEM27, and HNF4A* genes.

In addition to the above-mentioned genes, expression levels of others involved in the glycolytic pathway, TCA cycle, and mitochondrial oxidative phosphorylation were decreased in *Hnf1a* (−/−) knockout islets (Dukes et al., 1998; Servitja et al., 2009; Wang et al., 1998). This change is most likely due to indirect responses rather than the direct effect of an absence of HNF1α, but it is conceivable that further novel HNF1α target genes important for glucose-stimulated insulin secretion might exist.

4. HNF1α REGULATES β-CELL GROWTH

MODY3 patients display progressive loss of β-cell function, as shown by age-related deteriorating glucose tolerance. Mutant mice with loss of HNF1α function as well as transgenic mice expressing a naturally occurring human dominant negative mutation (P291fsinsC) in β-cells have both been shown to develop diabetes while exhibiting a progressive reduction of β-cell proliferation and numbers (Hagenfeldt-Johansson et al., 2001; Pontoglio et al., 1998; Yamagata et al., 2002, 1998). This suggests that some target genes of HNF1α are required for the maintenance of a normal β-cell mass. Although the precise molecular mechanisms underlying this regulation are still unknown, reduced insulin-like growth factor-1 (IGF-1) signaling might be involved in the β-cell growth failure by an HNF1α deficiency (Yang et al., 2002). One study suggested that collectrin is involved in the regulation of β-cell growth (Akpinar et al., 2005), although this has not been confirmed by other studies (Altirriba et al., 2010; Fukui et al., 2005).

In order to identify further target genes of HNF1α that are responsible for mediating β-cell growth, we established the MIN6 β-cell line that stably expresses HNF1α-specific shRNA (HNF1α KD-MIN6 cells) and compared the gene expression profile between control MIN6 cells and HNF1α KD-MIN6 cells (Ohki et al., 2012). We found that expression of the gene encoding HGF activator (Hgfac), a serine protease that efficiently activates HGF (Miyazawa, 2010), was decreased in HNF1α KD-MIN6 cells. Down-regulation of *Hgfac* expression was also found in the islets of HNF1α knockout mice. Reporter gene analysis and a chromatin immunoprecipitation (ChIP) assay confirmed that HNF1α directly regulates the expression of *Hgfac* in β-cells (Ohki et al., 2012).

HGF was originally identified as a potent mitogen for hepatocytes (Nakamura et al., 1989), and subsequent studies have shown that it has mitogenic and prosurvival effects on pancreatic β-cells. Transgenic overexpression of HGF in pancreatic β-cells increases their replication, mass, and function (Garcia-Ocaña et al., 2000), while loss of HGF signaling in β-cells during gestation leads to decreased replication and a decline of cell mass (Demirci et al., 2012; Mellado-Gil et al., 2011). HGF is secreted in a latent form, and proteolytic conversion by the serine protease Hgfac is required for its activation (Miyazawa, 2010). It is possible that HNF1α controls β-cell mass at least partly by regulating cellular Hgfac expression. However, further studies are necessary to understand how the reduction of HNF1α activity leads to a decline in β-cell mass and the onset of diabetes.

5. HNF4α GENE AND DIABETES

HNF4α is a member of the steroid hormone receptor superfamily and is expressed in the liver, kidney, small intestine, and pancreas (including β-cells) (Ihara et al., 2005; Nammo et al., 2008). HNF4α has multiple functional domains, including the N-terminal A/B domain associated with the transactivation domain (AF-1), a DNA-binding C domain, a functionally complex E domain that forms a ligand-binding domain, a dimerization interface and transactivation domain (AF-2), and an F domain with a negative regulatory function (Hadzopoulou-Cladaras et al., 1997; Ihara et al., 2005; Sladek, Zhong, Lai, & Darnell, 1990). Since genetic linkage studies identified that MODY1 is tightly linked with markers near *HNF4A* on chromosome 20 (Bell et al., 1991), we screened *HNF4A* for mutations in MODY1 patients and found that *MODY1* encodes HNF4α (Yamagata, Furuta, et al., 1996). HNF4α diabetes is relatively uncommon, but more than 50 mutations have been identified to date (Fig. 16.2). Clinical studies have shown that the primary cause of MODY1 is an impairment of insulin secretion by pancreatic β-cells, indicating that loss of HNF4α leads to β-cell dysfunction (Byrne et al., 1995). Although the diabetic phenotype in MODY1 is similar to that in MODY3, *MODY1* mutation carriers present a different prediabetic phenotype (transient neonatal hypoglycemia and increased body weight) that is not observed in MODY3 (Pearson et al., 2007).

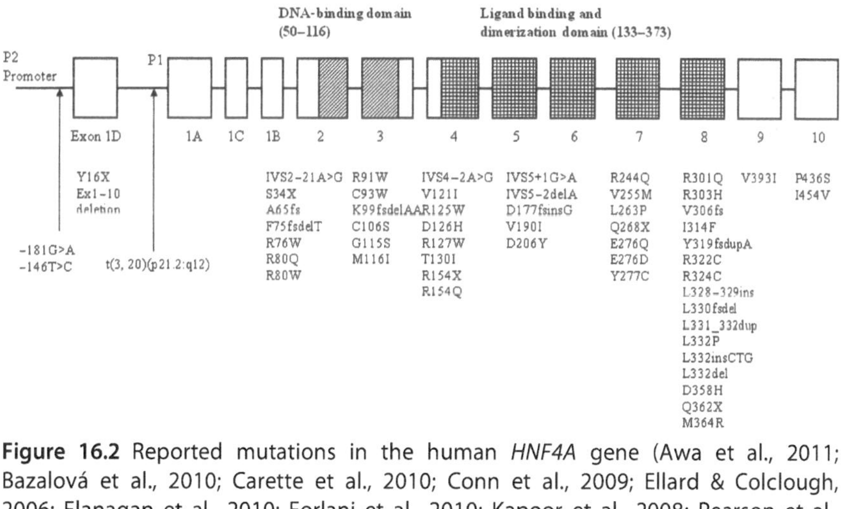

Figure 16.2 Reported mutations in the human *HNF4A* gene (Awa et al., 2011; Bazalová et al., 2010; Carette et al., 2010; Conn et al., 2009; Ellard & Colclough, 2006; Flanagan et al., 2010; Forlani et al., 2010; Kapoor et al., 2008; Pearson et al., 2007; Plengvidhya et al., 2009; Stanescu et al., 2012; Yamagata, Oda, et al., 1996; Yorifuji et al., 2012). Numbering, except for Y16X, is based on +1 as the A of the methionine codon of exon 1A. Y16X is a mutation in exon 1D. Mutations are shown as commonly used nomenclature.

The *HNF4A* gene has two distinct promoters (P1 and P2). Hepatocytes utilize the proximal P1 promoter and transcribe exon 1A, but pancreatic β-cells use the distal P2 promoter and transcribe exon 1D (Boj et al., 2001; Thomas et al., 2001). Common variants in the P2 promoter region are associated with common type 2 diabetes in some populations (Love-Gregory et al., 2004; Silander et al., 2004). In addition, recent studies have shown reduced expression levels of *HNF4α* mRNA in pancreatic islets of type 2 diabetic patients (Gunton et al., 2005). These findings suggest that HNF4α may be involved in the impaired insulin secretion seen in type 2 diabetes as well as MODY1 patients.

6. FUNCTIONAL ROLE OF HNF4α IN β-CELLS

Targeted disruption of *Hnf4a* in mice results in early embryonic death, while heterogeneous *Hnf4a* (+/−) knockout mice exhibit normal glucose tolerance (Chen et al., 1994; Stoffel & Duncan, 1997). We and others generated β-cell-specific HNF4α knockout mice to examine the role of this molecule in β-cells (Boj, Petrov, & Ferrer, 2010; Gupta et al., 2005; Miura et al., 2006). Although such mice did not develop overt diabetes, their glucose levels after intraperitoneal administration of glucose were significantly higher than wild-type mice. In addition, insulin secretion in response to glucose was significantly reduced in the knockout mice. Thus, β-cell specific *Hnf4a* knockout mice constitute a valid experimental model for MODY1, which provides further evidence that HNF4α plays a key role in the maintenance of normal insulin secretion in β-cells. Although the precise molecular mechanism of insulin secretion defects is unknown, an altered function of the K_{ATP} channel, a central component of the insulin secretion machinery, seems to be involved (Gupta et al., 2005; Miura et al., 2006).

As described above, pancreatic β-cell mass is markedly reduced in HNF1α mutant mice. By contrast, β-cell-specific *Hnf4a* knockout mice exhibit normal islet mass, islet number, and β-cell size (Miura et al., 2006). Although HNF4α has been shown to be required for β-cell mass expansion during pregnancy by regulating Ras/ERK signaling (Gupta et al., 2007), the β-cell mass of the *Hnf4a* knockout mice did not differ from that of control mice after high-fat diet feeding (another potent β-cell proliferation stimulus) (Fig. 16.3; our unpublished results) (Maestro et al., 2007). This suggests that the contribution of HNF4α to β-cell growth is limited.

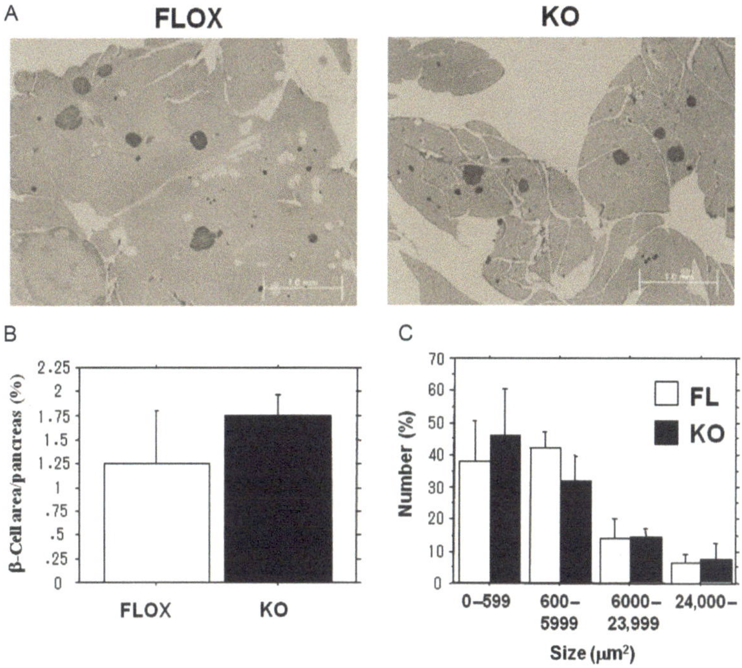

Figure 16.3 β-Cell growth in β-cell-specific HNF4α knockout (βHNF4α KO) mice. Mice were fed a high-fat diet for 8 weeks ($n = 3$, each genotype). (A) Insulin staining of control (FLOX) and βHNF4α KO mice. (B and C) Quantification of β-cell area and size distribution. Data are expressed as mean ± S.E. values. (See the color plate.)

7. Anks4b IS A NOVEL TARGET OF HNF4α IN β-CELLS

HNF4α plays a critical role in liver nutrient transport and metabolism by regulating target genes including phosphoenolpyruvate carboxykinase (PEPCK), glucose-6-phosphatase (G6Pase), apo-AII, and microsomal triglyceride transfer protein (MTP) (Sladek, 1993). However, little information is available about the target genes of HNF4α in pancreatic β-cells. The expression of pancreatic β-cell genes involved in insulin secretion is largely unchanged in β-cell-specific *Hnf4a* knockout islets. Then, we performed large-scale expression profiling analysis using *Hnf4a* knockout islets and identified that ankyrin repeat and sterile alpha motif domain containing 4b (Anks4b) is a direct target gene of HNF4α in β-cells (Sato et al., 2012).

Anks4b was originally cloned as a harmonin-interacting protein, although its function is completely unknown (Johnston et al., 2004). We found that Anks4b bound to glucose-regulated protein 78 (GRP78), a major

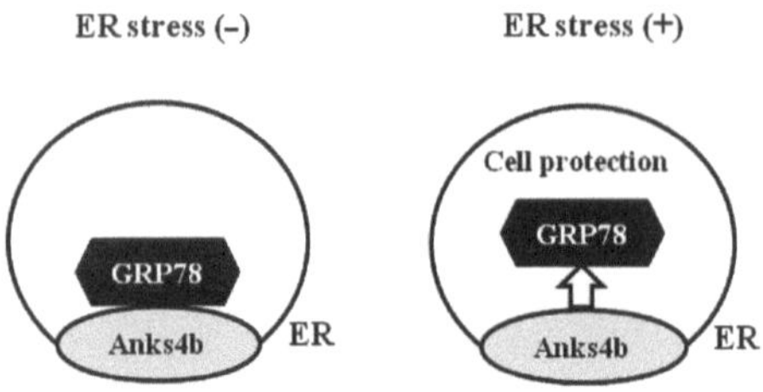

Figure 16.4 Schematic representation of binding between Anks4b and GRP78. ER stress decreases the binding of GRP78 to Anks4b, leading to cell protection from ER stress and apoptosis.

endoplasmic reticulum (ER) chaperone protein that protects cells from ER stress, by mass spectrometry analysis. We also found that its intracellular localization is adjacent to the ER membrane. Overexpression of Anks4b in MIN6 β-cells enhances ER stress responses and ER stress-associated apoptosis. Conversely, suppression of Anks4b reduces β-cell susceptibility to ER stress-induced apoptosis, indicating that Anks4b regulates the sensitivity to ER stress and apoptosis (Sato et al., 2012). Furthermore, induction of ER stress reduces the interaction between Anks4b and GRP78 (our unpublished results). Anks4b might therefore regulate ER stress in β-cells by controlling the pool size of free GRP78 (Fig. 16.4).

Since reduced expression of Anks4b is associated with a decrease, rather than an increase, of ER stress and apoptosis, its significance in the occurrence of diabetes in MODY1 patients is unclear. However, decreased expression of Anks4b may be involved in the hyperinsulinemic hypoglycemia of MODY1 patients at birth. Further studies are necessary to clarify the roles of Anks4b in MODY1. Interestingly, we also found that HNF4α and HNF1α synergistically activate Anks4b gene expression, suggesting that both are involved in the regulation of ER stress in β-cells (Sato et al., 2012).

8. CONCLUDING REMARKS

The identification of *HNF1A* and *HNF4A* as MODY genes has uncovered the importance of these transcription factors in β-cell function and growth (Fig. 16.5). However, we still do not understand the detailed mechanisms that control these processes. Nevertheless, genetic studies have identified that variants of *HNF1A* and *HNF4A* are also associated with common type 2 diabetes and that some environmental factors affect the

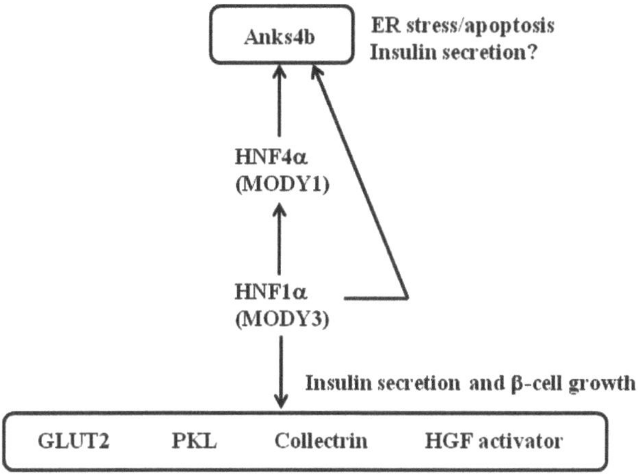

Figure 16.5 Schematic representation of HNF transcriptional cascade in pancreatic β-cells.

expression levels of these transcription factors in β-cells. A better understanding of the roles of HNF would be helpful in clarifying the molecular mechanism of type 2 diabetes and may lead to new therapeutic approaches.

ACKNOWLEDGMENTS

I thank members of the Yamagata laboratory for their helpful contribution on the manuscript. This work was supported by a Grant-in-Aid for Scientific Research (S), a Grant-in-Aid for Scientific Research on Innovative Areas, Health Labour Sciences Research Grant, and grants from Novo Nordisk Insulin Research Foundation, and Japan Diabetes Foundation.

REFERENCES

Akpinar, P., Kuwajima, S., Krützfeldt, J., & Stoffel, M. (2005). Tmem27: A cleaved and shed plasma membrane protein that stimulates pancreatic beta cell proliferation. *Cell Metabolism, 2*(6), 385–397.

Altirriba, J., Gasa, R., Casas, S., Ramírez-Bajo, M. J., Ros, S., Gutierrez-Dalmau, A., et al. (2010). The role of transmembrane protein 27 (TMEM27) in islet physiology and its potential use as a β cell mass biomarker. *Diabetologia, 53*(7), 1406–1414.

Awa, W. L., Thon, A., Raile, K., Grulich-Henn, J., Meissner, T., Schober, E., et al. (2011). Genetic and clinical characteristics of patients with HNF1A gene variations from the German-Austrian DPV database. *European Journal of Endocrinology, 164*(4), 513–520.

Bazalová, Z., Rypácková, B., Broz, J., Brunerová, L., Polák, J., Rusavý, Z., et al. (2010). Three novel mutations in MODY and its phenotype in three different Czech families. *Diabetes Research and Clinical Practice, 88*(2), 132–138.

Bell, G. I., Xiang, K. S., Newman, M. V., Wu, S. H., Wright, L. G., Fajans, S. S., et al. (1991). Gene for non-insulin-dependent diabetes mellitus (maturity-onset diabetes of the young subtype) is linked to DNA polymorphism on human chromosome 20q. *Proceedings of the National Academy of Sciences of the United States of America, 88*(4), 1484–1488.

Bellanné-Chantelot, C., Carette, C., Riveline, J. P., Valéro, R., Gautier, J. F., Larger, E., et al. (2008). The type and the position of HNF1A mutation modulate age at diagnosis of diabetes in patients with maturity-onset diabetes of the young (MODY)-3. *Diabetes, 57*(2), 503–508.

Bellanné-Chantelot, C., Chauveau, D., Gautier, J. F., Dubois-Laforgue, D., Clauin, S., Beaufils, S., et al. (2004). Clinical spectrum associated with hepatocyte nuclear factor-1β mutations. *Annals of Internal Medicine, 140*(7), 510–517.

Boj, S. F., Parrizas, M., Maestro, M. A., & Ferrer, J. (2001). A transcription factor regulatory circuit in differentiated pancreatic cells. *Proceedings of the National Academy of Sciences of the United States of America, 98*(25), 14481–14486.

Boj, S. F., Petrov, D., & Ferrer, J. (2010). Epistasis of transcriptomes reveals synergism between transcriptional activators Hnf1alpha and Hnf4alpha. *PLoS Genetics, 6*(5), e1000970.

Bonnefond, A., Philippe, J., Durand, E., Dechaume, A., Huyvaert, M., Montagne, L., et al. (2012). Whole-exome sequencing and high throughput genotyping identified KCNJ11 as the thirteenth MODY gene. *PLoS One*, 7(6), e37423.

Borowiec, M., Liew, C. W., Thompson, R., Boonyasrisawat, W., Hu, J., Mlynarski, W. M., et al. (2009). Mutations at the BLK locus linked to maturity onset diabetes of the young and β-cell dysfunction. *Proceedings of the National Academy of Sciences of the United States of America, 106*, 14460–14465.

Bowman, P., Flanagan, S. E., Edghill, E. L., Damhuis, A., Shepherd, M. H., Paisey, R., et al. (2012). Heterozygous ABCC8 mutations are a cause of MODY. *Diabetologia, 55*(1), 123–127.

Buchbinder, S., Zorn, M., Bierhaus, A., Nawroth, P. P., Müller, M., & Schilling, T. (2011). Maturity-onset diabetes of the young (MODY) caused by a novel nonsense mutation E41X in the HNF-1α gene. *Experimental and Clinical Endocrinology & Diabetes, 119*(3), 182–185.

Byrne, M. M., Sturis, J., Fajans, S. S., Ortiz, F. J., Stoltz, A., Stoffel, M., et al. (1995). Altered insulin secretory responses to glucose in subjects with a mutation in the MODY1 gene on chromosome 20. *Diabetes, 44*(6), 699–704.

Byrne, M. M., Sturis, J., Menzel, S., Yamagata, K., Fajans, S. S., Dronsfield, M. J., et al. (1996). Altered insulin secretory responses to glucose in diabetic and nondiabetic subjects with mutations in the diabetes susceptibility gene MODY3 on chromosome 12. *Diabetes, 45*(11), 1503–1510.

Cappelli, A., Tumini, S., Consoli, A., Carinci, S., Piersanti, C., Ruggiero, G., et al. (2009). Novel mutations in GCK and HNF1A genes in Italian families with MODY phenotype. *Diabetes Research and Clinical Practice, 83*(3), e72–e74.

Carette, C., Dubois-Laforgue, D., Saint-Martin, C., Clauin, S., Beaufils, S., Larger, E., et al. (2010). Familial young-onset forms of diabetes related to HNF4A and rare HNF1A molecular aetiologies. *Diabetic Medicine, 27*(12), 1454–1458.

Chen, W. S., Manova, K., Weinstein, D. C., Duncan, S. A., Plump, A. S., Prezioso, V. R., et al. (1994). Disruption of the HNF-4 gene, expressed in visceral endoderm, leads to cell death in embryonic ectoderm and impaired gastrulation of mouse embryos. *Genes and Development, 8*(20), 2466–2477.

Conn, J. J., Simm, P. J., Oats, J. J., Nankervis, A. J., Jacobs, S. E., Ellard, S., et al. (2009). Neonatal hyperinsulinaemic hypoglycaemia and monogenic diabetes due to a heterozygous mutation of the HNF4A gene. *Australian and New Zealand Journal of Obstetrics and Gynaecology, 49*(3), 328–330.

Demirci, C., Ernst, S., Alvarez-Perez, J. C., Rosa, T., Valle, S., Shridhar, V., et al. (2012). Loss of HGF/c-Met signaling in pancreatic β-cells leads to incomplete maternal β-cell adaptation and gestational diabetes mellitus. *Diabetes, 61*, 1143–1152.

Dukes, I. D., Sreenan, S., Roe, M. W., Levisetti, M., Zhou, Y. P., Ostrega, D., et al. (1998). Defective pancreatic β-cell glycolytic signaling in hepatocyte nuclear factor-1α-deficient mice. *Journal of Biological Chemistry*, *273*(38), 24457–24464.

Edghill, E. L., Flanagan, S. E., Patch, A. M., Boustred, C., Parrish, A., Shields, B., et al. (2008). Insulin mutation screening in 1,044 patients with diabetes: Mutations in the INS gene are a common cause of neonatal diabetes but a rare cause of diabetes diagnosed in childhood or adulthood. *Diabetes*, *57*, 1034–1042.

Eide, S. A., Raeder, H., Johansson, S., Midthjell, K., Søvik, O., Njølstad, P. R., et al. (2008). Prevalence of HNF1A (MODY3) mutations in a Norwegian population (the HUNT2 Study). *Diabetic Medicine*, *25*(7), 775–781.

Ellard, S., & Colclough, K. (2006). Mutations in the genes encoding the transcription factors hepatocyte nuclear factor 1 alpha (HNF1A) and 4 alpha (HNF4A) in maturity-onset diabetes of the young. *Human Mutation*, *27*(9), 854–869.

Ellard, S., Thomas, K., Edghill, E. L., Owens, M., Ambye, L., Cropper, J., et al. (2007). Partial and whole gene deletion mutations of the GCK and HNF1A genes in maturity-onset diabetes of the young. *Diabetologia*, *50*(11), 2313–2317.

Fajans, S. S., & Bell, G. I. (2011). MODY: History, genetics, pathophysiology, and clinical decision making. *Diabetes Care*, *34*(8), 1878–1884.

Flanagan, S. E., Kapoor, R. R., Mali, G., Cody, D., Murphy, N., Schwahn, B., et al. (2010). Diazoxide-responsive hyperinsulinemic hypoglycemia caused by HNF4A gene mutations. *European Journal of Endocrinology*, *162*(5), 987–992.

Forlani, G., Zucchini, S., Di Rocco, A., Di Luzio, R., Scipione, M., Marasco, E., et al. (2010). Double heterozygous mutations involving both HNF1A/MODY3 and HNF4A/MODY1 genes. *Diabetes Care*, *33*(11), 2336–2338.

Frain, M., Swart, G., Monaci, P., Nicosia, A., Stämpfli, S., Frank, R., et al. (1989). The liver-specific transcription factor LF-B1 contains a highly diverged homeobox DNA binding domain. *Cell*, *59*, 145–157.

Frayling, T. M., Evans, J. C., Bulman, M. P., Pearson, E., Allen, L., Owen, K., et al. (2001). β-Cell genes and diabetes: Molecular and clinical characterization of mutations in transcription factors. *Diabetes*, *50*(Suppl. 1), S94–S100.

Fukui, K., Yang, Q., Cao, Y., Takahashi, N., Hatakeyama, H., Wang, H., et al. (2005). The HNF-1 target collectrin controls insulin exocytosis by SNARE complex formation. *Cell Metabolism*, *2*(6), 373–384.

Garcia-Ocaña, A., Takane, K. K., Syed, M. A., Philbrick, W. M., Vasavada, R. C., & Stewart, A. F. (2000). Hepatocyte growth factor overexpression in the islet of transgenic mice increases beta cell proliferation, enhances islet mass, and induces mild hypoglycemia. *Journal of Biological Chemistry*, *275*, 1226–1232.

Gunton, J. E., Kulkarni, R. N., Yim, S., Okada, T., Hawthorne, W. J., Tseng, Y. H., et al. (2005). Loss of ARNT/HIF1β mediates altered gene expression and pancreatic-islet dysfunction in human type 2 diabetes. *Cell*, *122*(3), 337–349.

Gupta, R. K., Gao, N., Gorski, R. K., White, P., Hardy, O. T., Rafiq, K., et al. (2007). Expansion of adult β-cell mass in response to increased metabolic demand is dependent on HNF-4α. *Genes and Development*, *21*(7), 756–769.

Gupta, R. K., Vatamaniuk, M. Z., Lee, C. S., Flaschen, R. C., Fulmer, J. T., Matschinsky, F. M., et al. (2005). The MODY1 gene HNF-4α regulates selected genes involved in insulin secretion. *Journal of Clinical Investigation*, *115*(4), 1006–1015.

Hadzopoulou-Cladaras, M., Kistanova, E., Evagelopoulou, C., Zeng, S., Cladaras, C., & Ladias, J. A. (1997). Functional domains of the nuclear receptor hepatocyte nuclear factor 4. *Journal of Biological Chemistry*, *272*(1), 539–550.

Hagenfeldt-Johansson, K. A., Herrera, P. L., Wang, H., Gjinovci, A., Ishihara, H., & Wollheim, C. B. (2001). Beta-cell-targeted expression of a dominant-negative hepatocyte nuclear factor-1 alpha induces a maturity-onset diabetes of the young (MODY)3-like phenotype in transgenic mice. *Endocrinology, 142*(12), 5311–5320.

Hattersley, A. T., & Pearson, E. R. (2006). Minireview: Pharmacogenetics and beyond: The interaction of therapeutic response, β-cell physiology, and genetics in diabetes. *Endocrinology, 147*(6), 2657–2663.

Horikawa, Y., Iwasaki, N., Hara, M., Furuta, H., Hinokio, Y., Cockburn, B. N., et al. (1997). Mutation in hepatocyte nuclear factor-1 β gene (TCF2) associated with MODY. *Nature Genetics, 17*(4), 384–385.

Ihara, A., Yamagata, K., Nammo, T., Miura, A., Yuan, M., Tanaka, T., et al. (2005). Functional characterization of the HNF4α isoform (HNF4α8) expressed in pancreatic β-cells. *Biochemical and Biophysical Research Communications, 329*(3), 984–990.

Isomaa, B., Henricsson, M., Lehto, M., Forsblom, C., Karanko, S., Sarelin, L., et al. (1998). Chronic diabetic complications in patients with MODY3 diabetes. *Diabetologia, 41*(4), 467–473.

Iwasaki, N., Ogata, M., Tomonaga, O., Kuroki, H., Kasahara, T., Yano, N., et al. (1998). Liver and kidney function in Japanese patients with maturity-onset diabetes of the young. *Diabetes Care, 21*(12), 2144–2148.

Jesić, M. D., Sajić, S., Jesić, M. M., Maringa, M., Micić, D., & Necić, S. (2008). A case of new mutation in maturity-onset diabetes of the young type 3 (MODY 3) responsive to a low dose of sulphonylurea. *Diabetes Research and Clinical Practice, 81*(1), e1–e3.

Johnston, A. M., Naselli, G., Niwa, H., Brodnicki, T., Harrison, L. C., & Góñez, L. J. (2004). Harp (harmonin-interacting, ankyrin repeat-containing protein), a novel protein that interacts with harmonin in epithelial tissues. *Genes to Cells, 9*(10), 967–982.

Kapoor, R. R., Locke, J., Colclough, K., Wales, J., Conn, J. J., Hattersley, A. T., et al. (2008). Persistent hyperinsulinemic hypoglycemia and maturity-onset diabetes of the young due to heterozygous HNF4A mutations. *Diabetes, 57*(6), 1659–1663.

Karges, B., Bergmann, C., Scholl, K., Heinze, E., Rasche, F. M., Zerres, K., et al. (2007). Digenic inheritance of hepatocyte nuclear factor-1α and -1β with maturity-onset diabetes of the young, polycystic thyroid, and urogenital malformations. *Diabetes Care, 30*(6), 1613–1614.

Kooptiwut, S., Sujjitjoon, J., Plengvidhya, N., Boonyasrisawat, W., Chongjaroen, N., Jungtrakoon, P., et al. (2009). Functional defect of truncated hepatocyte nuclear factor-1α (G554fsX556) associated with maturity-onset diabetes of the young. *Biochemical and Biophysical Research Communications, 383*(1), 68–72.

Kuo, C. J., Conley, P. B., Chen, L., Sladek, F. M., Darnell, J. E., Jr., & Crabtree, G. R. (1992). A transcriptional hierarchy involved in mammalian cell-type specification. *Nature, 355*(6359), 457–461.

Kyithar, M. P., Bacon, S., Pannu, K. K., Rizvi, S. R., Colclough, K., Ellard, S., et al. (2011). Identification of HNF1A-MODY and HNF4A-MODY in Irish families: Phenotypic characteristics and therapeutic implications. *Diabetes & Metabolism, 37*(6), 512–519.

Lopez, A. P., Foscaldi, S. A., Perez, M. S., Rodriguez, M., Traversa, M., Puchulu, F. M., et al. (2011). HNF1 α gene coding regions mutations screening, in a Caucasian population clinically characterized as MODY from Argentina. *Diabetes Research and Clinical Practice, 91*(2), 208–212.

Lorini, R., Klersy, C., d'Annunzio, G., Massa, O., Minuto, N., Iafusco, D., et al. (2009). Maturity-onset diabetes of the young in children with incidental hyperglycemia: A multicenter Italian study of 172 families. *Diabetes Care, 32*(10), 1864–1866.

Love-Gregory, L. D., Wasson, J., Ma, J., Jin, C. H., Glaser, B., Suarez, B. K., et al. (2004). A common polymorphism in the upstream promoter region of the hepatocyte nuclear factor-4 alpha gene on chromosome 20q is associated with type 2 diabetes and appears to contribute to the evidence for linkage in an Ashkenazi Jewish population. *Diabetes, 53*(4), 1134–1140.

Maestro, M. A., Cardalda, C., Boj, S. F., Luco, R. F., Servitja, J. M., & Ferrer, J. (2007). Distinct roles of HNF1β, HNF1α, and HNF4α in regulating pancreas development, β-cell function and growth. *Endocrine Development, 12*, 33–45.

Malecki, M. T., Jhala, U. S., Antonellis, A., Fields, L., Doria, A., Orban, T., et al. (1999). Mutations in NEUROD1 are associated with the development of type 2 diabetes mellitus. *Nature Genetics, 23*, 323–328.

Maraschin, Jde F., Kannengiesser, C., Murussi, N., Campagnolo, N., Canani, L. H., Gross, J. L., et al. (2008). HNF1α mutations are present in half of clinically defined MODY patients in South-Brazilian individuals. *Arquivos Brasileiros de Endocrinologia e Metabologia, 52*(8), 1326–1331.

Mellado-Gil, J., Rosa, T. C., Demirci, C., Gonzalez-Pertusa, J. A., Velazquez-Garcia, S., Ernst, S., et al. (2011). Disruption of hepatocyte growth factor/c-Met signaling enhances pancreatic β-cell death and accelerates the onset of diabetes. *Diabetes, 60*, 525–536.

Mendel, D. B., & Crabtree, G. R. (1991). HNF-1, a member of a novel class of dimerizing homeodomain proteins. *Journal of Biological Chemistry, 266*, 677–680.

Miura, A., Yamagata, K., Kakei, M., Hatakeyama, H., Takahashi, N., Fukui, K., et al. (2006). Hepatocyte nuclear factor-4α is essential for glucose-stimulated insulin secretion by pancreatic β-cells. *Journal of Biological Chemistry, 281*(8), 5246–5257.

Miyazawa, K. (2010). Hepatocyte growth factor activator (HGFA): A serine protease that links tissue injury to activation of hepatocyte growth factor. *The FEBS Journal, 277*, 2208–2214.

Nakamura, T., Nishizawa, T., Hagiya, M., Seki, T., Shimonishi, M., Sugimura, A., et al. (1989). Molecular cloning and expression of human hepatocyte growth factor. *Nature, 342*, 440–443.

Nammo, T., Yamagata, K., Hamaoka, R., Zhu, Q., Akiyama, T. E., Gonzalez, F. J., et al. (2002). Expression profile of MODY3/HNF-1α protein in the developing mouse pancreas. *Diabetologia, 45*, 1142–1153.

Nammo, T., Yamagata, K., Tanaka, T., Kodama, T., Sladek, F. M., Fukui, K., et al. (2008). Expression of HNF-4α (MODY1), HNF-1β (MODY5), and HNF-1α (MODY3) proteins in the developing mouse pancreas. *Gene Expression Patterns, 8*(2), 96–106.

Neve, B., Fernandez-Zapico, M. E., Ashkenazi-Katalan, V., Dina, C., Hamid, Y. H., Joly, E., et al. (2005). Role of transcription factor KLF11 and its diabetes-associated gene variants in pancreatic β cell function. *Proceedings of the National Academy of Sciences of the United States of America, 102*, 4807–4812.

Ohki, T., Sato, Y., Yoshizawa, T., Yamamura, K., Yamada, K., & Yamagata, K. (2012). Identification of hepatocyte growth factor activator (Hgfac) gene as a target of HNF1α in mouse β-cells. *Biochemical and Biophysical Research Communications, 425*(3), 619–624.

Párrizas, M., Maestro, M. A., Boj, S. F., Paniagua, A., Casamitjana, R., Gomis, R., et al. (2001). Hepatic nuclear factor 1-α directs nucleosomal hyperacetylation to its tissue-specific transcriptional targets. *Molecular and Cellular Biology, 21*(9), 3234–3243.

Pearson, E. R., Boj, S. F., Steele, A. M., Barrett, T., Stals, K., Shield, J. P., et al. (2007). Macrosomia and hyperinsulinaemic hypoglycaemia in patients with heterozygous mutations in the HNF4A gene. *PLoS Medicine, 4*(4), e118.

Pearson, E. R., Starkey, B. J., Powell, R. J., Gribble, F. M., Clark, P. M., & Hattersley, A. T. (2003). Genetic cause of hyperglycaemia and response to treatment in diabetes. *Lancet, 362*(9392), 1275–1281.

Plengvidhya, N., Boonyasrisawat, W., Chongjaroen, N., Jungtrakoon, P., Sriussadaporn, S., Vannaseang, S., et al. (2009). Mutations of maturity-onset diabetes of the young (MODY) genes in Thais with early-onset type 2 diabetes mellitus. *Clinical Endocrinology, 70*(6), 847–853.

Plengvidhya, N., Kooptiwut, S., Songtawee, N., Doi, A., Furuta, H., Nishi, M., et al. (2007). PAX4 mutations in Thais with maturity onset diabetes of the young. *Journal of Clinical Endocrinology & Metabolism, 92*, 2821–2826.

Pontoglio, M., Barra, J., Hadchouel, M., Doyen, A., Kress, C., Bach, J. P., et al. (1996). Hepatocyte nuclear factor 1 inactivation results in hepatic dysfunction, phenylketonuria, and renal Fanconi syndrome. *Cell, 84*(4), 575–585.

Pontoglio, M., Sreenan, S., Roe, M., Pugh, W., Ostrega, D., Doyen, A., et al. (1998). Defective insulin secretion in hepatocyte nuclear factor 1α-deficient mice. *Journal of Clinical Investigation, 101*(10), 2215–2222.

Radha, V., Ek, J., Anuradha, S., Hansen, T., Pedersen, O., & Mohan, V. (2009). Identification of novel variants in the hepatocyte nuclear factor-1α gene in South Indian patients with maturity onset diabetes of young. *Journal of Clinical Endocrinology and Metabolism, 94*(6), 1959–1965.

Raeder, H., Johansson, S., Holm, P. I., Haldorsen, I. S., Mas, E., Sbarra, V., et al. (2006). Mutations in the CEL VNTR cause a syndrome of diabetes and pancreatic exocrine dysfunction. *Nature Genetics, 38*, 54–62.

Sato, Y., Hatta, M., Karim, M. F., Sawa, T., Wei, F. Y., Sato, S., et al. (2012). Anks4b, a novel target of HNF4α protein, interacts with GRP78 protein and regulates endoplasmic reticulum stress-induced apoptosis in pancreatic β-cells. *Journal of Biological Chemistry, 287*(27), 23236–23245.

Servitja, J. M., Pignatelli, M., Maestro, M. A., Cardalda, C., Boj, S. F., Lozano, J., et al. (2009). Hnf1α (MODY3) controls tissue-specific transcriptional programs and exerts opposed effects on cell growth in pancreatic islets and liver. *Molecular and Cellular Biology, 29*(11), 2945–2959.

Shih, D. Q., Screenan, S., Munoz, K. N., Philipson, L., Pontoglio, M., Yaniv, M., et al. (2001). Loss of HNF-1α function in mice leads to abnormal expression of genes involved in pancreatic islet development and metabolism. *Diabetes, 50*(11), 2472–2480.

Silander, K., Mohlke, K. L., Scott, L. J., Peck, E. C., Hollstein, P., Skol, A. D., et al. (2004). Genetic variation near the hepatocyte nuclear factor-4 alpha gene predicts susceptibility to type 2 diabetes. *Diabetes, 53*(4), 1141–1149.

Sladek, F. M. (1993). Orphan receptor HNF-4 and liver-specific gene expression. *Receptor, 3*(3), 223–232.

Sladek, F. M., Zhong, W. M., Lai, E., & Darnell, J. E., Jr. (1990). Liver-enriched transcription factor HNF-4 is a novel member of the steroid hormone receptor superfamily. *Genes and Development, 4*(12B), 2353–2365.

Stanescu, D. E., Hughes, N., Kaplan, B., Stanley, C. A., & De León, D. D. (2012). Novel presentations of congenital hyperinsulinism due to mutations in the MODY genes: HNF1A and HNF4A. *Journal of Clinical Endocrinology and Metabolism, 97*(10), E2026–E2030.

Stoffel, M., & Duncan, S. A. (1997). The maturity-onset diabetes of the young (MODY1) transcription factor HNF4alpha regulates expression of genes required for glucose transport and metabolism. *Proceedings of the National Academy of Sciences of the United States of America, 94*(24), 13209–13214.

Stoffers, D. A., Ferrer, J., Clarke, W. L., & Habener, J. F. (1997). Early-onset type-II diabetes mellitus (MODY4) linked to IPF1. *Nature Genetics, 17*(2), 138–139.

Tattersall, R. B. (1974). Mild familial diabetes with dominant inheritance. *Quarterly Journal of Medicine, 43*(170), 339–357.

Thomas, H., Jaschkowitz, K., Bulman, M., Frayling, T. M., Mitchell, S. M., Roosen, S., et al. (2001). A distant upstream promoter of the HNF-4α gene connects the transcription factors involved in maturity-onset diabetes of the young. *Human Molecular Genetics, 10*(19), 2089–2097.

Toaima, D., Näke, A., Wendenburg, J., Praedicow, K., Rohayem, J., Engel, K., et al. (2005). Identification of novel GCK and HNF1A/TCF1 mutations and polymorphisms in German families with maturity-onset diabetes of the young (MODY). *Human Mutation, 25*(5), 503–504.

Triggs-Raine, B. L., Kirkpatrick, R. D., Kelly, S. L., Norquay, L. D., Cattini, P. A., Yamagata, K., et al. (2002). HNF-1α G319S, a transactivation-deficient mutant, is associated with altered dynamics of diabetes onset in an Oji-Cree community. *Proceedings of the National Academy of Sciences of the United States of America, 99*(7), 4614–4619.

Vionnet, N., Stoffel, M., Takeda, J., Yasuda, K., Bell, G. I., Zouali, H., et al. (1992). Nonsense mutation in the glucokinase gene causes early-onset non-insulin-dependent diabetes mellitus. *Nature, 356*(6371), 721–722.

Voight, B. F., Scott, L. J., Steinthorsdottir, V., Morris, A. P., Dina, C., Welch, R. P., et al. (2010). Twelve type 2 diabetes susceptibility loci identified through large-scale association analysis. *Nature Genetics, 42*(7), 579–589.

Wang, H., Maechler, P., Hagenfeldt, K. A., & Wollheim, C. B. (1998). Dominant-negative suppression of HNF-1α function results in defective insulin gene transcription and impaired metabolism-secretion coupling in a pancreatic β-cell line. *The EMBO Journal, 17*(22), 6701–6713.

Yamagata, K., Furuta, H., Oda, N., Kaisaki, P. J., Menzel, S., Cox, N. J., et al. (1996). Mutations in the hepatocyte nuclear factor-4α gene in maturity-onset diabetes of the young (MODY1). *Nature, 384*(6608), 458–460.

Yamagata, K., Nammo, T., Moriwaki, M., Ihara, A., Iizuka, K., Yang, Q., et al. (2002). Overexpression of dominant-negative mutant hepatocyte nuclear fctor-1 α in pancreatic β-cells causes abnormal islet architecture with decreased expression of E-cadherin, reduced β-cell proliferation, and diabetes. *Diabetes, 51*(1), 114–123.

Yamagata, K., Nammo, T., Sato, Y., Saisho, K., Shoda, H., & Fukui, K. (2007). The HNF-1α-SNARE connection. *Diabetes, Obesity & Metabolism, 9*(Suppl. 2), 40–45.

Yamagata, K., Oda, N., Kaisaki, P. J., Menzel, S., Furuta, H., Vaxillaire, M., et al. (1996). Mutations in the hepatocyte nuclear factor-1α gene in maturity-onset diabetes of the young (MODY3). *Nature, 384*(6608), 455–458.

Yamagata, K., Yang, Q., Yamamoto, K., Iwahashi, H., Miyagawa, J., Okita, K., et al. (1998). Mutation P291fsinsC in the transcription factor hepatocyte nuclear factor-1alpha is dominant negative. *Diabetes, 47*(8), 1231–1235.

Yang, Q., Yamagata, K., Fukui, K., Cao, Y., Nammo, T., Iwahashi, H., et al. (2002). Hepatocyte nuclear factor-1α modulates pancreatic β-cell growth by regulating the expression of insulin-like growth factor-1 in INS-1 cells. *Diabetes, 51*(6), 1785–1792.

Yorifuji, T., Fujimaru, R., Hosokawa, Y., Tamagawa, N., Shiozaki, M., Aizu, K., et al. (2012). Comprehensive molecular analysis of Japanese patients with pediatric-onset MODY-type diabetes mellitus. *Pediatric Diabetes, 13*(1), 26–32.

Yoshiuchi, I., Yamagata, K., Yang, Q., Iwahashi, H., Okita, K., Yamamoto, K., et al. (1999). Three new mutations in the hepatocyte nuclear factor-1alpha gene in Japanese subjects with diabetes mellitus: Clinical features and functional characterization. *Diabetologia, 42*(5), 621–626.

Zhang, H., Wada, J., Hida, K., Tsuchiyama, Y., Hiragushi, K., Shikata, K., et al. (2001). Collectrin, a collecting duct-specific transmembrane glycoprotein, is a novel homolog of ACE2 and is developmentally regulated in embryonic kidneys. *Journal of Biological Chemistry, 276*(20), 17132–17139.

CHAPTER SEVENTEEN

Role of the Mammalian Target of Rapamycin (mTOR) Complexes in Pancreatic β-Cell Mass Regulation

Alberto Bartolome[*,†,‡], **Carlos Guillén**[*,†,‡,1]
[*]Departamento de Bioquímica y Biología Molecular II, Facultad de Farmacia, Universidad Complutense, Madrid, Spain
[†]Centro de Investigación Biomédica en Red de Diabetes y Enfermedades Metabólicas Asociadas (CIBERDEM), Barcelona, Spain
[‡]Instituto de Investigación Sanitaria del Hospital Clínico San Carlos de Madrid (IdISSC), Madrid, Spain
[1]Corresponding author: e-mail address: cguillen@farm.ucm.es

Contents

Vitamins and Hormones, Volume 95
ISSN 0083-6729
http://dx.doi.org/10.1016/B978-0-12-800174-5.00017-X

Abstract

Exquisite regulation of insulin secretion by pancreatic β-cells is essential to maintain metabolic homeostasis. β-Cell mass must be accordingly adapted to metabolic needs and can be largely modified under different situations. The mammalian target of rapamycin (mTOR) complexes has been consistently identified as key modulators of β-cell mass. mTOR can be found into two different complexes, mTORC1 and mTORC2. Under systemic insulin resistance, mTORC1/mTORC2 signaling in β-cells is needed to increase β-cell mass and insulin secretion. However, type 2 diabetes arises when these compensatory mechanisms fail, being the role of mTOR complexes still obscure in β-cell failure. In this chapter, we introduce the protein composition and regulation of mTOR complexes and their role in pancreatic β-cells. Furthermore, we describe their main signaling effectors through the review of numerous animal models, which indicate the essential role of mTORC1/mTORC2 in pancreatic β-cell mass regulation.

1. INTRODUCTION

Pancreatic β-cells are the main source of insulin, hormone required to maintain metabolic homeostasis. The major function of this cell type is the fine adjustment of insulin secretion in response to the organism's nutritional status. Accordingly, β-cell mass needs to be adapted to the insulin requirements of the organism and can be largely modified through life in response to pathophysiological circumstances (Bonner-Weir, Deery, Leahy, & Weir, 1989; Butler et al., 2003).

The mechanisms leading to increased β-cell mass and subsequently increased insulin synthesis and secretion are essential for adaptation to conditions of higher metabolic load. The failure of such mechanisms triggers the development of hyperglycemia and the characteristic complications of diabetes (Rhodes, 2005). That is why our better comprehension of these mechanisms and causes of their failure will be needed to establish new treatments and prevention strategies in order to delay or stop diabetes progression.

Recent breakthroughs in β-cell research have unraveled molecular signaling pathways that largely affect normal β-cell mass, as well as the compensatory mechanisms, leading to mass increase under certain circumstances. In this regard, β-cell autocrine insulin action and signaling through mammalian target of rapamycin (mTOR) complexes (mTORC1/mTORC2) have consistently been shown to be key regulators of β-cell mass. In this chapter, we introduce the central role of β-cell mass in diabetes pathophysiology and the structure and function of mTOR complexes, and then focus on β-cell-specific insulin and mTORC1/mTORC2 signaling and its impact on β-cell mass.

2. PANCREATIC β-CELL MASS

2.1. β-Cell mass in normal physiology

β-Cell mass results from the net balance between mechanisms that increase it: hyperplasia, hypertrophy, and generation of new β-cells from ductal precursors (neogenesis)—and those that decrease its mass—hypoplasia, atrophy, and cell death.

In normal individuals, β-cell mass increases during youth due to hyperplasia (Köhler et al., 2011; Meier et al., 2008) as opposed to neogenesis (Dor, Brown, Martinez, & Melton, 2004). Studies of lipofuscin accumulation reflect that the population of β-cells in healthy subjects is mainly established during youth, being proliferation during adulthood relatively low (Butler et al., 2003; Cnop et al., 2010). This "postmitotic" nature of the tissue was also found in other studies in humans (Köhler et al., 2011) and rodents (Teta, Long, Wartschow, Rankin, & Kushner, 2005). However, β-cell mass continues to be increased during adulthood dependent of cell hypertrophy (Montanya, Nacher, Biarnés, & Soler, 2000). β-Cell mass shows a high plasticity and can be adapted depending on the insulin demand of the organism. A good example of this plasticity is the adaptive changes observed in β-cell mass during pregnancy (Parsons, Brelje, & Sorenson, 1992; Van Assche, Aerts, & De Prins, 1978). Increased insulin resistance and maternal body weight sharply increase insulin demand; therefore, β-cell mass becomes hyperplasic and hypertrophic. In humans and rodents, β-cell mass can increase up to 150% during pregnancy (Brelje et al., 1993; Butler et al., 2010). However, after delivery, β-cell mass rapidly returns to normal due to enhanced apoptosis (Scaglia, Cahill, Finegood, & Bonner-Weir, 1997). Impaired adaptation of the β-cell mass is hypothesized to contribute to gestational diabetes (Zahr et al., 2007).

2.2. β-Cell mass in progression to type 2 diabetes

Type 2 diabetes is a complex disease arising from multiple factors, being main contributors of insulin resistance and β-cell dysfunction. Systemic insulin resistance results from genetic and environmental factors such as a hypercaloric diet or a sedentary life. However, insulin resistance can be compensated by an increase in the levels of circulating insulin. This is achieved by an increase in both β-cell mass and function. Diabetes mellitus will appear when insulin resistance exceeds insulin production capacity, or when β-cell function declines (commonly known as β-cell failure).

Systemic insulin resistance development sharply increases insulin demand. Several studies show how the β-cell mass is able to rely on hyperplasia to achieve compensatory hyperinsulinemia (Brüning et al., 1997; Escribano et al., 2009). Other studies indicate that this compensation, even under extreme insulin resistance (*ob/ob* mice), mainly occurs through cell hypertrophy (Bock, Pakkenberg, & Buschard, 2003). Increased islet neogenesis is also reported in various studies in rodents and humans, although its particular role in adult life is controversial (Butler et al., 2003; Dor et al., 2004). Still, interventions focused on increasing islet neogenesis in adults are promising (Juhl, Bonner-Weir, & Sharma, 2010). The specific contributions of β-cell hyperplasia, hypertrophy, or neogenesis to compensatory hyperinsulinemia are not yet clear. Even the possibility of increased function per given β-cell mass unit appears to play a role on the prediabetes stage. Several reports indicate the low replication capacity of human β-cells as compared with rodents, even after partial pancreatectomy or in insulin-resistant obese patients (Butler et al., 2003; Menge et al., 2008). Hence, evidences of increased β-cell mass in humans mainly rely on cell hypertrophy. Recent reports indicate how the major regulator of cell size, mTORC1, plays key roles in β-cell mass adaptation, as described below.

2.3. β-Cell failure

There is no doubt that reduction of β-cell mass and insulin deficiency lies behind type 1 diabetes pathophysiology. In fact, transplantation studies have shown that the metabolic defects that characterize type 1 diabetes can be restored if a functional β-cell mass is recovered (Keymeulen et al., 1998; Shapiro et al., 2000).

β-Cell dysfunction, and its relationship with type 2 diabetes, is also well documented (Del Guerra et al., 2005; Kahn, 1998). However, "β-cell mass decrease," as opposed to "impaired β-cell function" as the causative agent of β-cell dysfunction, began to gain importance during the past decade. This was in part due to the low accessibility of the pancreatic tissue and the absence of β-cell mass longitudinal studies in humans.

However, nowadays the paradigm has changed, mainly possible due to emerging evidences from postmortem studies showing decreased β-cell mass in hyperglycemic human patients (Butler et al., 2003; Sakuraba et al., 2002) or animal models (Larsen et al., 2006; Pick et al., 1998; Saisho et al., 2010). Recent studies in humans indicate that glucose intolerance appears after ~20% reduction in β-cell mass, while overt diabetes develops with ~65% reduction (Meier et al., 2012). Apoptosis has been considered as the underlying mechanism leading to decreased β-cell mass (Butler et al., 2003; Pick et al., 1998), although recent reports also point to the possibility of β-cell dedifferentiation as an important contributor to β-cell dysfunction and diabetes development (Talchai, Xuan, Lin, Sussel, & Accili, 2012).

3. STRUCTURE OF mTORC1/mTORC2 COMPLEXES

3.1. mTOR: Discovery, structure, properties

Two Tor genes sharing 67% homology (*tor1* and *tor2*) were first discovered in yeasts as the genes involved in rapamycin toxicity (Heitman, Movva, & Hall, 1991). Rapamycin (sirolimus) and FK506 (tacrolimus) are two structurally related molecules that bind to the same receptor, FK506-binding protein (known as FKBP12). Rapamycin was first isolated from *Streptomyces hygroscopicus* in a soil sample from Easter Island (known by natives as Rapa Nui) (Vézina, Kudelski, & Sehgal, 1975). Contrary to FK506–FKBP12–calcineurin interaction, the mammalian protein that directly associates with FKBP12–rapamycin complex was identified as the mTOR, and its encoding gene was cloned from both human (FRAP, FK506-binding protein 12–rapamycin-associated protein 1) (Brown et al., 1994) and rat (RAFT, rapamycin, and FKBP target) (Sabatini, Erdjument-Bromage, Lui, Tempst, & Snyder, 1994) cDNA. The full-length FRAP is a 289-kDa protein, currently known as the mechanistic target of rapamycin. mTOR is a serine/threonine kinase containing a putative phosphatidylinositol kinase domain that allows its inclusion in the family of phosphatidyl inositol-3′ kinase-related kinases (PIKKs) (Lempiäinen & Halazonetis, 2009). In humans, this family is formed by six members including ataxia–telangiectasia-mutated, ataxia- and Rad3-related, the catalytic subunit of DNA-dependent protein kinase, mTOR, and suppressor of morphogenesis in genitalia and transformation/transcription domain-associated protein (TRAAP).

The N-terminal region of mTOR contains a solenoid protein domain named HEAT repeats, acronym arising from the first identified proteins containing these repeats (Huntingtin, elongation factor 3, alpha-regulatory subunit of protein phosphatase 2A, and TOR1). HEAT repeats form a helical secondary structure involved in protein–protein interactions (Andrade,

Perez-Iratxeta, & Ponting, 2001). This motif allows the interaction of mTOR with regulatory-associated protein of mTOR (RAPTOR) or RICTOR (Kim et al., 2002; Sarbassov et al., 2004). Next domain is named FAT domain, which is also present in other PIKK proteins (Bosotti, Isacchi, & Sonnhammer, 2000). The FKBP12–rapamycin binding (FRB) domain is located in an N-terminal position with respect to the kinase domain (KD). This region interacts with FKBP12–rapamycin as well as FKBP38–Rheb (Fig. 17.1A) (Choi, Chen, Schreiber, & Clardy, 1996; Stan et al., 1994). The C-terminal domain of mTOR contains several important elements, including the kinase catalytic domain, structurally similar to the catalytic site of phosphatidylinositol 3-kinases (PI3Ks). The catalytic domain also contains a region with several phosphorylatable residues, named as the negative regulatory domain (NRD) or "repressor domain"

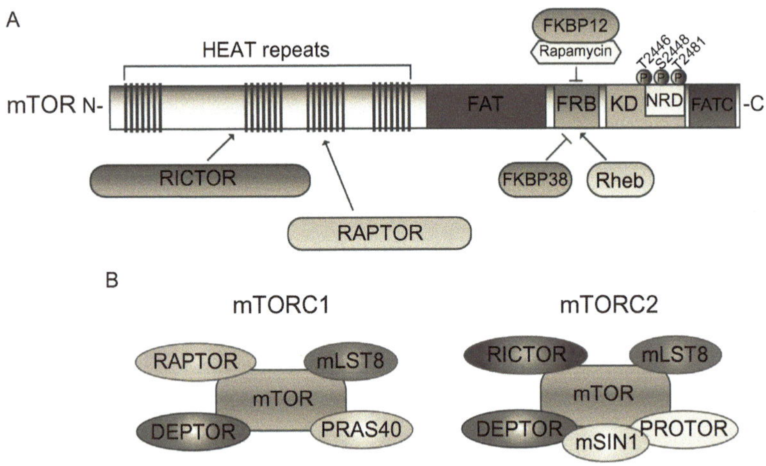

Figure 17.1 Structure of mTOR and mTOR complexes. (A) mTOR structural domains including the phosphorylation residues, regions for binding to RAPTOR or RICTOR as well as for rapamycin and Rheb interaction. The abbreviations used are the following: HEAT repeats (huntingtin, elongation factor 3, alpha-regulatory subunit of protein phosphatase 2A and TOR1); FAT domain (FRAP-ATM-TRAAP); FKBP12–rapamycin-binding domain (FRB); negative regulatory domain (NRD); kinase domain (KD); FATC domain (FRAP, ATM, TRRAP C-terminal). (B) Composition of mTORC1 and mTORC2 complexes. The regulatory-associated protein of mTOR (RAPTOR) and the 40-kDa proline-rich Akt substrate (PRAS40) are specific from mTORC1 complex. DEPTOR (DEP domain-containing mTOR-interacting protein) is present in both complexes as well as mammalian lethal with SEC13 protein 8 (mLST8). The rapamycin-insensitive companion of mTOR (RICTOR), the mammalian stress-activated MAP kinase-interacting protein 1 (mSIN1), and the protein observed with RICTOR (PROTOR) are specifically bound to mTORC2. (For color version of this figure, the reader is referred to the online version of this chapter.)

(Edinger & Thompson, 2004; Sekulić et al., 2000). Within this domain, there are phosphorylation sites conserved in kinases with similar structure. Ser^{2448} and Ser^{2481} phosphorylation are correlated with overall higher levels of mTOR activity. Of particular note was the identification of the mTORC1 downstream target, p70S6 kinase (S6K), as an mTOR kinase at Ser^{2448} site, this establishing a positive feedback loop (Chiang & Abraham, 2005; Holz & Blenis, 2005). mTOR Ser^{2481} was first reported as an autophosphorylation site in a rapamycin- and amino acid-insensitive manner. In contrast, the phosphorylation residue Thr^{2446} is a negative indicator of mTOR kinase activity, it becomes phosphorylated after nutrient deprivation, and it is reduced after insulin stimulation (Cheng, Fryer, Carling, & Shepherd, 2004).

The FATC region, corresponding to the C-terminal domain of mTOR, is a highly conserved domain with 30 amino acids of length (Bosotti et al., 2000). Several studies indicate that this domain is critical for the kinase activity of the different PIKKs and is very sensitive to mutagenesis. Deletion of 10–20 residues from the C-terminus of mTOR abolishes its kinase activity at the level of a kinase-inactive mutant (Peterson, Beal, Comb, & Schreiber, 2000).

3.2. mTORC1/mTORC2

According to the proteins that are associated with mTOR, it can be found in two different complexes, mTORC1 and mTORC2 (Fig. 17.1B). These complexes have both a characteristic protein essential for the assembly of the complex and interaction with other regulatory elements. The RAPTOR and the 40-kDa proline-rich Akt substrate (PRAS40) are specific from mTORC1 complex (Hara et al., 2002; Sabatini, 2006; Sancak et al., 2007; vander Haar, Lee, Bandhakavi, Griffin, & Kim, 2007). However, the rapamycin-insensitive companion of mTOR, known as RICTOR, the mammalian stress-activated MAP kinase-interacting protein 1 (mSIN1), and the protein observed with RICTOR are specifically bound to mTORC2 (Zoncu, Efeyan, & Sabatini, 2011). DEPTOR (DEP domain-containing mTOR interacting protein) (Peterson et al., 2009) is present in both complexes, and along with PRAS40 serve as negative regulator of mTOR catalytic activity. DEPTOR presents both two DEP (disheveled, egl-10, pleckstrin) domains and a PDZ (postsynaptic density 95, discs large, zonula occludens-1) domain (Peterson et al., 2009) and can bind either mTORC1 or mTORC2. mSIN1 is an important and characteristic component of mTORC2, and the protein is responsible for mTORC2 response to phosphatidylinositol (3,4,5)-trisphosphate (PIP_3) and its localization in membranes for complete activation Akt by phosphorylation in Ser^{473} (Sarbassov, Guertin, Ali, & Sabatini, 2005; Yang, Inoki, Ikenoue, & Guan, 2006). Another component of both mTOR complexes is mLST8. This component was first discovered as an mTOR element that binds to the KD stabilizing mTOR–RAPTOR interaction and stimulating mTOR activity. mLST8 interacts with mTOR within the KD, and different mLST8 mutants with reduced binding affinity to mTOR show decreased mTOR activation capacity (Kim et al., 2003). mLST8 is essential for mTOR–RICTOR association and the downstream phosphorylation of Akt and PKCα (Guertin et al., 2006).

While mTORC1 is inhibited by rapamycin through its interaction with FKBP12 (Brown et al., 1994), mTORC2 is unresponsive to the compound, at least after acute stimulation (Jacinto et al., 2004). However, in some cell lines including pancreatic β-cells, prolonged rapamycin treatment also impairs mTORC2 action (Barlow et al., 2012; Sarbassov et al., 2006), being this not as the consequence of rapamycin targeting mTORC2, but as the chronic effect of sequestering mTOR pool in rapamycin–FKBP12 complex. The best-characterized substrates of mTORC1 are S6 kinase 1 (S6K1) and eIF4E-binding protein 1 (4E-BP1), which control protein synthesis and ribosome biogenesis as described below (Ma & Blenis, 2009). mTORC2 was identified as PDK2, and its activation is needed for the full activation of Akt (García-Martínez et al., 2009; Ikenoue, Inoki, Yang, Zhou, & Guan, 2008; Sarbassov et al., 2005).

The mechanism leading to mTORC2 activation and Akt-Ser^{473} phosphorylation is not fully understood. However, mSIN1 is a critical component of mTORC2 which possess a PH-domain that could be interacting with PIP_3 in the plasmatic membrane, allowing Akt phosphorylation (Yang et al., 2006).

Apart from its kinase activity on Akt-Ser^{473}, mTORC2 can also phosphorylate Akt-Thr^{450} during Akt synthesis, while the nascent protein is still attached to the ribosome, favoring its stability (Oh et al., 2010). mTORC2 is regulated by signals acting through tyrosine kinase receptors. The TSC1–TSC2 complex was also found to be required for mTORC2 full activation (Huang, Dibble, Matsuzaki, & Manning, 2008). Apart from the metabolic effects mediated by insulin through Akt, mTORC2 is able to phosphorylate and activate PKC (Ikenoue et al., 2008), which mediate anabolic actions, cell-cycle progression, and survival. mTORC2 also plays a role in the organization of actin cytoskeleton, controlling cell polarity (Jacinto et al., 2004) (Fig. 17.2).

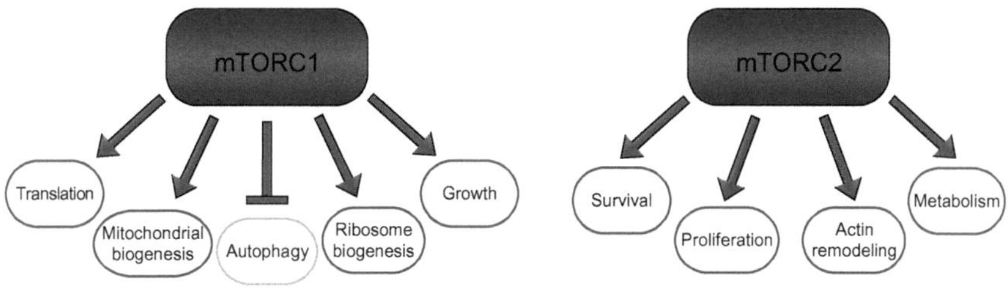

Figure 17.2 Positive and negative effects of both mTORC1 and mTORC2 complexes in different cellular actions. (For color version of this figure, the reader is referred to the online version of this chapter.)

4. INSULIN AND mTORC2 SIGNALING IN PANCREATIC β-CELLS

4.1. Insulin receptor and its isoforms

Insulin receptor (IR) is a heterotetramer composed of two extracellular α-subunits and two transmembrane β-subunits, bound together by disulfide bonds. These subunits arise from a single transcript, the proreceptor, later assembled after proteolytic cleavage (Ullrich et al., 1985). After insulin binding to its receptor, there is a conformational change that allows ATP binding and autophosphorylation of tyrosine residues of the β-subunits (Kasuga, Karlsson, & Kahn, 1982; Kasuga, Zick, Blithe, Crettaz, & Kahn, 1982), allowing IR interaction with its intracellular substrates.

The human *IR* gene contains 22 exons. By alternative splicing of exon 11, two different isoforms arise: IR_A (−ex. 11) or IR_B (+ex. 11). These two isoforms exclusively differ in 12 amino acids located on α-subunit C-terminus (Seino & Bell, 1989). IR isoform expression varies among tissues (McClain, 1991), being IR_A characteristic of fetal development and closely related to cancer (Denley, Wallace, Cosgrove, & Forbes, 2003). However, IR_A is also expressed in adult tissues. There is not a clear consensus between the relative affinities of these isoforms for insulin, as several authors indicate higher affinity of IR_A (Denley et al., 2004; McClain, 1991; Yamaguchi, Flier, Benecke, Ransil, & Moller, 1993), but others report identical affinities (Whittaker, Sørensen, Gadsbøll, & Hinrichsen, 2002). Higher IR_A affinity for IGF-II is reported by all authors, being relatively higher than for IGF-I reviewed in Belfiore, Frasca, Pandini, Sciacca, and Vigneri (2009).

Mice homozygous null for the IR ($Ir^{-/-}$) are born without apparent defects but die 48–72 h after delivery due to severe ketoacidosis (Accili et al., 1996). These report showed how the IR is dispensable for prenatal development but extremely important for metabolic homeostasis during independent life.

Tissue-specific IR knock-out models have allowed comprehension of insulin action in different tissues, and discovery of new elements of its signaling, reviewed in Kitamura, Kahn, and Accilii (2003). β-Cell-specific IR knock-out mice (βIRKO) show a small reduction of β-cell mass, and glucose intolerance due to impaired glucose-stimulated insulin secretion (GSIS) (Otani et al., 2004). However, IR is important for compensatory β-cell mass increase. βIRKO mice develop diabetes on high-fat diet, or in the background of liver-specific IR knock-out mice (LIRKO), as β-cell mass cannot be adapted to these conditions (Okada et al., 2007). Deletion of IR in β-cell lines also has a negative impact on cell proliferation (Bartolomé, Guillén, & Benito, 2010; Guillen, Navarro, Robledo, Valverde, & Benito, 2006).

IGF-I receptor in β-cells is important for the correct regulation of insulin secretion; βIGF1RKO mice do not display changes on β-cell mass but present impaired GSIS (Kulkarni et al., 2002). IGF-I is not essential for compensatory β-cell mass increase in the same way that IR is (Okada et al., 2007). However, total insulin/IGF-I resistance in the model βIRKO; βIGF1RKO results in β-cell hypoplasia and severe diabetes by 3 weeks of age (Ueki et al., 2006).

On the role of IR isoforms in β-cells, IR_B is predominantly expressed in adult pancreatic β-cells (Muller, Huang, Amiel, Jones, & Persaud, 2007). Hyperglycemia has been linked with increased IR_A expression in β-cell lines and human islets (Hribal et al., 2003). IR_A signaling is described to increase insulin synthesis, while IR_B mediates increased glucokinase transcription (Leibiger et al., 2001). Furthermore, increased IR_A expression in isolated islets is linked to β-cell hyperplasia in the model of inducible liver-specific IR knock-out mice (iLIRKO) (Escribano et al., 2009). *In vitro* expression of IR_A in β-cells increase proliferation capability and prolonged insulin signaling compared to IR_B expression (Bartolomé et al., 2010). These observations point to the role of IR_A expression in β-cells, leading to β-cell mass expansion and increased insulin synthesis and secretion under systemic insulin resistance conditions.

4.2. IR substrates

There are several IR substrates, which also have an important role on IGF1R signaling reviewed in Taniguchi, Emanuelli, and Kahn (2006). Among them, the best-characterized are the family of insulin receptor substrates

(IRSs), with at least six members showing high homology. IRSs have differential tissue distribution and function. IRS1 and IRS2 are widely distributed, being IRS2 fundamental for insulin signaling in hepatocytes and β-cells. IRS3 is expressed in the brain and adipocytes, while IRS4 is characteristic of fetal development. IRS5 and IRS6 have limited expression and known functions.

Irs1$^{-/-}$ mice show growing defects due to impaired IGF-I signaling, and skeletal muscle insulin resistance. In this scenario, insulin resistance is compensated by β-cell mass increase and hyperinsulinemia, and *Irs1*$^{-/-}$ mice do not develop diabetes (Araki et al., 1994; Tamemoto et al., 1994).

Irs2$^{-/-}$ mice display a diabetic phenotype due to liver insulin resistance and absence of compensatory hyperinsulinemia (Kubota et al., 2000; Withers et al., 1998), while β-cell mass is increased in mice overexpressing IRS2 in β-cells (Hennige et al., 2003). Decreased β-cell mass and glucose intolerance is also observed in young β-cell-specific IRS2 knock-out mice (Choudhury et al., 2005; Lin et al., 2004), although in these models, β-cells escaping Cre-mediated recombination are able to repopulate the pancreas, indicating the key role of IRS2 on insulin/IGF-I signaling for β-cell proliferation and survival.

Even in situations of extreme insulin resistance, such as in *Ir*$^{+/-}$ and *Irs1*$^{-/-}$ mice, β-cell mass can be enhanced in order to supply increased insulin requirements (Brüning et al., 1997), but this compensatory mechanism is dysfunctional in *Ir*$^{+/-}$; *Irs2*$^{-/-}$ mice (Kim, Kido, Scherer, White, & Accili, 2007).

IRS proteins contain multiple residues susceptible of phosphorylation. After phosphorylation, tyrosine residues (21 in IRS1, from which 14 are conserved in IRS2) serve as docking points for SH2 domain-containing proteins. Many of these proteins act as adaptor molecules, such as the regulatory subunit of PI3K, or Grb2 (growth factor receptor-bound protein 2). Tyrosine phosphorylation is counterbalanced by tyrosine-phosphatases, found upregulated in insulin resistance states (Goldstein, Li, Ding, Ahmad, & Zhang, 1998). Probably, the best-characterized tyrosine-phosphatase is PTP1B (protein tyrosine-phosphatase 1B); *Ptp1b*$^{-/-}$ mice show enhanced insulin responsiveness and are resistant to diet-induced obesity (Elchebly et al., 1999). These mice display decreased β-cell mass due to decreased insulin requirements of the organism. Combined *Ptp1b*$^{-/-}$; *Irs2*$^{-/-}$ mice are able to partially restore the expression of effectors of insulin signaling in β-cells such as pancreatic and duodenal homeobox-1 (Pdx1), although β-cell mass eventually capitulates due to IRS2 absence (Kushner et al., 2004).

In addition to tyrosine phosphorylation, IRSs can be phosphorylated in serine/threonine by different kinases (up to 30 residues). The kinase of the ribosomal S6 protein (S6K), a direct effector of mTORC1, is able to phosphorylate IRS1 and IRS2 in different residues (Shah, Wang, & Hunter, 2004; Tremblay et al., 2007; Um et al., 2004). Serine/threonine phosphorylation of IRSs is the cause of insulin and IGF-I resistance, also promoting IRS sequestration by 14-3-3 proteins (Craparo, Freund, & Gustafson, 1997; Ogihara et al., 1997). Phosphorylation of these residues is a contraregulatory mechanism of insulin signaling, activated after prolonged stimulus, and also serves as a link with other signaling pathways that negatively regulate insulin signaling (TNFα, JNK, IKKβ, etc.) (Hotamisligil et al., 1996).

4.3. PI3K and phosphoinositide-dependent protein kinases

PI3K is formed by a regulatory and a catalytic subunit, existing several isoforms for each of them reviewed in Engelman, Luo, and Cantley (2006). The regulatory subunits interact via their SH2-domain with phosphotyrosine-rich domains in IRS, leading to the activation of the catalytic subunit of PI3K (Myers et al., 1992). After stimulation of IR/IGF1R, there is a rapid activation of PI3K that leads to PIP_3 formation, class IA PI3K family accounts for the best part of its production. In β-cells, class IA PI3K is important mediators of autocrine insulin signaling. Mice lacking *Pi3kr2* systematically and *Pi3kr1* specifically in β-cells shows decreased β-cell mass due to impaired survival, although proliferation is enhanced probably owing to increased Ras-ERK signaling. These mice also showed impaired GSIS and glucose intolerance but do not develop overt diabetes (Kaneko et al., 2010).

PI3K action can be counterbalanced by PIP_3 phosphatases, Pten (phosphatase and tensin homolog; 3′-phosphatase of PIP_3) and SHIP2 (SH2-containing PIP_3 phosphatase 2; 5′-phosphatase). Mice models lacking these genes show improved insulin sensitivity and are resistant to diet-induced obesity (Sleeman et al., 2005; Wijesekara et al., 2005). β*Pten*$^{-/-}$ mice show β-cell mass expansion, hyperinsulinemia, hypoglycemia, improved glucose tolerance, and increased β-cell survival after streptozotocin treatment (Gu, Lindner, Kumar, Yuan, & Magnuson, 2011; Stiles et al., 2006). SHIP2 inhibition in β-cell lines also increases cell proliferation (Grempler, Leicht, Kischel, Eickelmann, & Redemann, 2007).

PIP_3 acts as a second messenger, allowing anchoring to the plasmatic membrane and activation of proteins with PH-domain (pleckstrin homology), such as the phosphoinositide-dependent protein kinase-1 (PDK1).

Activation of PDK1 by PIP_3 leads to Akt-Thr^{308} and PKCζ-Thr^{410} phosphorylation. For complete activation of Akt, phosphorylation in Ser^{473} is also required, and it is mediated by the Rictor-containing mTOR complex: mTORC2, as previously described (Sarbassov et al., 2005). This signaling pathway is essential for β-cell mass maintenance and metabolic homeostasis; β-cell-specific *Pdk1* knock-out mice develops diabetes due to drastic reduction in β-cell mass (Hashimoto et al., 2006), resembling other models previously mentioned such as *Irs2*$^{-/-}$ (Kubota et al., 2000; Withers et al., 1998) or βIRKO; βIGF1RKO (Ueki et al., 2006). In β*Pdk1*$^{-/-}$ mice, absence of Akt-Thr^{308} phosphorylation is observed, but Akt-Ser^{473} phosphorylation remains unchanged. On the other hand, β*Rictor*$^{-/-}$ mice show the opposite profile, and Akt-Ser^{473} phosphorylation is blunted but Akt-Thr^{308} is slightly increased (Gu et al., 2011). Noteworthy is that β*Rictor*$^{-/-}$ mice display mild glucose intolerance, with impaired GSIS and approximately 30% reduction in β-cell mass due to impaired proliferation, but no effect on cell size. While β*Pdk1*$^{-/-}$ mice develop severe diabetes with affected β-cell number and size and a total 80% reduction in β-cell mass (Hashimoto et al., 2006). These studies indicate how the contribution of Akt-Thr^{308} phosphorylation to β-cell maintenance is quantitatively higher than that mediated by Akt-Ser^{473}. β*Rictor*$^{-/-}$ phenotype can be rescued by Pten deletion, owing to the hyperphosphorylation of Akt-Thr^{308}, even in the absence of mTORC2 activity and Akt-Ser^{473} phosphorylation (Gu et al., 2011).

4.4. Akt and its downstream effectors

Akt is an important mediator of insulin actions on all tissues, therefore essential for metabolic homeostasis. Akt is a serine/threonine kinase present in three isoforms. Akt1 is ubiquitously expressed, while Akt2 is highly expressed in key tissues for the metabolic actions of insulin such as liver and adipose tissue, and Akt3 is preferentially found in nervous tissue reviewed in Gonzalez and McGraw (2009). Akt1 is required for normal growth, but mice lacking Akt1 show no disorders in glucose homeostasis (Cho, Thorvaldsen, Chu, Feng, & Birnbaum, 2001). However, Akt2 disruption leads to insulin resistance, but diabetes is not fully developed due to fourfold increase of β-cell mass and insulinemia (Cho, Mu, et al., 2001). Other authors using *Akt2*$^{-/-}$ mice describe a biphasic effect on β-cell mass, with early compensatory increase of β-cell mass followed by β-cell failure and diabetes onset (Garofalo et al., 2003). These results indicate that Akt isoforms in β-cells might play redundant roles, as compensatory mechanisms are not completely blunted in the absence of one isoform.

In vivo expression of a constitutive active form of Akt in β-cells results in hyperinsulinemia due to sixfold increase of β-cell mass. Hyperplasia and hypertrophy were observed with threefold increase in β-cell number and doubled cell size (Bernal-Mizrachi, Wen, Stahlhut, Welling, & Permutt, 2001). Akt is able to mediate β-cell proliferation through regulation of cell-cycle proteins such as cyclin D1, cyclin D2, p21, and Cdk4 (Fatrai et al., 2006).

Targets downstream Akt are diverse, and GSK3β (glycogen synthase kinase 3β) is an important player in cell-cycle progression that is phosphorylated and inhibited by Akt (Cross, Alessi, Cohen, Andjelkovich, & Hemmings, 1995). β-Cell-specific expression of a constitutive GSK3β form leads to β-cell hypoplasia and glucose intolerance (Liu, Tanabe, Bernal-Mizrachi, & Permutt, 2008), while β$Gsk3\beta^{-/-}$ mice display the inverse phenotype (Liu et al., 2010). Regeneration of pancreatic acini and β-cells was achieved in mice subjected to ~90% pancreatectomy, and subsequently treated locally with morpholino-oligonucleotides against GSK3β (Figeac, Ilias, Bailbe, Portha, & Movassat, 2012). GSK3 also connects insulin signaling with mTORC1 through direct phosphorylation of TSC2 (Inoki et al., 2006). *Ex vivo* treatment of human islets with GSK3 inhibitors promotes cell proliferation in an mTORC1-dependent manner (Liu et al., 2009).

Akt also interacts with transcription factors of the family forkhead box class O (FoxO) such as FoxO1, FoxO3a, or FoxO4 (Nakae et al., 2002). Phosphorylation of these factors by Akt inhibits their nuclear actions as they are excluded from nucleus. These factors strongly inhibit proliferation through positive transcriptional regulation of $p27^{Kip1}$ (Medema, Kops, Bos, & Burgering, 2000), an inhibitor of cyclin D4/Cdk4 complex formation, which is essential for β-cell proliferation (Rane et al., 1999). FoxO1 is an important regulator of proliferation and stress response. Under normal circumstances, autocrine insulin signaling maintains cytoplasmic FoxO1 location in β-cells. Insulin resistance and nuclear localization of FoxO1 strongly impair proliferation by suppressing Foxa2-dependent *Pdx1* transcription (Kitamura et al., 2002). FoxO1 haploinsufficiency is able to partially revert the phenotype of other models with severe insulin resistance in β-cells: $Irs2^{-/-}$ and $Foxo1^{+/-}$ (Kitamura et al., 2002), β$Pdk1^{-/-}$; $Foxo1^{+/-}$ (Hashimoto et al., 2006). However, FoxO1 is also important for stress response in β-cells, protecting against β-cell failure through the expression of transcription factors such as NeuroD and MafA (Kitamura et al., 2005). In fact, recent reports show how total absence of FoxO1 in β-cells impairs insulin production and even may promote cell dedifferentiation (Kobayashi et al., 2012; Talchai et al., 2012).

Pdx1 is a key transcription factor for β-cell identity and proliferation (McKinnon & Docherty, 2001). Pdx1 loss of function is related with early diabetes development in humans (Stoffers, Ferrer, Clarke, & Habener, 1997), and impaired proliferation together with β-cell failure in *Pdx1*$^{+/-}$ mice (Fujimoto et al., 2009; Sachdeva et al., 2009). Pdx1 is an important effector of autocrine insulin signaling in β-cells, and its forced expression is able to stop diabetes progression in *Irs2*$^{-/-}$ mice (Kushner et al., 2002).

Akt activation connects insulin signaling with mTORC1 through multiple mechanisms. As described, Akt phosphorylates and inhibits GSK3β and FoxOs, both negative regulators of mTORC1 signaling (Cao et al., 2006; Chen et al., 2010; Inoki et al., 2006). Moreover, Akt directly phosphorylates and inhibits TSC2 (Inoki, Li, Zhu, Wu, & Guan, 2002; Manning, Tee, Logsdon, Blenis, & Cantley, 2002), as well as the mTORC1 component PRAS40 (Sancak et al., 2007; vander Haar et al., 2007). Akt downstream actions are regulated differentially by phosphorylation in Ser^{473} or Thr^{308}. mTORC2 and Akt-Ser^{473} phosphorylation is required for Akt-mediated inhibition of FoxOs and PKCα phosphorylation, but not for Akt actions toward TSC2, GSK3β, and mTORC1 (Guertin et al., 2006). Akt has pleiotropic actions on β-cells, and although those mediated by mTORC1 are important for cell mass maintenance, β-cell mass is still increased in mice with constitutive activation of Akt and deletion of mTORC1 downstream effectors *βAkt-myr; S6k1*$^{-/-}$; *S6k2*$^{-/-}$ (Alliouachene et al., 2008) (Fig. 17.3 and Table 17.1).

5. INTEGRATION OF INSULIN, ENERGY, AND STRESS SIGNALS BY mTORC1

5.1. Glucose and energy signaling in β-cells

In β-cells, glucose is transported in an insulin-independent manner due to expression of a passive and very efficient glucose transporter (GLUT2) (Guillam et al., 1997). This peculiarity has allowed the exploration of insulin-independent glucose signaling in β-cells, where is capable of stimulating MEK–ERK pathway (Briaud, Lingohr, Dickson, Wrede, & Rhodes, 2003; Frödin et al., 1995). Although glucose-mediated MEK–ERK activation is not fully understood, it is dependent on Ca^{2+} and AMPc (Briaud

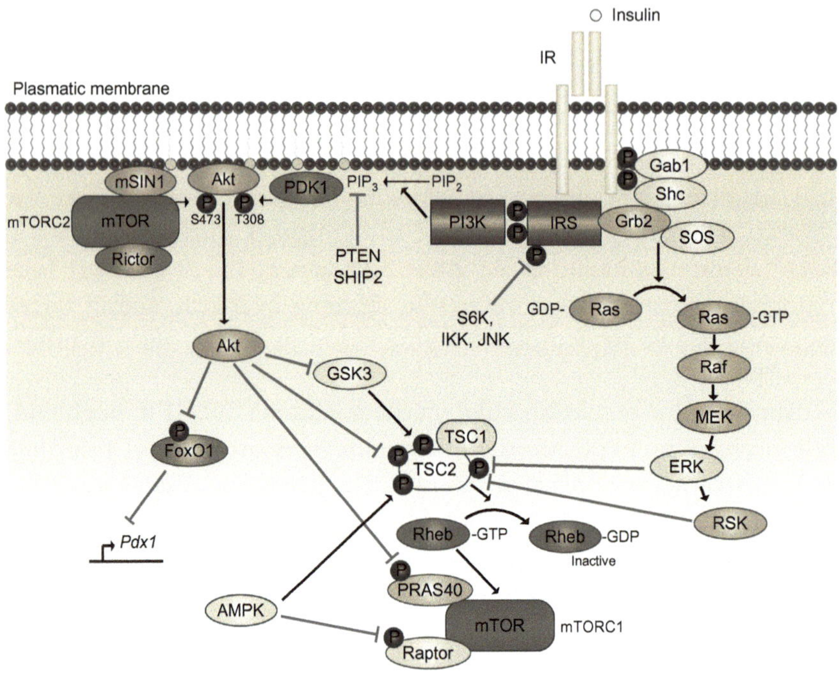

Figure 17.3 Insulin and mTORC1/mTORC2 signaling pathway. Some of the elements introduced in this section are shown. After insulin binding to IR and tyrosine autophosphorylation, substrates of the IR are recruited: IRS, Shc (SH2-domain-containing protein), Gab2 (Grb2-associated-binding protein), Grb2 (growth factor receptor-bound protein 2), and SOS (son of sevenless) are required for Ras (rat sarcoma protein) GTPase domain activation, and subsequent activation of Raf (v-raf murine sarcoma viral oncogene homolog B1) and the MEK-ERK signaling pathway; MEK (mitogen extracellular signal-regulated kinase), ERK (extracellular signal-regulated kinase). On the other hand, PI3K/Akt signaling pathway is depicted. (For color version of this figure, the reader is referred to the online version of this chapter.)

et al., 2003). We previously showed how this activation is totally independent of autocrine insulin signaling, as studies with β-cells lacking IR supported this observation (Guillen et al., 2006). Glucose in β-cells is able to stimulate ERK-dependent TSC2 Ser^{664} phosphorylation (Bartolomé et al., 2010), which leads to mTORC1 activation (Ma, Chen, Erdjument-Bromage, Tempst, & Pandolfi, 2005). Other studies showed that glucose-mediated ERK activation influences β-cell proliferation but had no effect on insulin secretion (Khoo & Cobb, 1997).

Other β-cell lines-based studies also describe how glucose is able to modulate both basal and IGF-I or growth hormone-stimulated cell proliferation

Table 17.1 Insulin signaling in β-cells: mouse models

Model	β-Cell mass			β-Cell	Phenotype	References
	Total	Cell number	Cell size	function		
$\beta Ir^{-/-}$	↓ 50%	Hypoplasia	N/D	↓ GSIS	25% develop diabetes, 75% normal glucose tolerance	Otani et al. (2004)
$\beta Ir^{-/-}$; LIRKO/HFD	Compensatory increase impaired	No hyperplasia	N/D	↓ GSIS	Severe glucose intolerance Early death	Okada et al. (2007)
$\beta Igf1r^{-/-}$	↔	N/D	N/D	↓ GSIS	Glucose intolerance	Kulkarni et al. (2002)
$\beta Igf1r^{-/-}$; HFD	↑ Threefold (compensatory)	Hyperplasia	N/D	N/D	Insulin resistance, glucose intolerance	Okada et al. (2007)
$\beta Ir^{-/-}$; $\beta Igf1r^{-/-}$	↓ >50%	Hypoplasia and apoptosis	N/D	↓ GSIS	Hypoinsulinemia, severe diabetes and death	Ueki et al. (2006)
$Ir^{+/-}$; $Irs1^{-/-}$	↑ 10-fold (compensatory)	Hyperplasia	N/D	N/D	Hyperinsulinemia, severe insulin resistance. 40% develop diabetes	Brüning et al. (1997)
$Ir^{+/-}$; $Irs2^{-/-}$	↓ 50–75%	N/D	N/D	↑ Temporary	Severe diabetes	Kim et al. (2007)
$Irs1^{-/-}$	↑ 1.5-fold (compensatory)	N/D	N/D	N/D	Grow defect, insulin resistance in muscle	Araki et al. (1994), Tamemoto et al. (1994), and Withers et al. (1998)

Continued

Table 17.1 Insulin signaling in β-cells: mouse models—cont'd

Model	β-Cell mass			β-Cell function	Phenotype	References
	Total	Cell number	Cell size			
Irs2$^{-/-}$	↓ 50%	Hypoplasia	N/D	N/D	Hypoinsulinemia, severe diabetes	Withers et al. (1998) and Kubota et al. (2000)
Irs2$^{-/-}$; Pdx1-tg	↔[a]	↔	↔	↔	Mild glucose intolerance	Kushner et al. (2002)
Irs2$^{-/-}$; *Foxo1*$^{+/-}$	↓ 20%[b]	↓	N/D	N/D	Glucose intolerance, diabetes not developed	Kitamura et al. (2002)
β*Pik3r1*$^{-/-}$; *Pik3r2*$^{-/-}$	↓ (32 weeks)	↑ Proliferation ↑ Apoptosis	N/D	↓	Glucose intolerance	Kaneko et al. (2010)
β*Pten*$^{-/-}$	↑ 4.5-fold	↑	↔	↔	Hypoglycemia Enhanced glucose tolerance	Stiles et al. (2006)
β*Rictor*$^{-/-}$	↓ 30%	Hypoplasia	↔	↓ GSIS	Glucose intolerance, hyperglycemia	Gu et al. (2011)
β*Rictor*$^{-/-}$; β*Pten*$^{-/-}$	↔[c]	↑	↑	↔	Normal	Gu et al. (2011)
β*Pdk1*$^{-/-}$	↓ 80%	Hypoplasia	↓	N/D	Hypoinsulinemia, severe diabetes	Hashimoto et al. (2006)
β*Pdk1*$^{-/-}$; *Foxo1*$^{+/-}$	↓ 50%[d]	Hypoplasia[d]	↓	N/D	Diabetes not developed	Hashimoto et al. (2006)

Akt1$^{-/-}$	N/D	N/D	N/D	N/D	Normal glucose tolerance	Cho, Thorvaldsen, et al. (2001)
Akt2$^{-/-}$	↑ Fourfold (compensatory) Biphasic[e]	N/D	N/D	N/D	Severe insulin resistance, glucose intolerance, diabetes development[e]	Cho, Mu, et al. (2001) and Garofalo et al. (2003)
β*Akt1-myr*	↑ Sixfold	↑ Threefold	↑ Two- to fivefold[f]	N/D	Hyperinsulinemia, insulinoma	Bernal-Mizrachi et al. (2001)
β*Akt1-myr*; *S6k1*$^{-/-}$/ *S6k2*$^{-/-}$	N/D	N/D	↓[g]	N/D	Insulinoma not developed	Alliouachene et al. (2008)
β*Gsk3β*-CA	↓ 40%	Hypoplasia	N/D	N/D	Glucose intolerance	Liu et al. (2008)
β*Gsk3β*$^{-/-}$	↑ 25%	Hyperplasia	N/D	N/D	Enhanced glucose tolerance	Liu et al. (2010)
β*Foxo1*$^{-/-}$	↓[h]	Dediferentiation[h]	N/D	↓ GSIS	Hypoinsulinemia, hyperglycemia	Talchai et al. (2012) and Kobayashi et al. (2012)
Pdx1$^{+/-}$; HFD	Compensatory increase impaired	↑ Apoptosis	No increase	↓ GSIS	Hypoinsulinemia, severe diabetes	Sachdeva et al. (2009)

[a]Normal β-cell mass when compared with WT, improved when compared with *Irs2*$^{-/-}$.
[b]Decreased 20% when compared with WT, improved when compared with *Irs2*$^{-/-}$.
[c]Normal β-cell mas when compared with WT, improved when compared with β*Pten*$^{-/-}$.
[d]Reduced β-cell mass due to hypoplasia, but much improved when compared with β*Pdk1*$^{-/-}$.
[e]Biphasic response of β cell mass and diabetes development only described by Garofalo and cols.
[f]Twofold size increase is described in Bernal-Mizrachi et al. (2001), but fivefold in Alliouachene et al. (2008).
[g]Decreased when compared with β*Akt1-myr*, but still increased compared with WT.
[h]Mice submitted to stress (aged males, multipareae females: Talchai and cols; diet or *Lepr*$^{-/-}$ background; Kobayashi and cols.). Dedifferentiation reported by Talchai and cols.

(Cousin et al., 1999; Hügl, White, & Rhodes, 1998). A study in a model of streptozotozin-induced diabetes showed how β-cell proliferation is positively related to glycemia (Pechhold et al., 2009). Others specifically show how increased β-cell glucose metabolism, rather than glycemia, is responsible for β-cell regeneration (Porat et al., 2011). In β-cell-specific glucokinase haploinsufficient mice, β-cell mass cannot be increased under high-fat diet, and diabetes is developed. Being glucokinase essential for glucose metabolism and signaling in β-cells, this work proves the key role of glucose on β-cell mass (Terauchi et al., 2007). Authors attribute this effect to IRS2 downregulation, observation in agreement with others showing positive role of glucose on IRS2 expression in β-cell lines or isolated islets (Lingohr et al., 2006).

Still, glucose effect on β-cell mass is insufficient under conditions where insulin/IGF-I is disrupted, as shown in βIRKO; βIGFIRKO mice, which develop diabetes with severe hyperglycemia and no compensatory β-cell mass increase (Ueki et al., 2006). GLP-1 enhancer effect on β-cell mass is glucose dependent (Buteau, Roduit, Susini, & Prentki, 1999). GLP-1 acts through AMPc as secondary messenger, which synthesized by adenylate cyclase in a manner dependent of ATP. GLP-1 is able to activate mTORC1 in a fashion dependent of Ca^{2+} and AMPc (Kwon, Marshall, Pappan, Remedi, & McDaniel, 2004). This supports the notion of glucose and GLP-1 synergic action, as glucose action on MEK–ERK/mTORC1 is also AMPc and Ca^{2+} dependent (Briaud et al., 2003; Guillen et al., 2006).

Glucose metabolism increases ATP:AMP ratio, hence influencing the quintessential energy sensor of the cell, the AMP-activated protein kinase (AMPK).

AMPK is a heterotrimeric complex composed of three subunits (α, β, γ), conserved in all eukaryotes. In mammals, there are two genes encoding different isoforms for the α catalytic subunit (α_1 and α_2), two of β (β_1 and β_2), and three of γ (γ_1, γ_2, and γ_3). All 12 possible combinations can exist, being some preferably found, reviewed in Hardie (2011). Although some isoforms are ubiquitously expressed, others do it in a tissue-specific manner. In β-cells, AMPKα_1 catalytical isoform is predominantly expressed (Da Silva Xavier et al., 2000; Sun et al., 2010). AMPK is activated by an increase in the AMP:ATP ratio, caused by metabolic stresses interfering with ATP production, scarcity of fuel or oxidizer (i.e., nutrient deprivation or hypoxia), or increased ATP consumption. AMP promotes the allosteric activation of AMPK, allowing phosphorylation of its Thr^{172} residue by LKB1 (liver kinase B1), thus increasing 100-fold AMPK catalytic activity (Jenne et al., 1998).

There is a plethora of proteins targeted by AMPK downstream action. AMPK constitutes one of the most important nodes of cell metabolism regulation, and the activation of the kinase leads to inhibition of ATP-consuming biosynthetic processes. Some of the AMPK targets are (1) on lipidic metabolism: ACC, HMG-CoA reductase. (2) On carbohydrate metabolism and transport: glycogen synthase, phosphofructokinase, AS160. (3) On protein synthesis and autophagy: TSC2, RAPTOR, ULK1. AMPK inhibits cell growth and proliferation by the inhibition of lipid, carbohydrate, and protein biosynthesis. Importance of AMPK in type 2 diabetes is evidenced, as this molecule is a target of biguanides such as metformin, one of the most commonly prescribed antidiabetic drugs. Although biguanides main effect is hepatic gluconeogenesis inhibition, the precise outcome of their specific action in β-cells is still obscure.

AMPK role on β-cell physiology has been extensively studied. AMPK plays an important role on insulin secretion, artificial activation of AMPK blocks GSIS (Leclerc et al., 2004; Salt, Johnson, Ashcroft, & Hardie, 1998), as it downregulates proinsulin expression (Da Silva Xavier et al., 2000; Kim et al., 2008) and secretory vesicles dynamics (Tsuboi, 2003). On the other hand, chronic AMPK activation mediated by AICAR or metformin can lead to β-cell apoptosis (Kefas et al., 2003, 2004), in a fashion dependent of JNK and caspase-3 (Kefas et al., 2003). *In vivo* effects of AMPK on β-cells were elegantly showed using streptozotozin-induced diabetic mice as islet transplantation recipients. Mice were divided in three groups and received islets expressing a control gene or either a constitutive active or a dominant-negative form of AMPK. Mice recipient of islets expressing a dominant-negative form of AMPK achieved a more efficient glycemic control, just the opposite as those expressing AMPK constitutive active form (Richards, Parton, Leclerc, Rutter, & Smith, 2005). Specific knockout mice of *Lkb1* in β-cells show enhanced glucose tolerance due to increased β-cell mass (hyperplasia and hypertrophy), and also enhanced insulin secretion (Fu et al., 2009; Granot et al., 2009). Loss of LKB1 impairs AMPK activity and consequently drives mTORC1-dependent cell hypertrophy, reversed by rapamycin treatment. Consistent with these data, β-cell-specific overexpression of a constitutive active form of AMPK results in 25% reduction in β-cell mass and glucose intolerance, while no major changes were reported on mice expressing dominant-negative AMPK

(Sun et al., 2010). Surprisingly, mice βAMPK-DKO (*Ampkα1*$^{-/-}$; β*Ampkα2*$^{-/-}$) does not show increased β-cell mass (Sun et al., 2010). An expected effect would be increased mTORC1 activity and hypertrophy, but authors show the opposite as these mice develop β-cell atrophy as well as severely compromised insulin secretion. These mice also developed AMPK deletion in hypothalamic neurons, due to RIP2 (rat insulin promoter)-driven Cre recombinase expression. Therefore, the increase in parasympathetic tone observed may obscure interpretation of results.

5.2. TSC1–TSC2 complex

TSC1 and *TSC2* genes were identified in 1997 and 1993 as the genetic loci mutated in the disease known as tuberous sclerosis complex (TSC) (European TSC Consortium, 1993; van Slegtenhorst et al., 1997). These genes' products are two proteins, TSC1 and TSC2, which do not share any homology between them, and very little with any other. Apparently, the only active domain within the two proteins is the C-terminal region of TSC2, showing GAP (GTPase-activating protein) activity (Zhang et al., 2003). TSC1 and TSC2 associate, establishing a heterodimer complex. TSC1 is required to stabilize TSC2 and prevent its ubiquitin-mediated proteasomal degradation or its sequestration by 14-3-3 binding (Li, Inoki, Yeung, & Guan, 2002; Shumway, Li, & Xiong, 2003). There is no other known downstream function for TSC1 apart from stabilizing TSC2; therefore, mutations in the *TSC1* locus affect TSC2 activity (Hodges et al., 2001).

The complex principal action is to serve as a brake of mTORC1 activity. In conditions in which TSC2 is stabilized by TSC1, and a proper status of phosphorylation, GAP activity toward Rheb (Ras-homolog enriched in brain) promotes Rheb GTPase activity and Rheb-GTP is hydrolyzed to Rheb-GDP, shutting off mTORC1 activity (Inoki, Li, Xu, & Guan, 2003; Zhang et al., 2003). The GEF (guanine exchange factor) that should be loading Rheb again with GTP is still unknown in mammals, although identified in *Drosophila* as dTCTP (translationally controlled tumor protein) (Hsu, Chern, Cai, Liu, & Choi, 2007).

TSC1 and TSC2 proteins are regulated by phosphorylation, mainly on TSC2 although TSC1 can also be phosphorylated by IKKβ (inhibitor of nuclear factor kappa-B kinase β) (Lee et al., 2007), Cdk1 (Astrinidis, Senapedis, Coleman, & Henske, 2003), and GSK3 (Mak, Kenerson, Aicher, Barnes, & Yeung, 2005). TSC2-GAP activity is maximal in low energy status and in the absence of growth factors.

Insulin signaling mediates TSC2 phosphorylation and inhibition in a manner dependent of Akt (Inoki et al., 2002; Manning et al., 2002) and ERK (Ma et al., 2005), promoting mTORC1 activation. Growth factors can also promote RSK-, DAPK-, and MK2-mediated TSC2 phosphorylation and inhibition (Li, Inoki, Vacratsis, & Guan, 2003; Roux, Ballif, Anjum, Gygi, & Blenis, 2004; Stevens et al., 2009).

But TSC2 can also be phosphorylated by AMPK in conditions of low ATP:AMP ratio, or other stress signals that activate the kinase. AMPK-mediated phosphorylation leads to TSC1–TSC2 complex stabilization, increasing GAP activity toward Rheb and allowing turning off mTORC1 signaling (Inoki, Zhu, & Guan, 2003). Wnt signaling can also regulate mTORC1 through GSK3-mediated phosphorylation of TSC2, which acts synergistically with AMPK to block mTORC1 signaling (Inoki et al., 2006). Other stress signals such as reactive oxygen species or hypoxia can also affect TSC2 activity and downregulate mTORC1 signaling (Alexander et al., 2010; Brugarolas et al., 2004).

Recently, another partner of the TSC1–TSC2 complex was identified, the TBC domain family member 7 (TBC1D7). This protein stabilizes the complex through interaction with TSC1 and increases complex activity toward Rheb (Dibble et al., 2012).

FoxO1 and TSC2 are phosphorylated and inhibited by Akt. After Akt-mediated phosphorylation, FoxO1 is excluded from nucleus and localized in cytoplasm, where is able to interact with TSC2 C-terminal region. This interaction impairs TSC2-GAP activity, promoting mTORC1 activation (Cao et al., 2006). TSC2 can also associate with the NAD^+-dependent deacetylase SIRT1 (Ghosh, McBurney, & Robbins, 2010). Although evidences of TSC1–TSC2 regulation by acetylation have not yet been found, this possibility is currently under our investigation. Another possibility would be that sirtuins might be modulating TSC2 interaction with FoxO transcription factors, as the latest are well-characterized targets of sirtuin deacetylase activity (Brunet et al., 2004; Nemoto, Fergusson, & Finkel, 2004).

5.3. mTORC1 regulation

TSC1–TSC2 complex, through TSC2-GAP domain, is the main regulator of mTORC1 activity. Rheb-GTP is able to free mTORC1 from its interaction with FKBP38. When FKBP38 is complexed with mTORC1, it inhibits its activity in similar fashion as rapamycin–FKBP12 does (Bai et al., 2007). However, TSC2-GAP promotes Rheb GTPase activity and

Rheb-GDP can no longer promote mTORC1 activation (Inoki, Li, et al., 2003).

Rheb-mediated mTORC1 activation is more complex, as Rheb-GTP is located in endomembranes. In order to localize mTORC1 with Rheb, the action of Rag-GTPases is needed. In the presence of amino acids, Rag-GTPases form heterodimers directly interacting with RAPTOR and relocate mTORC1 complex in the surface of endomembranes, where Rheb resides (Kim, Goraksha-Hicks, Li, Neufeld, & Guan, 2008; Sancak et al., 2008). In order to activate mTORC1, these two events must converge, TSC2 has to be inhibited so Rheb can be in its active GTP form, but also amino acid availability is important for Rag-GTPases-mediated relocation of mTORC1 as reviewed in Zoncu et al. (2011).

Other proteins can mediate Rheb-independent regulation of mTORC1. PRAS40, an inhibitor of mTORC1, can be phosphorylated and inhibited by Akt, therefore activating mTORC1 (Sancak et al., 2007). RAPTOR can also be modulated by phosphorylation, and AMPK mediates RAPTOR phosphorylation in $Ser^{727/792}$, promoting 14-3-3 binding and dissociation from mTORC1 (Gwinn et al., 2008). As RAPTOR is essential for mTORC1 functioning, AMPK-mediated phosphorylation has a negative impact on mTORC1 activity.

5.4. Downstream mTORC1 targets

mTORC1 is the major regulator of protein synthesis and ribosomal biogenesis, allowing fine coupling of cell size to cell-cycle progression. These processes are controlled by mTOR kinase activity-dependent phosphorylations. 4E-BP1 is phosphorylated and inhibited by mTORC1. Under growth limiting conditions, 4E-BP1 is repressing protein synthesis by binding to the transcription initiation factor eIF4E. mTORC1 promotes multiple phosphorylation of 4E-BP1, releasing eIF4E which binds to the translation initiation complex, allowing protein synthesis (Hara, 1997). mTORC1 also activates S6K by phosphorylation. S6K (present in two isoforms, S6K1 and S6K2) is one of the major effectors of cell growth. S6K directly phosphorylates the 40S ribosomal protein S6 (rpS6), activating protein synthesis and ribosomal biogenesis (Kuo et al., 1992). Phosphorylation of S6 allows selective translation of mRNA encoding for ribosomal proteins, which are identified by an oligopyrimidine signal in 5′ (5′-TOP) (Montagne et al., 1999). S6K activates multiple proteins of the mRNA translation machinery by phosphorylation or direct interaction, playing a role in both translation initiation and elongation reviewed in Ma and Bleniss (2009). As mTORC1 directs protein synthesis, hyperactivation of this pathway has been related with endoplasmic reticulum (ER) stress. This is observed in *Tsc1*$^{-/-}$ or *Tsc2*$^{-/-}$ fibroblasts, and in tumors from TSC patients (Ozcan et al., 2008).

S6K, as effector of mTORC1 signaling, mediates a negative feedback loop by phosphorylation of IRS proteins in serine, causing a desensitization of the pathway (Shah et al., 2004). Consistent with these findings, *S6k1*$^{-/-}$ mice are insulin hypersensitive and protected against obesity development on high-fat diet (Ozcan et al., 2004). *Lepr*$^{-/-}$ or wild type under high-fat diet shows hyperactivation of S6K and insulin resistance due to IRS1-Ser^{1101} phosphorylation in the liver (Tremblay et al., 2007).

5.5. mTORC1 and autophagy

mTORC1 is involved in protein catabolism as it negatively modulates autophagy. Rapamycin is a classical autophagy inducer (Noda & Ohsumi, 1998; Ravikumar et al., 2004). In yeast, under TORC1 inactivity, the complex formed by Atg1, Atg13, and Atg17 controls autophagy induction (Kamada et al., 2000). In mammals, there are two proteins with Atg1 homology: ULK1 and ULK2 (uncoordinated 51-like kinase); there are not clear mammal homologues of Atg17, although FIP200 seems to play its role (Hara et al., 2008). mTORC1 associates with ULK:Atg13:FIP200 complex through direct interaction with ULK1. When mTORC1 is active, it phosphorylates ULK1 and Atg13, inhibiting autophagy. Instead, lack of mTORC1 activity is a signal for autophagy induction (Ganley, Wong, Gammoh, & Jiang, 2011; Hosokawa et al., 2009; Kim, Kundu, Viollet, & Guan, 2011).

Inhibition of mTORC1 stimulates autophagy, but the lysosomal digestion of proteins generates free amino acids, which are able to reactivate mTORC1 signaling. Under these conditions, mTORC1 is responsible for the final destination of autolysosomes; since in an mTORC1-dependent manner, the lysosomal content of the cell is replenished (Yu et al., 2010). Hence, from these observations, we can evidence that mTORC1, besides being essential in autophagy induction, is also important for autophagy termination.

Mice with β-cell-specific autophagic impairment show the essentiality of this process for β-cell mass maintenance (Ebato et al., 2008; Jung et al., 2008). We have also recently showed how autophagy is important for β-cell survival under ER stress (Bartolomé, Guillén, & Benito, 2012), and how mTORC1 hyperactivation might be playing a negative effect on β-cell survival due to autophagy downregulation both *in vitro* and *in vivo* (Bartolomé et al., 2012) and unpublished results.

5.6. mTORC1 and mitochondria

mTORC1-mediated regulation of mitochondria can take place at multiple levels. In HEK293 cells, mTORC1 increases mitochondrial oxidative function, while rapamycin treatment diminishes mitochondrial membrane potential, oxygen consumption, and ATP production (Schieke et al., 2006). The mechanism responsible for these effects seems to be related with the formation of a ternary complex of mTORC1 with the peroxisome proliferator-activated receptor gamma coactivator 1α (PGC1α) and ying-yang-1 (YY1) transcription factors (Cunningham et al., 2007), leading to a transcriptional increase of key genes for mitochondrial metabolism.

Interestingly, young mice with mTORC1 hyperactivation in β-cells due to *Tsc2* deletion (β*Tsc2*$^{-/-}$) show increased expression of mitochondrial genes, mitochondrial number, and ATP content, this leading to increased GSIS (Koyanagi et al., 2011).

The role of mTORC1 in the selective autophagy of mitochondria (mitophagy) and mitochondrial dynamics is understudied, although mTORC1 inhibition has been recently reported to be required for mitophagy of mitochondria with mtDNA mutations (Gilkerson et al., 2012). Our data show how mTORC1 hyperactivation in β-cells impairs mitophagy and might contribute to mitochondrial dysfunction, oxidative stress, and β-cell failure (unpublished results).

5.7. TSC1–TSC2 and mTORC1 signaling in pancreatic β-cells

5.7.1 TSC1–TSC2 complex

Proof of the great interest aroused by the role of the TSC1–TSC2 complex in β-cells was the parallel emergence of four tissue-specific mice models in just over a year. There are two β-cell-specific *Tsc2* knock-out mice models (β*Tsc2*$^{-/-}$). Shigeyama and collaborators described the biphasic consequences of mTORC1 hyperactivation in β-cells, showing β-cell mass increase mediated by hypertrophy in young animals, together with hyperinsulinemia and hypoglycemia. However, insulin resistance was also found due to increased S6K activity, and β-cell mass regression occurred from weeks 30 to 35, followed by decreased insulinemia and severe diabetes. β-Cell failure was prevented by rapamycin treatment from week

18 (Shigeyama et al., 2008). This work also showed how increase of mTORC1 signaling in β-cells is a common feature of progression to type 2 diabetes, as also occurred in wild-type mice fed high-fat diet or *Lepr*$^{-/-}$ mice. We have recently unraveled some of the mechanisms that might be accounting for β-cell failure under mTORC1 hyperactivity in β*Tsc2*$^{-/-}$ mice, as β-cell ER stress develops in an age-dependent manner, and autophagy impairment is also found (unpublished results).

Surprisingly, other group working with β*Tsc2*$^{-/-}$ mice did only report β-cell mass increase, hyperinsulinemia, and hypoglycemia, but not followed by β-cell mass failure (Rachdi et al., 2008). In parallel, β*Tsc1*$^{-/-}$ was also generated and also showed β-cell hypertrophy, increased cell mass, hyperinsulinemia, and hypoglycemia. However, older β*Tsc1*$^{-/-}$ mice could not be studied as they die before week 30 due to neuroendocrine tumors arising from RIP2-Cre expression in the nervous system (Mori, Inoki, Münzberg, et al., 2009; Mori, Inoki, Opland, et al., 2009). Finally, another mouse model, expressing in β-cells a constitutive active form of Rheb, showed similar phenotype as TSC complex-deficient mice, but in a more limited fashion (Hamada et al., 2009), probably as TSC2-GAP activity remains intact in these mice.

5.7.2 mTORC1 and rapamycin treatment

Rapamycin is used as immunosuppressant after islet transplantation, following Edmonton Protocol (Shapiro et al., 2000). Although this protocol has provided the best results up to date, largely avoiding graft rejection (Shapiro et al., 2006); there are certain doubts about the possible toxicity of rapamycin for islets, and how this could be affecting progressive β-cell dysfunction observed in transplanted patents (Desai et al., 2003). Rapamycin toxicity was proved in mice recipient for islet transplantation (Zhang et al., 2006); its deleterious effect on isolated islets and β-cell lines is also well known (Aronovitz et al., 2008; Bartolomé et al., 2010; Bell et al., 2003; Tanemura et al., 2012). Some authors propose that long-term toxicity of rapamycin on β-cells is consequence of mTORC2 inhibition (Barlow et al., 2012).

Rapamycin therapy also impairs β-cell mass adaptation during pregnancy in mice (Zahr et al., 2007). Rapamycin is able to increase systemic insulin sensitivity through mTORC1/S6K1 blockade, which short circuits feedback loop on IRS (Shah et al., 2004; Um et al., 2004). Yet the attempts to use it as to improve the metabolic parameters of *Psammomys obesus* feed high-fat diet were unsuccessful (Fraenkel et al., 2008). As rapamycin blocks compensatory β-cell mass increase under high-fat diet, hyperinsulinemia does not take place in rapamycin-treated animals, which develop severe diabetes. Other study also found how mTORC1 activity is also important for cell-cycle progression, as it directly stabilizes cyclin D2. Rapamycin treatment of mice reduced cyclin D2 synthesis and stability as well as Cdk4 activity, impairing β-cell proliferation (Balcazar et al., 2009).

5.7.3 mTORC1 downstream targets

Downstream mTORC1 targets such as S6K have also been found to largely impact β-cell mass. *S6k1*$^{-/-}$ mice present a characteristic phenotype highly influenced from β-cell-derived effects (Pende et al., 2000). *S6k1*$^{-/-}$ mice are insulin hypersensitive due to reduced S6K-mediated IRS serine phosphorylation, but these mice are also display atrophic β-cells, hypoinsulinemia, and glucose intolerance derived from reduced β-cell mass. On the other hand, β-cell-specific overexpression of a constitutive active form of S6K (β*S6kCA*) does not lead to overall β-cell mass increase, as hypertrophy and hypoplasia are observed. Although Ki67 reactivity in β*S6kCA* islets is higher, β-cells are not fully able to progress through cell-cycle and hypoplasia results from increased apoptosis. Authors indicate that chronic insulin resistance in these mice, leading to enhanced expression of cell-cycle inhibitors such as p21 and p27$^{\mathrm{Kip1}}$ may account for increased apoptosis in β*S6kCA* mice (Elghazi et al., 2010).

A systemic knock-in model of the ribosomal protein S6 (rpS6), with its five phosphorylatable residues substituted by alanine, showed specific β-cell atrophy, followed by hypoinsulinemia and glucose intolerance (Ruvinsky et al., 2005). The fact that other cell types showed normal cell size indicates the central role of rpS6 in pancreatic β-cells.

The obesity model lacking leptin receptor (*Lepr*$^{-/-}$), previously found to display mTORC1 hyperactivation in β-cells (Shigeyama et al., 2008), also shows increased ribosomal biogenesis in β-cells. However, this observation was connected to ER stress and β-cell failure developed in *Lepr*$^{-/-}$ mice (Asahara, Matsuda, Kido, & Kasuga, 2009).

Up to date, most of the research conducted on mTORC1 signaling in β-cells indicates the positive role of this pathway. However, some data also indicate negative effects derived from chronic mTORC1/S6K hyperactivation and insulin resistance. Other aspects of mTORC1 hyperactivation such as ER stress and autophagy inhibition have not been fully explored, and this remains a field of potential interest (Table 17.2).

Table 17.2 mTORC1 signaling in β-cells: mouse models

Model	β-Cell mass: Total	β-Cell mass: Cell number	β-Cell mass: Cell size	β-Cell function	Phenotype	References
β*Lkb1*$^{-/-}$	↑ 37%	N/D	Hyperthrophy	↑ GSIS	Hyperinsulinemia, enhanced glucose tolerance	Fu et al. (2009) and Granot et al. (2009)
β*Ampkα1*$^{-/-}$; β*Ampkα2*$^{-/-a}$	↔	Hyperplasia	Atrophy	↓ GSIS	Glucose intolerance	Sun et al. (2010)
β*Ampkα1*-CA	↓ 25%	N/D	N/D	↓ GSIS	Mild glucose intolerance	Sun et al. (2010)
β*Ampkα1*-DN	↔	N/D	N/D	↑ GSIS	Normal	Sun et al. (2010)
β*Tsc1*$^{-/-a}$	↑ Twofold	↔	↑	↑ GSIS	Hyperinsulinemia	Mori, Inoki, Münzberg, et al. (2009) and Mori, Inoki, Opland, et al. (2009)
β*Tsc2*$^{-/-}$ (I)	↑ 2.5-fold (8 weeks) ↓ 75% (40 weeks)	↔ (8 weeks) ↑ Apoptosis (older)	↑ 4.5-fold (volume)[b]	↑ GSIS	Hyperinsulinemia. β-cell failure in older mice, hyperglycemia	Shigeyama et al. (2008) and Koyanagi et al. (2011)
β*Tsc2*$^{-/-}$ (II)	↑ 2.5 fold	Hyperplasia	↑ 1.6-fold	↑ GSIS	Hyperinsulinemia, enhanced glucose tolerance	Rachdi et al. (2008)
β*Rheb*-CA	↑ 25%	↔	↑ 1.3-fold	↑ GSIS	Hyperinsulinemia, enhanced glucose tolerance	Hamada et al. (2009)

Continued

Table 17.2 mTORC1 signaling in β-cells: mouse models—cont'd

Model	β-Cell mass			β-Cell function	Phenotype	References
	Total	Cell number	Cell size			
S6k1$^{-/-}$	↓	↔	Atrophy	↓ GSIS	Glucose intolerance, insulin hypersensitivity, hypoinsulinemia	Pende et al. (2000)
β*S6k1*-CA	↔	↑ Apoptosis	↑ Twofold	↑ GSIS	Hyperinsulinemia, enhanced glucose tolerance	Elghazi et al. (2010)
Rps6$^{P-/-}$	↓	N/D	Atrophy	↓ GSIS	Mild glucose intolerance	Ruvinsky et al. (2005)

[a] Also show deletion in hypothalamic neurons due to RIP2-Cre expression.
[b] Volume analysis, our unpublished data.

6. CONCLUSIONS AND FUTURE DIRECTIONS

In pancreatic β-cells, insulin signaling and activation of mTOR complexes are positive players in β-cell mass regulation. Integration of nutritional and hormonal signals through TSC1–TSC2 complex and mTORC1 is important for β-cell mass adaptation under different pathophysiological circumstances. Enhanced mTORC1/mTORC2 signaling is essentially required for β-cell mass increase under higher metabolic load (Fraenkel et al., 2008; Otani et al., 2004). However, recent evidences suggest that chronic mTORC1 hyperactivity in β-cells may also be having negative consequences on β-cell lifespan, and thus promoting type 2 diabetes onset (Elghazi et al., 2010; Shigeyama et al., 2008). mTORC1 hyperactivity is a well-known cause of insulin resistance and ER stress (Ozcan et al., 2008; Um et al., 2004). Also, mTORC1 negatively modulates autophagy, an essential process with important homeostatic and cytoprotective effects in β-cells (Ebato et al., 2008; Jung et al., 2008). In fact, mTOR is considered a master regulator of aging in mammals and other organisms (Harrison et al., 2009; Vellai et al., 2003), and evidences link the beneficial effects of dietary restriction with mTORC1 inhibition (Selman et al., 2009). Future studies focused on these processes, and the possible connection of mTORC1 hyperactivation leading to β-cell dysfunction would be needed to further clarify the role of mTOR in β-cells.

REFERENCES

Accili, D., Drago, J., Lee, E. J., Johnson, M. D., Cool, M. H., Salvatore, P., et al. (1996). Early neonatal death in mice homozygous for a null allele of the insulin receptor gene. *Nature Genetics, 12*, 106–109.

Alexander, A., Cai, S.-L., Kim, J., Nanez, A., Sahin, M., MacLean, K. H., et al. (2010). ATM signals to TSC2 in the cytoplasm to regulate mTORC1 in response to ROS. *Proceedings of the National Academy of Sciences of the United States of America, 107*, 4153–4158.

Alliouachene, S., Tuttle, R. L., Boumard, S., Lapointe, T., Berissi, S., Germain, S., et al. (2008). Constitutively active Akt1 expression in mouse pancreas requires S6 kinase 1 for insulinoma formation. *The Journal of Clinical Investigation, 118*, 3629–3638.

Andrade, M. A., Perez-Iratxeta, C., & Ponting, C. P. (2001). Protein repeats: Structures, functions, and evolution. *Journal of Structural Biology, 134*, 117–131.

Araki, E., Lipes, M. A., Patti, M.-E., Brüning, J. C., Haag, B., III., Johnson, R. S., et al. (1994). Alternative pathway of insulin signalling in mice with targeted disruption of the IRS-1 gene. *Nature, 372*, 186–190.

Aronovitz, A., Josefson, J., Fisher, A., Newman, M., Hughes, E., Chen, F., et al. (2008). Rapamycin inhibits growth factor-induced cell cycle regulation in pancreatic beta cells. *Journal of Investigative Medicine: The Official Publication of the American Federation for Clinical Research, 56*, 985–996.

Asahara, S.-I., Matsuda, T., Kido, Y., & Kasuga, M. (2009). Increased ribosomal biogenesis induces pancreatic beta cell failure in mice model of type 2 diabetes. *Biochemical and Biophysical Research Communications, 381*, 367–371.
Astrinidis, A., Senapedis, W., Coleman, T. R., & Henske, E. P. (2003). Cell cycle-regulated phosphorylation of hamartin, the product of the tuberous sclerosis complex 1 gene, by cyclin-dependent kinase 1/cyclin B. *The Journal of Biological Chemistry, 278*, 51372–51379.
Bai, X., Ma, D., Liu, A., Shen, X., Wang, Q. J., Liu, Y., et al. (2007). Rheb activates mTOR by antagonizing its endogenous inhibitor FKBP38. *Science (New York, NY), 318*, 977–980.
Balcazar, N., Sathyamurthy, A., Elghazi, L., Gould, A., Weiss, A., Shiojima, I., et al. (2009). mTORC1 activation regulates beta-cell mass and proliferation by modulation of cyclin D2 synthesis and stability. *The Journal of Biological Chemistry, 284*, 7832–7842.
Barlow, A. D., Xie, J., Moore, C. E., Campbell, S. C., Shaw, J. A. M., Nicholson, M. L., et al. (2012). Rapamycin toxicity in MIN6 cells and rat and human islets is mediated by the inhibition of mTOR complex 2 (mTORC2). *Diabetologia, 55*, 1355–1365.
Bartolomé, A., Guillén, C., & Benito, M. (2010). Role of the TSC1-TSC2 complex in the integration of insulin and glucose signaling involved in pancreatic beta-cell proliferation. *Endocrinology, 151*, 3084–3094.
Bartolomé, A., Guillén, C., & Benito, M. (2012). Autophagy plays a protective role in endoplasmic reticulum stress-mediated pancreatic β cell death. *Autophagy, 8*, 1757–1768.
Belfiore, A., Frasca, F., Pandini, G., Sciacca, L., & Vigneri, R. (2009). Insulin receptor isoforms and insulin receptor/insulin-like growth factor receptor hybrids in physiology and disease. *Endocrine Reviews, 30*, 586–623.
Bell, E., Cao, X., Moibi, J. A., Greene, S. R., Young, R., Trucco, M., et al. (2003). Rapamycin has a deleterious effect on MIN-6 cells and rat and human islets. *Diabetes, 52*, 2731–2739.
Bernal-Mizrachi, E., Wen, W., Stahlhut, S., Welling, C. M., & Permutt, M. A. (2001). Islet beta cell expression of constitutively active Akt1/PKB alpha induces striking hypertrophy, hyperplasia, and hyperinsulinemia. *The Journal of Clinical Investigation, 108*, 1631–1638.
Bock, T., Pakkenberg, B., & Buschard, K. (2003). Increased islet volume but unchanged islet number in ob/ob mice. *Diabetes, 52*, 1716–1722.
Bonner-Weir, S., Deery, D., Leahy, J. L., & Weir, G. C. (1989). Compensatory growth of pancreatic beta-cells in adult rats after short-term glucose infusion. *Diabetes, 38*, 49–53.
Bosotti, R., Isacchi, A., & Sonnhammer, E. L. (2000). FAT: A novel domain in PIK-related kinases. *Trends in Biochemical Sciences, 25*, 225–227.
Brelje, T. C., Scharp, D. W., Lacy, P. E., Ogren, L., Talamantes, F., Robertson, M., et al. (1993). Effect of homologous placental lactogens, prolactins, and growth hormones on islet B-cell division and insulin secretion in rat, mouse, and human islets: Implication for placental lactogen regulation of islet function during pregnancy. *Endocrinology, 132*, 879–887.
Briaud, I., Lingohr, M. K., Dickson, L. M., Wrede, C. E., & Rhodes, C. J. (2003). Differential activation mechanisms of Erk-1/2 and p70(S6K) by glucose in pancreatic beta-cells. *Diabetes, 52*, 974–983.
Brown, E. J., Albers, M. W., Shin, T. B., Ichikawa, K., Keith, C. T., Lane, W. S., et al. (1994). A mammalian protein targeted by G1-arresting rapamycin-receptor complex. *Nature, 369*, 756–758.
Brugarolas, J., Lei, K., Hurley, R. L., Manning, B. D., Reiling, J. H., Hafen, E., et al. (2004). Regulation of mTOR function in response to hypoxia by REDD1 and the TSC1/TSC2 tumor suppressor complex. *Genes & Development, 18*, 2893–2904.

Brunet, A., Sweeney, L. B., Sturgill, J. F., Chua, K. F., Greer, P. L., Lin, Y., et al. (2004). Stress-dependent regulation of FOXO transcription factors by the SIRT1 deacetylase. *Science (New York, NY)*, *303*, 2011–2015.

Brüning, J. C., Winnay, J., Bonner-Weir, S., Taylor, S. I., Accili, D., & Kahn, C. R. (1997). Development of a novel polygenic model of NIDDM in mice heterozygous for IR and IRS-1 null alleles. *Cell*, *88*, 561–572.

Buteau, J., Roduit, R., Susini, S., & Prentki, M. (1999). Glucagon-like peptide-1 promotes DNA synthesis, activates phosphatidylinositol 3-kinase and increases transcription factor pancreatic and duodenal homeobox gene 1 (PDX-1) DNA binding activity in beta (INS-1)-cells. *Diabetologia*, *42*, 856–864.

Butler, A. E., Cao-Minh, L., Galasso, R., Rizza, R. A., Corradin, A., Cobelli, C., et al. (2010). Adaptive changes in pancreatic beta cell fractional area and beta cell turnover in human pregnancy. *Diabetologia*, *53*, 2167–2176.

Butler, A. E., Janson, J., Bonner-Weir, S., Ritzel, R., Rizza, R. A., & Butler, P. C. (2003). Beta-cell deficit and increased beta-cell apoptosis in humans with type 2 diabetes. *Diabetes*, *52*, 102–110.

Cao, Y., Kamioka, Y., Yokoi, N., Kobayashi, T., Hino, O., Onodera, M., et al. (2006). Interaction of FoxO1 and TSC2 induces insulin resistance through activation of the mammalian target of rapamycin/p70 S6K pathway. *The Journal of Biological Chemistry*, *281*, 40242–40251.

Chen, C.-C., Jeon, S.-M., Bhaskar, P. T., Nogueira, V., Sundararajan, D., Tonic, I., et al. (2010). FoxOs inhibit mTORC1 and activate Akt by inducing the expression of Sestrin3 and Rictor. *Developmental Cell*, *18*, 592–604.

Cheng, S. W. Y., Fryer, L. G. D., Carling, D., & Shepherd, P. R. (2004). Thr2446 is a novel mammalian target of rapamycin (mTOR) phosphorylation site regulated by nutrient status. *The Journal of Biological Chemistry*, *279*, 15719–15722.

Chiang, G. G., & Abraham, R. T. (2005). Phosphorylation of mammalian target of rapamycin (mTOR) at Ser-2448 is mediated by p70S6 kinase. *The Journal of Biological Chemistry*, *280*, 25485–25490.

Cho, H., Mu, J., Kim, J. K., Thorvaldsen, J. L., Chu, Q., Crenshaw, E. B., et al. (2001). Insulin resistance and a diabetes mellitus-like syndrome in mice lacking the protein kinase Akt2 (PKB beta). *Science (New York, NY)*, *292*, 1728–1731.

Cho, H., Thorvaldsen, J. L., Chu, Q., Feng, F., & Birnbaum, M. J. (2001). Akt1/PKBalpha is required for normal growth but dispensable for maintenance of glucose homeostasis in mice. *The Journal of Biological Chemistry*, *276*, 38349–38352.

Choi, J., Chen, J., Schreiber, S. L., & Clardy, J. (1996). Structure of the FKBP12-rapamycin complex interacting with the binding domain of human FRAP. *Science (New York, NY)*, *273*, 239–242.

Choudhury, A. I., Heffron, H., Smith, M. A., Al-Qassab, H., Xu, A. W., Selman, C., et al. (2005). The role of insulin receptor substrate 2 in hypothalamic and beta cell function. *The Journal of Clinical Investigation*, *115*, 940–950.

Cnop, M., Hughes, S. J., Igoillo-Esteve, M., Hoppa, M. B., Sayyed, F., van de Laar, L., et al. (2010). The long lifespan and low turnover of human islet beta cells estimated by mathematical modelling of lipofuscin accumulation. *Diabetologia*, *53*, 321–330.

Cousin, S. P., Hügl, S. R., Myers, M. G., White, M. F., Reifel-Miller, A., & Rhodes, C. J. (1999). Stimulation of pancreatic beta-cell proliferation by growth hormone is glucose-dependent: Signal transduction via janus kinase 2 (JAK2)/signal transducer and activator of transcription 5 (STAT5) with no crosstalk to insulin receptor substrate-mediated mitogenic signalling. *The Biochemical Journal*, *344*(Pt. 3), 649–658.

Craparo, A., Freund, R., & Gustafson, T. A. (1997). 14-3-3 (Epsilon) interacts with the insulin-like growth factor I receptor and insulin receptor substrate I in a phosphoserine-dependent manner. *The Journal of Biological Chemistry, 272*, 11663–11669.

Cross, D. A., Alessi, D. R., Cohen, P., Andjelkovich, M., & Hemmings, B. A. (1995). Inhibition of glycogen synthase kinase-3 by insulin mediated by protein kinase B. *Nature, 378*, 785–789.

Cunningham, J. T., Rodgers, J. T., Arlow, D. H., Vazquez, F., Mootha, V. K., & Puigserver, P. (2007). mTOR controls mitochondrial oxidative function through a YY1-PGC-1alpha transcriptional complex. *Nature, 450*, 736–740.

Da Silva Xavier, G., Leclerc, I., Salt, I. P., Doiron, B., Hardie, D. G., Kahn, A., et al. (2000). Role of AMP-activated protein kinase in the regulation by glucose of islet beta cell gene expression. *Proceedings of the National Academy of Sciences of the United States of America, 97*, 4023–4028.

Del Guerra, S., Lupi, R., Marselli, L., Masini, M., Bugliani, M., Sbrana, S., et al. (2005). Functional and molecular defects of pancreatic islets in human type 2 diabetes. *Diabetes, 54*, 727–735.

Denley, A., Bonython, E. R., Booker, G. W., Cosgrove, L. J., Forbes, B. E., Ward, C. W., et al. (2004). Structural determinants for high-affinity binding of insulin-like growth factor II to insulin receptor (IR)-A, the exon 11 minus isoform of the IR. *Molecular Endocrinology (Baltimore, Md), 18*, 2502–2512.

Denley, A., Wallace, J. C., Cosgrove, L. J., & Forbes, B. E. (2003). The insulin receptor isoform exon 11-(IR-A) in cancer and other diseases: A review. *Hormone and Metabolic Research Hormon- und Stoffwechselforschung Hormones et métabolisme, 35*, 778–785.

Desai, N. M., Goss, J. A., Deng, S., Wolf, B. A., Markmann, E., Palanjian, M., et al. (2003). Elevated portal vein drug levels of sirolimus and tacrolimus in islet transplant recipients: Local immunosuppression or islet toxicity? *Transplantation, 76*, 1623–1625.

Dibble, C. C., Elis, W., Menon, S., Qin, W., Klekota, J., Asara, J. M., et al. (2012). TBC1D7 is a third subunit of the TSC1-TSC2 complex upstream of mTORC1. *Molecular Cell, 47*, 535–546.

Dor, Y., Brown, J., Martinez, O. I., & Melton, D. A. (2004). Adult pancreatic beta-cells are formed by self-duplication rather than stem-cell differentiation. *Nature, 429*, 41–46.

Ebato, C., Uchida, T., Arakawa, M., Komatsu, M., Ueno, T., Komiya, K., et al. (2008). Autophagy is important in islet homeostasis and compensatory increase of beta cell mass in response to high-fat diet. *Cell Metabolism, 8*, 325–332.

Edinger, A. L., & Thompson, C. B. (2004). An activated mTOR mutant supports growth factor-independent, nutrient-dependent cell survival. *Oncogene, 23*, 5654–5663.

Elchebly, M., Payette, P., Michaliszyn, E., Cromlish, W., Collins, S., Loy, A. L., et al. (1999). Increased insulin sensitivity and obesity resistance in mice lacking the protein tyrosine phosphatase-1B gene. *Science (New York, NY), 283*, 1544–1548.

Elghazi, L., Balcazar, N., Blandino-Rosano, M., Cras-Méneur, C., Fatrai, S., Gould, A. P., et al. (2010). Decreased IRS signaling impairs beta-cell cycle progression and survival in transgenic mice overexpressing S6K in beta-cells. *Diabetes, 59*, 2390–2399.

Engelman, J. A., Luo, J., & Cantley, L. C. (2006). The evolution of phosphatidylinositol 3-kinases as regulators of growth and metabolism. *Nature Reviews Genetics, 7*, 606–619.

Escribano, O., Guillén, C., Nevado, C., Gómez-Hernández, A., Kahn, C. R., & Benito, M. (2009). Beta-Cell hyperplasia induced by hepatic insulin resistance: Role of a liver-pancreas endocrine axis through insulin receptor A isoform. *Diabetes, 58*, 820–828.

European TSC Consortium (1993). Identification and characterization of the tuberous sclerosis gene on chromosome 16. *Cell, 75*, 1305–1315.

Fatrai, S., Elghazi, L., Balcazar, N., Cras-Méneur, C., Krits, I., Kiyokawa, H., et al. (2006). Akt induces beta-cell proliferation by regulating cyclin D1, cyclin D2, and p21 levels and cyclin-dependent kinase-4 activity. *Diabetes, 55*, 318–325.

Figeac, F., Ilias, A., Bailbe, D., Portha, B., & Movassat, J. (2012). Local in vivo GSK3β knockdown promotes pancreatic β cell and acinar cell regeneration in 90% pancreatectomized rat. *Molecular Therapy: The Journal of the American Society of Gene Therapy, 20*, 1944–1952. http://dx.doi.org/10.1038/mt.2012.112.

Fraenkel, M., Ketzinel-Gilad, M., Ariav, Y., Pappo, O., Karaca, M., Castel, J., et al. (2008). mTOR inhibition by rapamycin prevents beta-cell adaptation to hyperglycemia and exacerbates the metabolic state in type 2 diabetes. *Diabetes, 57*, 945–957.

Frödin, M., Sekine, N., Roche, E., Filloux, C., Prentki, M., Wollheim, C. B., et al. (1995). Glucose, other secretagogues, and nerve growth factor stimulate mitogen-activated protein kinase in the insulin-secreting beta-cell line, INS-1. *The Journal of Biological Chemistry, 270*, 7882–7889.

Fu, A., Ng, A. C.-H., Depatie, C., Wijesekara, N., He, Y., Wang, G.-S., et al. (2009). Loss of Lkb1 in adult beta cells increases beta cell mass and enhances glucose tolerance in mice. *Cell Metabolism, 10*, 285–295.

Fujimoto, K., Hanson, P. T., Tran, H., Ford, E. L., Han, Z., Johnson, J. D., et al. (2009). Autophagy regulates pancreatic beta cell death in response to Pdx1 deficiency and nutrient deprivation. *The Journal of Biological Chemistry, 284*, 27664–27673.

Ganley, I. G., Wong, P.-M., Gammoh, N., & Jiang, X. (2011). Distinct autophagosomal-lysosomal fusion mechanism revealed by thapsigargin-induced autophagy arrest. *Molecular Cell, 42*, 731–743.

García-Martínez, J. M., Moran, J., Clarke, R. G., Gray, A., Cosulich, S. C., Chresta, C. M., et al. (2009). Ku-0063794 is a specific inhibitor of the mammalian target of rapamycin (mTOR). *The Biochemical Journal, 421*, 29–42.

Garofalo, R. S., Orena, S. J., Rafidi, K., Torchia, A. J., Stock, J. L., Hildebrandt, A. L., et al. (2003). Severe diabetes, age-dependent loss of adipose tissue, and mild growth deficiency in mice lacking Akt2/PKB beta. *The Journal of Clinical Investigation, 112*, 197–208.

Ghosh, H. S., McBurney, M., & Robbins, P. D. (2010). SIRT1 negatively regulates the mammalian target of rapamycin. *PloS One, 5*, e9199.

Gilkerson, R. W., de Vries, R. L. A., Lebot, P., Wikstrom, J. D., Torgyekes, E., Shirihai, O. S., et al. (2012). Mitochondrial autophagy in cells with mtDNA mutations results from synergistic loss of transmembrane potential and mTORC1 inhibition. *Human Molecular Genetics, 21*, 978–990.

Goldstein, B. J., Li, P. M., Ding, W., Ahmad, F., & Zhang, W. R. (1998). Regulation of insulin action by protein tyrosine phosphatases. *Vitamins and Hormones, 54*, 67–96.

Gonzalez, E., & McGraw, T. E. (2009). The Akt kinases: Isoform specificity in metabolism and cancer. *Cell Cycle (Georgetown, Tex), 8*, 2502–2508.

Granot, Z., Swisa, A., Magenheim, J., Stolovich-Rain, M., Fujimoto, W., Manduchi, E., et al. (2009). LKB1 regulates pancreatic beta cell size, polarity, and function. *Cell Metabolism, 10*, 296–308.

Grempler, R., Leicht, S., Kischel, I., Eickelmann, P., & Redemann, N. (2007). Inhibition of SH2-domain containing inositol phosphatase 2 (SHIP2) in insulin producing INS1E cells improves insulin signal transduction and induces proliferation. *FEBS Letters, 581*, 5885–5890.

Gu, Y., Lindner, J., Kumar, A., Yuan, W., & Magnuson, M. A. (2011). Rictor/mTORC2 is essential for maintaining a balance between beta-cell proliferation and cell size. *Diabetes, 60*, 827–837.

Guertin, D. A., Stevens, D. M., Thoreen, C. C., Burds, A. A., Kalaany, N. Y., Moffat, J., et al. (2006). Ablation in mice of the mTORC components raptor, rictor, or mLST8 reveals that mTORC2 is required for signaling to Akt-FOXO and PKCalpha, but not S6K1. *Developmental Cell, 11*, 859–871.

Guillam, M. T., Hümmler, E., Schaerer, E., Yeh, J. I., Birnbaum, M. J., Beermann, F., et al. (1997). Early diabetes and abnormal postnatal pancreatic islet development in mice lacking Glut-2. *Nature Genetics, 17*, 327–330.
Guillen, C., Navarro, P., Robledo, M., Valverde, A. M., & Benito, M. (2006). Differential mitogenic signaling in insulin receptor-deficient fetal pancreatic beta-cells. *Endocrinology, 147*, 1959–1968.
Gwinn, D. M., Shackelford, D. B., Egan, D. F., Mihaylova, M. M., Mery, A., Vasquez, D. S., et al. (2008). AMPK phosphorylation of raptor mediates a metabolic checkpoint. *Molecular Cell, 30*, 214–226.
Hamada, S., Hara, K., Hamada, T., Yasuda, H., Moriyama, H., Nakayama, R., et al. (2009). Upregulation of the mammalian target of rapamycin complex 1 pathway by Ras homolog enriched in brain in pancreatic beta-cells leads to increased beta-cell mass and prevention of hyperglycemia. *Diabetes, 58*, 1321–1332.
Hara, K. (1997). Regulation of eIF-4E BP1 phosphorylation by mTOR. *Journal of Biological Chemistry, 272*, 26457–26463.
Hara, K., Maruki, Y., Long, X., Yoshino, K.-I., Oshiro, N., Hidayat, S., et al. (2002). Raptor, a binding partner of target of rapamycin (TOR), mediates TOR action. *Cell, 110*, 177–189.
Hara, T., Takamura, A., Kishi, C., Iemura, S.-I., Natsume, T., Guan, J.-L., et al. (2008). FIP200, a ULK-interacting protein, is required for autophagosome formation in mammalian cells. *The Journal of Cell Biology, 181*, 497–510.
Hardie, D. G. (2011). AMP-activated protein kinase: An energy sensor that regulates all aspects of cell function. *Genes & Development, 25*, 1895–1908.
Harrison, D. E., Strong, R., Sharp, Z. D., Nelson, J. F., Astle, C. M., Flurkey, K., et al. (2009). Rapamycin fed late in life extends lifespan in genetically heterogeneous mice. *Nature, 460*, 392–395.
Hashimoto, N., Kido, Y., Uchida, T., Asahara, S.-I., Shigeyama, Y., Matsuda, T., et al. (2006). Ablation of PDK1 in pancreatic beta cells induces diabetes as a result of loss of beta cell mass. *Nature Genetics, 38*, 589–593.
Heitman, J., Movva, N. R., & Hall, M. N. (1991). Targets for cell cycle arrest by the immunosuppressant rapamycin in yeast. *Science (New York, NY), 253*, 905–909.
Hennige, A. M., Burks, D. J., Ozcan, U., Kulkarni, R. N., Ye, J., Park, S., et al. (2003). Upregulation of insulin receptor substrate-2 in pancreatic beta cells prevents diabetes. *The Journal of Clinical Investigation, 112*, 1521–1532.
Hodges, A. K., Li, S., Maynard, J., Parry, L., Braverman, R., Cheadle, J. P., et al. (2001). Pathological mutations in TSC1 and TSC2 disrupt the interaction between hamartin and tuberin. *Human Molecular Genetics, 10*, 2899–2905.
Holz, M. K., & Blenis, J. (2005). Identification of S6 kinase 1 as a novel mammalian target of rapamycin (mTOR)-phosphorylating kinase. *The Journal of Biological Chemistry, 280*, 26089–26093.
Hosokawa, N., Hara, T., Kaizuka, T., Kishi, C., Takamura, A., Miura, Y., et al. (2009). Nutrient-dependent mTORC1 association with the ULK1-Atg13-FIP200 complex required for autophagy. *Molecular Biology of the Cell, 20*, 1981–1991.
Hotamisligil, G. S., Peraldi, P., Budavari, A., Ellis, R., White, M. F., & Spiegelman, B. M. (1996). IRS-1-mediated inhibition of insulin receptor tyrosine kinase activity in TNF-alpha- and obesity-induced insulin resistance. *Science (New York, NY), 271*, 665–668.
Hribal, M. L., Perego, L., Lovari, S., Andreozzi, F., Menghini, R., Perego, C., et al. (2003). Chronic hyperglycemia impairs insulin secretion by affecting insulin receptor expression, splicing, and signaling in RIN beta cell line and human islets of Langerhans. *The FASEB Journal: Official Publication of the Federation of American Societies for Experimental Biology, 17*, 1340–1342.

Hsu, Y.-C., Chern, J. J., Cai, Y., Liu, M., & Choi, K.-W. (2007). Drosophila TCTP is essential for growth and proliferation through regulation of dRheb GTPase. *Nature*, *445*, 785–788.

Huang, J., Dibble, C. C., Matsuzaki, M., & Manning, B. D. (2008). The TSC1-TSC2 complex is required for proper activation of mTOR complex 2. *Molecular and Cellular Biology*, *28*, 4104–4115.

Hügl, S. R., White, M. F., & Rhodes, C. J. (1998). Insulin-like growth factor I (IGF-I)-stimulated pancreatic beta-cell growth is glucose-dependent. Synergistic activation of insulin receptor substrate-mediated signal transduction pathways by glucose and IGF-I in INS-1 cells. *The Journal of Biological Chemistry*, *273*, 17771–17779.

Ikenoue, T., Inoki, K., Yang, Q., Zhou, X., & Guan, K.-L. (2008). Essential function of TORC2 in PKC and Akt turn motif phosphorylation, maturation and signalling. *The EMBO Journal*, *27*, 1919–1931.

Inoki, K., Li, Y., Xu, T., & Guan, K.-L. (2003). Rheb GTPase is a direct target of TSC2 GAP activity and regulates mTOR signaling. *Genes & Development*, *17*, 1829–1834.

Inoki, K., Li, Y., Zhu, T., Wu, J., & Guan, K.-L. (2002). TSC2 is phosphorylated and inhibited by Akt and suppresses mTOR signalling. *Nature Cell Biology*, *4*, 648–657.

Inoki, K., Ouyang, H., Zhu, T., Lindvall, C., Wang, Y., Zhang, X., et al. (2006). TSC2 integrates Wnt and energy signals via a coordinated phosphorylation by AMPK and GSK3 to regulate cell growth. *Cell*, *126*, 955–968.

Inoki, K., Zhu, T., & Guan, K.-L. (2003). TSC2 mediates cellular energy response to control cell growth and survival. *Cell*, *115*, 577–590.

Jacinto, E., Loewith, R., Schmidt, A., Lin, S., Rüegg, M. A., Hall, A., et al. (2004). Mammalian TOR complex 2 controls the actin cytoskeleton and is rapamycin insensitive. *Nature Cell Biology*, *6*, 1122–1128.

Jenne, D. E., Reimann, H., Nezu, J., Friedel, W., Loff, S., Jeschke, R., et al. (1998). Peutz-Jeghers syndrome is caused by mutations in a novel serine threonine kinase. *Nature Genetics*, *18*, 38–43.

Juhl, K., Bonner-Weir, S., & Sharma, A. (2010). Regenerating pancreatic beta-cells: Plasticity of adult pancreatic cells and the feasibility of in-vivo neogenesis. *Current Opinion in Organ Transplantation*, *15*, 79–85.

Jung, H. S., Chung, K. W., Won Kim, J., Kim, J., Komatsu, M., Tanaka, K., et al. (2008). Loss of autophagy diminishes pancreatic beta cell mass and function with resultant hyperglycemia. *Cell Metabolism*, *8*, 318–324.

Kahn, B. B. (1998). Type 2 diabetes: When insulin secretion fails to compensate for insulin resistance. *Cell*, *92*, 593–596.

Kamada, Y., Funakoshi, T., Shintani, T., Nagano, K., Ohsumi, M., & Ohsumi, Y. (2000). Tor-mediated induction of autophagy via an Apg1 protein kinase complex. *The Journal of Cell Biology*, *150*, 1507–1513.

Kaneko, K., Ueki, K., Takahashi, N., Hashimoto, S., Okamoto, M., Awazawa, M., et al. (2010). Class IA phosphatidylinositol 3-kinase in pancreatic β cells controls insulin secretion by multiple mechanisms. *Cell Metabolism*, *12*, 619–632.

Kasuga, M., Karlsson, F. A., & Kahn, C. R. (1982). Insulin stimulates the phosphorylation of the 95,000-dalton subunit of its own receptor. *Science (New York, NY)*, *215*, 185–187.

Kasuga, M., Zick, Y., Blithe, D. L., Crettaz, M., & Kahn, C. R. (1982). Insulin stimulates tyrosine phosphorylation of the insulin receptor in a cell-free system. *Nature*, *298*, 667–669.

Kefas, B. A., Cai, Y., Kerckhofs, K., Ling, Z., Martens, G., Heimberg, H., et al. (2004). Metformin-induced stimulation of AMP-activated protein kinase in beta-cells impairs their glucose responsiveness and can lead to apoptosis. *Biochemical Pharmacology*, *68*, 409–416.

Kefas, B. A., Cai, Y., Ling, Z., Heimberg, H., Hue, L., Pipeleers, D., et al. (2003). AMP-activated protein kinase can induce apoptosis of insulin-producing MIN6 cells through stimulation of c-Jun-N-terminal kinase. *Journal of Molecular Endocrinology*, *30*, 151–161.

Kefas, B. A., Heimberg, H., Vaulont, S., Meisse, D., Hue, L., Pipeleers, D., et al. (2003). AICA-riboside induces apoptosis of pancreatic beta cells through stimulation of AMP-activated protein kinase. *Diabetologia*, *46*, 250–254.

Keymeulen, B., Ling, Z., Gorus, F. K., Delvaux, G., Bouwens, L., Grupping, A., et al. (1998). Implantation of standardized beta-cell grafts in a liver segment of IDDM patients: Graft and recipients characteristics in two cases of insulin-independence under maintenance immunosuppression for prior kidney graft. *Diabetologia*, *41*, 452–459.

Khoo, S., & Cobb, M. H. (1997). Activation of mitogen-activating protein kinase by glucose is not required for insulin secretion. *Proceedings of the National Academy of Sciences of the United States of America*, *94*, 5599–5604.

Kim, J.-W., Cho, J.-H., Ko, S.-H., Park, H.-S., Ha, J., Song, K.-H., et al. (2008). Transcriptional mechanism of suppression of insulin gene expression by AMP-activated protein kinase activator 5-amino-4-imidazolecarboxamide riboside (AICAR) in beta-cells. *Biochemical and Biophysical Research Communications*, *365*, 614–620.

Kim, E., Goraksha-Hicks, P., Li, L., Neufeld, T. P., & Guan, K.-L. (2008). Regulation of TORC1 by Rag GTPases in nutrient response. *Nature Cell Biology*, *10*, 935–945.

Kim, J. J., Kido, Y., Scherer, P. E., White, M. F., & Accili, D. (2007). Analysis of compensatory beta-cell response in mice with combined mutations of Insr and Irs2. *American Journal of Physiology Endocrinology and Metabolism*, *292*, E1694–E1701.

Kim, J., Kundu, M., Viollet, B., & Guan, K.-L. (2011). AMPK and mTOR regulate autophagy through direct phosphorylation of Ulk1. *Nature Cell Biology*, *13*, 132–141.

Kim, D.-H., Sarbassov, D. D., Ali, S. M., King, J. E., Latek, R. R., Erdjument-Bromage, H., et al. (2002). mTOR interacts with raptor to form a nutrient-sensitive complex that signals to the cell growth machinery. *Cell*, *110*, 163–175.

Kim, D.-H., Sarbassov, D. D., Ali, S. M., Latek, R. R., Guntur, K. V. P., Erdjument-Bromage, H., et al. (2003). GbetaL, a positive regulator of the rapamycin-sensitive pathway required for the nutrient-sensitive interaction between raptor and mTOR. *Molecular Cell*, *11*, 895–904.

Kitamura, T., Kahn, C. R., & Accili, D. (2003). Insulin receptor knockout mice. *Annual Review of Physiology*, *65*, 313–332.

Kitamura, Y. I., Kitamura, T., Kruse, J.-P., Raum, J. C., Stein, R., Gu, W., et al. (2005). FoxO1 protects against pancreatic beta cell failure through NeuroD and MafA induction. *Cell Metabolism*, *2*, 153–163.

Kitamura, T., Nakae, J., Kitamura, Y., Kido, Y., Biggs, W. H., Wright, C. V. E., et al. (2002). The forkhead transcription factor Foxo1 links insulin signaling to Pdx1 regulation of pancreatic beta cell growth. *The Journal of Clinical Investigation*, *110*, 1839–1847.

Kobayashi, M., Kikuchi, O., Sasaki, T., Kim, H.-J., Yokota-Hashimoto, H., Lee, Y.-S., et al. (2012). FoxO1 as a double-edged sword in the pancreas: Analysis of pancreas- and β-cell-specific FoxO1 knockout mice. *American Journal of Physiology. Endocrinology and Metabolism*, *302*, E603–E613.

Köhler, C. U., Olewinski, M., Tannapfel, A., Schmidt, W. E., Fritsch, H., & Meier, J. J. (2011). Cell cycle control of β-cell replication in the prenatal and postnatal human pancreas. *American Journal of Physiology. Endocrinology and Metabolism*, *300*, E221–E230.

Koyanagi, M., Asahara, S.-I., Matsuda, T., Hashimoto, N., Shigeyama, Y., Shibutani, Y., et al. (2011). Ablation of TSC2 enhances insulin secretion by increasing the number of mitochondria through activation of mTORC1. *PloS One*, *6*, e23238.

Kubota, N., Tobe, K., Terauchi, Y., Eto, K., Yamauchi, T., Suzuki, R., et al. (2000). Disruption of insulin receptor substrate 2 causes type 2 diabetes because of liver insulin resistance and lack of compensatory beta-cell hyperplasia. *Diabetes*, *49*, 1880–1889.

Kulkarni, R. N., Holzenberger, M., Shih, D. Q., Ozcan, U., Stoffel, M., Magnuson, M. A., et al. (2002). beta-Cell-specific deletion of the Igf1 receptor leads to hyperinsulinemia and glucose intolerance but does not alter beta-cell mass. *Nature Genetics*, *31*, 111–115.

Kuo, C. J., Chung, J., Fiorentino, D. F., Flanagan, W. M., Blenis, J., & Crabtree, G. R. (1992). Rapamycin selectively inhibits interleukin-2 activation of p70 S6 kinase. *Nature*, *358*, 70–73.

Kushner, J. A., Haj, F. G., Klaman, L. D., Dow, M. A., Kahn, B. B., Neel, B. G., et al. (2004). Islet-sparing effects of protein tyrosine phosphatase-1b deficiency delays onset of diabetes in IRS2 knockout mice. *Diabetes*, *53*, 61–66.

Kushner, J. A., Ye, J., Schubert, M., Burks, D. J., Dow, M. A., Flint, C. L., et al. (2002). Pdx1 restores beta cell function in Irs2 knockout mice. *The Journal of Clinical Investigation*, *109*, 1193–1201.

Kwon, G., Marshall, C. A., Pappan, K. L., Remedi, M. S., & McDaniel, M. L. (2004). Signaling elements involved in the metabolic regulation of mTOR by nutrients, incretins, and growth factors in islets. *Diabetes*, *53*(Suppl. 3), S225–S232.

Larsen, M. O., Rolin, B., Sturis, J., Wilken, M., Carr, R. D., Pørksen, N., et al. (2006). Measurements of insulin responses as predictive markers of pancreatic beta-cell mass in normal and beta-cell-reduced lean and obese Göttingen minipigs in vivo. *American Journal of Physiology Endocrinology and Metabolism*, *290*, E670–E677.

Leclerc, I., Woltersdorf, W. W., da Silva Xavier, G., Rowe, R. L., Cross, S. E., Korbutt, G. S., et al. (2004). Metformin, but not leptin, regulates AMP-activated protein kinase in pancreatic islets: Impact on glucose-stimulated insulin secretion. *American Journal of Physiology Endocrinology and Metabolism*, *286*, E1023–E1031.

Lee, D.-F., Kuo, H.-P., Chen, C.-T., Hsu, J.-M., Chou, C.-K., Wei, Y., et al. (2007). IKK beta suppression of TSC1 links inflammation and tumor angiogenesis via the mTOR pathway. *Cell*, *130*, 440–455.

Leibiger, B., Leibiger, I. B., Moede, T., Kemper, S., Kulkarni, R. N., Kahn, C. R., et al. (2001). Selective insulin signaling through A and B insulin receptors regulates transcription of insulin and glucokinase genes in pancreatic beta cells. *Molecular Cell*, *7*, 559–570.

Lempiäinen, H., & Halazonetis, T. D. (2009). Emerging common themes in regulation of PIKKs and PI3Ks. *The EMBO Journal*, *28*, 3067–3073.

Li, Y., Inoki, K., Vacratsis, P., & Guan, K.-L. (2003). The p38 and MK2 kinase cascade phosphorylates tuberin, the tuberous sclerosis 2 gene product, and enhances its interaction with 14-3-3. *The Journal of Biological Chemistry*, *278*, 13663–13671.

Li, Y., Inoki, K., Yeung, R., & Guan, K.-L. (2002). Regulation of TSC2 by 14-3-3 binding. *The Journal of Biological Chemistry*, *277*, 44593–44596.

Lin, X., Taguchi, A., Park, S., Kushner, J. A., Li, F., Li, Y., et al. (2004). Dysregulation of insulin receptor substrate 2 in beta cells and brain causes obesity and diabetes. *The Journal of Clinical Investigation*, *114*, 908–916.

Lingohr, M. K., Briaud, I., Dickson, L. M., McCuaig, J. F., Alárcon, C., Wicksteed, B. L., et al. (2006). Specific regulation of IRS-2 expression by glucose in rat primary pancreatic islet beta-cells. *The Journal of Biological Chemistry*, *281*, 15884–15892.

Liu, H., Remedi, M. S., Pappan, K. L., Kwon, G., Rohatgi, N., Marshall, C. A., et al. (2009). Glycogen synthase kinase-3 and mammalian target of rapamycin pathways contribute to DNA synthesis, cell cycle progression, and proliferation in human islets. *Diabetes*, *58*, 663–672.

Liu, Y., Tanabe, K., Baronnier, D., Patel, S., Woodgett, J., Cras-Méneur, C., et al. (2010). Conditional ablation of Gsk-3β in islet beta cells results in expanded mass and resistance to fat feeding-induced diabetes in mice. *Diabetologia*, *53*, 2600–2610.

Liu, Z., Tanabe, K., Bernal-Mizrachi, E., & Permutt, M. A. (2008). Mice with beta cell overexpression of glycogen synthase kinase-3beta have reduced beta cell mass and proliferation. *Diabetologia*, *51*, 623–631.

Ma, X. M., & Blenis, J. (2009). Molecular mechanisms of mTOR-mediated translational control. *Nature Reviews. Molecular Cell Biology*, *10*, 307–318.
Ma, L., Chen, Z., Erdjument-Bromage, H., Tempst, P., & Pandolfi, P. P. (2005). Phosphorylation and functional inactivation of TSC2 by Erk implications for tuberous sclerosis and cancer pathogenesis. *Cell*, *121*, 179–193.
Mak, B. C., Kenerson, H. L., Aicher, L. D., Barnes, E. A., & Yeung, R. S. (2005). Aberrant beta-catenin signaling in tuberous sclerosis. *The American Journal of Pathology*, *167*, 107–116.
Manning, B. D., Tee, A. R., Logsdon, M. N., Blenis, J., & Cantley, L. C. (2002). Identification of the tuberous sclerosis complex-2 tumor suppressor gene product tuberin as a target of the phosphoinositide 3-kinase/akt pathway. *Molecular Cell*, *10*, 151–162.
McClain, D. A. (1991). Different ligand affinities of the two human insulin receptor splice variants are reflected in parallel changes in sensitivity for insulin action. *Molecular Endocrinology (Baltimore, Md)*, *5*, 734–739.
McKinnon, C. M., & Docherty, K. (2001). Pancreatic duodenal homeobox-1, PDX-1, a major regulator of beta cell identity and function. *Diabetologia*, *44*, 1203–1214.
Medema, R. H., Kops, G. J., Bos, J. L., & Burgering, B. M. (2000). AFX-like forkhead transcription factors mediate cell-cycle regulation by Ras and PKB through p27kip1. *Nature*, *404*, 782–787.
Meier, J. J., Breuer, T. G. K., Bonadonna, R. C., Tannapfel, A., Uhl, W., Schmidt, W. E., et al. (2012). Pancreatic diabetes manifests when beta cell area declines by approximately 65% in humans. *Diabetologia*, *55*, 1346–1354.
Meier, J. J., Butler, A. E., Saisho, Y., Monchamp, T., Galasso, R., Bhushan, A., et al. (2008). Beta-cell replication is the primary mechanism subserving the postnatal expansion of beta-cell mass in humans. *Diabetes*, *57*, 1584–1594.
Menge, B. A., Tannapfel, A., Belyaev, O., Drescher, R., Müller, C., Uhl, W., et al. (2008). Partial pancreatectomy in adult humans does not provoke beta-cell regeneration. *Diabetes*, *57*, 142–149.
Montagne, J., Stewart, M. J., Stocker, H., Hafen, E., Kozma, S. C., & Thomas, G. (1999). Drosophila S6 kinase: A regulator of cell size. *Science (New York, NY)*, *285*, 2126–2129.
Montanya, E., Nacher, V., Biarnés, M., & Soler, J. (2000). Linear correlation between beta-cell mass and body weight throughout the lifespan in Lewis rats: Role of beta-cell hyperplasia and hypertrophy. *Diabetes*, *49*, 1341–1346.
Mori, H., Inoki, K., Münzberg, H., Opland, D., Faouzi, M., Villanueva, E. C., et al. (2009). Critical role for hypothalamic mTOR activity in energy balance. *Cell Metabolism*, *9*, 362–374.
Mori, H., Inoki, K., Opland, D., Münzberg, H., Villanueva, E. C., Faouzi, M., et al. (2009). Critical roles for the TSC-mTOR pathway in β-cell function. *American Journal of Physiology Endocrinology and Metabolism*, *297*, E1013–E1022.
Muller, D., Huang, G. C., Amiel, S., Jones, P. M., & Persaud, S. J. (2007). Gene expression heterogeneity in human islet endocrine cells in vitro: The insulin signalling cascade. *Diabetologia*, *50*, 1239–1242.
Myers, M. G., Backer, J. M., Sun, X. J., Shoelson, S., Hu, P., Schlessinger, J., et al. (1992). IRS-1 activates phosphatidylinositol 3′-kinase by associating with src homology 2 domains of p85. *Proceedings of the National Academy of Sciences of the United States of America*, *89*, 10350–10354.
Nakae, J., Biggs, W. H., Kitamura, T., Cavenee, W. K., Wright, C. V. E., Arden, K. C., et al. (2002). Regulation of insulin action and pancreatic beta-cell function by mutated alleles of the gene encoding forkhead transcription factor Foxo1. *Nature Genetics*, *32*, 245–253.
Nemoto, S., Fergusson, M. M., & Finkel, T. (2004). Nutrient availability regulates SIRT1 through a forkhead-dependent pathway. *Science (New York, NY)*, *306*, 2105–2108.

Noda, T., & Ohsumi, Y. (1998). Tor, a phosphatidylinositol kinase homologue, controls autophagy in yeast. *The Journal of Biological Chemistry*, *273*, 3963–3966.

Ogihara, T., Isobe, T., Ichimura, T., Taoka, M., Funaki, M., Sakoda, H., et al. (1997). 14-3-3 Protein binds to insulin receptor substrate-1, one of the binding sites of which is in the phosphotyrosine binding domain. *The Journal of Biological Chemistry*, *272*, 25267–25274.

Oh, W. J., Wu, C.-C., Kim, S. J., Facchinetti, V., Julien, L.-A., Finlan, M., et al. (2010). mTORC2 can associate with ribosomes to promote cotranslational phosphorylation and stability of nascent Akt polypeptide. *The EMBO Journal*, *29*, 3939–3951.

Okada, T., Liew, C. W., Hu, J., Hinault, C., Michael, M. D., Krtzfeldt, J., et al. (2007). Insulin receptors in beta-cells are critical for islet compensatory growth response to insulin resistance. *Proceedings of the National Academy of Sciences of the United States of America*, *104*, 8977–8982.

Otani, K., Kulkarni, R. N., Baldwin, A. C., Krutzfeldt, J., Ueki, K., Stoffel, M., et al. (2004). Reduced beta-cell mass and altered glucose sensing impair insulin-secretory function in betaIRKO mice. *American Journal of Physiology Endocrinology and Metabolism*, *286*, E41–E49.

Ozcan, U., Cao, Q., Yilmaz, E., Lee, A.-H., Iwakoshi, N. N., Ozdelen, E., et al. (2004). Endoplasmic reticulum stress links obesity, insulin action, and type 2 diabetes. *Science (New York, NY)*, *306*, 457–461.

Ozcan, U., Ozcan, L., Yilmaz, E., Düvel, K., Sahin, M., Manning, B. D., et al. (2008). Loss of the tuberous sclerosis complex tumor suppressors triggers the unfolded protein response to regulate insulin signaling and apoptosis. *Molecular Cell*, *29*, 541–551.

Parsons, J. A., Brelje, T. C., & Sorenson, R. L. (1992). Adaptation of islets of Langerhans to pregnancy: Increased islet cell proliferation and insulin secretion correlates with the onset of placental lactogen secretion. *Endocrinology*, *130*, 1459–1466.

Pechhold, K., Koczwara, K., Zhu, X., Harrison, V. S., Walker, G., Lee, J., et al. (2009). Blood glucose levels regulate pancreatic beta-cell proliferation during experimentally-induced and spontaneous autoimmune diabetes in mice. *PloS One*, *4*, e4827.

Pende, M., Kozma, S. C., Jaquet, M., Oorschot, V., Burcelin, R., Le Marchand-Brustel, Y., et al. (2000). Hypoinsulinaemia, glucose intolerance and diminished beta-cell size in S6K1-deficient mice. *Nature*, *408*, 994–997.

Peterson, R. T., Beal, P. A., Comb, M. J., & Schreiber, S. L. (2000). FKBP12-rapamycin-associated protein (FRAP) autophosphorylates at serine 2481 under translationally repressive conditions. *The Journal of Biological Chemistry*, *275*, 7416–7423.

Peterson, T. R., Laplante, M., Thoreen, C. C., Sancak, Y., Kang, S. A., Kuehl, W. M., et al. (2009). DEPTOR is an mTOR inhibitor frequently overexpressed in multiple myeloma cells and required for their survival. *Cell*, *137*, 873–886.

Pick, A., Clark, J., Kubstrup, C., Levisetti, M., Pugh, W., Bonner-Weir, S., et al. (1998). Role of apoptosis in failure of beta-cell mass compensation for insulin resistance and beta-cell defects in the male Zucker diabetic fatty rat. *Diabetes*, *47*, 358–364.

Porat, S., Weinberg-Corem, N., Tornovsky-Babaey, S., Schyr-Ben-Haroush, R., Hija, A., Stolovich-Rain, M., et al. (2011). Control of pancreatic β cell regeneration by glucose metabolism. *Cell Metabolism*, *13*, 440–449.

Rachdi, L., Balcazar, N., Osorio-Duque, F., Elghazi, L., Weiss, A., Gould, A., et al. (2008). Disruption of Tsc2 in pancreatic beta cells induces beta cell mass expansion and improved glucose tolerance in a TORC1-dependent manner. *Proceedings of the National Academy of Sciences of the United States of America*, *105*, 9250–9255.

Rane, S. G., Dubus, P., Mettus, R. V., Galbreath, E. J., Boden, G., Reddy, E. P., et al. (1999). Loss of Cdk4 expression causes insulin-deficient diabetes and Cdk4 activation results in beta-islet cell hyperplasia. *Nature Genetics*, *22*, 44–52.

Ravikumar, B., Vacher, C., Berger, Z., Davies, J. E., Luo, S., Oroz, L. G., et al. (2004). Inhibition of mTOR induces autophagy and reduces toxicity of polyglutamine expansions in fly and mouse models of Huntington disease. *Nature Genetics*, *36*, 585–595.

Rhodes, C. J. (2005). Type 2 diabetes-a matter of beta-cell life and death? *Science (New York, NY)*, *307*, 380–384.

Richards, S. K., Parton, L. E., Leclerc, I., Rutter, G. A., & Smith, R. M. (2005). Over-expression of AMP-activated protein kinase impairs pancreatic {beta}-cell function in vivo. *The Journal of Endocrinology*, *187*, 225–235.

Roux, P. P., Ballif, B. A., Anjum, R., Gygi, S. P., & Blenis, J. (2004). Tumor-promoting phorbol esters and activated Ras inactivate the tuberous sclerosis tumor suppressor complex via p90 ribosomal S6 kinase. *Proceedings of the National Academy of Sciences of the United States of America*, *101*, 13489–13494.

Ruvinsky, I., Sharon, N., Lerer, T., Cohen, H., Stolovich-Rain, M., Nir, T., et al. (2005). Ribosomal protein S6 phosphorylation is a determinant of cell size and glucose homeostasis. *Genes & Development*, *19*, 2199–2211.

Sabatini, D. M. (2006). mTOR and cancer: Insights into a complex relationship. *Nature Reviews Cancer*, *6*, 729–734.

Sabatini, D. M., Erdjument-Bromage, H., Lui, M., Tempst, P., & Snyder, S. H. (1994). RAFT1: A mammalian protein that binds to FKBP12 in a rapamycin-dependent fashion and is homologous to yeast TORs. *Cell*, *78*, 35–43.

Sachdeva, M. M., Claiborn, K. C., Khoo, C., Yang, J., Groff, D. N., Mirmira, R. G., et al. (2009). Pdx1 (MODY4) regulates pancreatic beta cell susceptibility to ER stress. *Proceedings of the National Academy of Sciences of the United States of America*, *106*, 19090–19095.

Saisho, Y., Butler, A. E., Manesso, E., Galasso, R., Zhang, L., Gurlo, T., et al. (2010). Relationship between fractional pancreatic beta cell area and fasting plasma glucose concentration in monkeys. *Diabetologia*, *53*, 111–114.

Sakuraba, H., Mizukami, H., Yagihashi, N., Wada, R., Hanyu, C., & Yagihashi, S. (2002). Reduced beta-cell mass and expression of oxidative stress-related DNA damage in the islet of Japanese Type II diabetic patients. *Diabetologia*, *45*, 85–96.

Salt, I. P., Johnson, G., Ashcroft, S. J., & Hardie, D. G. (1998). AMP-activated protein kinase is activated by low glucose in cell lines derived from pancreatic beta cells, and may regulate insulin release. *The Biochemical Journal*, *335*(Pt. 3), 533–539.

Sancak, Y., Peterson, T. R., Shaul, Y. D., Lindquist, R. A., Thoreen, C. C., Bar-Peled, L., et al. (2008). The Rag GTPases bind raptor and mediate amino acid signaling to mTORC1. *Science (New York, NY)*, *320*, 1496–1501.

Sancak, Y., Thoreen, C. C., Peterson, T. R., Lindquist, R. A., Kang, S. A., Spooner, E., et al. (2007). PRAS40 is an insulin-regulated inhibitor of the mTORC1 protein kinase. *Molecular Cell*, *25*, 903–915.

Sarbassov, D. D., Ali, S. M., Kim, D.-H., Guertin, D. A., Latek, R. R., Erdjument-Bromage, H., et al. (2004). Rictor, a novel binding partner of mTOR, defines a rapamycin-insensitive and raptor-independent pathway that regulates the cytoskeleton. *Current Biology: CB*, *14*, 1296–1302.

Sarbassov, D. D., Ali, S. M., Sengupta, S., Sheen, J.-H., Hsu, P. P., Bagley, A. F., et al. (2006). Prolonged rapamycin treatment inhibits mTORC2 assembly and Akt/PKB. *Molecular Cell*, *22*, 159–168.

Sarbassov, D. D., Guertin, D. A., Ali, S. M., & Sabatini, D. M. (2005). Phosphorylation and regulation of Akt/PKB by the rictor-mTOR complex. *Science (New York, NY)*, *307*, 1098–1101.

Scaglia, L., Cahill, C. J., Finegood, D. T., & Bonner-Weir, S. (1997). Apoptosis participates in the remodeling of the endocrine pancreas in the neonatal rat. *Endocrinology*, *138*, 1736–1741.

Schieke, S. M., Phillips, D., McCoy, J. P., Aponte, A. M., Shen, R.-F., Balaban, R. S., et al. (2006). The mammalian target of rapamycin (mTOR) pathway regulates mitochondrial oxygen consumption and oxidative capacity. *The Journal of Biological Chemistry*, *281*, 27643–27652.

Seino, S., & Bell, G. I. (1989). Alternative splicing of human insulin receptor messenger RNA. *Biochemical and Biophysical Research Communications*, *159*, 312–316.

Sekulić, A., Hudson, C. C., Homme, J. L., Yin, P., Otterness, D. M., Karnitz, L. M., et al. (2000). A direct linkage between the phosphoinositide 3-kinase-AKT signaling pathway and the mammalian target of rapamycin in mitogen-stimulated and transformed cells. *Cancer Research*, *60*, 3504–3513.

Selman, C., Tullet, J. M. A., Wieser, D., Irvine, E., Lingard, S. J., Choudhury, A. I., et al. (2009). Ribosomal protein S6 kinase 1 signaling regulates mammalian life span. *Science (New York, NY)*, *326*, 140–144.

Shah, O. J., Wang, Z., & Hunter, T. (2004). Inappropriate activation of the TSC/Rheb/mTOR/S6K cassette induces IRS1/2 depletion, insulin resistance, and cell survival deficiencies. *Current Biology: CB*, *14*, 1650–1656.

Shapiro, A. M., Lakey, J. R., Ryan, E. A., Korbutt, G. S., Toth, E., Warnock, G. L., et al. (2000). Islet transplantation in seven patients with type 1 diabetes mellitus using a glucocorticoid-free immunosuppressive regimen. *The New England Journal of Medicine*, *343*, 230–238.

Shapiro, A. M. J., Ricordi, C., Hering, B. J., Auchincloss, H., Lindblad, R., Robertson, R. P., et al. (2006). International trial of the Edmonton protocol for islet transplantation. *The New England Journal of Medicine*, *355*, 1318–1330.

Shigeyama, Y., Kobayashi, T., Kido, Y., Hashimoto, N., Asahara, S.-I., Matsuda, T., et al. (2008). Biphasic response of pancreatic beta-cell mass to ablation of tuberous sclerosis complex 2 in mice. *Molecular and Cellular Biology*, *28*, 2971–2979.

Shumway, S. D., Li, Y., & Xiong, Y. (2003). 14-3-3Beta binds to and negatively regulates the tuberous sclerosis complex 2 (TSC2) tumor suppressor gene product, tuberin. *The Journal of Biological Chemistry*, *278*, 2089–2092.

Sleeman, M. W., Wortley, K. E., Lai, K.-M. V., Gowen, L. C., Kintner, J., Kline, W. O., et al. (2005). Absence of the lipid phosphatase SHIP2 confers resistance to dietary obesity. *Nature Medicine*, *11*, 199–205.

Stan, R., McLaughlin, M. M., Cafferkey, R., Johnson, R. K., Rosenberg, M., & Livi, G. P. (1994). Interaction between FKBP12-rapamycin and TOR involves a conserved serine residue. *The Journal of Biological Chemistry*, *269*, 32027–32030.

Stevens, C., Lin, Y., Harrison, B., Burch, L., Ridgway, R. A., Sansom, O., et al. (2009). Peptide combinatorial libraries identify TSC2 as a death-associated protein kinase (DAPK) death domain-binding protein and reveal a stimulatory role for DAPK in mTORC1 signaling. *The Journal of Biological Chemistry*, *284*, 334–344.

Stiles, B. L., Kuralwalla-Martinez, C., Guo, W., Gregorian, C., Wang, Y., Tian, J., et al. (2006). Selective deletion of Pten in pancreatic beta cells leads to increased islet mass and resistance to STZ-induced diabetes. *Molecular and Cellular Biology*, *26*, 2772–2781.

Stoffers, D. A., Ferrer, J., Clarke, W. L., & Habener, J. F. (1997). Early-onset type-II diabetes mellitus (MODY4) linked to IPF1. *Nature Genetics*, *17*, 138–139.

Sun, G., Tarasov, A. I., McGinty, J., McDonald, A., Da Silva Xavier, G., Gorman, T., et al. (2010). Ablation of AMP-activated protein kinase alpha1 and alpha2 from mouse pancreatic beta cells and RIP2.Cre neurons suppresses insulin release in vivo. *Diabetologia*, *53*, 924–936.

Talchai, C., Xuan, S., Lin, H. V., Sussel, L., & Accili, D. (2012). Pancreatic β cell dedifferentiation as a mechanism of diabetic β cell failure. *Cell*, *150*, 1223–1234.

Tamemoto, H., Kadowaki, T., Tobe, K., Yagi, T., Sakura, H., Hayakawa, T., et al. (1994). Insulin resistance and growth retardation in mice lacking insulin receptor substrate-1. *Nature*, *372*, 182–186.
Tanemura, M., Ohmura, Y., Deguchi, T., Machida, T., Tsukamoto, R., Wada, H., et al. (2012). Rapamycin causes upregulation of autophagy and impairs islets function both in vitro and in vivo. *American Journal of Transplantation: Official Journal of the American Society of Transplantation and the American Society of Transplant Surgeons*, *12*, 102–114.
Taniguchi, C. M., Emanuelli, B., & Kahn, C. R. (2006). Critical nodes in signalling pathways: Insights into insulin action. *Nature Reviews Molecular Cell Biology*, *7*, 85–96.
Terauchi, Y., Takamoto, I., Kubota, N., Matsui, J., Suzuki, R., Komeda, K., et al. (2007). Glucokinase and IRS-2 are required for compensatory beta cell hyperplasia in response to high-fat diet-induced insulin resistance. *The Journal of Clinical Investigation*, *117*, 246–257.
Teta, M., Long, S. Y., Wartschow, L. M., Rankin, M. M., & Kushner, J. A. (2005). Very slow turnover of cells in aged adult mice. *Diabetes*, *54*, 2557–2567.
Tremblay, F., Brûlé, S., Hee Um, S., Li, Y., Masuda, K., Roden, M., et al. (2007). Identification of IRS-1 Ser-1101 as a target of S6K1 in nutrient- and obesity-induced insulin resistance. *Proceedings of the National Academy of Sciences of the United States of America*, *104*, 14056–14061.
Tsuboi, T. (2003). 5′-AMP-activated protein kinase controls insulin-containing secretory vesicle dynamics. *Journal of Biological Chemistry*, *278*, 52042–52051.
Ueki, K., Okada, T., Hu, J., Liew, C. W., Assmann, A., Dahlgren, G. M., et al. (2006). Total insulin and IGF-I resistance in pancreatic beta cells causes overt diabetes. *Nature Genetics*, *38*, 583–588.
Ullrich, A., Bell, J. R., Chen, E. Y., Herrera, R., Petruzzelli, L. M., Dull, T. J., et al. (1985). Human insulin receptor and its relationship to the tyrosine kinase family of oncogenes. *Nature*, *313*, 756–761.
Um, S. H., Frigerio, F., Watanabe, M., Picard, F., Joaquin, M., Sticker, M., et al. (2004). Absence of S6K1 protects against age- and diet-induced obesity while enhancing insulin sensitivity. *Nature*, *431*, 200–205.
Van Assche, F. A., Aerts, L., & De Prins, F. (1978). A morphological study of the endocrine pancreas in human pregnancy. *British Journal of Obstetrics and Gynaecology*, *85*, 818–820.
van Slegtenhorst, M., de Hoogt, R., Hermans, C., Nellist, M., Janssen, B., Verhoef, S., et al. (1997). Identification of the tuberous sclerosis gene TSC1 on chromosome 9q34. *Science (New York, NY)*, *277*, 805–808.
vander Haar, E., Lee, S. I., Bandhakavi, S., Griffin, T. J., & Kim, D. H. (2007). Insulin signalling to mTOR mediated by the Akt/PKB substrate PRAS40. *Nature Cell Biology*, *9*, 316–323.
Vellai, T., Takács-Vellai, K., Zhang, Y., Kovács, A. L., Orosz, L., & Müller, F. (2003). Genetics: Influence of TOR kinase on lifespan in C. elegans. *Nature*, *426*, 620.
Vézina, C., Kudelski, A., & Sehgal, S. N. (1975). Rapamycin (AY-22,989), a new antifungal antibiotic. I. Taxonomy of the producing streptomycete and isolation of the active principle. *The Journal of Antibiotics*, *28*, 721–726.
Whittaker, J., Sørensen, H., Gadsbøll, V. L., & Hinrichsen, J. (2002). Comparison of the functional insulin binding epitopes of the A and B isoforms of the insulin receptor. *The Journal of Biological Chemistry*, *277*, 47380–47384.
Wijesekara, N., Konrad, D., Eweida, M., Jefferies, C., Liadis, N., Giacca, A., et al. (2005). Muscle-specific Pten deletion protects against insulin resistance and diabetes. *Molecular and Cellular Biology*, *25*, 1135–1145.
Withers, D. J., Gutierrez, J. S., Towery, H., Burks, D. J., Ren, J. M., Previs, S., et al. (1998). Disruption of IRS-2 causes type 2 diabetes in mice. *Nature*, *391*, 900–904.

Yamaguchi, Y., Flier, J. S., Benecke, H., Ransil, B. J., & Moller, D. E. (1993). Ligand-binding properties of the two isoforms of the human insulin receptor. *Endocrinology, 132*, 1132–1138.

Yang, Q., Inoki, K., Ikenoue, T., & Guan, K.-L. (2006). Identification of Sin1 as an essential TORC2 component required for complex formation and kinase activity. *Genes & Development, 20*, 2820–2832.

Yu, L., McPhee, C. K., Zheng, L., Mardones, G. A., Rong, Y., Peng, J., et al. (2010). Termination of autophagy and reformation of lysosomes regulated by mTOR. *Nature, 465*, 942–946.

Zahr, E., Molano, R. D., Pileggi, A., Ichii, H., Jose, S. S., Bocca, N., et al. (2007). Rapamycin impairs in vivo proliferation of islet beta-cells. *Transplantation, 84*, 1576–1583.

Zhang, Y., Gao, X., Saucedo, L. J., Ru, B., Edgar, B. A., & Pan, D. (2003). Rheb is a direct target of the tuberous sclerosis tumour suppressor proteins. *Nature Cell Biology, 5*, 578–581.

Zhang, N., Su, D., Qu, S., Tse, T., Bottino, R., Balamurugan, A. N., et al. (2006). Sirolimus is associated with reduced islet engraftment and impaired beta-cell function. *Diabetes, 55*, 2429–2436.

Zoncu, R., Efeyan, A., & Sabatini, D. M. (2011). mTOR: From growth signal integration to cancer, diabetes and ageing. *Nature Reviews. Molecular Cell Biology, 12*, 21–35.

INDEX

Note: Page numbers followed by "*f*" indicate figures and "*t*" indicate tables.

A

D

O

P

U

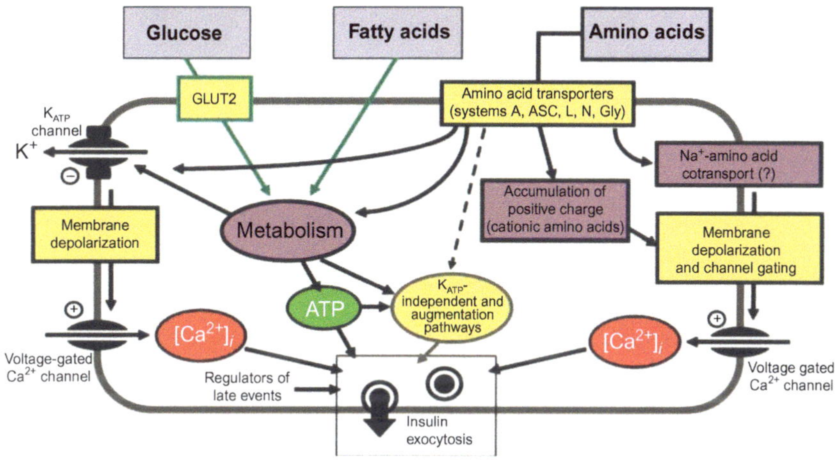

Kevin Keane and Philip Newsholme, Figure 1.1 Mechanisms of nutrient-stimulated insulin secretion. Glucose metabolism is essential for stimulation of insulin secretion (impacting on K^{+}_{ATP} channel closure prompting membrane depolarization). Amino acid metabolism enhances insulin secretion via (a) direct depolarization of the plasma membrane (e.g., cationic amino acid, L-arginine); (b) metabolism (e.g., alanine, glutamine, leucine); and (c) cotransport with Na^{+} and cell membrane depolarization (e.g., alanine). Fatty acid metabolism enhances basal insulin secretion in glucose absence through generation of ATP. *Taken from Newsholme, Gaudel, and McClenaghan (2010).*

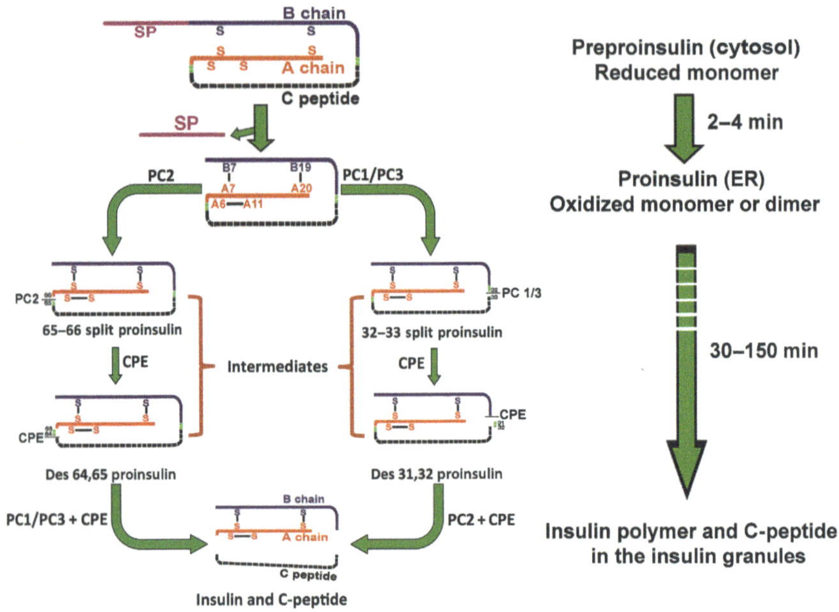

Ming Liu *et al.*, Figure 2.1 Insulin biosynthesis in pancreatic beta cells. Insulin biosynthesis begins as a precursor, preproinsulin, within the cytosol. Preproinsulin is comprised of sequentially as signal peptide (magenta), insulin B-chain (blue), C-peptide (black), and insulin A-chain (red). Newly synthesized preproinsulin undergoes co- and posttranslational translocation into the endoplasmic reticulum (ER), where it is cleaved by signal peptidase, forming proinsulin. The proinsulin folds in the ER, forming three evolutionarily conserved disulfide bonds, including two interchain disulfide bonds B7–A7 and B19–A20 and one intrachain disulfide bond A6–A11. Properly folded proinsulin forms dimers and exits from the ER, trafficking through Golgi complex into secretory granules where prohormone convertases (PC1/3 and PC2) in concert with carboxypeptidase E (CPE) to process proinsulin to C-peptide and two-chain mature insulin stored in the insulin granules. *Liu et al.*

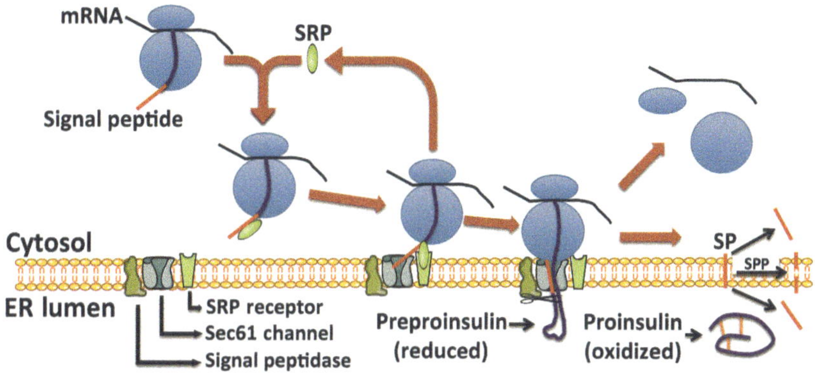

Ming Liu *et al.*, Figure 2.2 The earliest events of insulin biosynthesis: cotranslational translocation of newly synthesized preproinsulin from the cytosol to the ER. The signal peptide (SP) of newly synthesized preproinsulin is first recognized and bound by signal recognition particle (SRP) as it emerges from the ribosome. This binding results in a slowing down or pause of preproinsulin translation known as "elongation arrest." SRP then targets the entire ribosome–preproinsulin complex to the Sec61 translocon by docking to SRP receptor (SR) on the ER membrane. SP interacts with Sec61 channel, SRP is released, preproinsulin translation resumes and its proinsulin domain begins to be translocated into the ER, where SP is cleaved by signal peptidase at the ER luminal side, forming proinsulin, which rapidly folds in the ER. *Figures were produced using Servier Medical Art www.servier.com; Liu et al.*

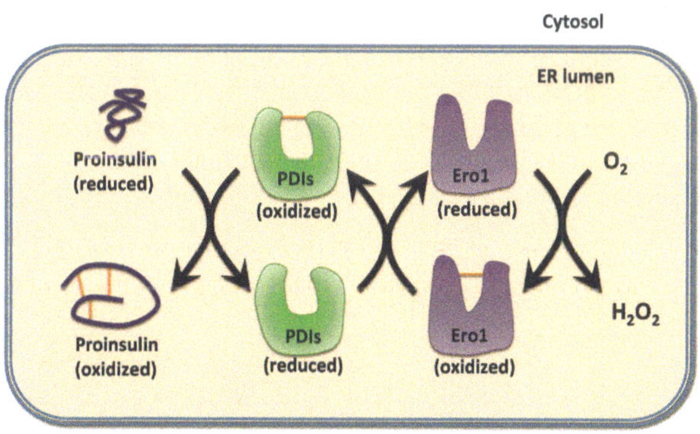

Ming Liu *et al.*, Figure 2.4 Proinsulin disulfide bond formation. Within the ER, proinsulin must form three intramolecular disulfide bonds. Members of the PDI protein family (green) transfer disulfide bonds (orange line) to the proinsulin molecule, and then must be reoxidized by Ero1 (purple). Ero1 in turn forms *de novo* disulfide bonds by reducing molecular oxygen. This cycle must repeat three times to form the required proinsulin disulfide bonds. *Liu et al.*

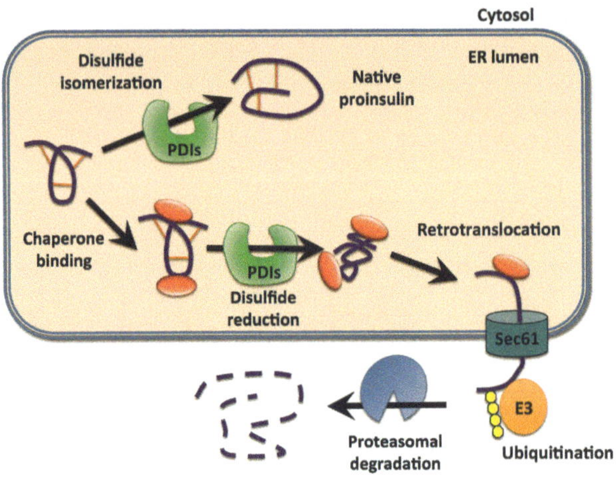

Ming Liu *et al.*, Figure 2.5 Disposal of misfolded proinsulin: isomerization and ERAD. When proinsulin misfolds and forms nonnative disulfide bonds, PDI family proteins act as isomerases to shuffle the disulfide bonds and allow the molecule to potentially reach its native conformation. When molecules remain misfolded, they are targeted for ERAD. Chaperones such as BiP (red) recognize the misfolded protein, and PDI family proteins (green) reduce the disulfide bonds prior to proinsulin retrotranslocation through the Sec61 translocon. During retrotranslocation, E3 ligases (orange) ubiquitinate the reduced proinsulin, targeting it for proteasomal degradation in the cytosol. *Liu et al.*

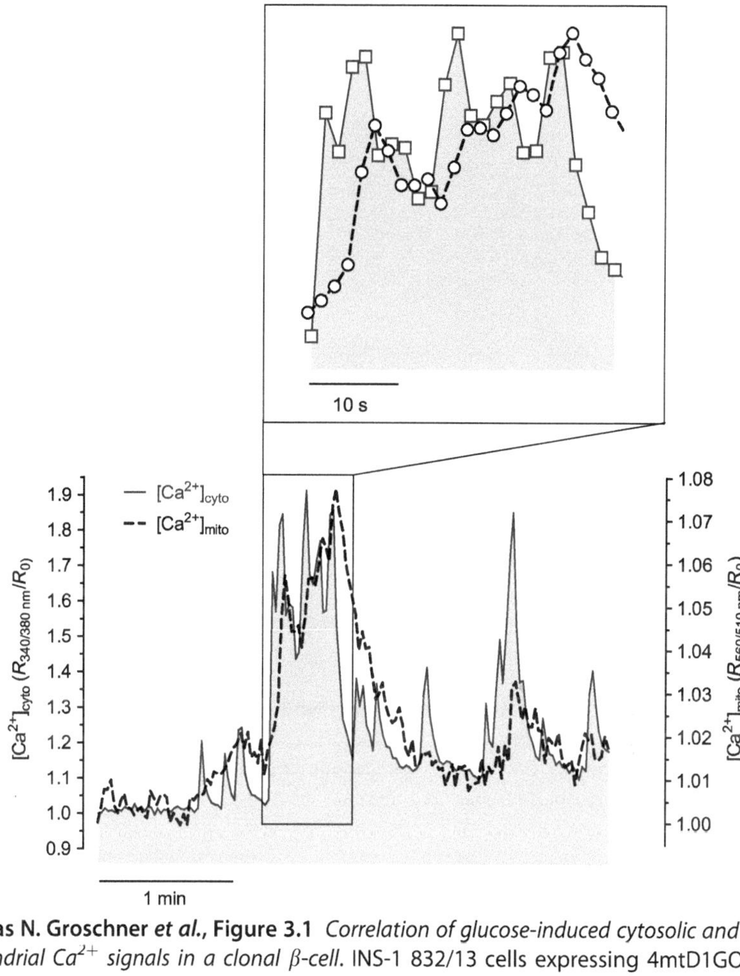

Lukas N. Groschner *et al.*, Figure 3.1 *Correlation of glucose-induced cytosolic and mitochondrial Ca^{2+} signals in a clonal β-cell.* INS-1 832/13 cells expressing 4mtD1GO-Cam were loaded with Fura-2 AM and fluorescence was recorded in response to 16 mM glucose. Glucose evokes cytosolic Ca^{2+} spikes (blue trace) followed by respective peaks in mitochondrial Ca^{2+} (black-dashed trace) with a delay of only 3–6 s. Ca^{2+} clearance from the mitochondrial matrix is slower as compared to the cytosolic compartment. The inset is showing a zoom-in image of the marked section.

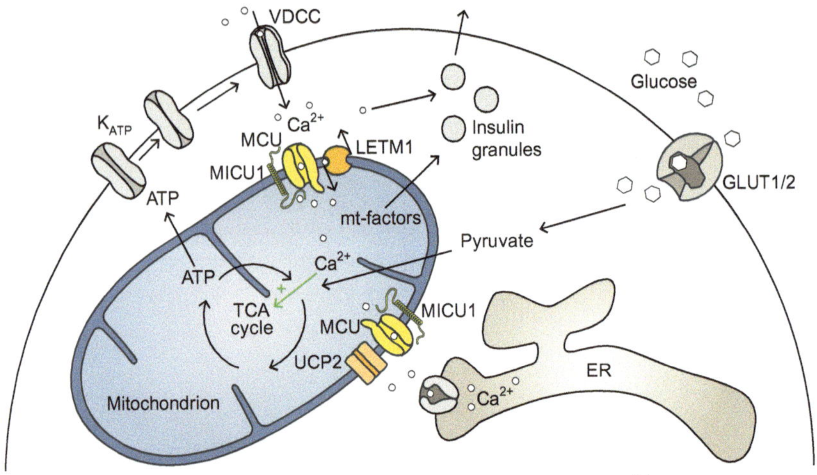

Lukas N. Groschner *et al.*, Figure 3.2 *Pathways of mitochondrial Ca^{2+} uptake in the pancreatic β-cell.* Glucose taken up by the β-cell via glucose transporter 1 or 2 (GLUT1/2) enters glycolysis to yield pyruvate. Pyruvate is transported into the mitochondrion where it fuels the TCA cycle and thereby oxidative metabolism to generate ATP and other mitochondrial coupling factors (mt-factors). ATP in turn causes K_{ATP} channels (K_{ATP}) to close triggering Ca^{2+} influx via voltage-dependent Ca^{2+} channels (VDCC). Ca^{2+} entering the cytosol does not only mediate insulin granule exocytosis, but is also transferred to the mitochondrial matrix. Proteins involved in this critical step are MICU1, MCU, and to some extent also LETM1, whereas Ca^{2+} released from the endoplasmic reticulum (ER) is taken up in a MICU1-, MCU-, and UCP2-dependent manner. Matrix-free Ca^{2+} activates mitochondrial dehydrogenases and thus acts as a feed-forward mechanism boosting the production of ATP and other factors required for a sustained amplifying phase of insulin secretion.

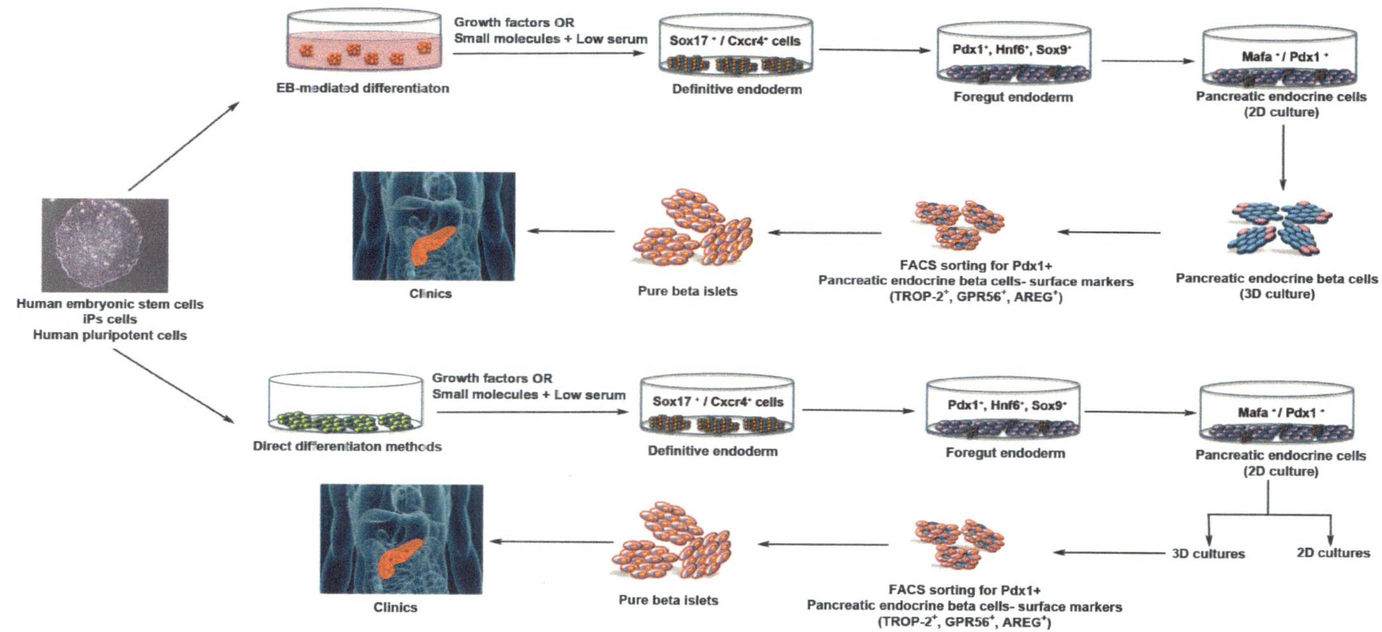

Bipasha Bose *et al.*, Figure 9.1 Strategies for *in vitro* pancreatic beta cell differentiation.

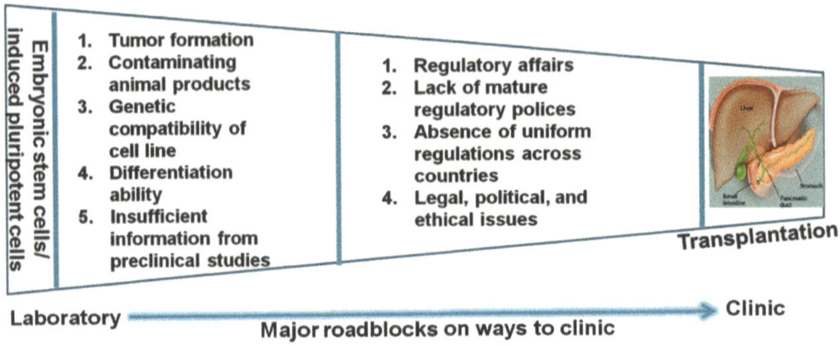

Bipasha Bose *et al.*, Figure 9.2 Schematic representation of major roadblocks for clinical application of embryonic and induced pluripotent cells.

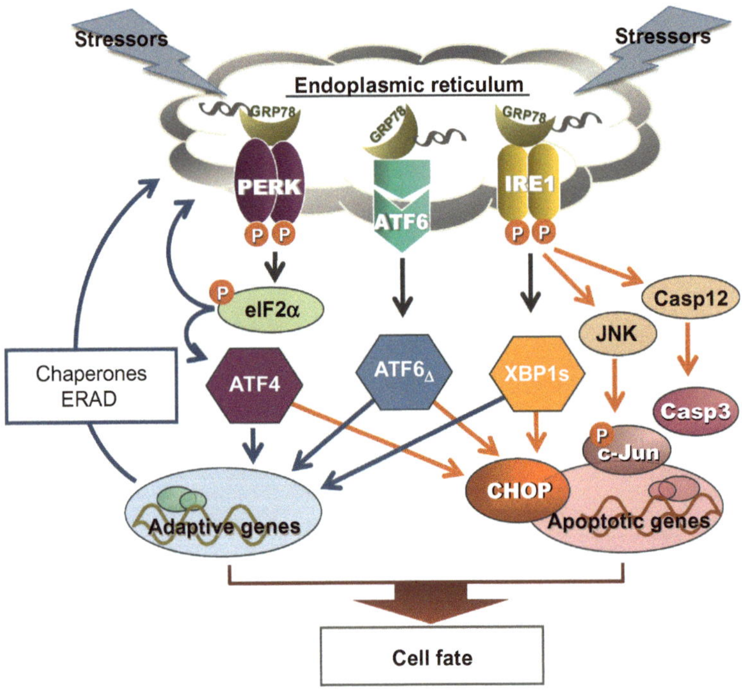

Pu Xia and Yanfei Qi, Figure 11.1 ER stress response—the UPR. Upon the challenges from various stressors on ER causing accumulation of unfolded and/or misfolded proteins in the ER lumen, the chaperone GRP78 dissociates from the luminal domain of the three ER transmembrane stress sensors: PERK, ATF6, and IRE1, leading to their activation. Both IRE1 and PERK are oligomerized and autophosphorylated. PERK induces phosphorylation of eIF2a, which blocks new protein synthesis and enables translation of ATF4 transcription factor, promoting the transcription of genes required to restore ER homeostasis. Activated ATF6 is cleaved as a cytosolic fragment that migrates to the nucleus, which regulates the expression of ER chaperones and X-box-binding protein 1 (XBP1). XBP1 mRNA spliced by IRE1 codes for the active transcription factor XBP1s that controls the transcription of chaperones and ERAD components. This concerted action of the UPR pathways restores the folding capacity of the ER by blocking further buildup of client proteins, enhancing its folding capacity and eliminating terminally misfolded proteins. Sustained or unresolved ER stress activates apoptotic mechanisms, including activation of JNK, caspase-12, and induction of CHOP, leading to cell death.

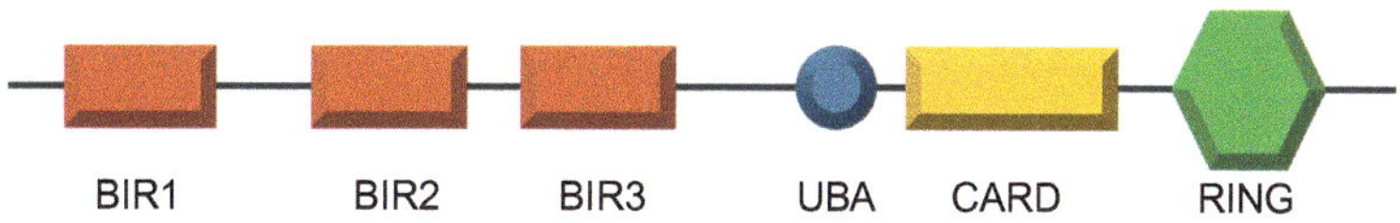

Pu Xia and Yanfei Qi, Figure 11.2 Domain structure of cIAP1. Three baculovirus IAP repeat (BIR) domains are located at the N-terminal of cIAP1 (indicated by red boxes). Along with the BIR domains, cIAP1 contains really interesting new gene (RING) domain at its C-terminus (indicated by green hexagon). cIAP1 also possesses a caspase activation and recruitment domain (CARD; indicated by yellow box) and a ubiquitin-associated (UBA) domain (indicated by blue circle) in the linker region between BIRs and CARD.

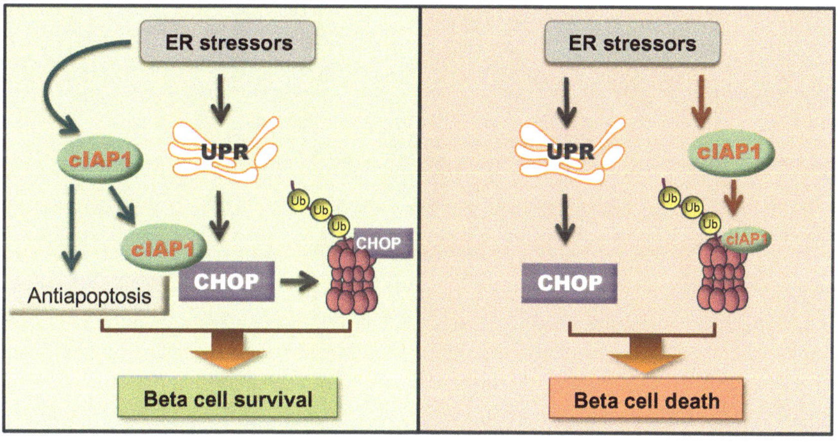

Pu Xia and Yanfei Qi, Figure 11.3 Model depicting the role of cIAP1 in determining beta cell fate under ER stress. For adaptation to ER stress, the UPR (e.g., induced by palmitoleate) activates survival pathways and increases the expression of cIAP1. cIAP1 functions through its antiapoptotic properties and the E3 ligase activity causing CHOP ubiquitination and degradation, ultimately leading to cell survival. Under certain ER stress conditions (e.g., exposure to palmitate), cIAP1 is quickly degraded through the apoptotic pathways, which relieves CHOP degradation and preserves its proapoptotic activity, resulting in cell death.

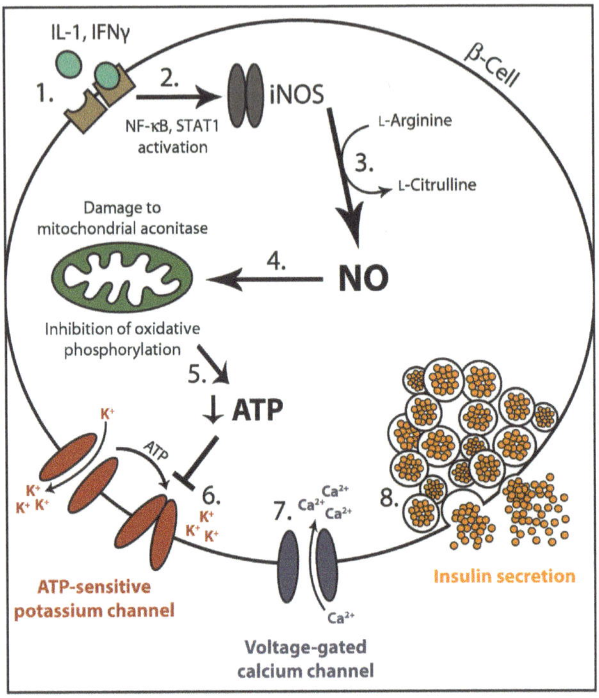

Katarzyna A. Broniowska *et al.*, Figure 12.3 The inhibitory effects of nitric oxide on β-cell insulin secretion. Cytokines (IL-1 and IFNγ) bind to their receptors on the β-cell (1) and activate NF-κB and STAT1-signaling cascades, stimulating expression of iNOS (2). iNOS generates micromolar levels of nitric oxide in β-cells via conversion of arginine to nitric oxide and citrulline (3). Nitric oxide mediates the damaging effects of cytokines on β-cells, causing damage to mitochondrial aconitase and resulting in the inhibition of oxidative phosphorylation (4) and a decrease in cellular ATP levels (5). The decrease in ATP prevents closure of ATP-sensitive potassium channels, preventing membrane depolarization (6) and calcium influx (7). The net effect is an inhibition of calcium-dependent secretion of insulin (8).

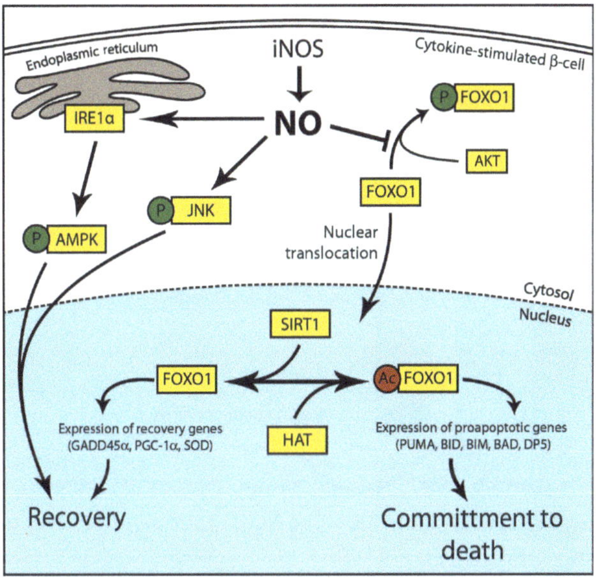

Katarzyna A. Broniowska *et al.*, Figure 12.4 Cellular mechanisms that control the β-cell responses to nitric oxide. Cytokines stimulate iNOS expression in β-cells, resulting in the production of micromolar levels of nitric oxide. Nitric oxide stimulates nuclear translocation of FOXO1. Once in the nucleus, FOXO1 can direct the expression of recovery genes or proapoptotic genes. The acetylation state of FOXO1 dictates which transcriptional program is activated. SIRT1-mediated deacetylation of FOXO1 promotes β-cell recovery, while acetylation of FOXO1 by a HAT (such as p300) activates a death cascade. AMPK and JNK are also rapidly activated by nitric oxide and participate in β-cell recovery.

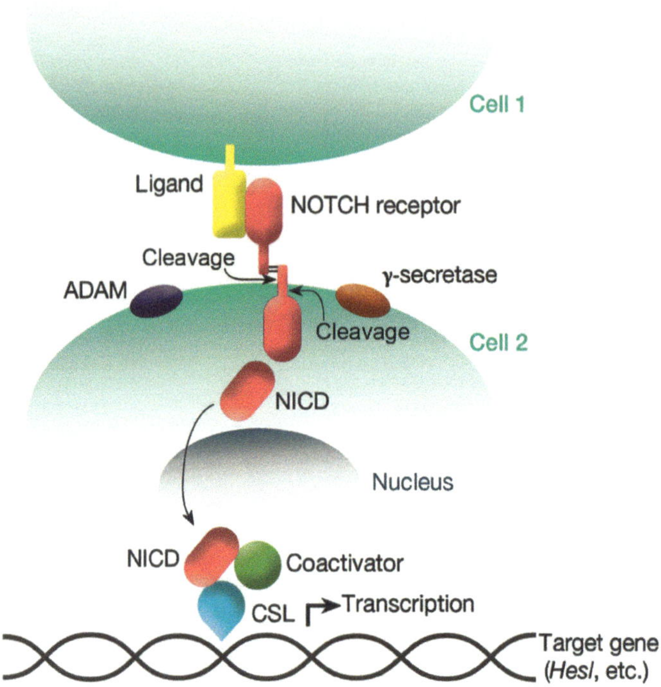

Yael Bar and Shimon Efrat, Figure 15.1 The NOTCH pathway. NOTCH signaling is triggered by ligands expressed on the surface of neighboring cells. Upon ligand binding, NOTCH receptors undergo successive proteolytic cleavages by an ADAM family protease and γ-secretase. The released NOTCH intracellular domain (NICD) translocates to the nucleus and associates with CSL and additional coactivators to form a transcription activation complex at target genes, such as *Hes1*.

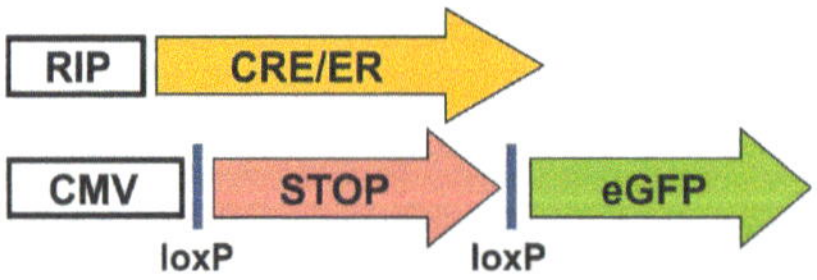

Yael Bar and Shimon Efrat, Figure 15.2 β-cell-specific labeling system. Schematic representation of the two lentivirus vectors used for β-cell-lineage tracing. *Reproduced from Russ, Ravassard, Kerr-Conte, Pattou, and Efrat (2009).*

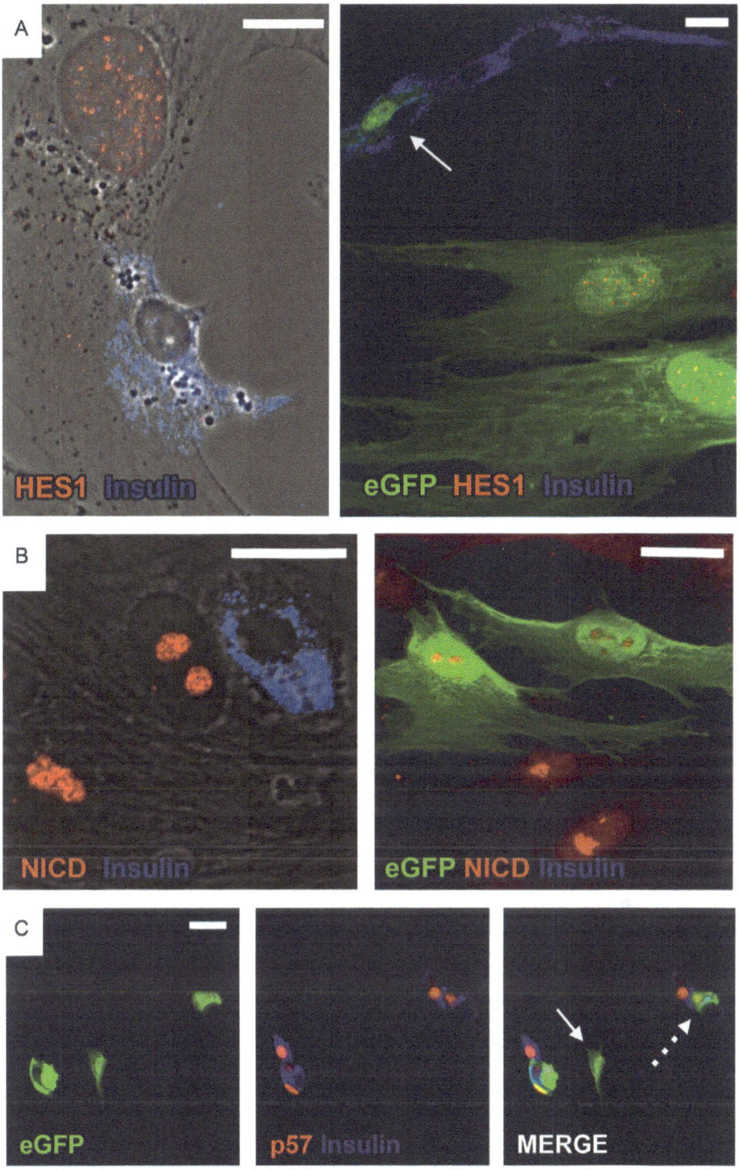

Yael Bar and Shimon Efrat, Figure 15.3 Notch pathway activation in BCD cells. (A, B) Immunofluorescence analysis of islet cells (left panels) and eGFP$^+$ cells derived from β cells following 10 days in culture (right panels). The left panels are merged with phase contrast images. Arrow points to a β cell that still expresses insulin and is not labeled for HES1. eGFP is detected in both cytoplasm and nucleus. (C) Immunofluorescence analysis of eGFP$^+$ cells derived from β cells following 10 days in culture. Solid arrow points to an eGFP$^+$ cell that has lost both insulin and p57 expression; dashed arrow points to an eGFP$^+$ β cell that maintains both insulin and p57 expression. Bar = 20 μm. *Reproduced from Bar et al. (2008).*

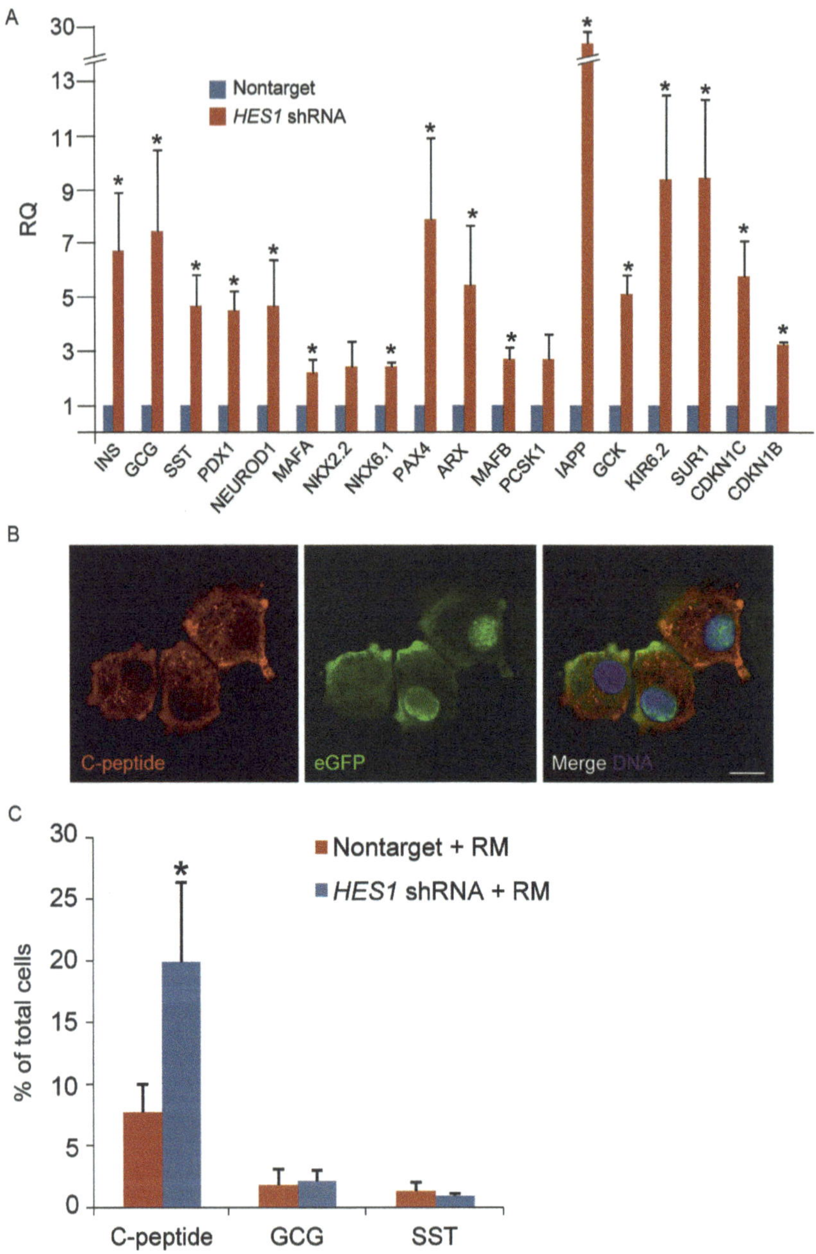

Yael Bar and Shimon Efrat, Figure 15.4 Effects of NOTCH pathway inhibition on BCD cell redifferentiation *in vitro*. (A) qPCR analyses of cultured islet cells at passage 4, 9 days following infection with *HES1* shRNA or nontarget viruses. RQ, relative quantification compared to nontarget virus. Values are mean ± SE ($n = 3$–4 donors). Asterisks mark significant changes ($p < 0.01$). (B) Coimmunofluorescence analysis for C-peptide and eGFP in labeled islet cells infected at passage 5 with *HES1* shRNA, and seeded 2 days later in medium with soluble differentiation factors (redifferentiation medium, RM) for 4 days. Bar = 10 μm. (C) Quantitation of 2000 cells in each group in the experiment in (B). Values are mean ± SE ($n = 3$ donors). No hormone-positive cells were found in untreated cells. Asterisk marks significant difference ($p < 0.05$). *Reproduced from Bar et al. (2012).*

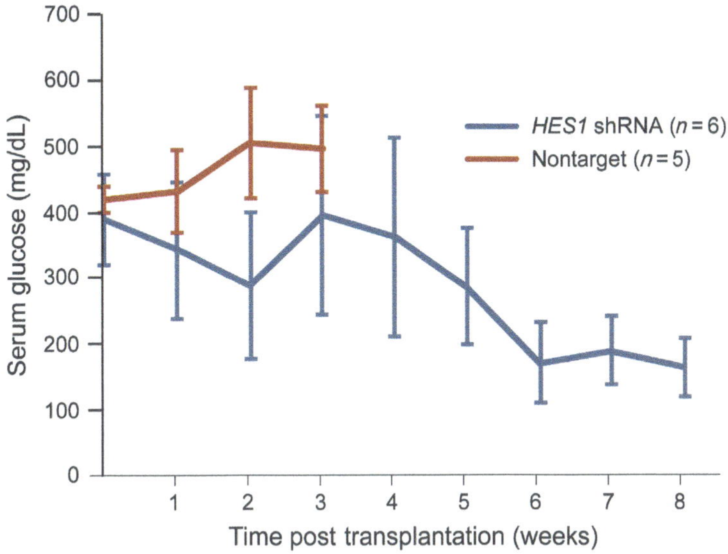

Yael Bar and Shimon Efrat, Figure 15.5 Effects of NOTCH pathway inhibition on BCD cell redifferentiation *in vivo*. Changes in blood glucose levels in immunodeficient mice made diabetic by treatment with streptozotocin and transplanted with 2×10^6 expanded islet cells infected at passage 5 with *HES1* shRNA or nontarget virus. Values are mean ± SE. *Reproduced from Bar et al. (2012).*

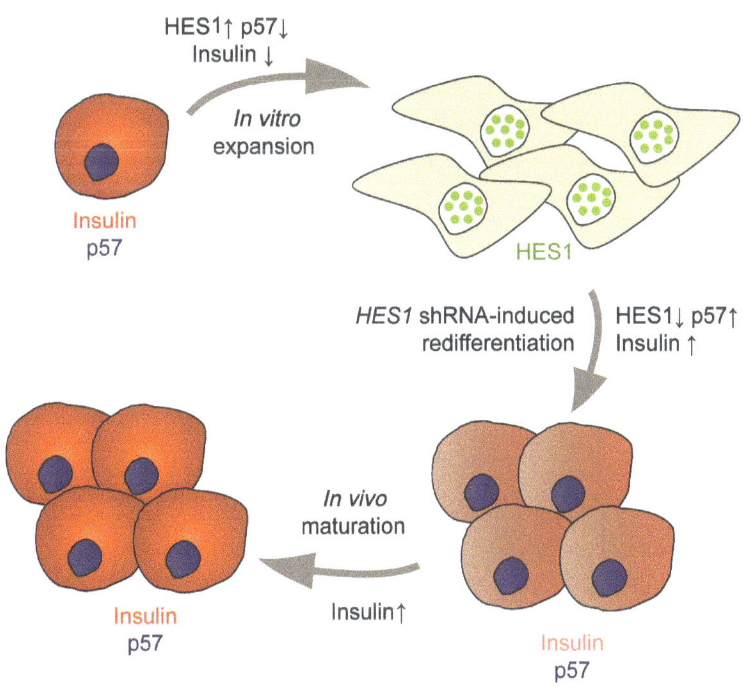

Yael Bar and Shimon Efrat, Figure 15.6 Model of HES1 involvement in proliferation, dedifferentiation, and redifferentiation of cultured human BCD cells. *Reproduced from Bar et al. (2012).*

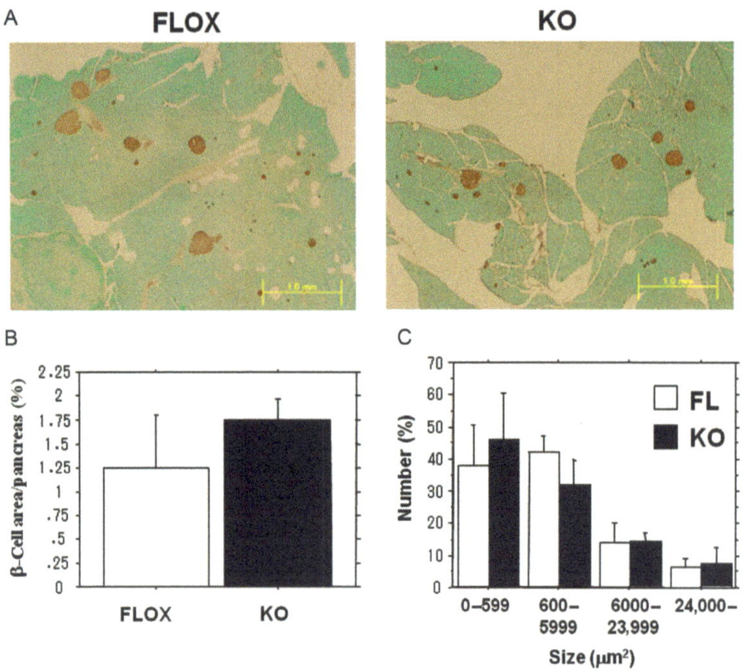

Kazuya Yamagata, Figure 16.3 β-Cell growth in β-cell-specific HNF4α knockout (βHNF4α KO) mice. Mice were fed a high-fat diet for 8 weeks ($n=3$, each genotype). (A) Insulin staining of control (FLOX) and βHNF4α KO mice. (B and C) Quantification of β-cell area and size distribution. Data are expressed as mean ± S.E. values.

Kolibri 360 GmbH
Ferdinand-Jühlke-Straße 7
99095 Erfurt, Deutschland
produktsicherheit@kolibri360.de